Craniofacial Malformations

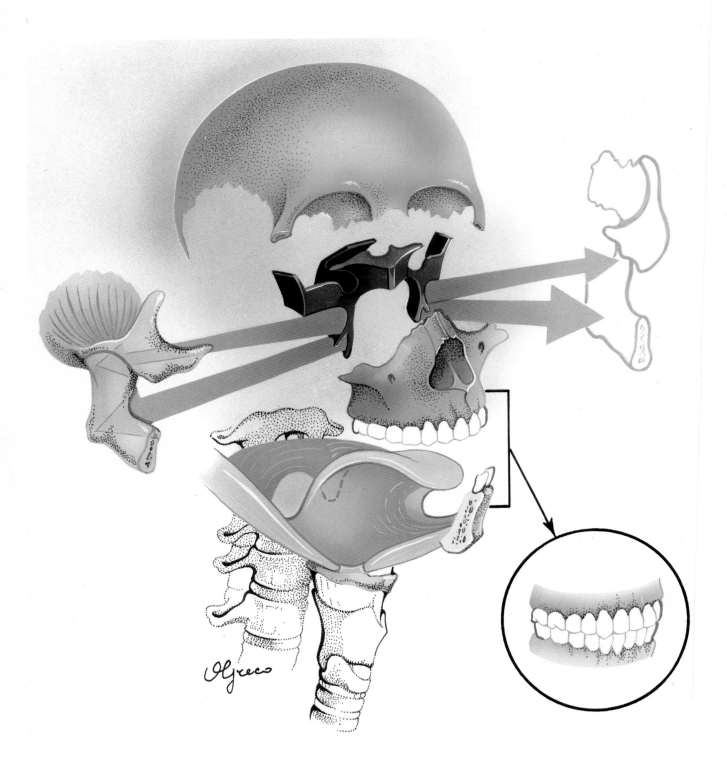

Craniofacial Malformations

EDITED BY

M. Stricker MD
Professor and Head of the Department of Plastic and Maxillofacial Surgery, University of Nancy, France

J. C. Van der Meulen MD
Professor and Head of the Department of Plastic and Reconstructive Surgery, Erasmus University, Rotterdam, The Netherlands

B. Raphael MD
Professor and Head of the Department of Plastic and Maxillofacial Surgery, University of Grenoble, France

R. Mazzola MD
Assistant Professor, Postgraduate School of Maxillofacial Surgery, University of Milan; Consultant, Plastic and Maxillofacial Surgery, Bassini Hospital, Milan, Italy

Linguistic editor

D. E. Tolhurst FRCS
Professor of Plastic and Reconstructive Surgery, University of Leiden, The Netherlands

Foreword by

Joseph E. Murray MD
Professor of Surgery, Emeritus, Harvard Medical School; Chief of Plastic Surgery, Emeritus, The Children's Hospital and Brigham and Women's Hospital, Boston, Massachusetts, USA

CHURCHILL LIVINGSTONE

EDINBURGH LONDON MELBOURNE AND NEW YORK 1990

CHURCHILL LIVINGSTONE
Medical Division of Longman Group UK Limited

Distributed in the United States of America by Churchill Livingstone
Inc., 1560 Broadway, New York, N.Y. 10036, and by associated
companies, branches and representatives throughout the world.

First published 1990

ISBN 0 443 03924 0

British Library Cataloguing in Publication Data
Craniofacial malformations.
  1. Man. Head. Congenital abnormalities
  I. Stricker, M.
  617'.51043

Library of Congress Cataloging-in-Publication Data
Craniofacial malformations/edited by M. Stricker . . . [et al.].
    Includes index.
    1. Skull — Abnormalities. 2. Face — Abnormalities. I. Stricker,
M. (Michel)
    [DNLM: 1. Face — abnormalities. 2. Skull — abnormalities. WE
705
    C89043]
    PD529.C7   1989
    617'.371 — dc19

Produced by Longman Singapore Publishers (Pte) Ltd
Printed in Singapore

Foreword

The course of medical progress is unpredictable. Therapeutic advances may result gradually from the accumulation of a critical mass of knowledge, e.g. body composition and metabolism, or suddenly from the development of new principles, drugs or techniques, e.g. asepsis, antibiotics, blood vessel anastomoses.

Craniofacial surgery started haltingly in the 1950s, grew slowly in the 60s, became vigorous in the 70s, and propagated in the 80s. As a result, surgeons today can safely operate in practically every anatomical area of the head and neck in order to remove disease or repair deformity. The last major fortress to withstand surgical penetration was the cranio-orbital-facial complex which had been a 'No-man's Land' between neurosurgery, ophthalmology, and plastic and maxillofacial surgery.

This major breakthrough was mainly due to Dr Paul Tessier's study, skill and persistence. He developed models for preoperative planning and established surgical techniques for wide exposure, hemostasis, firm fixation and elimination of dead space. His teaching sessions, in Paris and world-wide, spread the news rapidly. As a result a solid core of craniofacial surgeons on every continent quickly established their own teams. Currently major centres exist around the world and increasing numbers of patients with varieties of congenital, neoplastic and traumatic deformities are being treated successfully.

In addition to improving the appearance, function and psychology of these afflicted patients the craniofacial surgeon and his team have widened the scope and vision of the involved specialties. Specialty barriers as well as anatomical ones have dissolved; members of the craniofacial team must work together harmoniously and be prepared to evaluate and handle expertly all the tissues and organs of this complex anatomical area.

This carefully documented volume integrates and synthesizes a ten year experience of four surgical scholars from active centres in three European countries. The authors and their contributors have presented far more than their surgical experiences. They have enriched the volume with carefully prepared and well illustrated chapters on Embryology, Growth, Comparative Anatomy and Genetics.

Every major surgical advance impinges unexpectedly on other branches of medicine. No one could have predicted the vast impact of organ transplantation and cardiac surgery. Similarly, craniofacial surgery has already had a wide influence on other scientific disciplines. There is a healthy renewed dialogue and understanding with the disciplines of genetics, embryology and anatomy.

This 'biological revolution' has been well summarized by one of the contributors, Dr Slavkin: 'Traditional concepts and methods now merge within a new intellectual and methodological synthesis in cellular, molecular and developmental biology.'

In this era of diminishing respect for the medical profession, the escalating cost of medical care, increasing patient complaints, and the heavier burden of government interference with the doctor–patient relationship, it is healthy for us to stand back and consider the broad picture. What finer way to spend the one life we have been given than to care for these patients born with birth deformities. We can combine the best of surgery with the best of science and offer the product to a fellow human being. Now, for the first time, we can really help improve their condition; indeed, in many instances we can give them the chance of a normal life.

I am privileged to be part of such a talented and caring group of surgeons, physicians, and scientists. I thank the authors for the time, thought, and work they have woven together for the ultimate benefit of all of our patients.

Boston, Mass.,   J. E. M.
USA
1990

Dedication

This book is dedicated to Nicolette, Dolly, Luz and Carola
with gratitude.

They have done so much for so long.

Preface

This book presents the result of a confrontation that continued 10 long years between four persons of different language, cultural background, and way of thinking. The excellent quality of the professional and academic relationship that grew out of this made possible the harmonization of our views. It is this common philosophy that forms the basis of this book.

The ideas expressed in the book have gained in value by their graphic representation. The drawings, conceived by the main authors, prepared by **J. Lebeau** (Grenoble) and H. de Vries (Rotterdam) and produced by **Mrs O. Greco** (Milan) have enriched the text considerably.

The book has been written for cranio-maxillo-facial surgeons and for other surgeons involved in the treatment of cranio-facial malformations, but we also hope that the book will be of interest to paediatricians, gynaecologists, and all those participating in the study, examination, and treatment of cranio-maxillo-facial malformations: that is, all those sharing our concern for the well-being of these unfortunate children.

1990

MS
JVDM
BR
RM

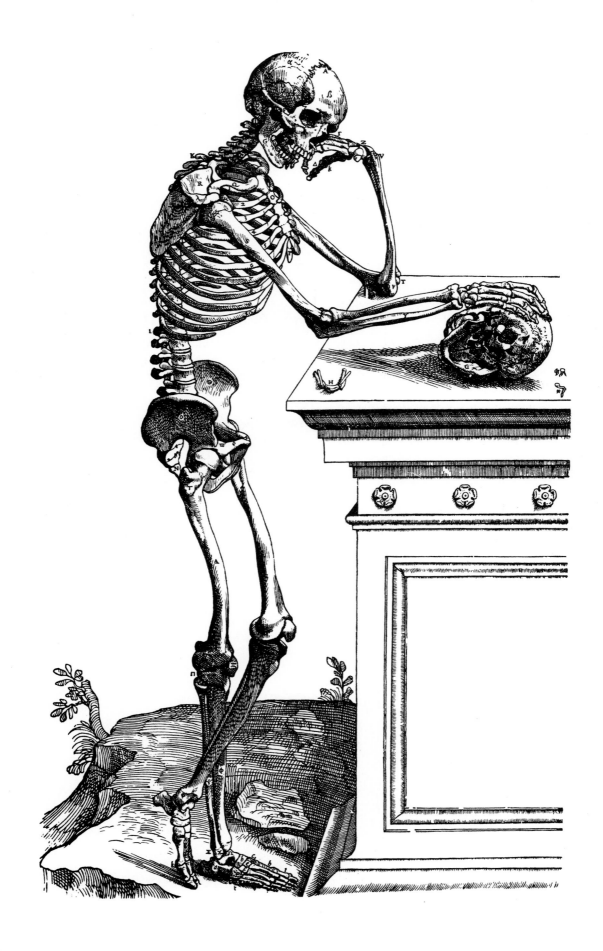

Acknowledgements

The writing of a book has many aspects, most important among these is the attempt to create order out of chaos. In this particular attempt, many people have helped. We are extremely grateful to:

our secretaries, Annemarie Thiebaul in Nancy, Marie Jeanne Belin, Odile Bruel in Grenoble, Paola Romagnani in Milan, and Yvonne van Neutegem and Judith Thirion in Rotterdam. The search for references, the typing of the manuscript, the repeated corrections made by Judith and her wordprocessor, all took many, many hours;

the photographers Christian Coin in Nancy, Christian Moreau in Grenoble and Sandor Lazlo and Lex Doff and the other members of the staff in the audiovisual department of the University Hospital in Rotterdam for their efforts to produce the best at short notice;

the medical artists J. Lebeau in Grenoble, H. de Vries in Rotterdam, Henri Desnoyer in Nancy and the *prima interpares*, Mrs O. Greco in Milan, who deserves special mention for her excellent work;

our linguistic editor David Tolhurst in Leyden, who had the difficult task of reading original translations from the French and the Dutch into Franglais or Anglo-Dutch and turning these into proper English;

the engineers F. Zonneveld and S. Lobregt in Eindhoven, who were responsible for many of the 3D reconstructions in this book;

our colleagues in the different surgical teams J. Montaut (in memoriam), A. Czorny and H. Hepner in Nancy, M. Vaandrager and D. Paz Geuze in Rotterdam and J. P. Chirossel and J. Lebeau in Grenoble;

and finally our sponsors, the Dean of the Medical Faculty in Grenoble, the Secretary of the Foundation for the Sick Child in Rotterdam, and the Director of Philips Medical Systems in Eindhoven, whose generous contribution made it possible to reproduce many illustrations in colour.

Contributors

A. Th. M. van Balen, MD, PhD
Professor and Chairman Department of Ophthalmology, Free University of Amsterdam, The Netherlands

L. Barinka, MD, CSc.,
Professor and Head of the Department of Plastic and Reconstructive Surgery, University of J. Ev. Purkyne, Brno, Czechoslovakia

S. Bracard, MD
Ancien Interne des Hopitaux, Praticien Hospitalier Universitaire, Service de Neuroradiologie, Centre Hospitalier Regional et Universitaire de Nancy, France

A. R. Chancholle, MD
Chirurgien Plasticien, Toulouse, France

R. J. Dambrain, MD
First assistant in maxillo-facial surgery, Associate of Anatomy, Catholic University of Louvain, Brussels, Belgium

P. Forlodou, MD
Assistant des Hopitaux en Neuroradiologie, Assistant d'Anatomie a la Faculté, Centre Hospitalier Regional et Universitaire de Nancy, France

N. M. Hilgevoord, MD
Senior Staff consultant anaesthesiology, University Hospital, Rotterdam, Sophia Children's Hospital, Rotterdam, The Netherlands

E. H. Huizing, MD
Professor and Head of Department of Otorhinolaryngology, University Hospital Utrecht, The Netherlands

I. T. Jackson, MB, Ch.B., FRCS (E), FRCS (G), FACS
Director, Institute for Craniofacial and Reconstructive Surgery, Providence Hospital, Southfield, Michigan, USA

M. Jupa, MD
Senior Consultant anesthesiologist, Department of Anesthesiology, University Hospital Rotterdam, Erasmus University, Rotterdam, The Netherlands

J. L. Marsh, MD, FACS
Professor of Surgery, Plastic and Reconstructive Medical Director, Cleft Palate and Craniofacial Deformities Institute, Washington University School of Medicine, St. Louis, Missouri, USA

R. F. Mazzola, MD
Assistant Professor, Postgraduate School of Maxillofacial Surgery, University of Milan; Consultant, Plastic and Maxillofacial Surgery, Bassini Hospital, Milan, Italy

C. Mentre, MD
Docteur ES Sciences, Diplome d'Etat 1978, Service de Chirurgie maxillo-faciale, Centre Regional et Universitaire de Nancy, France

J. C. Van der Meulen, MD
Professor and Head of the Department of Plastic and Reconstructive Surgery, Erasmus University, Rotterdam, The Netherlands

C. Moret, MD
Ancien Attache-Consultant des Hopitaux de Nancy, Praticien Hospitalier en Neuroradiologie au Centre Hospitalier Regional et Universitaire de Nancy, France

M. F. Niermeyer, MD
Professor of Genetics, Clinical geneticist, Department of Clinical Genetics, Erasmus University and University Hospital Rotterdam, Rotterdam, The Netherlands

L. Picard, MD
Professeur de Neuroradiologie Diagnostique et Therapeutique Radiologiste des Hopitaux, Chef de

Service de Neuroradiologie au Centre Hospitalier
Regional de Universitaire de Nancy, France

B. Raphael, MD
Professor and Head of the Department of Plastic and
Maxillo-Facial Surgery, University of Grenoble, France

H. C. Slavkin, DDs
Professor of Biochemistry, Department of Basic Sciences
and Laboratory Chief, Laboratory of Developmental
Biology, School of Dentistry, University of Southern
California, Los Angeles, USA

M. Stricker, MD
Professor and Head of the Department of Plastic and
Maxillofacial Surgery, Centre Regional et Universitaire
de Nancy, France

D. Tibboel, MD
Consultant Paediatric Intensivist, Paediatric Surgical
Intensive Care Unit, Sophia Children's Hospital,
Rotterdam, The Netherlands

P. Tridon, MD
Professor Titulaire Neuropsychiatrie Infantile, Directeur
Institut J. B. Thierry, Maxeville, France

M. W. Vannier, MD
Mallinckrodt Institute of Radiology, Washington
University School of Medicine, St Louis, Missouri, USA

C. Vermeij-Keers, MD
Associate Professor of Anatomy, Department of Anatomy
and Embryology, University of Leiden, The Netherlands

W. R. Marsh, MD
Associate Professor, Department of Neurosurgery, Mayo
Clinic, Rochester, Minnesota, USA

Contents

1. Evolving concepts in the understanding and treatment of craniofacial malformations

R. Mazzola, M. Stricker, J. Van der Meulen, B. Raphael

INTRODUCTION

A normal birth is always regarded as a logical, natural event. But when, for any reason, a deviation occurs, the malformation is received with a sense of fear and horror, but at the same time as an evincing example of the power of God.

The emotional reaction has varied according to education, civilization and religion: in some cultures the malformed baby is overprotected and adored, in others eliminated. However, in both events the malformed baby, or 'monster' as it was called in the past, symbolized the presence of a superior Being, the herald of mysterious warnings and prophecies.

When considering that in almost every civilization mythological deities are represented by dramatic figures borrowed partly from the animal world and partly from grotesque, malformed human creatures, we have reason to say that a relationship exists between malformation and the sense of fear it determines.

In ancient Egypt, for instance, there is an extreme prolificity of these examples. The Sphinx, an impossible being with a human head and a lion's body, manifested wisdom and power; the god Thot, symbol of the mind, possessed a human body with the head of a griffon. Similar figures are found in the Assyrian, Greek (the clover-hoofed Pan) and Roman mythologies (the two-headed Janus, Fig. 1.1).

THE MALFORMED AS PORTENTS

'Monstra, ostenta, portenta appellantur, quoniam monstrant, ostendunt, portendunt et praedicunt' — They are called monsters, ostents, portents, because they warn, ostend, portend and predict. This quotation from *De Divinatione* by Cicero summarizes the role played by the malformed for predicting future events.

Indeed the concept is very old. Babylonian clay tablets (early seventh century BC) are in this sense the oldest

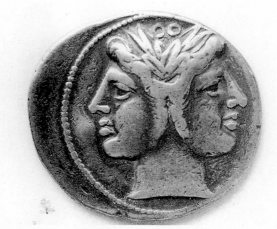

Fig. 1.1 Janus, as depicted on a Roman coin.

written records in our hands. They contain a list of 62 examples of human abnormalities with the related divination (Fig. 1.2). We report here those pertaining to the face (the numbers correspond to the original progressive order):

When a woman gives birth to an infant . . .
(15) whose nostrils are absent the country will be in affliction and the house of the man ruined;
(18) that has no tongue, the house of the man will be ruined;
(20) that has no nose, affliction will strike the country and the master of the house will die;
(22) whose upper lip overrides the lower, the people of the world will rejoice;
(23) that has no lips, affliction will strike the land and the house of the man will be destroyed.

In another tablet there is mention of a monster with a single eye in the forehead (cyclops), which will bring calamity to the country. As can be seen, none of the malformations described can be regarded as mythical, and, although rare, are well known and recorded in medical literature.

Although the Chaldean civilization disappeared, the importance of monsters in predicting the future and determining the course of events was essential in many cultures.

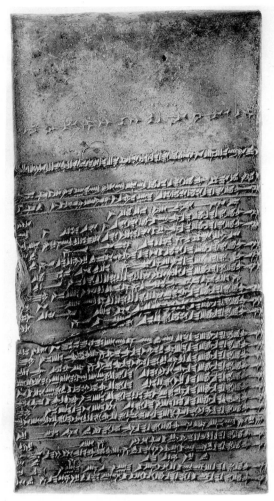

Fig. 1.2 Babylonian tablet: seventh century BC. (Reproduced with permission from the British Museum, London.)

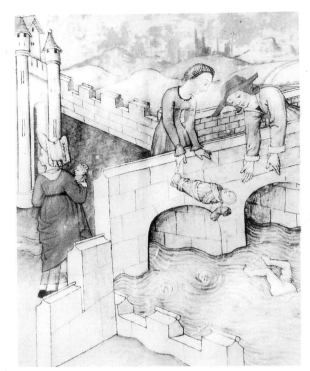

Fig. 1.3 Malformed infant being thrown into the Tiber.

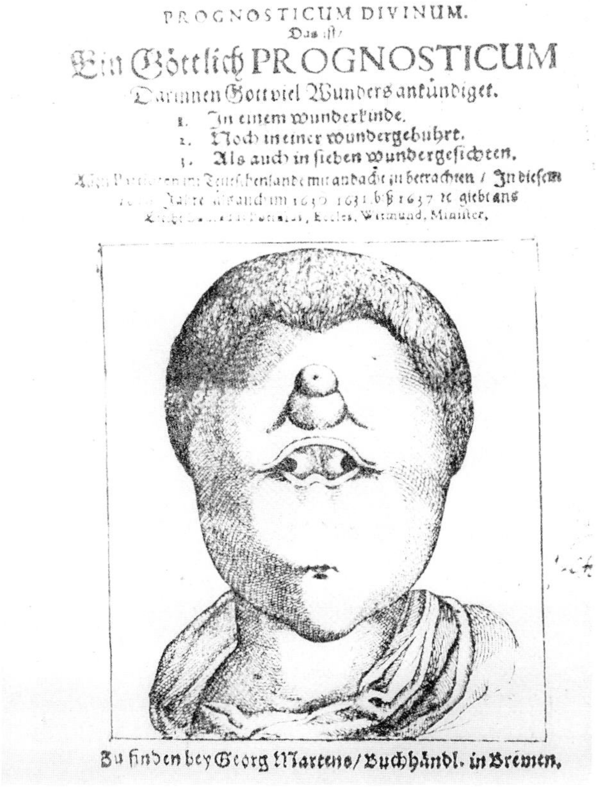

PROGNOSTICUM DIVINUM.
Das ist/
Ein Göttlich PROGNOSTICUM
Darinnen Gott viel Wunders ankündiget.
1. In einem wunderkinde.
2. Noch in einer wundergebuhrt.
3. Als auch in sieben wundergesichten.

Zu finden bey Georg Martens/ Buchhändl. in Bremen.

Fig. 1.4 Potinius: title page of his *Prognosticum Divinum* (1629).

In Greece and Rome they were identified as the cause of disasters and were therefore abandoned. Plato in his *Republic* suggested the elimination of malformed children, not only because they were considered responsible for misfortune, but also with a view to keeping the race as perfect and as strong as possible: it is well known that in Sparta they were thrown from Mount Taygetus. In Rome they had to undergo an inspection by five priests, although this formality was considered unnecessary, according to the Laws of the Twelve Tables. After that they were sacrificed or thrown into the Tiber (Fig. 1.3).

The concept that malformed children were to be taken as a warning was very popular not only in ancient civilizations but also later, in the period from the Middle Ages to the eighteenth century. Many pamphlets and leaflets were published on this subject (Fig. 1.4). It is, however, very interesting to note that this idea is still deeply rooted in some populations of Africa and Latin America.

THE MALFORMED: A CONTINUING CONFLICT BETWEEN FANTASY, SUPERSTITION AND SCIENCE

Probably the first writings on teratology were those of Aristotle (384–322 BC). His knowledge and detailed description of malformations is the result of careful observations: 'Monstrosity is contrary to nature. Nothing, in fact, can be produced contrary to that nature which is both eternal and essential . . . Monsters, i.e. where form did not tame matter.' Aristotle's report of hermaphroditism perfectly integrates with modern observations. He considered it impossible for a human to bear the head of a sheep and dismissed as unlikely the fantastic accounts of monsters described in ancient mythology.

After Aristotle the literature contains few descriptions of these phenomena: only sporadic examples of anomalies occur, in extravagant and ridiculous language, while Aristotle's statements were repeated for generations.

Pliny the Elder in his *Historia Naturalis* (AD 78) compiled an accurate report of some observations intermingled with a collection of mythological cases. He did not produce any order or explanation for the anomalies he described.

A number of incredible cases were illustrated during the following centuries and throughout the Middle Ages, with little resemblance to scientific truth. The principal aim was to create fright and horror for mankind and to describe the incredible wonders of God. The great majority of examples are a typical product of fantasy. The same type of deformity is tediously repeated by different artists, the only difference being the artistic quality of the woodcuts and plates. There are very few, sporadic personal observations.

Lychostenes is the author of a fascinating *Chronicle on Prodigies and Miracles on Earth and Heaven* from the origin of the world to the present time (1557). Among these miracles there is an extraordinary collection of congenital deformities: some realistic, others fantastic, some of them pertaining to the head and face (Fig. 1.5).

The great majority of these curiosities appear again 20 years later in a book by the French surgeon Ambroise Pare, specifically devoted to monsters (1575) (Fig. 1.8). Here the author gives a list of possible causes of monstrosities:

There are reckoned to be many causes of monsters; the first whereof is the glory of God, that his immense power may be manifested to those that are ignorant of it . . . Another cause is that God may punish men's wickedness, or show sign of punishment at hand . . . The third cause is an abundance of seed and overflowing matter . . . If, on the contrary, there be anything deficient in quantity, some or more members will be wanting, or more short and decrepite . . . The ancients have marked other causes of the generation of monsters . . . the force of imagination hath much power over the infant . . . Monsters are bred and caused by streightnesse of the womb . . . by the ill placing of the

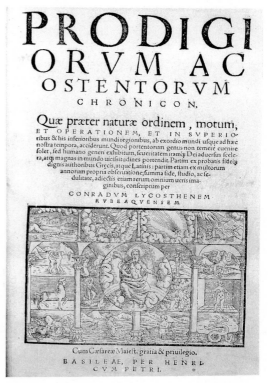

Fig. 1.5 Lychostenes: title page of his book on *prodigies* (1557).

mother in sitting, lying down or any other site of the body in the time of her being with child . . . by the injury of hereditary diseases, infants grow monstrous, for crookebakt produce crookebakt, lame produce lame, flat nosed their like . . . . Monsters are occasioned by the craft and subtlety of the Devill.

Hence, according to Pare the causes of congenital abnormalities may be summarized as follows: religious, environmental and hereditary. Apart from the first, these are still valid today. Pare's ideas represent the current concepts during the Middle Ages for explaining the origin of monsters.

Inspired, or even abundantly copied from Lychostenes, are the works on monsters by Schenk (1609), Licetus (1634), Aldrovandus (1642) and Schott (1667) (Fig. 1.6). More authentic and closer to reality are the reports on craniofacial anomalies by Bartholin (1654), van Meekeren (1682) and Tulp (1652) (Fig. 1.7).

An endless list of giants, dwarfs, conjoined twins, cyclops and anencephalic creatures fill the literature of the sixteenth and seventeenth centuries. Numerous reports on semihuman beings were invented as the result of bestiality and sexual perversions. Mothers of deformed children were considered witches and burnt at the stake for having an affair with the devil.

Finally, that maternal impressions had an important bearing on child formation was a popular belief all over the world (Ballantyne 1904). In Greece, pregnant women were recommended to look at beautiful statues and pictures to

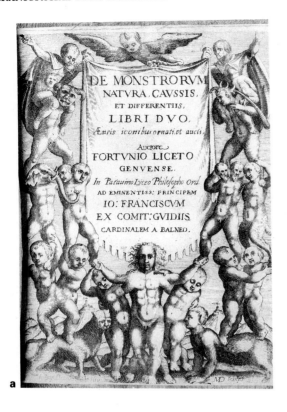

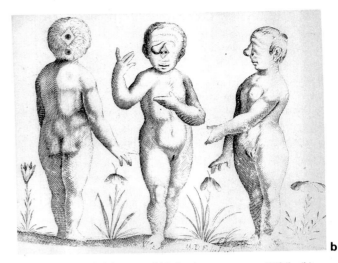

Fig. 1.6 Licetus: (a) title page of his book on monsters (1634); (b) some examples of cyclopia.

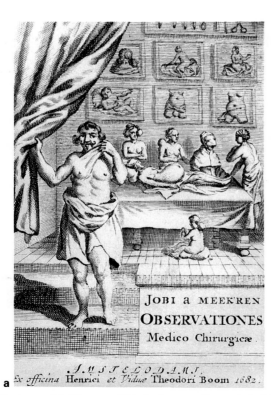

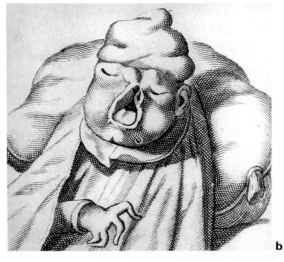

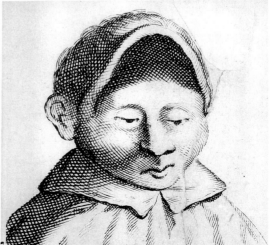

Fig. 1.7 van Meekeren: (a) title page of his book on medicosurgical observations (1682); (b) example of facial cleft; (c) example of craniostenosis.

deliver strong and perfect babies; in Sparta, they were obliged to observe the statues of Castor and Pollux. Pliny the Elder in his *Historia Naturalis* wrote that maternal and paternal thoughts at conception were determinant in shaping the child.

Conversely, a pregnant woman should not look at a monkey to avoid giving birth to anencephalic or microcephalic babies. Paré refers to the story of a monster born with a head shaped like that of a frog, because the mother in the first month of pregnancy held a frog in her hands (Fig. 1.8). The same story was later reported by Aldrovandus. Keating's *Cyclopaedia of the Diseases of Children* (1889) contains a chapter by Dabney on 'Maternal Impressions', which abounds with examples, such as the birth of a child with four fingers, because every day the mother saw a milkman with one finger amputated, or the birth of a child with a harelip, because the mother observed a man with that deformity, or the congenital absence of the auricle in a baby, because the mother at the fourth month of pregnancy was attacked by a man whose ear had been cut.

For centuries congenital malformations remained a field of superstition, fantasy and even of fraud in the sense that people exhibited freaks in order to make money out of them (Fig. 1.9).

Certainly behind the fantastic approach to the problem of congenital deformities lies the complete ignorance of any

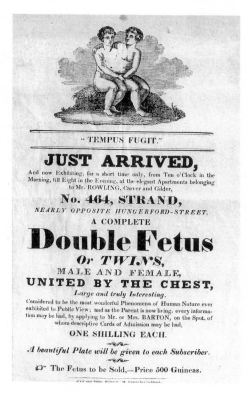

Fig. 1.9 Example of a nineteenth-century poster.

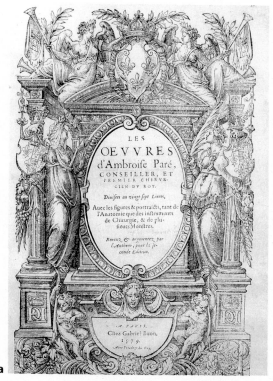

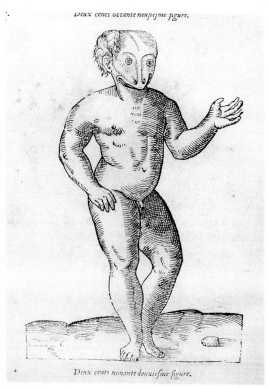

Fig. 1.8 Paré: (a) title page of his book on surgery (1575); (b) example of a monster.

concept of embryological formation. An important step forward in the history of congenital anomalies has been taken by the growing knowledge of embryology. Among the first contributions in this field mention should be made of *De Formato Fetu*, published in 1600 by Fabricius ab Aquapendente (1537–1619). Even more important is the *Exercitatio de Generatione Animalium*, published in 1651 by William Harvey (1578–1657), a disciple of Fabricius. For the first time appears the concept of developmental arrest during embryonic evolution as an explanation of congenital malformations. Harvey considered responsible for inducing malformation factors such as faulty maternal posture and the narrowness of the uterus:

In the foetuses of all animals, indeed that of man inclusive, the oral aperture without lips or cheeks is seen stretching from ear to ear, and this is the reason, unless I much mistake, why so many are born with the upper lip divided as it is seen in the hare and camel, whence the common name of harelip for the deformity. In the development of the human foetus the upper lip only coalesces in the middle line at a very late period.

By then, the development of embryology made certain deviations from the normal more understandable, and at the same time made it possible to face new problems, such as the medicolegal aspects posed by malformation.

The Italian Paolo Zacchia (1584–1659), one of the founders of medical jurisprudence, in his treatise *Quaestiones Medico-legales* (1655) includes a wide section on the medicolegal considerations of monsters.

The contribution by Albert von Haller (1708–1777) to the study of malformations is extremely important. In Volume 3 of his *Opuscula Minora* published in 1768, while giving a survey of the literature on congenital anomalies he attempts the first comprehensive classification of them. Other outstanding works about the same period are those published by the Netherlander W. van Doeveren (1765) and by the German Soemmerring (1791). While the former gives a detailed description of a case of bifid nose (Fig. 9.59), the latter tries to set up a classification of the midline and oblique facial clefts (Fig. 9.1).

The nineteenth century represents the beginning of a new era in the field of teratological science. Malformations were accurately studied in man and attempts to produce them artificially in animals were carried out.

Attempts were also made to treat some of them surgically. While at the turn of the century some works are still a blend of scientific and fantastic observations (Moreau de la Sarthe) (Fig. 1.10), others should be considered a reference point in this field for their accuracy. J.F. Meckel (1781–1833) compiled a detailed atlas of pathology, a couple of plates of which deal with facial deformities (1822–1828). Geoffroy St Hilaire not only described congenital anomalies but also set up a classification. He tried to reproduce them experimentally in chicken embryos, and his studies are elucidated in his

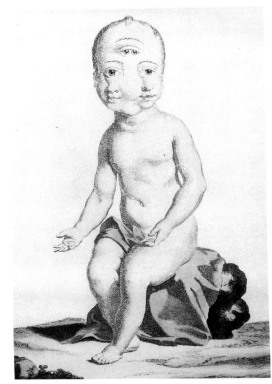

Fig. 1.10 Moreau de la Sarthe: case of facial duplication from his *Atlas* (1804) — fantasy and reality.

Traité de Teratologie, published in 1832, where the word teratology appears for the first time.

Many authors about this period produced remarkable works and well-documented monographs devoted to congenital anomalies, some of them specifically concerning craniofacial deformities. Those interested in this field of research are recommended to consult them, if possible, for the amount of information they possess. We quote here the most important:

Otto (1841): *Monstrorum Sexcentorum Descriptio*. A well-documented work.

von Ammon (1842): *Die Angeborenen Chirurgischen Krankheiten des Menschen*. His atlas is a collection of cases of malformations and is specifically concerned with their surgical treatment. An ample section is dedicated to the head and face.

Leukart (1845): *De Monstris*. This has a remarkable illustration of a craniofacial deformity.

Vrolik (1849): *Tabulae ad Illustrandam Embryogenesin*. Probably the most important atlas on this subject, with hundreds of observations, both personal and drawn from the literature, systematically arranged. There is the first report of a case of cloverleaf skull, with its autopsy (Fig. 9.154).

Spring (1853): *Monographie sur la Hernie du Cerveau*. The

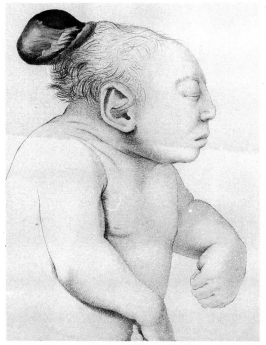

Fig. 1.11 Spring: hernia cerebri, a case from his *Monograph* (1853).

first monograph on meningoencephaloceles. It remains a reference point on this subject (Fig. 1.11).

von Bruns (1857): *Chirurgischer Atlas.* Another extraordinary collection of malformations and their surgical treatment.

Foerster (1865): *Die Missbildungen der Menschen.* A mine of information regarding the history of human congenital malformations and their classification.

Ahlfeld (1880): *Die Missbildungen der Menschen.* Another reference point in the field of congenital malformations, with a superb atlas containing hundreds of cases. The section on craniofacial deformities is well expounded (Figs. 1.12 and 9.112).

Stupka (1938): *Die Missbildungen der Nase.* The first monograph entirely dedicated to centrofacial deformities.

Other authors that deserve attention are: Taruffi (1881), Lannelongue & Menard (1891), Ballantyne (1904), Schwalbe (1906) and Hollaender (1921).

In the nineteenth century and the first three decades of the twentieth, pathologists had a good knowledge of morphology, pathogenesis and the classification of congenital malformations, but knew very little about the causative

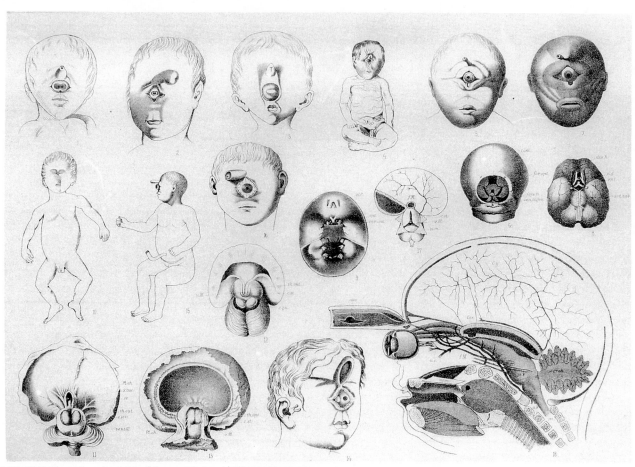

Fig. 1.12 Ahlfeld: a plate from his *Atlas on Human Malformations* (1880).

factors. Posture and amnios (oligohydramnios), the so-called mechanical factors, were considered the explanations for many malformations.

Other theories currently reported were the amniotic bands and the arrest of development. Probably Harvey, as we have seen, was the first to compare the cleft of the lip and cheek (i.e. macrostomia) with the arrest of lip and cheek formation at an early stage of development.

Some of these theories must not be entirely discarded and today, thanks to the investigations on animals with both spontaneous and induced defects, we have acquired a better understanding of the mechanism of anomalies. Careful extrapolation of these results to similar situations in man and the increasing knowledge in the pathogenesis of malformation have helped us to distinguish between different craniofacial defects and to classify them more accurately. From a practical point of view these findings provide the surgeon with a guide to planning the timing of appropriate reconstruction as related to growth.

THE SURGEON FACED WITH CONGENITAL CRANIOFACIAL MALFORMATIONS

As we have seen, in most ancient societies the way of treating newborns affected by congenital malformations was rather dramatic. In Sparta they were thrown from Mount Taygetus, while in Rome they were drowned in the Tiber. However, even nowadays a similar practice is still carried on in some Eastern Asian and Central African populations: the malformed is immediately exposed after birth. If for any reason it is not exposed or it survives, the untreated child is kept completely secluded from the rest of the population, society being reluctant to accept individuals that are not perfectly normal.

In the evolution of concepts for repairing congenital facial deformities, some steps should be mentioned. The first and easiest way to carry out the repair and to offer an immediate effective solution was to correct the cutaneous defect. The operation for cleft lip repair was already practised by Celsus (20 BC) and his plan for reconstructions was followed for centuries. For minor clefts he used to freshen the margins, while for the wider ones he carried out relaxing incisions on the cheek to facilitate closure. As for the cleft palate, it seems that prior to the first decade of the nineteenth century nobody dared to operate on it because it was considered to be caused by syphilis. Moreover, technical difficulties involving intense bleeding and lack of anaesthesia made any closure of the palate impossible. Von Graefe (1820) and Roux (1819) in the second decade of the nineteenth century were pioneers in carrying out this operation, which was later refined by von Langenbeck (1861).

Myelomeningocele was certainly known before Tulp (1652), who gave a full description of the anomaly and

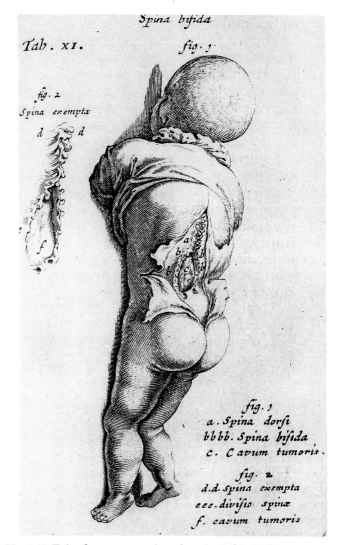

Fig. 1.13 Tulp: first representation of a spina bifida (1652).

coined the term spina bifida, still used today (Fig. 1.13). But for any surgical attempt to correct it, we have to await Bayer (1892), who, apparently for the first time, had the idea of using a flap containing muscle and fascia, so as to guarantee a satisfactory closure of the defect. Something similar can be said about anterior and posterior meningoencephaloceles. In the past attempted treatment consisted of compressions, repeated punctures and aspirations, and ligatures, obviously with little success.

Other examples of cutaneous correction of congenital facial defects during the nineteenth century are reported by Delpech (1828), a nasoschizis repaired by rotation of a trilobed forehead flap (Fig. 1.14); by von Ammon (1842), epicanthal folds by a Z-plasty; von Bruns (1857) and Warren (1867), facial haemangiomas by their excision; and Jalaguier (1909), bilateral oblique facial cleft by rotation of multiple local flaps (Fig. 1.15).

Major craniofacial anomalies were palliatively treated

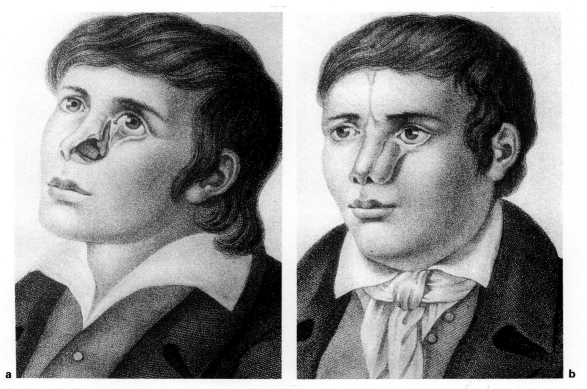

Fig. 1.14 Delpech: repair of a nasal malformation by a forehead flap (1828).

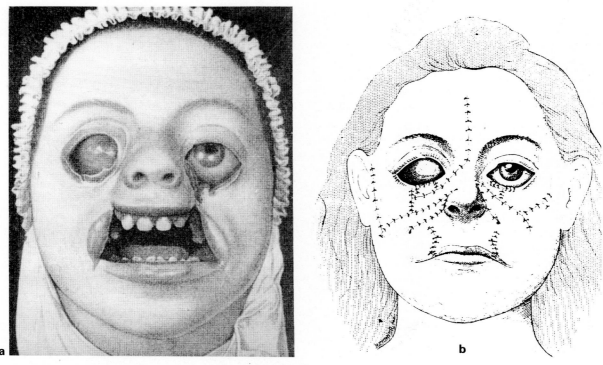

Fig. 1.15 Jalaguier: repair of oblique facial cleft by a series of flaps (1909).

until recently. Hypertelorism was modified by medial advancement of the eyebrows, modification of epicanthal folds and nasal bifidity, as suggested by Webster & Deming (1950). Midface retrusion in acrocephaly was modified, either with onlay bone grafts to enhance the hypoplastic infraorbital area (Lewin 1952), or with split-rib grafts extracranially placed to improve the contour (Longacre 1968).

The second step in surgery for malformations was the anatomical restoration of those structures severely distorted from birth and reorientation of inborn errors towards normality. For example, cleft lip and palate operations greatly improved in terms of results when muscular surgery, already advocated by Victor Veau in 1931, was recently introduced. It involves detachment of muscle fibres from their insertions at the alar base for cleft of the lip and at the posterior nasal spine for cleft of the palate, and their suture with the contralateral.

Repair of congenital craniofacial deformities represents one of the major breakthroughs of plastic surgery in the past twenty years. The Le Fort III osteotomy now currently used in craniofacial surgery is the result of a progressive evolution of techniques. Gillies & Harrison, in fact, borrowed the idea from the correction of a sequela of traumatism, i.e. to advance those midfacial structures brought in by the impact of trauma. They used this type of osteotomy in 1950 to advance the midface in a patient with craniofacial dysostosis, demonstrating how it was possible to extrapolate a technique from one field of surgery, i.e. traumatism, to another, i.e. malformations.

Tessier et al (1967) demonstrated that the intracranial approach was the sole solution in treating the problem of hypertelorism in a logical way, mobilizing the abnormally distant orbits and wiring them along the midline.

The third step includes correct timing for surgery. As emphasized above, better knowledge of embryology and growth provides the surgeon with a guide to plan the appropriate timing for surgery. Early surgery is a prerequisite to orientate growth towards normality in the presence of structures possessing an intrinsic growth potential, while late surgery is recommendable when this growth potential is minimal and approaches zero.

Finally, the last step includes preventive surgery, to correct malformation prior to birth. Intrauterine surgery, still experimental at present, will possibly become a reality in the future.

REFERENCES

Ahlfeld F 1880–1882 Die Missbildungen des Menschen. Grunow, Leipzig

Aldrovandus U 1642 Monstrorum historia. Tebaldino, Bologna

Ballantyne J W 1894 The teratological records of Chaldea. Teratologia 1: 130

Ballantyne J W 1904 Manual of antenatal pathology and hygiene. The embryo. Green, Edinburgh

Bartholin T 1654–1661 Historiarum anatomicarum Centuriae. Hauboldt, Copenhagen

Bayer L 1892 Zur Technik der Operation der Spina Bifida und Encephalocele. Prager Medizinische Wochenschrift 17: 317, 332, 345

Celsus A C 1478 De Medicina. Lorenzi, Florence

Delpech J M 1828 Chirurgie clinique de Montpellier. Vol II. Gabon, Paris

Fabricius ab Aquapendente G 1600 De formato foetu. Pasquati, Padua

Foerster A 1865 Die Missbildungen der Menschen systematisch dargestellt. Mauke, Jena

Geoffroy St Hilaire E 1822 Philosophie anatomique. Vol II. Publ author, Paris

Geoffroy St Hilaire I 1832 Histoire generale et particulière des anomalies en l'organisation chez l'homme et les animaux . . . ou traité de teratologie. Baillière, Paris

Gillies H, Harrison S H 1950 Operative correction by osteotomy of recessed malar maxillary compound in a case of oxycephaly. British Journal of Plastic Surgery 3: 123

Harvey W 1651 Exercitationes de generatione animalium. Pulleyn, London

Hollaender E 1921 Wundergeburt und Wundergestalt. Enke, Stuttgart

Jalaguier A 1909 Coloboma faciale bilaterale. Double fente congenitale bucco-orbitaire. Autoplasties successive. Guerison. Revue Orthopédique 25: 481

Keating J M (ed) 1889 Cyclopaedia of the diseases of children. Lippincott, Philadelphia

Lannelongue O M, Menard V 1891 Affections congenitales. Asselin & Houseau, Paris

Leukart, R 1845 De Monstris eorumque causis. Schweitzerbart, Gottingen

Lewin M L 1952 Facial deformity in acrocephaly and its surgical correction. Archives of Ophthalmology 47: 321

Licetus F 1634 De monstrorum natura, causis et differentiis. Frambotto, Padua

Longacre J J 1968 Craniofacial anomalies: pathogenesis and repair. Lippincott, Philadelphia

Lychostenes C 1557 Prodigiorum ac ostentorum chronicon. Petrus, Basel

Meckel J F jr 1817–1826 Tabulae anatomico-pathologicae. Gleditsch, Leipzig

Moreau de la Sarthe L J 1808 Description des principales monstruosités dans l'homme et dans les animaux. Fournier, Paris

Otto A W 1841 Monstrorum sexcentorum descriptio anatomica. Hirt, Wratislaw

Paré A 1575 Les oeuvres. Ch. 24. Buon, Paris

Potinius C 1629 Prognosticum divinum. Mateus, Bremen

Roux P J 1819 Observation sur une division congenitale du voile du palais et de la luette, guerie au moyen d'une operation analogue a celle du bec-de-lievre. Journal Universel des Sciences Médicales 15: 356

Schenk J G 1609 Monstrorum historia memorabilis. Becker, Frankfurt

Schott G 1667 Physica curiosa, sive mirabilia naturae et artis. Herzt, Wuerzburg

Schwalbe E 1906 Die Morphologie der Missbildungen des Menschen und der Tiere. Fischer, Jena

Soemmerring S 1791 Abbildungen und beschreibungen einiger Missgeburten. Universitaetsbuchhandlung, Mainz

Spring A 1853 Monographie sur la hernie du cerveau et de quelques lesions voisines. de Mortier, Brussels

Stupka W 1938 Die Missbildungen und Anomalien der Nase und des Nasenrachenraumes. Springer, Vienna

Taruffi C 1881 Storia della teratologia. Regia Tipografia, Bologna

Tessier P, Guiot G, Rougerie J, Delbet J P, Pastoriza J 1967 Osteotomies cranio-naso-orbital-faciales. Hypertélorisme. Annales de Chirurgie Plastique 12: 103

Tulp N 1652 Observationes medicae. Elzevir, Amsterdam

van Doeveren W 1765 Specimen observationum academicarum ad monstrorum historiam. Bolt & Luchmans, Gröningen

van Meekeren J J 1682 Observationes medico-chirurgicae. Boom, Amsterdam

Veau V 1931 Division palatine. Masson, Paris

von Ammon F A 1842 Die angeborenen chirurgischen Krankheiten des Meschen. Herbig, Berlin

von Bruns V 1857–1860 Chirurgischer Atlas. II. Abt: Kau- und Geschmachsorgan. Laupp & Siebeck, Tübingen

von Graefe C F 1820 Die Gaumennaht, ein neuentdecktes Mittel gegen angeborene Fehler der Sprache. Graefe und Walther's Journal der Chirurgie und Augenheilkunde 1: 1

von Haller A 1768 Opuscula anatomici argumenti minorum. Vol. III. Grasset, Lausanne

von Langenbeck B R 1861 Die Uranoplastik mittelst Abloesung des mucosperiostalen Gaumeueberzuges. Hirschwald, Berlin

Vrolik W 1849 Tabulae ad illustrandam embryogenesin hominis et mammalium. Londonck, Amsterdam

Warren J M 1867 Surgical observations with cases and operations. Ticknor & Fields, Boston

Webster J P, Deming E G 1950 Surgical treatment of the bifid nose. Plastic and Reconstructive Surgery 6: 1

Zacchia P 1655 Quaestiones medico-legales. Ch VII. Piot, Avignon

Craniofacial development

2. Cellular and molecular determinants during craniofacial development

H. C. Slavkin

INTRODUCTION

One of the most fascinating and significant problem areas in contemporary developmental biology concerns how differential gene activity is regionally regulated — when, where and how are genes expressed and how is differential gene regulation associated with specific patterns of morphogenesis? This is a core problem in craniofacial developmental biology.

During the last thirty years we have witnessed the genesis of the so-called 'biological revolution' (Crick 1982). In 1953 James Watson and Francis Crick published their seminal article on the structure and possible functional implications of DNA (deoxyribonucleic acid). Since that time incredible advances have continuously been reported, ranging from the identification, isolation and characterization of DNA polymerase, DNA ligase, RNA polymerases and restriction nucleases, to the structure and function of ribosomal RNA (rRNA), transfer RNA (tRNA), messenger RNA (mRNA), regulatory genes, structural genes and the protein–nucleic acid interactions which regulate differential gene expression during development (for example see Alberts et al 1983, Crick 1982, Judson 1979, Lewin 1985, Steinmetz & Hood 1983). These results have led to the 'new biology', a biological revolution in which traditional concepts and methods now merge within a new intellectual and methodological synthesis in the fields of cellular, molecular and developmental biology.

This chapter is designed to highlight the new biology as related to selected problems in normal and abnormal craniofacial developmental biology. A number of contemporary challenges in research now utilize recombinant DNA technology directed towards understanding the molecular basis of craniofacial morphogenesis. These studies offer significant promise towards enhanced diagnosis, treatment and prevention of inherited craniofacial malformations (see recent reviews such as Cohen & Rollnick 1985, Melnick et al 1982, Slavkin 1979, 1988, in press, Slavkin et al 1988).

GENE CONTROLS DURING CRANIOFACIAL DEVELOPMENTAL BIOLOGY

One of the most significant problems in craniofacial development concerns the processes by which specific gene activities are regionally and temporally controlled. The key issue is to understand how cells in different regions of the developing organism, and at different stages in the sequence of development, become committed to a specific phenotype (see critical discussion by Goodman et al 1984). When, where and how do cells acquire unique phenotypes during the sequence of gastrulation, neurulation, embryogenesis, fetal and neonatal development, and throughout the subsequent stages of the life process? (Fig. 2.1.)

In order to decipher this fascinating puzzle, it becomes essential to discriminate between several possibilities: (1) that cells are committed intrinsically for a particular pattern of cell differentiation according to a predetermined cell lineage; and/or (2) that cells become committed extrinsically according to positional and temporal instructions.

To pursue this problem, therefore, it becomes useful to

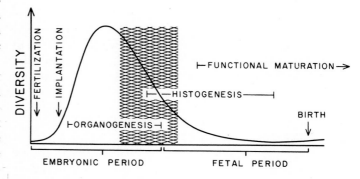

Fig. 2.1 The process of craniofacial development is initiated during early embryogenesis and continues throughout the human lifespan. Major determinants for craniofacial morphogenesis, histogenesis and cytodifferentiation are established during the embryonic period of human development.

obtain highly specific probes with which to ascertain a cell's phenotype in situ (e.g. in situ hybridization and immunocytochemical localization methods), as well as other experimental techniques which enable one to change the position of a cell during the process of development. These experimental approaches thereby provide for a dissection between inherited genetic information on the one hand, and cell–cell and cell–extracellular matrix (ECM) interactions on the other (see excellent reviews by Reddi 1984, Slavkin & Greulich 1975, Trelstad 1984).

It is clear that following fertilization and the first cleavages blastoderm cells are ionically and metabolically coupled — each blastoderm cell derived from the 2- and 4-cell zygote is capable of giving rise to an entire organism. Subsequent cleavages result in cells which are not capable of giving rise to an entire organism. Rather, cell groupings found within the blastocyst, gastrula and subsequent stages of development become increasingly restricted and thereafter constrain their influence to unique patterns of regional specification activity.

During the initial stages of development following fertilization, blastoderm cells within the 2- and 4-cell stages of the zygote are essentially equivalent. During subsequent development small 'differences' seem to appear and these differences become enhanced as increasing cell division and positional changes result in more complex patterns of embryogenesis. It is also assumed that these differences result from subtle alterations in the chemomechanical interactions between the nucleus, the cytoplasm and the plasma membrane within each cell, as well as the ionic and metabolic cooperativity between individual cells (Fig. 2.2).

Thereafter, individual differences become associated with regional aggregates of cells (i.e. tissues), and these regional differences serve to cue temporal and positional information during development. Of course, the critical question is how gene regulatory molecules become unequally distributed within and between emerging cell populations. Determinants for differences allegedly are localized either (1) within the fertilized egg, (2) progressively partitioned as cytoplasmic determinants, and/or (3) represented as small molecular signals within or between individual cells that mediate differential gene regulation during development (Fig. 2.3).

REGIONAL SPECIFICATION OF CELL TYPE-SPECIFIC GENE CONTROL

When, where and how does regional specification regulate cell type-specific gene control? It is now readily apparent that individual cells are not preprogrammed for subsequent cell differentiation. Intrinsic factors do not seem to regulate cell type-specific gene expression; rather extrinsic or environmental cues appear to mediate cell differentiation.

When and where cell type-specific gene expression takes

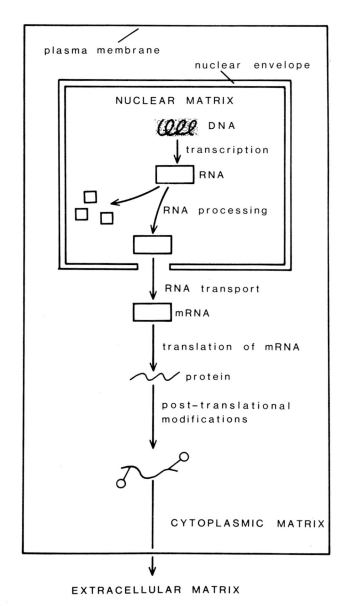

Fig. 2.2 A generalized scheme for gene expression. Eucaryotic cell types possess three major compartments or matrices which are closely coupled: (i) nuclear matrix, (ii) cytoplasmic matrix and (iii) extracellular matrix. Interactions between these matrices appear to mediate regional specification of *de novo* cell-specific gene expression.

place during development can now be evaluated at either (1) the production of specific transcripts (e.g. mRNA) level using cDNA or RNA probes directed against a unique nucleic acid sequence and the technique of in situ hybridization, or (2) the production of translated protein (i.e. translation level) using monoclonal or polyclonal antibodies against specific epitopes of the protein and the technique of immunocytochemistry. Each of these techniques is sufficient to provide the resolution to identify and localize discrete cells within the developing organism that have become determined for a particular phenotype — for example, mammary gland epithelial acinar cells producing

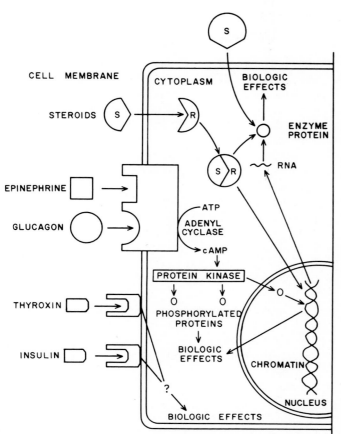

Fig. 2.3 Differential gene expression is regulated by epigenetic factors, ranging from polypeptide growth factors (e.g. tumour growth factor, platelet-derived growth factor, fibroblast growth factor, epidermal growth factor), steroid (S) and polypeptide hormone (e.g. cortisol, progesterone, insulin, thyroxin), trace elements and vitamins, to distinct molecules produced by adjacent and metabolically cooperative cell types. These mediators bind either to the cell surfaces or to intracytoplasmic binding proteins (R, receptors) which subsequently interact with chromatin DNA and thereby regulate gene expression.

casein, chick oviduct follicular epithelial cells producing ovalbumin, lung alveolar type II epithelial cells producing pulmonary surfactant protein, tooth enamel organ-derived epithelial cells producing enamel proteins, tooth ectomesenchyme cells becoming odontoblasts and producing dentine phosphoprotein, chondroblasts producing type II collagen, and neural crest-derived cells in the dorsal root ganglia producing a specific cytoplasmic polypeptide associated with the neuronal phenotype. How regional specification invokes the acquisition of a determined phenotype remains as yet unknown.

SEVERAL CRANIOFACIAL PARADIGMS FOR REGIONAL SPECIFICATION OF CELL TYPE-SPECIFIC GENE CONTROLS

The cranial neural crest

The cranial neural crest of the vertebrate embryo provides an excellent paradigm with which to dissect putative

controls for cell differentiation (see excellent reviews by Le Douarin 1982, 1986). The neural crest is a profoundly transitory embryonic structure which arises from the lateral ridges of the forming neural tube when they unite mediodorsally during the closure of the neural tube. Cells within the cranial neural crest are heterogeneous and possess varying potentials prior to their striking migration patterns from the neural tube throughout the forming embryo (Le Douarin 1986). Crest cells migrate from the tube at precise times and at precise locations, and subsequently follow precise pathways of migration resulting in the determination of specific phenotypes (Davis et al 1985) (Fig. 2.4). Of particular interest is that these cranial neural crest cells give rise to a large number of different phenotypes, including a number of neuronal cell types and the mesenchymal cells that differentiate into the brain meninges, the entire facial and visceral arch skeleton and dermis, the musculoconnective wall of the large arterial trunks arising from the aortic arches, and the connective tissues of the buccal and pharyngeal region including that of the teeth, mandible and maxillae, salivary glands, thyroid glands, parathyroid glands and thymus gland (see

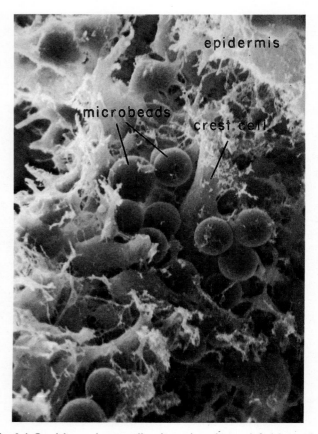

Fig. 2.4 Cranial neural crest cells migrate into the craniofacial complex and differentiate into many different phenotypes, including ectomesenchyme (e.g. cementoblasts, chrondroblasts, fibroblasts, osteoblasts, odontoblasts). Injection of microbeads into regions of premigratory cranial neural crest had been successfully used to trace the migratory pathways (see example by Davis et al 1985).

Edelman et al 1985, Goodman et al 1984, Le Douarin 1982, 1986, Slavkin 1979, Slavkin et al 1988). Cranial neural crest development involves the clear determination of different cell lineages.

What has now been established are a number of generalizations which directly relate to the theme of our discussion. Migrating cranial neural crest cell populations are not composed of homogeneous cell types that are all endowed with the entire range of developmental capacities expressed in the various crest-derived phenotypes. Within the premigratory cranial neural crest the individual cells are heterogeneous and many have already been restricted before migration. Further, during the migratory process, cranial crest cells are highly labile and respond to environmental cues from the extracellular matrix and/or other cell populations. Therefore, the cranial neural crest can be considered to represent a mixture of neuroepithelial cells with variable degrees of determination for particular phenotypes.

These dissimilar cells migrate along predetermined pathways which in turn have been developed according to temporal and positional patterns resulting from major embryonic morphogenesis (Thiery et al 1985a). Environmental cues representing neuronal- and non-neuronal-derived signals mediate the cranial neural crest progressive process of cell differentiation. The specific domains of the fibronectin molecule have recently been implicated in the process of crest cell migrations and the determination of specific phenotypes (see Thiery et al 1985b). Alterations in any level of this complex biological organization can result in major craniofacial malformations (see Cohen & Rollnick 1985, Melnick et al 1982, Noden 1988). Available evidence would suggest that definite regulatory genes may operate in the architecture of the forming craniofacial complex, and that these homoeotic genes may soon be identified and characterized in terms of the cranial neural crest-related processes (Fig. 2.5).

Severe congenital craniofacial malformations have been reported in association with the use of a new dermatological drug, isotretinoin (13-cis-retinoic acid or Accutane) (see Lammer et al 1985). Recent studies by Webster et al report a striking association between isotretinoin embryopathy and the cranial neural crest during in vivo and in vitro animal model studies. These authors suggest that many congenital craniofacial malformations allegedly induced in humans and other mammals by isotretinoin and its metabolite, 4-oxo-isotretinoin, result from drug effects on initial differentiation and migration of cranial neural crest cells.

Despite these interpretations regarding cranial neural

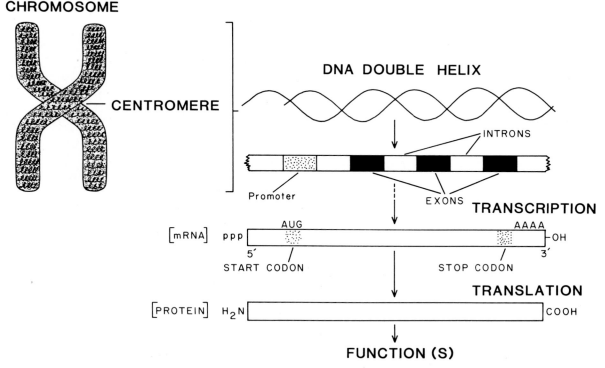

Fig. 2.5 Schematic drawing of a typical metaphase chromosome and several different levels of functional genetic constituents: (i) the double helix of DNA is approximately 2 nm wide and contains several hundred thousand gene sequences that are expressed during development; and (ii) a schematic representation of a DNA sequence or gene indicating a promoter, start codon signal, exons (genetic code resulting in protein primary structure), intron (spacer sequence) and stop codon signal sequences. Whereas a great deal of information is known regarding DNA replication (mitosis), transcription, reverse transcription and translation, very little is known as to how discrete sequences of DNA are activated and then transcribed under regional specification during embryogenesis.

crest migrations, the preponderance of the data being derived from chick and quail embryonic studies, other descriptions and interpretations have been put forward regarding the putative role of neurulation processes with subsequent craniofacial morphogenesis (see excellent discussions by Vermeij-Keers et al 1983, Smits-van Prooije 1986, Lumsden 1988). These authors suggest that primary craniofacial malformations originate from defects occurring during the cephalic neurological changes associated with facial morphogenesis. Evidence has been recently interpreted to challenge the notion of cranial neural crest-derived ectomesenchyme cell migrations during mammalian embryogenesis, in contrast to the information available for amphibian and avian embryos (see Smits-van Prooije 1986). Advances in microtechniques applied to mammalian embryos should provide clarification in the not too distant future.

The tooth organ

Recent studies have determined that ectodermal-derived oral epithelium, associated with first branchial arch morphogenesis, determines the timing, position and number of tooth organs (see excellent review by Lumsden 1988). It is now known that mesenchyme tissue provides regional specification for associated epithelial cell type-specific gene expression (see reviews by Dhouailly 1983, Kollar 1983, Slavkin 1978, 1979, 1984, 1985, Slavkin et al 1984a,b). Regional mesenchyme specification is a major feature of the integument development, resulting in exquisite patterns of epidermal differentiation (e.g. squamous, columnar, cuboidal, stratified squamous) and histogenesis (e.g. hair follicles, nail formation, sebaceous gland formation) (see extensive review by Dhouailly 1984). Of particular interest has been the recent results showing

that heterotypic tissue recombinations, such as between non-dental epithelial and dental mesenchyme tissues, resulted in the formation of tooth organs with the sequence of ameloblast cell differentiation and the expression of enamel genes with production of the enamel extracellular matrix (see review by Kollar 1983).

How mesenchyme regional specification mediates epithelial differentiation has been illustrated in the now classical experiment by Kollar & Fisher (1980). In their studies avian chick embryonic pharyngeal epithelial tissue was isolated and recombined with mouse fetal dental mesenchyme tissue and cultured as a heterotypic tissue recombinant within a permissive environment. These unorthodox tissue recombinants produced tooth-like organs with the apparent production of enamel extracellular matrix. Whereas modern birds do not express teeth nor do they express enamel genes, how can mesenchymal regional specification of cell type-specific gene expression be explained? (Fig. 2.6.)

How could the cranial neural crest-derived ectomesenchymal cells of the mouse fetal dental organ provide signals to activate avian quiescent enamel structural genes? Are there enamel genes in the chick genomic DNA? What are the putative ectomesenchyme-derived signals which activate the enamel organ epithelial developmental programme? How are these putative signals received by the epithelial cells? (Fig. 2.7.)

In order to investigate further this fascinating model for mesenchyme regional specification for cell type-specific gene expression, methods are required which can identify enamel-specific nucleic acid sequences as well as enamel polypeptides, and additional methods are required to seek putative mesenchyme-derived signals and their receptors within responding epithelial cells. This strategy requires the new biology and the integration of different disciplines

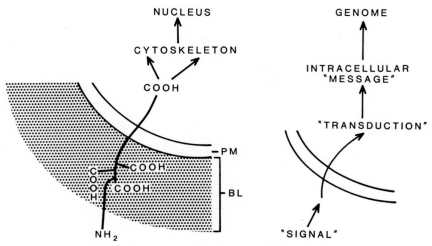

Fig. 2.6 Intercellular communication has been established as a major influence on differential gene expression. Extracellular 'signals' (e.g. platelet-derived growth factor) bind to transmembrane integral protein receptors which are often related to phosphorylation processes. These molecular interactions mediate transduction and a pathway by which signals influence gene activities during craniofacial development.

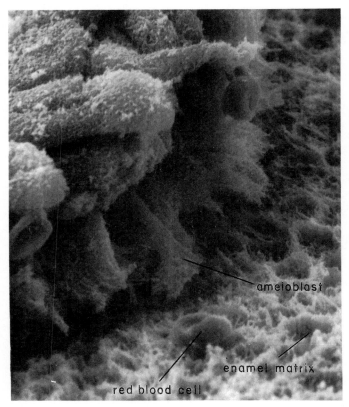

Fig. 2.7 Mesenchyme-derived instructions induce adjacent epithelial cells to differentiate into secretory ameloblasts with the production of enamel extracellular matrix and subsequent biomineralization. In this scanning electron photomicrograph red blood cells (7 μm in diameter) are present, associated with this topographical view of secretory ameloblasts.

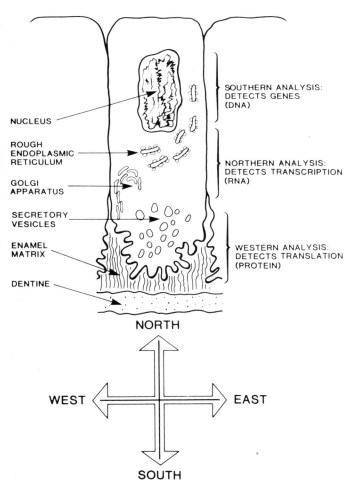

Fig. 2.8 Methods of studying the molecular biology of ameloblast cell function.

to focus on the complexity of this problem — recombinant DNA technology, immunocytochemistry, computer graphic analyses, protein chemistry, evolutionary biology, in vitro culture techniques using serumless and chemically defined media, embryology, morphology and additional types of scientific inquiry have become essential (Fig. 2.8). In this context, the construction and identification of a complementary DNA proble directed against the major mouse amelogenin has been completed (Snead et al 1983), the predicted primary structure of this major amelogenin polypeptide has been reported (Snead et al 1985), and the initial detection of nascent mRNA transcripts for this major amelogenin have been identified during the developmental sequence of epithelial differentiation in mouse molar tooth organs (Slavkin et al 1984a,b, Snead et al 1984, 1988) (Fig. 2.9).

THE NEW BIOLOGY AND CRANIOFACIAL DEVELOPMENTAL BIOLOGY

The major focus of the new biology is to investigate genes and how they function during biological processes. For example, what are the genes which regulate morphogenesis? Our challenge is to identify what are the genes which regulate morphogenesis, what is the language or code of these genes, what regulates the activation and silencing of these genes, and how we can investigate these questions using the knowledge of recombinant DNA technology (Figs. 2.10, 2.11).

The history of the new biology is short, interesting, readily accessible and clearly a product of the twentieth century. Whereas DNA was discovered in the sperm of trout found in the Rhine in 1871, it was not until 1943 that Oswald Avery and his colleagues experimentally demonstrated that DNA likely served to transmit inheritance within microorganisms. Then in 1953 James Watson and Francis Crick published their critical scientific paper indicating the physical structure of DNA and suggested functions in biological systems. Thereafter followed the biological revolution of the 1960s, 1970s and the 1980s — physics, chemistry, biology and mathematics converged into a new intellectual arrangement with a new syntax — a cellular, molecular and developmental biological strategy

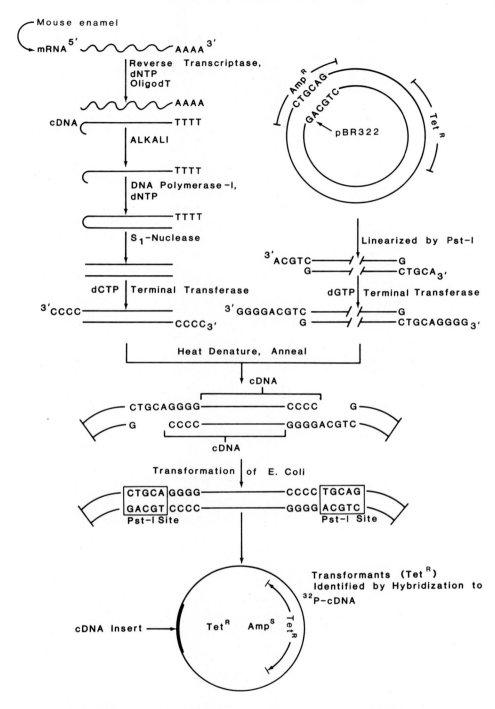

Fig. 2.9 The cloning of enamel genes involves a complex scheme in which messenger RNAs (mRNA) for enamel proteins are used as templates to produce double-stranded complementary DNA (cDNA) (shown at the left of this diagram). The steps require energy and specific enzymes such as reverse transcriptase, DNA polymerase-I, nuclease and, subsequently, terminal transferase. In turn, specific sites in the DNA of a unique bacterial source (i.e. pBR322) are used for enamel cDNA insertion, resulting in a specific transformant bacterium.

for investigations of problems ranging from virus assembly to the intricate complexities of craniofacial morphogenesis. The limited space of this chapter does not permit a detailed description of these numerous advances. There-

fore, the curious reader is encouraged to pursue these issues in such excellent primers as Alberts et al (1983), Crick (1982), Judson (1979), Lewin (1985) and Slavkin (1979).

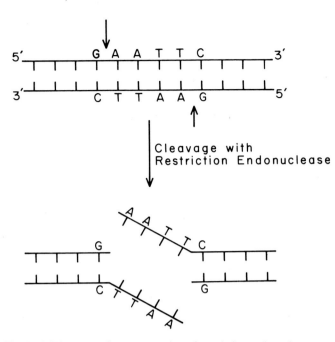

Fig. 2.10 Diagrammatic representation of restriction endonuclease enzyme cleavage of double-stranded DNA at one specific site or at staggered sites, and a suggested process by which cut ends can join or be annealed together to form unorthodox recombinations between foreign DNA (e.g. human insulin) and host DNA (*Escherichia coli* bacterial DNA).

GENES AND MORPHOGENESIS: CHALLENGES FOR CRANIOFACIAL BIOLOGY

The author has selected recent progress made at different levels of biological organization which relate to the theme of this chapter and which highlight what is now state-of-the-art investigations in the field of craniofacial developmental biology: (1) the discovery of the homoeo box in fruitflies and human beings; (2) the suggested function of gap junctions in establishing bilateral symmetry during neurulation; (3) the discovery of gene expression alternatives to type I collagen expression during mammalian organ formations; (4) the discovery that a single fibronectin gene is expressed through post-transcriptional processing into three different messenger RNAs; and (5) the utilization of transgenic methods to discover when, where and how specific genes are expressed during mammalian development.

Homoeo box in fruit-flies and human beings

Are there specific genes which control morphogenesis? Recently, different laboratories performed a critical genetic dissection of pattern formation processes which take place during embryogenesis in *Drosophila melanogaster* resulting

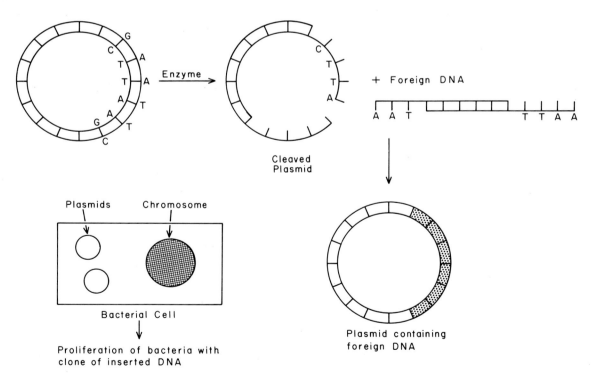

Fig. 2.11 Diagrammatic representation of the cloning of a gene to illustrate several features of a complex process. The insertion of fragments of eucaryotic DNA (e.g. mouse amelogenin cDNA) into bacterial plasmids (i.e. a small circular DNA found in bacterial cells, capable of autonomous self-replication), followed by cloning (bacterial cell multiplication), facilitates the growing of bacterial cell cultures of any size containing a unique foreign DNA sequence (e.g. mouse amelogenin DNA sequence, human insulin, chick collagen type I cDNA sequences).

in the discovery of regulatory or homoeotic genes (i.e. termed homoeo box) (see Gehring 1978, 1985, Hafen et al 1984, Kaufman 1983, Kuroiwa et al 1984, North 1984).

Within the four chromosomes of the fruitfly a discrete regulatory gene has been identified and cloned consisting of 180 nucleotides which code for a protein of 60 amino acids. There appears to be at least seven copies of this homoeo box gene sequence in the fruitfly genome. The homoeo box gene sequence is expressed in those creatures which generate segmentation along the anteroposterior axis of the organism (from fruitfly to philosopher). Mutation of this homoeo box gene expression results in gross aberrations in the morphogenesis of the organism.

This discovery has stimulated international scientific efforts to focus upon the possibility of linking discrete regulatory genes with specific stages of embryonic morphogenesis in creatures ranging from the invertebrates to human beings (see excellent review by Gehring 1985). These efforts are being brought to focus upon the regional specification of mammalian body-forming regions such as the central nervous system (Awgulewitsch et al 1986), branchial arch, somite and limb formations (see recent review by Gehring 1985).

If mouse and human homoeo box genes direct specific morphogenetic functions during craniofacial development, one would predict spatial and temporal localization of their expression to specific craniofacial regions (e.g. branchial arches, maxilla, mandible, dentition, tooth organs) of the developing organism (Holland 1988). Rapid progress has been possible in the fruitfly because of the extensive genetic knowledge available for *Drosophila melanogaster*, and the large number of mutations. Comparable advances are more difficult in mammals in that few mutations are known to disrupt morphogenesis without being lethal. However, the descriptive and comparative homology amongst invertebrate and vertebrate homoeo box genes (e.g. fruitfly, frog, chick, mouse and human) now provides a basis for future experimental analyses beyond conjecture.

Bilateral symmetry and intercellular communication

It is well established that gap junctions represent a specialized form of intercellular communication representing electrical, ionic and/or metabolic coupling amongst homotypic cells (e.g. epithelia). Gap junctions are visualized by transmission electron microscopy and appear to consist of open channels connecting adjacent similar cells. These junctions appear to facilitate the passage of ions and molecules of no greater than 1000 molecular weight.

Of particular interest are the recent findings which illustrate that gap junction proteins regulate intercellular communication during early embryogenesis (Warner et al 1984, Gutherie 1984, Fraser et al 1988). The major 27 000 molecular weight gap junction proteins from rat liver cells have been isolated and sequenced and affinity purified

polyclonal antibodies have been produced. These antibodies have been used to determine the putative functions of gap junctions during early amphibian embryogenesis following injection of antibodies into 2-, 4- and 8-cell stage embryos and then examining the subsequent consequences of this procedure. Preimmune antibodies were used as controls.

Antibodies injected into 8-cell stage embryos resulted in major aberrations in the establishment of bilateral symmetry during amphibian neurulation, thereby indicating that gap junction proteins serve a major function in the determination of symmetry prior to and during neurulation in the amphibian. Control injections with preimmune antibodies did not cause abnormal development ruling out possible effects of techniques of injection and suggesting allosteric hindrance from a non-specific antibody interaction during early development.

Collagen gene expression during embryogenesis

How does the extracellular matrix influence gene expression (Reddi 1984, Slavkin and Greulich 1975, Trelstad 1984)? Do secreted extracellular matrix macromolecules (e.g. collagens, fibronectin, glycosaminoglycans, laminin, phosphoproteins, proteoglycans) produced by specific cell types influence subsequent events during development? A number of significant advances have been made in the isolation, characterization and functional significance of tissue-specific collagen molecules (see Table 2.1).

More recently, the gene for type I collagen has been

Table 2.1 Collagen genetic heterogeneity

Collagen type	Chain organization	Tissue location
I	$[a1(I)]_2 \, a2(I)$	All connective tissues including skin, tendon, bone, cementum, dentine, cornea, fascia, periodontal ligament
I Trimer	$[a1(I)]_3$	Cells in culture, tumors, rapidly growing tissues.
II	$[a1(II)]_3$	Hyaline cartilage, vitreous humor, notochord
III	$[a1(III)]_3$	Lung, liver, cementum (not detected in bone or dentine)
IV	$[a1(IV)]_2 a2(IV)$	Basal lamina
V	$\alpha(V)$	All connective tissues
VI	$\alpha(VI)$	Microfibrils in blood vessels, uterus, placenta
VII	$\alpha(VII)$	Amnion
VIII	?	Hyaline cartilage
IX a1(IX), a2 (IX)	$\alpha3(IX)$	Fetal cartilage (maybe a proteoglycan)
X	?	Cultured fetal cartilage
XI	$\alpha1, \alpha2, \alpha3(XI)$	Cartilage
XII	?	Tendon fibroblasts and periodontal ligament fibroblasts

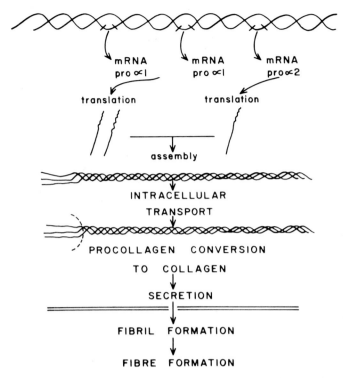

Fig. 2.12 Scheme for type I collagen transcription and translation in dentine, bone, cementum and connective tissue formation during craniofacial morphogenesis.

identified and sequenced, resulting in the ability to investigate a number of inherited connective tissue disorders such as Ehlers–Danlos syndrome, osteogenesis imperfecta and dentinogenesis imperfecta (see recent and comprehensive assessment edited by Fleischmajer et al 1985).

Metabolic perturbations of collagen using inhibitors of protein synthesis, hydroxylation of lysine and proline amino acids, glycosylation, intracellular transport of protein, removal of both amino- and carboxy-terminal peptides, secretion and intra- and intermolecular cross-linking have resulted in abnormalities of development. These results have been interpreted to mean that collagen (perhaps type I collagen) has major morphogenetic influences on the development of many biological systems such as tooth organs, dermal-epidermal interactions of the integument, bone formation, and the formation of many organs (e.g. salivary gland, lung organ, mammary glands, thymus gland) (see recent discussions by Hay 1984). Of particular clinical interest are the genetic defects associated with Ehlers–Danlos syndrome type VII, osteogenesis imperfecta, dentinogenesis imperfecta, dermatosparaxis, keloids, lung and kidney fibrosis and scleroses (Fig. 2.12).

In order to test the suggestion that type I collagen plays a major role in embryogenesis, an animal model system has been identified in which a provirus becomes incorporated into the genome of a mouse strain ('Move-13') in a position within DNA which blocks the transcription of the type I collagen gene; specifically, a Moloney murine leukaemia provirus becomes inserted into the first intron of the collagen a1 (I) gene, resulting in the complete block of the type 1 collage gene transcription during embryonic development (see Jaenisch 1985). The consequence of this engineered event is the production of a mouse strain which transmits this unique genetic defect according to classical Mendelian conventions. One striking feature of the homozygotes is that these embryos develop 'normally' until 12 days' gestation and then appear to die of major haemorrhage resulting from vascular defects. No type I collagen is produced by the homozygotes!

One fascinating derivative from these significant observations has been that taken experimentally by Klaus Kratochwil in collaboration with Rudie Jaenisch and Jurgen Lohler (1984). These scientists removed initial embryonic organ rudiments from 11-day gestation homozygotes and then cultured these organ primordia in vitro for extended periods of time (e.g. lung, kidney, heart, thymus gland, salivary gland, skin).

Whereas advanced morphogenesis, histogenesis and cell differentiation were observed in these extended cultures using serum supplementation, immunolocalization of type I collagen using monospecific antibodies was negative. Presumably, adaptive collagen gene expression resulted both in vivo using the animal model system as well as in vitro by producing other tissue-specific types of collagen other than type I collagen under these experimental conditions. These results have stimulated a number of approaches towards understanding when, where and how type I collagen influences morphogenesis.

Fibronectin gene expression

During craniofacial development cell-cell and cell-interactions appear to determine when and where developmental events take place. Fibronectin (FN) is a major ECM macromolecule implicated in how and where cells migrate (see excellent review by Yamada et al 1984). This glycoprotein consists of a dimer of two subunits; each subunit of approximately 250 000 molecular weight can be identical or similar. The allosteric features and the primary sequence information of FN provide additional information regarding FN functions in mediating cell–cell and cell–ECM interactions (see Thiery et al 1985a,b).

The recent advent of microchemical laboratories capable of obtaining the primary sequence of remarkably small amounts of purified protein, the utility of both monoclonal and polyclonal antibodies, advances in the production of cDNA probes with exquisite specificity, and a number of other techniques have resulted in a quantum leap in understanding the molecular biology of FN (see Hynes 1985). From these studies of the molecular biology of FN we now understand that there are multiple forms of FN subunits, that these subunits have varying structures and functions, and that these variations within the functional FN macromolecule are produced via intricate alterations during the transcription process of a single FN gene resulting in multiple and functional mRNAs. This example of yet another level of biological organization and control operant during craniofacial morphogenesis has been learned from the new biology of the 1980s.

Transgenic models in development

When, where and how specific genes are activated and expressed during developmet is being investigated using transgenic models. By a transgenic model the author describes a methodology now being used in the new biology which enables the insertion of a specific gene into the germ line of a complex species such as a mouse. The paradigm for this methodology was clearly established by Richard Palmiter, Ralph Brinster and their colleagues in their now classical scientific paper of 1982 where they demonstrated that isolated rat growth hormone ($\sim$ 10–13 M) could be injected into newly fertilized mouse eggs, become inserted into the mouse genome and subsequently be expressed, resulting in much larger mice. The methods to discriminate between genes and gene products of different species (e.g. rat and mouse) are being used to determine when, where and how selected genes are expressed during normal as well as abnormal development. These methods are also useful for studies of either structural (e.g. keratin, collagens, myosin, actin, enamel, dentine phosphoproteins) or regulatory (e.g. homoeo box) genes.

PROSPECTUS

The recent advent of the 'biological revolution' is nothing short of remarkable. Approaches to complex developmental biological questions unrealized but a few years ago have become mainstream cellular, molecular and developmental biological strategies in the 1980s. Mouse embryos are now cultured in vitro, structural and regulatory genes are being introduced into the germ line of murine species (see excellent summary by Pedersen 1988), and regulatory molecules are being defined which mediate exquisite biological processes (see recent example of McNeish et al 1988). A unity has been discovered which unites the effort between scientists curious about procaryotic as well as eucaryotic cells. Genes have been linked with specific phases of development as well as with specific inherited diseases. Moreover, there is an increased desire within the international biomedical research community to focus upon biotechnological issues and reduce the transfer time from fundamental laboratory research to applications for health care. It should be readily apparent, therefore, that we are on the threshold of a new biology which offers both unlimited promise as well as uncertainty to all of us engaged in craniofacial biology.

ACKNOWLEDGEMENTS

I wish especially to acknowledge my colleagues Joseph Bonner, Pablo Bringas, Richard Croissant, Jefferson Davis, Tina Jaskoll, Lawrence Honig, Mark Ferguson, Alan Fincham, Mary MacDougall, Michael Melnick, Sam Pruzansky, Malcolm Snead, Libby Wilson and Maggie Zeichner-David, with whom so much was learned about normal and abnormal craniofacial developmental biology. Many concepts as well as information was acquired through the generous support provided by the National Institutes of Health research grants DE-02848 and DE-07006.

REFERENCES

Alberts B, Bray D, Lewis J, Raff M, Roberts K, Watson J D 1983 Molecular Biology of the Cell. Garland, New York

Awgulewitsch A, Utset M F, Hart C P, McGinnis W, Ruddle F H 1986 Spatial restriction in expression of a mouse homoeo box locus within the central nervous system. Nature 320: 328–336

Cohen M M, Rollnick B R (eds) 1985 Craniofacial dysmorphology. Journal of Craniofacial Genetics and Developmental Biology (suppl

Crick F 1982 DNA today. Perspectives in Biology and Medicine 25: 512–517

Davis J U, Bringas P, Slavkin H C 1985 Quantitative localization of polystyrene microspheres following microinjection in the avian metencephalic neural crest pathway. Journal of Craniofacial Genetics and Developmental Biology 5: 11–19

Dhouailly D 1983 Feather forming properties of the foot integument in avian embryos. In: Sawyer R M, Fallow J F (eds) Epithelial–mesenchymal interactions in development. Praeger, New York

Dhouailly D 1984 Specification of feather and scale patterns. In: Malacinski S M, Bryant S V (eds) Pattern formation. Collier Macmillan, London. pp 581–602

Edelman G M, Hoffman S, Chuong C M, Cunningham B A 1985 The molecular bases and dynamics of cell adhesion in embryogenesis. In: Edelman G M (ed) Molecular determinants of animal form. Liss, New York. pp 195–222

Fleischmajer R, Olsen B R, Kuhn K (eds) 1985 Biology, chemistry, and pathology of collagen. Annals of the New York Academy of Science 460: 1–537

Fraser S E, Green C R, Bode H R, Bode P M, Gilula N B 1988 A perturbation analysis of the role of gap junctional communication in developmental patterning. In: Hertzberg E L, Johnson R G (eds) Gap Junctions. New York, Alan R. Liss, pp 515–526

Gehring W J (ed) 1978 Genetic mosaics and cell differentiation. Vol 9: Results and problems in cell differentiation. Springer-Verlag, Berlin

Gehring W J 1985 Homeotic genes and the control of cell

determination. In: Davidson E H, Firtel R A (eds) Molecular biology of development. Liss, New York. pp 3–22

Goodman C S, Bastiani M J, Doe C Q et al 1984 Cell recognition during neuronal development. Science 225: 1271–1279

Gutherie S C 1984 Patterns of junctional communication in the early amphibian embryo. Nature 311: 149–151

Hafen E, Kuroiwa A, Gehring W J 1984 Spatial distribution of transcripts from the segmentation gene Fushi Tarazu during *Drosophila* embryonic development. Cell 37: 833–841

Hay E D 1984 Cell–matrix interaction in the embryo: cell shape, cell surface, cell skeletons, and their role in differentiation. In: Trelstad R L (ed) The role of extracellular matrix in development. Liss, New York. pp 1–32

Holland P W H 1988 Homeobox genes and the vertebrate head. Development 103 Supplement 17–24

Hynes R 1985 Molecular biology of fibronectin. Annual Review of Cell Biology 1: 67–90

Jaenisch R 1985 Retroviruses and insertional mutagenesis in mice. In: Edelman G M (ed) Molecular determinants of animal form. Liss, New York. pp 47–58

Judson H F 1979 The eighth day of creation. Simon & Schuster, New York

Kaufman T 1983 The genetic regulation of segmentation in *Drosophila melangaster*. In: Jeffery W R, Raff R A (eds) Time, space, and pattern in embryonic development. Liss, New York. pp 365–384

Kollar E J 1983 Epithelial–mesenchymal interactions in the mammalian integument: tooth development as a model for instructive induction. In: Sawyer R H, Fallon J F (eds), Epithelial–mesenchymal interactions in development. Praeger, New York. pp 27–50

Kollar E J, Fisher C 1980 Tooth induction in chick epithelium: expression of quiescent genes for enamel synthesis. Science 207: 993–995

Kratochwil K, Lohler J, Jaenisch R 1984 Normal epithelial morphogenesis in the absence of collagen I. Journal of Embryology and Experimental Morphology 82: 30

Kuroiwa A, Hafen E, Gehring W J 1984 Cloning and transcriptional analysis of the segmentation gene Fushi Tarazu of *Drosophila*. Cell 37: 825–831

Lammer E J, Chen D T, Hoar R M et al 1985 Retinoic acid embryopathy. New England. Journal of Medicine 313: 837–841

Le Douarin N M 1982 The Neural Crest. Cambridge University Press, Cambridge

Le Douarin N M 1986 Cell line segregation during peripheral nervous system ontogeny. Science 231: 1515–1522

Lewin B 1985 Genes II. Wiley, New York

Lumsden A G S 1988 Spatial organization of the epithelium and the role of neural crest cells in the initiation of the mammalian tooth germ. Development 103 Supplement 155–169

McNeish J D, Scott W J, Potter S S 1988 Legless, a novel mutation found in PHT 1–1 transgenic mice. Science 241: 837–839

Mayne R 1984 The different types of collagen and collagenous peptides. In: Trelstad R L (ed) The role of extracellular matrix in development. Liss, New York. pp: 33–42

Melnick M, Shields E D, Burzynski N J (eds) 1982 Clinical dysmorphology of oral-facial structures. Wright, Boston

Noden D M 1988 Interactions and fates of avian craniofacial mesenchyme. Development 103 Supplement 121–140

North G 1984 How to make a fruitfly? Nature 311: 214–216

Palmiter R D, Brinster R L, Hammer R E et al 1982 Dramatic growth of mice that develop from eggs microinjected with metallothionein-growth hormone fusion genes. Nature 300: 611–615

Pedersen R A 1988 Early mammalian embryogenesis. In: Knobil E, Neill J et al (eds) The Physiology of Reproduction. New York, Raven Press, pp 187–230

Reddi A H (ed) 1984 Extracellular matrix: structure and function. Liss, New York

Slavkin H C 1978 The nature and nurture of epithelio-mesenchymal interactions during tooth morphogenesis. Journal de Biologie Buccale 6: 189–204

Slavkin H C 1979 Developmental craniofacial biology. Lea & Febiger, Philadelphia

Slavkin H C 1984 Morphogenesis of a complex organ: vertebrate palate development. In: Zimmerman E (ed) Current topics in developmental biology. Academic Press, New York. pp 1–16

Slavkin H C 1985 Regional specification of cell-specific gene expression during craniofacial development. Journal of Craniofacial Genetics and Developmental Biology (suppl) 1: 57–66

Slavkin H C 1988 Gene regulation in the development of oral tissues. Journal of Dental Research 67: 1142–1149

Slavkin H C, Greulich R C (eds) 1975 Extracellular matrix influences on gene expression. Academic Press, New York

Slavkin H C (in press) Molecular determinants during dental morphogenesis and cytodifferentiation: a review. In: Townsley J, Johnston M (eds) Research Advances in Prenatal Craniofacial Development. New York, Alan R. Liss

Slavkin H C, Snead M L, Zeichner-David M, Bringas P, Greenberg G L 1984a Amelogenin gene expression during epithelial–mesenchymal interactions. In: Trelstad R L (ed) The role of extracellular matrix in development. Liss, New York. pp 221–254

Slavkin H C, Snead M L, Zeichner-David M, Jaskoll T F, Smith B T 1984b Concepts of epithelial–mesenchymal interactions during development: tooth and lung organogenesis. Journal of Cellular Biochemistry 26: 117–125

Slavkin H C, MacDougall M, Zeichner-David M, Oliver P, Nakamura M, Snead M L 1988 Molecular determinants of cranial neural crest-derived odontogenic ectomesenchyme during dentinogenesis. American Journal of Medical Genetics 4: 7–22

Smits-van Prooije A E 1986 Processes involved in normal and abnormal fusion of the neural walls in murine embryos. PhD Thesis, University of Leiden, Netherlands

Snead M L, Zeichner-David M, Chandra T, Robson K J H, Woo S L C, Slavkin H C 1983 Construction and identification of mouse amelogenin cDNA clones. Proceedings of the National Academy of Science USA 80: 7254–7258

Snead M L, Bringas P, Bessem C, Slavkin H C 1984 De novo gene expression detected by amelogenin transcript analysis. Developmental Biology 104: 255–258

Snead M L, Lau E C, Zeichner-David M, Fincham A G, Woo S L C, Slavkin H C 1985 DNA sequence for cloned cDNA for murine amelogenin reveal the amino acid sequence for enamel-specific protein. Biochemical and Biophysical Research Communications. 129: 812–818

Snead M L, Luo W, Lau E C, Slavkin H C 1988 Spatial- and temporal-restricted pattern for amelogenin gene expression during mouse molar tooth organogenesis. Development 104: 77–85

Steinmetz M, Hood L 1983 Genes of the major histocompatibility complex in mouse and man. Science 222: 727–733

Thiery J P, Boucaut J C, Yamada K M 1985a Cell migration in the vertebrate embryo. In: Edelman G M (ed) Molecular determinants of animal form. Liss, New York. pp 167–194

Thiery J P, Duband J L, Tucker G C 1985b Cell migration in the vertebrate embryo. Annual Review of Cell Biology 1: 91–114

Trelstad R L (ed) 1984 The role of extracellular matrix in development. Liss, New York

Vermeij-Keers C, Mazzola R F, Van der Meulen J C, Strickler M 1983 Cerebro-craniofacial and craniofacial malformations: an embryological analysis. Cleft Palate Journal 20: 128–145

Warner A E, Gutherie S C, Gilula N B 1984 Antibodies to gap-junctional protein selectively disrupt junctional communication in the early amphibian embryo. Nature 311: 127–131

Watson J D, Crick F H C 1953 Molecular structure of deoxypentose nucleic acids. Nature 171: 738–739

Webster W S, Johnston M C, Lammer E J, Sulik K K 1986 Isotretinoin embryopathy and the cranial neural crest: an in vivo and in vitro study. Journal of Craniofacial Genetics and Developmental Biology 6: 3: 211–222

Yamada K M, Hayashi M, Hirano H, Akiyama S K 1984 Fibronectin and cell surface interactions. In: Trelstad R L (ed) The role of extracellular matrix in development. Liss, New York. pp 89–122

3. Craniofacial embryology and morphogenesis: normal and abnormal

C. Vermeij-Keers

INTRODUCTION

The morphogenetic development of the brain, cranium and face of mammalian embryos, including man, is generally well known but for the developmental processes playing a part in morphogenesis.

From a histological point of view cell proliferation, cell degeneration, cell differentiation and the extracellular matrix are most important. These four elements occur up to the final developmental stage of the fetus. The extent of their influence on morphogenesis is unknown, although there has to be a perfect interconnected system between these elements, leading to a normal specimen.

The morphogenesis of the head region is brought about by the neuroectoderm, the surface ectoderm, the mesoderm and the endoderm together. In the early embryonic stages — ≤ 17 mm crown–rump length (C–RL) — the most striking morphogenetic changes, such as the formation of the neural and nasal tubes, are taking place. These changes can be described as caused by outgrowth of swellings that approach and contact each other. The swellings are composed of mesoderm covered with an epithelium, i.e. neuroectoderm and/or surface ectoderm. At the contact places epithelial plates develop. These remain or disappear as a result of cell degeneration. During the degeneration of the epithelial plates the mesoderm of the swellings fuses gradually. Although the fusion process of the swellings is obvious the mechanism responsible for this process needs explanation.

In the mesoderm of postimplantation embryonic stages local differences in the amount of cell proliferation are common (Poelmann 1980). This can explain the outgrowth of the facial swellings around the nasal placode (Vermeij-Keers & Poelmann 1980). The proliferation of the covering epithelia and the increase in the extracellular matrix keep place with this local phenomenon. Between the outgrowing facial swellings, grooves, such as the internasal groove, develop.

In later embryonic stages (≥17 mm C–RL) these grooves are squeezed out in a process called merging (cf. Minkoff 1980, Patten 1961). In the same stages differentiation of the cells of the mesodermal compartment into cartilage, bone centres and muscles takes place. Outgrowth of bone centres towards one another, within cartilage or intramembranous, resulting in fusion of bone centres or suture formation, is very important to the normal development of the skull.

The origin and migration of the cells in the mesodermal compartment of the head region are thought to be essential in normal and abnormal development (e.g. Johnston 1975, Weston 1981). It is generally accepted that the cells from the cephalic neural crest form the major part of this mesodermal compartment (Johnston 1975, Le Douarin 1975, 1982). The mesodermal cores are present before the cephalic neural crest starts its activity. According to the current opinion this is during the neural groove stage. The mesoderm of the cores is indicated as prechordal (endo) mesoderm (e.g. Adelmann 1936, De Myer et al 1964, Sulik et al 1984) and its origin is thought to be the prechordal plate (Müller and O'Rahilly 1983, O'Rahilly and Müller 1981).

In accordance with this concept, migration of neural crest derived cells (mesectodermal cells) is necessary in order to reach target organs and structures, such as the branchial arches and facial swellings, via specific pathways. These specific pathways are described as cell-free spaces, filled with extracellular matrix, on one side between the neuroectoderm and mesoderm, and on the other side between the surface ectoderm and the mesoderm. These data are obtained by experiments performed on amphibian (Hörstadius 1950, Raven 1937) and chicken embryos (Johnston 1966, Noden 1975, Weston 1963) and extrapolated to mammals (Johnston 1975, Le Douarin 1982), without knowledge of the normal development and activity of their neural crest.

However, recent microscopic studies on murine embryos revealed that the cephalic neural crest starts its activity in presomite stages, before the neural plate develops (Smits-van Prooije et al 1985, Smits-van Prooije 1986, Vermeij-Keers & Poelmann 1980). These authors

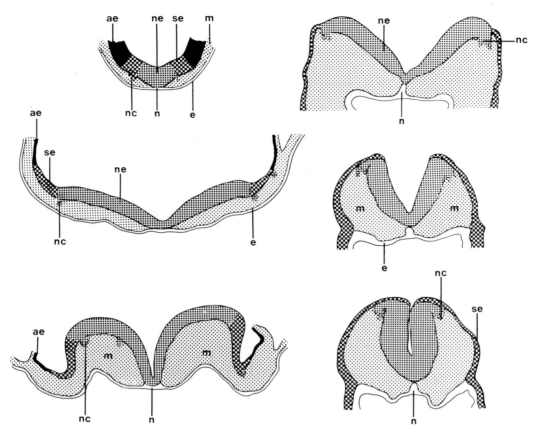

Fig. 3.1 Schematic representation of the cephalic region of mouse embryos in six stages — 7.3, 7.5, 7.8 (1 somite), 8.3, 8.4 and 8.5 (11 somites) days p.c. — based on transversely oriented 1 μm microscopic sections at the same magnification. n = notochordal plate; m = mesodermal compartment; ne = neuroectoderm; ae = amniotic epithelium; nc = neural crest; se = surface ectoderm; e = endoderm.

never found cell-free spaces in properly fixed murine embryos, indicating that migration of mesectodermal cells via specific pathways (long-distance migration), does not take place. It is postulated that in presomite murine embryos the neural crest starts to drop cells directly between the ectoderm and endoderm (Fig. 3.1). During the outgrowth of the neuroectoderm from the neural plate, via the neural groove into the neural tube, the cephalic neural crest shifts first laterally and then dorsally and medially relative to the notochordal plate (Fig. 3.1).

Throughout this transformation the neural crest drops cells that retain their position and divide there. The term 'dropping' was introduced by Vermeij-Keers & Poelmann (1980) and has been replaced by 'deposition' and 'migration' (Smits-van Prooije et al 1985). These terms only indicate that cells leave their epithelial configuration.

The above results are confirmed and further developed by an experimental approach performed on murine embryos cultured in vitro. A gold label, wheatgerm agglutinin-gold (WGA-Au; Smits-van Prooije et al 1986) is injected in the amniotic cavity by microinjection. All cells surrounding the amniotic cavity, i.e. cells of the neuro-ectoderm, surface ectoderm and the amniotic epithelium,

endocytose gold particles, that subsequently stay within the cells as gold-containing vacuoles. Among these cells are those of the neural crest and of the supposed surface ecto-derm placodes (Smits-van Prooije et al 1985, Smits-van Prooije 1986). When cells of these structures migrate from their epithelial configuration into the underlying meso-derm, they can be detected by these gold-filled vacuoles (Smits-van Prooije et al 1986). Injecting embryos of presomite to late somite stages and using different survival times, it is possible to obtain an overall view of the activity of the neural crest and the surface ectoderm placodes in the head region. These findings can be visualized using a three-dimensional microcomputer reconstruction technique (Kontron-MOP videoplan; Poelmann & Verbout 1985, Smits-van Prooije 1986). This study shows that in early presomite embryos the entire ectoderm, a columnar epithelium, has the capacity to deposit cells (Smits-van Prooije et al 1987), as was suggested by Vermeij-Keers & Poelmann (1980). In the late presomite stages this capacity remains only rostrally in the developing headfolds and caudally in the neural crest and in the primitive streak. The neural crest is defined as the margin of the neuroecto-derm, in neural plate and groove stages, and as the dorsal part of the neural tube when the neural walls have adhered. When rat embryos have four somites (9.3 days post coitum, p.c.) the lateral part of the ectoderm of the headfolds thins to a cuboidal and squamous epithelium and eventually becomes the surface ectoderm of the head region (Fig. 3.1). The medial part of the head region develops into the neuroectoderm. At the transition of surface and neuroectoderm, the neuroectoderm still deposits mesectodermal cells; this is the cephalic neural crest (Smits-van Prooije et al 1985). In developmental stages before four somites the lateral part of each headfold can be considered to be a surface ectoderm placode. According to Smits-van Prooije (1986) cells derived from both the neural crest and from the surface ectoderm placodes are mesectodermal cells. The cephalic neural crest is active in embryos from four up to about 20 somites, when the anterior neuropore is already closed. Another source of mesectodermal cells is the dorsorostral part of the optic vesicles, called the optic neural crest (Bartelmez & Blount 1954, Smits-van Prooije 1986).

From the 16-somite stage onwards placodal activity is seen in the branchial arches, called epibranchial placodes (Adelmann 1925, Smits-van Prooije 1986), in the nasal groove, called the nasal placodes (Smits-van Prooije 1986) and in the otic vesicles, called acoustic placodes (Batten 1958, Smits-van Prooije 1986).

From the experiments using gold as a marker performed on murine embryos cultured in vitro, it can be concluded that the mesodermal compartment of the head region is formed by the neural crest, the optic neural crest and the surface ectoderm placodes.

Before the mesectodermal cells are deposited in the mesodermal compartment, they have to lose their epithelial configuration. In other words, the onset of migration involves disruption of the basal lamina (Erickson & Weston 1983, Morriss & Thorogood 1978). Vermeij-Keers & Poelmann (1980) and Vermeij-Keers et al (1983a) suggest that a high frequency of cell degeneration in the neural crest is related to the loss of cell junctions, enlargement of the intercellular spaces and finally to disruption of its basal lamina. As a result the neural crest cells lose their epithelial configuration.

In contradiction to Geelen (1980) Smits-van Prooije (1986) has found that degenerating cells are present in the neural crest before, during and after the transformation of the neural plate into the tube. Moreover cell degeneration is found during the transformation of the surface ectoderm placodes, such as the nasal placodes (Vermeij-Keers, unpublished data). This suggests that cell degeneration must have a relevant function in normal development, as is also seen in the disappearance of epithelial plates during fusion processes (Poelmann & Vermeij-Keers 1976).

From present knowledge the normal development of the brain, cranium and face can be explained by local cell proliferation, cell degeneration and differentiation, including the formation of the extracellular matrix. Therefore abnormal development in the head region can be attributed to local derailments in one or more of these cell properties.

Until recently nearly all the experimental investigations concerning neural crest activity were done on non-mammalian vertebrates. The results of these studies are extrapolated to normal and abnormal development in human embryos (e.g. Johnston 1975). Some conclusions, however, for example the explanation of the development of cyclopia and hypertelorism, were not in agreement with the observations on human embryos (Vermeij-Keers et al 1983a, 1984, 1987). Human embryos of presomite and early somite stages are hardly available in serial sections and they cannot be used for experimental purposes. Murine embryos were chosen as a 'stand in' because murine and human embryos have many developmental similarities in the field of neural crest activity and transformation and fusion processes.

NORMAL CRANIOFACIAL DEVELOPMENT

The early development of the brain and face (≤17 mm C–RL)

The early development of the brain and face is characterized by the formation and transformation of the headfolds: first the neural walls with the eye primordia, than the otic disc and placode, the branchial arches, and finally the lens and nasal placodes. All these transformations show a rather basic principle: outgrowth of swellings forming and surrounding a cavity or groove that subsequently is closed partly or totally as a result of the fusion of the swellings (Fig. 3.2). The outgrowing swellings cause a three-dimensional increase of the embryo, especially in transverse and ventrodorsal directions. These time-overlapping transformation processes take place in developmental stages up to about 17 mm C–RL. The first slightly lordotic shape of the human embryo facilitates the initial fusion process of the neural groove into the neural tube. Later on the lordosis changes into a kyphosis, enabling the transformation of the branchial arches and resulting in the formation of the neck. The distance between the tops of the swellings decreases owing to the curvature of the embryo (Fig. 3.3). The location of the highest point of the curve is opposite that of the first contact between the swellings involved.

THE HEADFOLDS

The development of the headfolds in human and murine embryos is comparable. In human embryos the development of the headfolds takes place around 18–20 days p.c. (stage 8–9, O'Rahilly and Müller 1981), in mouse embryos around 7.5 days p.c. and in rat embryos around 8.5 days p.c. (Smits-van Prooije 1986). At that stage the neural crest and surface ectoderm placodes of the headfolds of

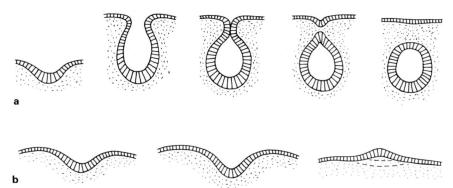

Fig. 3.2 Schematic representation of phases (a) of the fusion process and (b) of merging. During the fusion process an epithelial plate or stalk is formed that disappears by cell degeneration.

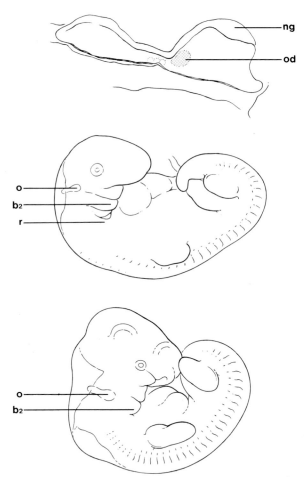

Fig. 3.3 Schematic representation of three human embryos of 2.7 (drawing after Fig. 62, O'Rahilly, 1973), 6.2 and 8 mm C–RL, seen in profile. b_2 = second branchial arch; r = retrobranchial ridge; od = otic disc; o = otic vesicle; ng = neural groove. All stages are drawn to the same total length.

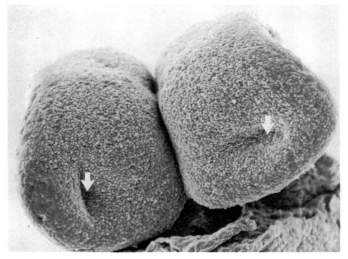

Fig. 3.4 Scanning electron micrograph of a mouse embryo aged about 8.0 days p.c., showing the optic sulci (↓) as bilateral grooves in head-folds (frontal view, heart removed).

murine embryos are depositing mesectodermal cells. O'Rahilly and Müller indicate in their article of 1981 that the headfolds are neural folds (stage 8). The headfolds are covered with columnar epithelium. They are the first

structures to appear rostrally in the embryo, and continue caudally as the neural plate (Fig. 3.4). In 1- to 7-somite mouse embryos the headfolds are growing out rapidly and elevate from the visceral yolk-sac (Fig. 3.5). During this developmental period the ectoderm of the lateral part of the headfolds is thinning gradually from a pseudostratified columnar epithelium into a cuboidal and, later in development, locally into a squamous epithelium. This lateral part of the headfolds becomes the surface ectoderm in the head-neck region. The otic disc, the nasal fields and surface ectoderm placodes localized on the branchial arches retain a cuboidal to low columnar epithelium. The transition of the medial (neuroectoderm) and lateral (surface ectoderm) part of the headfolds becomes visible at this stage. Here the neuroectoderm remains active in deposition of mesectodermal cells and is indicated as cephalic neural crest (Fig. 3.1). The border of the headfolds appears to be the transition of the surface ectoderm and

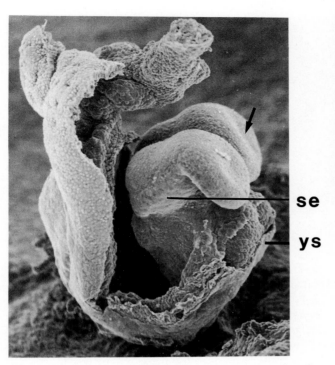

Fig. 3.5 Scanning electron micrograph of a mouse embryo aged 8.1 days p.c. (6 somites). The headfolds with the optic sulci (↓) in profile. ys = yolk sac; se = surface ectoderm.

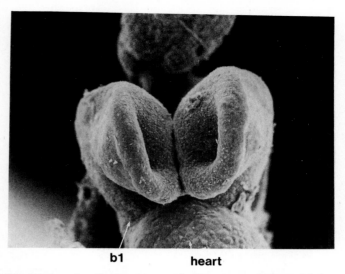

Fig. 3.6 Scanning electron micrograph of a mouse embryo aged 8.3 days p.c. Prosencephalon (forebrain) with the evaginating optic vesicles (frontal view). b_1 = first branchial arch.

the amnion (Smits-van Prooije et al 1985, Smits-van Prooije 1986).

During the transformation of the headfolds into the cephalic neural walls, also called neural folds (O'Rahilly & Müller 1981), the optic primordia (optic sulci) develop within the neuroectoderm as two separate shallow grooves (rat embryo 5-somite stage, mouse embryo 7 somites, Smits-van Prooije et al 1985; human embryo stage 10, 8 somites, O'Rahilly 1966) (Fig. 3.4). Close to the margin of the neuroectoderm the otic disc develops as a concavity of columnar epithelium in the surface ectoderm (3-somite mouse embryo, Verwoerd & Van Oostrom 1979; 1–3-somite human embryos stage 9, Müller & O'Rahilly 1983, O'Rahilly 1966) (Fig. 3.3). Moreover, the first branchial arch is taking shape (7-somite mouse embryo, Smits-van Prooije et al 1985; 8–10-somite human embryos, Starck 1955) (Fig. 3.6).

Meanwhile the neural plate located more caudally in the embryo changes via the neural groove into the neural tube. According to Müller & O'Rahilly (1985) the initial contact between the neural walls takes place in the caudal part of the rhombencephalic folds (at the level of the first four somites) or in the upper cervical neural folds (at the level of somites 5–7) in embryos of approximately 5 somites. In a 5-somite mouse embryo (Smits-van Prooije et al 1985) the neural groove narrows at the level of somites 3 and 4, the walls appose in a 6-somite embryo and adhere in a 7-somite embryo, the surface ectoderm making the first

contact. In the caudal direction the neural groove closes like a zipper and the closure of the posterior neuropore occurs when the murine embryo has 30 somites (Smits-van Prooije et al 1985) and 25–27 somites in human embryos (O'Rahilly & Gardner 1979).

Rostrally, in the head extra points of closure occur both in the mouse embryo (Geelen & Langman 1977) and in the human embryo (Müller & O'Rahilly 1985). The final closure of the anterior neuropore is located between two areas of ectodermal thickenings composed of cuboidal to columnar epithelium, the nasal fields (15-somite mouse embryos, Vermeij-Keers et al 1983a; 20-somite human embryos, O'Rahilly 1967; O'Rahilly & Gardner 1971) (Fig. 3.7). In later developmental stages, a certain part of both nasal fields transforms into the nasal placodes and nasal grooves, respectively. The location of the final closure of the anterior neuropore corresponds with the presumptive internasal groove (Fig. 3.8).

Cell degeneration is observed in the epithelium all along the fusion zone, before, during and after closure of the neural groove to form the neural tube (Fig. 3.2).

CEPHALIC NEURAL CREST

As mentioned before, the entire ectoderm of early presomite embryos and the ectoderm of the headfolds in late presomite and early somite murine embryos is able to deposit mesectodermal cells into the mesodermal compartment. From 4-somite murine embryos and older the cephalic neural crest (the margin of the neuroectoderm in neural plate and groove stages and the dorsal part of the neural tube) is active up to about the 20-somite stage, i.e. after the closure of the anterior neuropore (Figs. 3.1, 3.9). In human embryos of stage 9 (1–3 somites) Müller & O'Rahilly (1983) describe deposition of mesectodermal

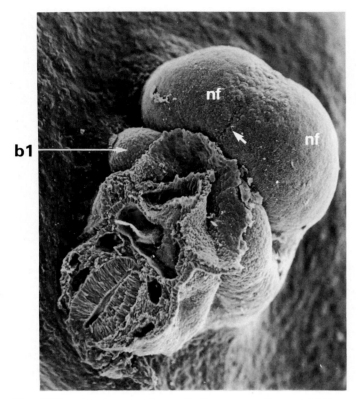

Fig. 3.7 Scanning electron micrograph of a mouse embryo aged 8.7 days p.c. Prosencephalon is fused except for the anterior neuropore (↑), which has practically closed, and which separates the two nasal fields (nf); b₁ = first branchial arch (frontal view, heart removed).

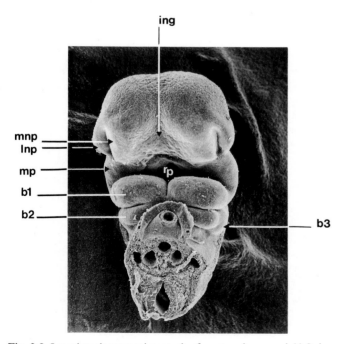

Fig. 3.8 Scanning electron micrograph of a rat embryo aged 11.9 days p.c. (heart removed). Nasal placodes have been transformed into nasal grooves by the medial nasal (mnp), lateral nasal (lnp) and maxillary processes (mp). b = branchial arch 1–3; rp = Rathke's pouch; ing = internasal groove.

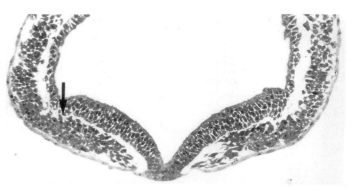

Fig. 3.9 Transverse 1-μm section at the level of the first somite of a 3-somite mouse embryo aged 7.9 days p.c., showing neural crest cells in contact with the underlying mesoderm (↑) (×275).

cells from parts of the headfolds being probably the rostral crest and the facial crest. According to these authors, some embryos of stage 9 are the earliest examples of the initial formation of the neural crest in humans. The neural crest continues its activity in stage 10 (4–12 somites; Müller & O'Rahilly 1985, and own observations).

It is most likely that the mesectoderm formation in the headfolds of the two species is comparable. The only difference between the two species is that in murine embryos mesectoderm formation starts earlier. This discrepancy might be explained by the difference in preparation of the sections and the histological quality of the embryos used for microscopic investigations in early developmental stages. The murine embryos are dissected out of the uterus, directly fixed in half-strength Karnovsky's fixative (Karnovsky 1965), embedded in Epon 812 and sectioned semithin (1 μm). The human embryos are fixed in formalin or Bouin, embedded in celloidin and paraffin and the sections were 5–12 μm thick. The period between abortion and fixation is unknown. The histological quality of human embryos is in all cases worse than that of the murine embryos and semithin sections provide a better insight into the local cell arrangements of the epithelia, and into migration of cells out of their epithelial configuration.

Mesectoderm formation by the neural crest takes place before, during and even some period after the transformation process of the neuroectoderm. Along the neural crest itself crest activity is not a regular process. The number of cells produced varies between embryos of the same and of different developmental stages and between the various places in the embryo proper (Smits-van Prooije 1986, Vermeij-Keers & Poelmann 1980) (Fig. 3.1). For example, the neural crest is not active at the level of the otic discs during its transformation up to the 20-somite stage, when the otic vesicles are nearly separated from the surface ectoderm (Smits-van Prooije 1986). In the literature it is generally accepted (e.g. Adelmann 1925) that the most rostral part of the head region does not produce mesectodermal cells. Recently it was observed using WGA-Au as a label that in presomite and early somite embryos the ectoderm of this rostral part is active in deposition of mesectodermal cells (Smits-van Prooije et al 1987). This activity continues as neural crest activity, during the transformation of the optic sulcus into the optic vesicle up to the 20-somite stage (Smits-van Prooije 1986). In addition the optic neural crest, the dorsorostral part of the neuroectoderm of the optic vesicles, is also producing mesectodermal cells (Bartelmez & Blount 1954, Smits-van Prooije 1986). The neural crest in the rostral part of the head, reaching halfway to the optic sulci/vesicles, is, however, less active in cell production than its caudal part. The neural crest at the level of the caudal half of the optic sulci/vesicles up to the otic disc, and caudally from the otic disc to the level of the fourth somite, produces a considerable number of cells that form the mesodermal area of a prospective facial swelling, the maxillary process, and of the successive branchial arches. The cells of the mesodermal areas of the other prospective facial swellings, the medial and lateral nasal processes (Fig. 3.8), are produced by the neural crest of the rostral part of the head.

From the WGA-Au experiments it was concluded that the cells within the mesodermal areas of the three facial swellings and of the branchial arches are distributed at random (Smits-van Prooije 1986). Mesodermal cores, consisting of unlabelled cells derived from the prechordal plate, surrounded by a sheet of labelled mesectodermal cells (cf. chicken embryos, Le Douarin 1982) are not found in murine embryos. The localization of these sheets should correspond to that of the cell-free spaces in which the mesectodermal cells are supposed to migrate, according to the theory of long-distance migration. Moreover the cell-free spaces that are present in chicken embryos between the (neuro)ectoderm and mesoderm are never seen in properly fixed murine embryos.

SURFACE ECTODERM PLACODES

The mesodermal compartment of the head region is not only supplied by mesectodermal cells derived from the cephalic neural crest but also by cells deposited by the surface ectoderm placodes. The following surface ectoderm placodes are suggested: the nasal placodes (Verwoerd & Van Oostrom 1979), the acoustic placode (Batten 1958) and the epibranchial placodes at the branchial arches (Adelmann 1925). All these placodes are active in mesectodermal cell production during transformation processes (Smits-van Prooije 1986). In other words they add cells to the prospective and/or outgrowing swellings.

EYE DEVELOPMENT

The first appearance of the optic primordia is seen in 8-somite human embryos (Bartelmez & Blount 1954, O'Rahilly 1966) as a thickened area of each neural wall in which a shallow sulcus is present. During the outgrowth and transformation of the neural walls into the neural tube of the forebrain, each sulcus widens and changes into an optic vesicle (Figs. 3.4, 3.6). This process is called evagination (Glücksmann, 1951). The surface ectoderm in early developmental stages that forms part of the headfolds and is located over each optic vesicle is composed of cuboidal to low columnar epithelium and represents the nasal fields. Both fields are separated initially by the anterior neuropore. At the site of its closure, the surface ectoderm is cuboidal to squamous. The remainder of the surroundings of the nasal fields is composed of squamous epithelium.

Within each nasal field two placodes develop as a result of local thickening of the ectoderm: the lens placode (mouse embryos 8.8 days p.c., 15–16 somites; human embryos about 4.2–4.5 mm C–RL, 32–34 somites, stage 13, O'Rahilly 1966) and the nasal placode (mouse embryos 9.8 days p.c.; human embryos 6.0–6.5 mm C–RL) (Figs. 3.10–3.12). The lens placode is more or less in contact with the optic vesicle. The structures are at later developmental stages simultaneously transformed into lens vesicle and optic cup, respectively (Fig. 3.13). Subsequently the walls of the short stalk of the lens vesicle make contact. In human embryos of about 7 mm C–RL the lens vesicle detaches from the surface ectoderm by cell degeneration in its stalk (Fig. 3.14). This fusion process has finished when the surface ectoderm is separated from the lens vesicle and mesectoderm moves between both epithelia (Fig. 3.2). Both structures have their own epithelial continuity with their own basement membrane (mouse embryo, over 45 somites, Theiler 1972), 6–7 mm C–RL, human embryos.

The cavity of the optic vesicle communicates via the lumen of the initially short optic stalk with that of the

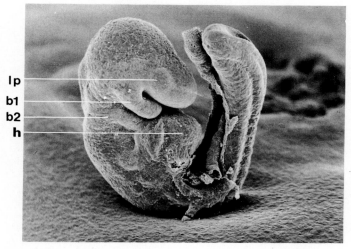

lp
b1
b2
h

Fig. 3.10 Scanning electron micrograph of a rat embryo aged 10.8 days p.c., in profile (20 somites). The lens placode (lp) has developed in the nasal field. $b_{1,2}$ = branchial arches; h = heart.

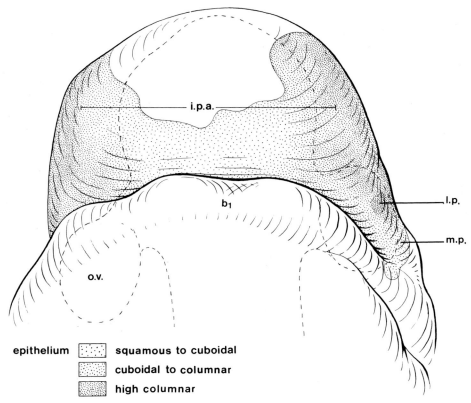

epithelium [....] squamous to cuboidal

[:::] cuboidal to columnar

[▓] high columnar

Fig. 3.11 Graphic reconstruction of a 6.5-mm C–RL human embryo showing the prosencephalon with the optic vesicles (ov), lens (lp) and nasal placodes, in frontal view. High columnar epithelium = lens and nasal placodes. ipa = interplacodal area; b₁ = first branchial arch: mp = maxillary process.

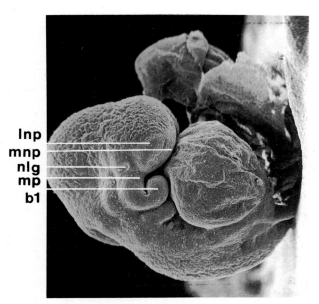

Fig. 3.12 Scanning electron micrograph of a mouse embryo aged 9.8 days p.c., in profile. The nasal placode (np) has developed and the lens placode evaginates into lens vesicle (lv). b₁ = first branchial arch; ipa = interplacodal area; mp = maxillary process.

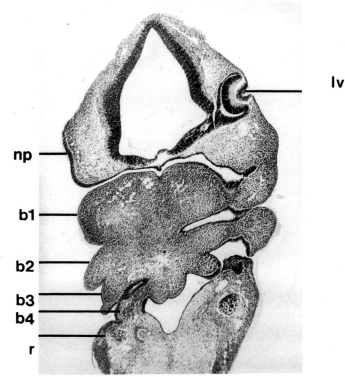

Fig. 3.13 Frontal 10-μm section through the nasal placode (np) and the optic cup and lens vesicle (lv) of a human embryo of 6.5 mm C–RL. b = branchial arch 1–4; r = retrobranchial ridge.

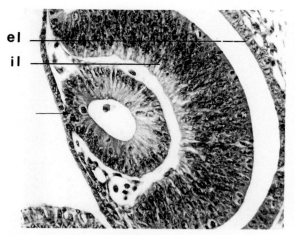

Fig. 3.14 Frontal 10-μm section through the stalk of the lens vesicle. Cell degeneration is indicated (↑). (Mouse embryo 10.5 days p.c.). el = external layer optic cup; il = internal layer optic cup.

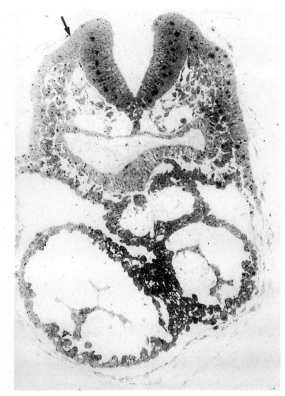

Fig. 3.15 Transverse 1-μm section through the otic discs (↑) of a mouse embryo of 8 somites (8.3 days p.c.).

forebrain. During the transformation of the vesicle into the optic cup, the external layer of the optic cup grows out in the direction of its internal layer (Fig. 3.14). The direction is determined by the localization of the lens placode. The lens placode transforms asymmetrically (Fig. 3.12) as well as the optic cup forming the optic or choroid fissure. During these transformations, accompanied by cell degeneration, the cavity of the optic vesicle, cup and stalk is obliterated finally by apical cell adherence of the internal and external layers. The optic stalk has lengthened. The optic fissure closes in human embryos of 17 mm C–RL without cell degeneration (Silver & Hughes 1974) and with fusion of its basement membranes, i.e. basal intraepithelial fusion (Vermeij-Keers et al 1983a).

EAR DEVELOPMENT

The otic disc or the prospective otic placode is the first ill-defined appearance of the developing ear (3-somite mouse embryo, Verwoerd & Van Oostrom 1979; 5-somite rat embryo, Smits-van Prooije 1986; 1–3-somite human embryos, stage 9, Müller & O'Rahilly 1983, O'Rahilly 1966) (Fig. 3.3). Its localization in the surface ectoderm close to the margin of the neuroectoderm is characterized by the basement membranes of the neuroectodermal and disc cells making contact (Fig. 3.15). This contact persists during further transformation of the inner ear. The initial sign of the transformation is a concavity in the disc developing in all species (Fig. 3.16). In the human embryo it is seen towards the end of stage 10, 10–12 somites (Müller & O'Rahilly 1985). During the transformation of the otic disc into the otic vesicle (Fig. 3.17) the ectoderm of the disc thickens and is then called a placode (mouse embryo 17-somite stage, Verwoerd & Van Oostrom 1979; human embryo 17-somite stage, Wen 1928). The margins of the

placode grow out, probably induced by the mesectoderm formation of the neural crest rostrally and caudally of the placode (Smits-van Prooije et al 1985). A vesicle is formed, and subsequently the walls of its short stalk make contact (mouse embryo 20-somite stage, Smits-van Prooije et al 1985; human embryo 4.4 mm C–RL, Vermeij-Keers 1967) and the now solid stalk disappears by cell degeneration (Fig. 3.18). In this way the surface ectoderm and the ectoderm of the otic vesicle are separated. Later, mesectodermal cells move between these ectodermal layers (human embryo 6.2 mm C–RL, Vermeij-Keers 1967), finishing the fusion process (Fig. 3.2). Meanwhile the ventrorostral side of the otic vesicle produces mesectodermal cells (35-somite rat embryo, Smits-van Prooije 1986) forming the primitive facial-acoustic ganglion. From the development described above, especially with respect to the contact of the basement membranes that persists all through the transformation of the inner ear, it can be concluded that the otic placode evaginates rather than invaginates (cf. Müller & O'Rahilly 1985). In human embryos of about 7 mm C–RL the otic vesicle transforms into the prospective endolymph duct and sac, the duct portion for the developing semicircular ducts, and utriculosaccular and cochlear portions (Arey 1965). During this transformation the walls of the vesicle, surrounded by condensed mesoderm of the otic capsule, are locally

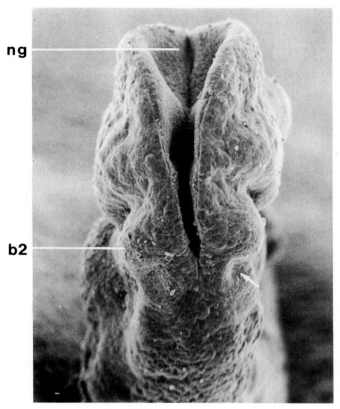

Fig. 3.16 Scanning electron micrograph of a mouse embryo aged 8.5 days p.c. (12 somites). The otic discs are visible as shallow concavities (↑) (dorsal view). ng = neural groove; b₂ = second branchial arch.

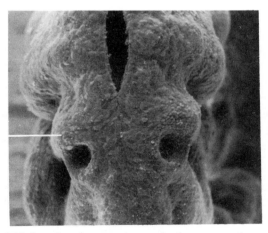

Fig. 3.17 Scanning electron micrograph of a mouse embryo of 8.8 days p.c. (15 somites). Both otic discs are evaginating into otic vesicles (dorsal view). b₂ = second branchial arch.

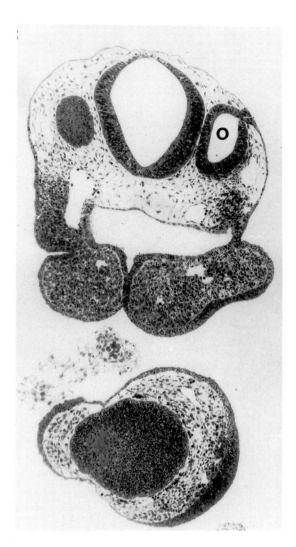

Fig. 3.18 Transverse 1-μm section through the otic vesicle (o) with its stalk. Mouse embryo of 24 somites, aged 9.5 days p.c.

growing out into the lumen. In this way the cavity narrows at some places into ducts: the cochlear duct and the endolymph duct. The latter is determined by its close contact with the neuroectoderm. The asymmetrical outgrowth of the duct portion gives rise to three epithelial plates orientated perpendicularly to each other. Semicircular ducts are the result of cell degeneration in the centre of these plates (see stage 18, 13–17 mm C–RL, O'Rahilly 1983). The utriculosaccular portion widens and separates subsequently by local outgrowth resulting in grooves and swellings. The otic capsule is precartilaginous in stage 18 (13–17 mm C–RL, O'Rahilly 1983).

The middle and external ear develop from the first pharyngeal pouch and first branchial groove, respectively. Pouch and groove are on the same level, and are separated by the first branchial membrane (Fig. 3.19) (e.g. Poelmann et al 1985), that develops into the tympanic membrane. The first pharyngeal pouch is transformed into the auditory tube and tympanic cavity. This transformation is caused by local outgrowth of swellings into the pharyngeal cavity. Simultaneously, the first branchial groove deepens by the outgrowing first and second branchial arches in a lateral direction, forming the external acoustic meatus (11–14 mm C–RL, stage 17, O'Rahilly 1983).

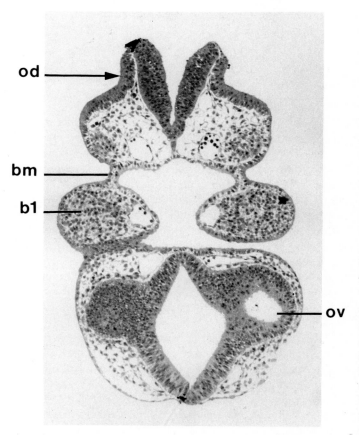

Fig. 3.19 Transverse 1-μm section of the head–neck region of a mouse embryo aged 8.6 days p.c. (12 somites). ov = optic vesicles; b_1 = first branchial arch; bm = first branchial membrane; od = otic disc.

BRANCHIAL ARCHES

The foregut, a relatively wide tube in the head region of late presomite mouse embryos (Poelmann et al 1985) and late presomite or early somite human embryos (stage 8 and 9, O'Rahilly 1973), is the prospective pharynx and part of the mouth. The lateral wall of the foregut is composed of endoderm (originally the yolk-sac), a small layer of mesectodermal cells (deposited by the ectoderm of the headfolds) and ectoderm of the lateral parts of the headfolds, the future surface ectoderm. The rostral extension of the foregut is formed by the buccopharyngeal membrane, consisting of only ectoderm (stomodeum) and endoderm (foregut), with their fused basement membranes in between. The heart primordium and notochordal plate are situated ventrally and dorsally of the foregut, respectively. Caudally, the foregut is in continuity with the yolk-sac. In fact, the embryo grows out over the yolk-sac. In other words the yolk-sac is incorporated gradually in the embryo. During this process the wide tube is transformed into pharyngeal pouches by outgrowing swellings into the lumen of the foregut. The first pharyngeal pouch develops in the early somite stages. The endoderm of its lateral wall makes contact via cell protrusions with those of the surface ectoderm (4-somite stage). The few mesectodermal cells in between are enclosed or pushed aside. At this location the first pharyngeal membrane starts to develop, lying between the first pharyngeal pouch and its complementary branchial groove (Fig. 3.19). Initially the groove is shallow and wide but deepens subsequently when the first branchial arch grows out. At the outside of the embryo this arch is visible in 7-somite murine embryos and 8–10-somite human embryos. In human embryos five branchial arches, separated by four grooves, develop in succession. The first one is the biggest, and develops cranially of the heart primordium on both sides of the embryo, forming only the mandibular processes of the facial swellings. (Vermeij-Keers et al 1983a). The last arch is poorly developed. The transformation of the branchial arches starts in about 6 mm C–RL human embryos (Vermeij-Keers 1967). The mandibular processes keep their positions and grow out, forming a groove in the midline between the two swellings. These swellings do not fuse (cf. Patten 1953), because no epithelial plate is formed. These swellings merge (Fig. 3.2). The second arch begins to grow from the side of the second branchial groove in a caudal and lateral direction, covering the third and fourth arches (Figs. 3.3, 3.13). The third branchial arch does the same with respect to the fourth. The retrobranchial ridge, incorporating the fifth arch, grows out in the direction of the second branchial arch (Starck 1955). Via contacts with the fourth and third arch, respectively, this swelling adheres and fuses with the second branchial arch. Initially, slit-like cavities, remnants of the branchial grooves, remain present between these contact places. In the literature these cavities are indicated

Swellings at either side of the widening orifice of the first branchial groove, the auricular hillocks, become visible in embryos of 7–9 mm C–RL (stage 15, O'Rahilly 1983, Hinrichsen 1985). In stage 18 (13–17 mm C–RL, O'Rahilly 1983) the wide shallow grooves between the swellings, including the dorsal extension of the first branchial groove, are smoothed out in a process called merging (Fig. 3.2), to form the primordium of the definite auricle.

A condensed mesenchymal mass in the second branchial arch, the preliminary stapes in which the stapedial artery is present, is the first indication of the auditory ossicles (7 mm C–RL, Vermeij-Keers 1967). This condensation is localized between the ear vesicle surrounded by the mesenchym of the otic capsule and the tympanic cavity of the first pharyngeal pouch. The stapes can be identified as a dark ring caused by the loose mesenchymal sheet around the stapedial artery in the 12 mm C–RL embryo (Vermeij-Keers 1967). Condensations in the first branchial arch (11–14 mm C–RL) are the primordial malleus and incus (O'Rahilly 1983).

The transformation of the middle and external ear takes place exactly in the same developmental period.

erroneously as one triangular cavity, the cervical sinus. As a result of the combined outgrowth, the fourth arch obtains a medial position, the third one an intermedial, and the second branchial arch with the retrobranchial ridge a lateral position (Figs. 3.13, 3.20). In this way, the width of the embryo in the neck region increases and the branchial arches disappear as such at the outside of the embryo (12 mm C–RL human embryos, Vermeij-Keers 1967). Inside the embryo the slit-like cavities obliterate and ectodermal epithelial plates are formed at the contact places between the swellings (Fig. 3.20). These plates disappear by cell degeneration. The outgrowing branchial arches and their attendant shiftings cause not only transformations of the branchial grooves but also of their corresponding pharyngeal pouches. The successive organs developing out of the pharyngeal pouches, except for the first one, do not migrate to their permanent positions as indicated in the literature (Moore 1982), but in the first instance they attain these positions during the above-described outgrowth of the branchial arch system. Thereafter they differentiate to form, for example, the thymus (derivative of the third pouch) and the superior (fourth pouch) and inferior (third pouch) parathyroid glands. In addition, local differences

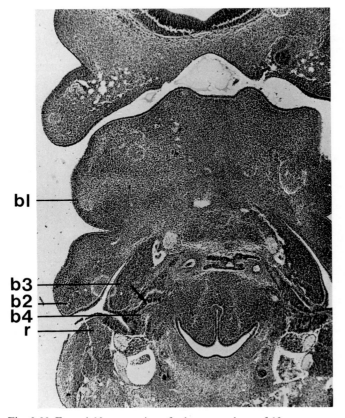

Fig. 3.20 Frontal 10-μm section of a human embryo of 12 mm C–RL. The head–neck area with epithelial plate formation between the branchial arches (↑). b = branchial arch 1–4; r = retrobranchial ridge.

in proliferation rate cause a relative shift of the organs (Gasser 1979, Smits-van Prooije 1986).

DEVELOPMENT OF THE NOSE

The nasal fields are outlined after differentiation of the ectoderm of the headfolds into neuroectoderm and surface ectoderm. This differentiation starts bilaterally in 4-somite murine embryos (Smits-van Prooije 1986) and continues gradually during the transformation of the neural walls into the neural tube by flattening of the surface ectoderm (Figs. 3.5, 3.10). Some areas of the surface ectoderm, including (among others) the nasal fields, keep cuboidal to low columnar epithelium (murine embryos, 11 somites, 8.5 days p.c., Vermeij-Keers et al 1983a). The final fusion of the forebrain, i.e. the closure of the anterior neuropore, takes place in 15-somite murine embryos (Smits-van Prooije et al 1985) and in 20-somite human embryos, and is localized between the two nasal fields (Fig. 3.7) (murine embryos, Vermeij-Keers et al 1983a; human embryos, O'Rahilly 1967, O'Rahilly & Gardner 1971). Before, during and after closure of the anterior neuropore a high frequency of cell degeneration is seen (Geelen & Langman 1979, Smits-van Prooije 1986), followed by breakdown of the basement membranes (Vermeij-Keers et al 1983a). In the area between the nasal fields, the surface ectoderm is cuboidal to squamous. The nasal fields are in continuity with the prospective lens placodes (Fig. 3.11).

In human embryos of 6.0–6.5 mm C–RL and mouse embryos of 9.8 days p.c., the nasal placodes develop laterally within the nasal fields frontocaudally to the optic cup as oval areas of thickening epithelium. The nasal fields are much bigger than the nasal placodes. The frontal area between the nasal placodes is called the interplacodal area (Vermeij-Keers et al 1983a) (Fig. 3.11). In the current literature this area is called the frontonasal process. This term is, however, unacceptable because in this area there is no swelling. Around each nasal placode three facial swellings — definable as mesenchymal proliferations covered by ectoderm and separated from each other by grooves — will grow out. They transform the nasal placode via the nasal groove into the nasal tube, resulting in the formation of the primary palate and primitive mouth cavity (Figs. 3.8, 3.12, 3.21, 3.22). At the medial side of each placode the medial nasal process and laterally the lateral nasal and maxillary processes develop. Between the outgrowing lateral nasal and maxillary processes a narrow groove, the nasolacrimal groove, becomes visible (Fig. 3.21). It extends to the optic cup. The outgrowth of the maxillary processes is not coupled with changes in the shape of the first branchial arch. Therefore the maxillary process must represent a separate swelling and does not form part of the mandibular arch. Both medial nasal processes grow out in the interplacodal area, separated by a wide shallow groove,

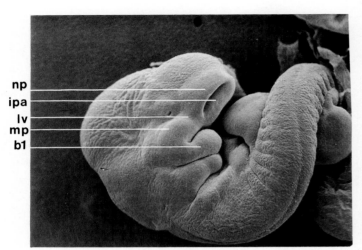

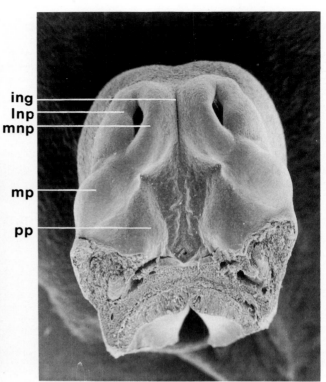

Fig. 3.21 Scanning electron micrograph of a mouse embryo aged 10.1 days p.c., in profile. The nasal groove is visible and formed by the lateral nasal (lnp), medial nasal (mnp) and maxillary processes (mp). b_1 = first branchial arch; nlg = nasolacrimal groove.

Fig. 3.22 Scanning electron micrograph of a rat embryo aged 13 days p.c. (mandible and heart removed). Caudal view of the primitive palate with both developing palatine processes (pp). ing = internasal groove; mnp = medial nasal process; lnp = lateral nasal process; mp = maxillary process.

the internasal groove (Vermeij-Keers et al 1983a) (Figs 3.8, 3.22). Actually in early developmental stages the nose can be considered as two separate organs, which can develop asymmetrically.

At either side of the prosencephalon the facial swellings grow out. The nasal placodes do not invaginate, as indicated in the current literature, but evaginate. The oval nasal placode is turned over in the first instance by outgrowth of the lateral nasal and maxillary processes. Subsequently the closure of the nasal groove takes place in an occipital to frontal direction. The first contact between the swellings is made between the maxillary and medial nasal processes (7 mm C–RL human embryos, Vermeij-Keers 1972a) and not between both nasal processes as is often indicated (Hochstetter 1891, 1950, Hinrichsen 1985, Kosaka et al 1985, Töndury 1950, 1964). Later (11 mm C–RL) the lateral nasal process will contact the medial process (Fig. 3.23). Complete adhesion occurs at the 12 mm C–RL stage (Vermeij-Keers 1972a) (Fig. 3.24). These two nasal processes form the external nostrils.

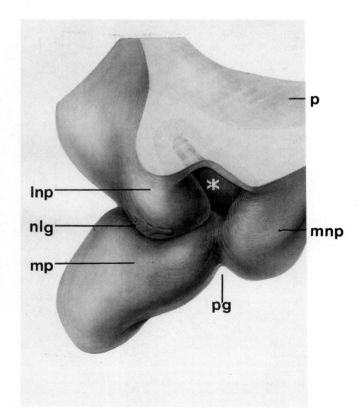

Fig. 3.23 (right) Artist's impression of the nasal groove (⋆) of a human embryo of 11 mm C–RL. lnp = lateral nasal process; mp = maxillary process; mnp = medial nasal process; nlg = nasolacrimal groove; pg = palatine groove; p = prosencephalon.

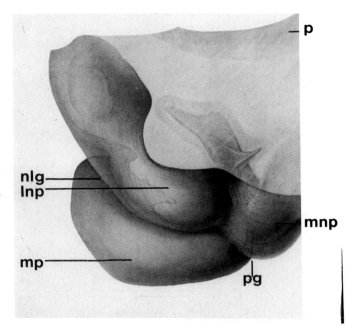

Fig. 3.24 Artist's impression of the nasal tube of a human embryo of 12 mm C–RL. lnp = lateral nasal process; mp = maxillary process; mnp = medial nasal process; nlg = nasolacrimal groove; pg = palatine groove; p = prosencephalon.

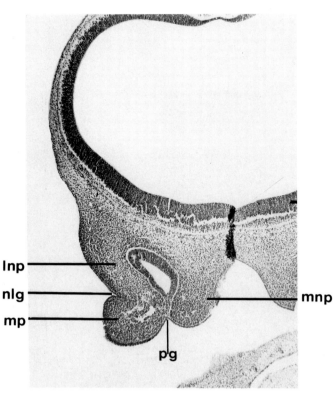

Fig. 3.25 Frontal 10-μm section of the epithelial plate of Hochstetter of a 11-mm C–RL human embryo. lnp = lateral nasal process; mp = maxillary process; mnp = medial nasal process; pg = palatine groove; p = prosencephalon; nlg = nasolacrimal groove.

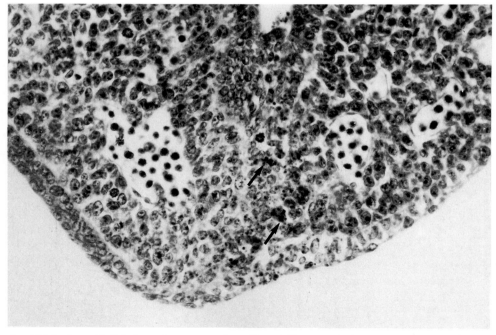

Fig. 3.26 Cell degeneration (↑) in the epithelial plate of a mouse embryo (frontal 10-μm section).

At the place of contact between the three facial swellings an epithelial plate develops: the epithelial plate or membrane of Hochstetter (the nasal fin). Cell degeneration is observed before, during and after formation of this epithelial plate (Figs. 3.25, 3.26). Subsequently the first disruption in that plate appears halfway, right above the primitive oral cavity (Fig. 3.27). Cell degeneration continues (Vermeij-Keers 1972a,b, Poelmann & Vermeij-Keers 1976, Gaare & Langmann 1980) and gradually the fusion of the three swellings becomes a fact, resulting in formation of the primitive palate (11–17 mm C–RL). Laterally in the primitive oral cavity the palatine grooves are visible, representing the fusion zone of these swellings (7–17 mm C–RL; Figs. 3.23–3.25, 3.27, 3.28).

Slightly later in this developmental period the bucconasal membrane unfolds from the posterior part of the epithelial plate of Hochstetter (Fig. 3.27) and, subsequently disappears by cell degeneration (12–17 mm C–RL). Occipitally the nasal tube opens now into the primitive oral cavity. The opening between the primitive nasal and oral cavities is bounded by the maxillary and medial nasal processes and is called the primitive choana.

The above-described transformation is not only accompanied by considerable morphogenetic changes in the developing facial region itself, but also by changes in the nasal lumen and the anlage of the nasolacrimal duct (Figs. 3.23, 3.24, 3.28). Grooves can be found in the nasal lumen, as in the developing face. In the lateral wall of the nasal groove and nasal tube, the lateral nasal and maxillary processes are separated at both sides by grooves. Because of outgrowth of these processes in the lateral as well as the medial directions, both grooves deepen and at the same time narrow so much that the ectoderm of their walls come into contact with each other (Figs. 3.27, 3.29, 3.30). At the areas of contact, epithelial plates consisting of a

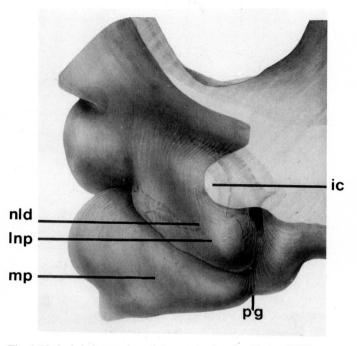

Fig. 3.28 Artist's impression of the nasal tube of a 15-mm C–RL human embryo with formation of the nasolacrimal duct (nld). lnp = lateral nasal process, mp = maxillary process; ic = inferior concha; pg = palatine groove.

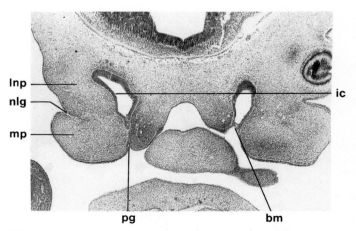

Fig. 3.27 Frontal 10-μm section of the nasal tubes of a 12-mm C–RL human embryo. The epithelial plate of Hochstetter has disappeared and the bucconasal membrane (bm) has developed. lnp = lateral nasal process; mp = maxillary process; ic = inferior concha; pg = palatine groove; nlg = nasolacrimal groove.

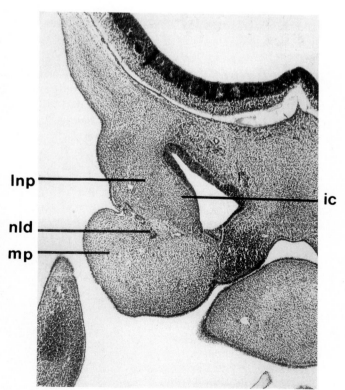

Fig. 3.29 Frontal 10-μm section of the nasal tube of a 15-mm C–RL human embryo (see Fig. 3.28). The epithelial plate between the lateral nasal (lnp) and maxillary processes (mp) has lost its continuity, resulting in formation of the nasolacrimal duct (nld). ic = inferior concha.

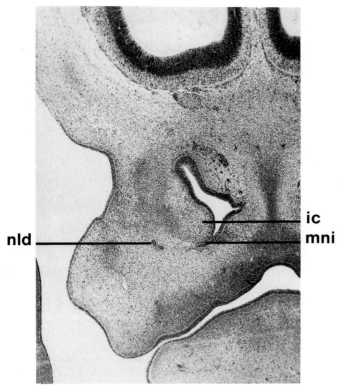

Fig. 3.30 Frontal 10-μm section of the nasal tube of a 17-mm C–RL human embryo. Outgrowth of the inferior concha (ic) into the nasal lumen. nld = nasolacrimal duct; mni = future meatus nasi inferior.

lateral plate is isolated by cell degeneration in the rest of the plate and forms the nasolacrimal duct (12–15 mm C–RL; Vermeij-Keers 1972a, 1975a). In the medial epithelial plate, cell degeneration is never observed. This plate opens again in the fetal period on the side of the nasal lumen, and becomes the meatus nasi inferior. The future inferior concha is caused by the swelling in the nasal lumen of the lateral nasal process. Outgrowth of the lateral nasal process into the nasal lumen narrows this cavity (Figs. 3.29, 3.30).

In the course of fetal development both the nasolacrimal duct and the meatus nasi inferior make contact. The initial solid duct opens by cell degeneration.

Apart from the nasolacrimal and internasal grooves the interorbital groove develops gradually by outgrowth of the lateral nasal processes and the telencephalic vesicles bulging out the forehead (Fig. 3.31). This groove runs from one eye-cup to the other over the nasal root, which can now be distinguished (Vermeij-Keers 1972a). The groove indicates on both sides the localization of the future medial angle of the eye. Slightly laterally, the nasolacrimal groove ends in the fold of the developing lower eyelid. In this way the area between these two grooves is formed by the lateral nasal process. As a consequence the lower eyelid develops out of the maxillary and lateral nasal processes. The area between the internasal and interorbital grooves is indicated as the triangular area (Fig. 3.31).

double layer of ectoderm develop. The nasolacrimal duct evolves from the epithelial plate of the lateral groove, the nasolacrimal groove; the meatus nasi inferior develops from the medial groove. The solid medial border of the

DEVELOPMENT OF THE MOUTH

After rupture of the buccopharyngeal membrane in human embryos of 2.5 mm C–RL (Arey 1965) by cell degeneration (murine embryos 18–29 somites, Poelmann et al 1985) the stomodeum communicates with the foregut. At

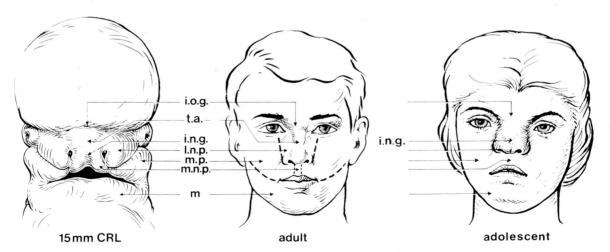

Fig. 3.31 An artist's impression of the face of a 15-mm C–RL human embryo with the facial swellings indicated in relation to an adult face and an adolescent one with orbital hypertelorism. All stages are drawn to the same total height. Localization of the dotted lines in the adult face correspond with the grooves and epithelial plates between the facial swellings of the embryo. Physiologically embryos of this stage show hypertelorism. iog = interorbital groove; ing = internasal groove; ta = triangular area; lnp = lateral nasal process; mp = maxillary process; mnp = medial nasal process; m = mandible (in Vermeij-Keers et al, Ophthalmic Paediatrics and Genetics, 4: 97–105, 1984).

this transition the ectoderm passes into the endoderm. The biggest part of the primitive oral cavity, however, is derived from the stomodeum and is therefore covered with ectoderm. The roof of the stomodeum makes contact with the floor of the prosencephalon, just in front of the still intact buccopharyngeal membrane. After rupture of this membrane the surrounding tissues grow out into the primitive oral cavity, resulting in the formation of Rathke's pouch (Figs. 3.32, 3.33). Subsequently the walls of the pouch make contact and eventually form a solid stalk that disappears by cell degeneration in the 17 mm C–RL stage (Fig. 3.34). During this process the shape of the primitive oral cavity changes and its size reduces relatively.

The stomodeum, and in later stages the primitive oral cavity, is bounded by the first branchial arches (or mandibular processes), the maxillary processes and the interplacodal area (Figs. 3.11, 3.12). In later stages the medial nasal processes grow out within this area. After the formation of both the primitive nasal cavities, the primitive oral cavity remains bounded by the same swellings in combination with the lateral nasal processes, considering the primitive palate as the area from the external nostril to the bucconasal membrane or primitive choana, respectively (Peter 1950, Vermeij-Keers 1972a) (Fig. 3.22).

After the formation of the primitive palate the transformation of the primitive oral cavity continues by outgrowth of swellings into this cavity (12–17 mm C–RL, 6–7 weeks). On both sides the maxillary and mandibular processes are growing out towards each other and a rather narrow epithelial plate is formed. This plate extends forwards from the vicinity of the ear anlage to the corner of the primitive mouth opening (Fig. 3.31). An epithelial

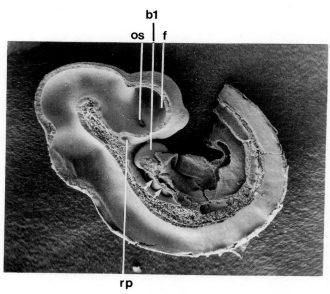

Fig. 3.32 Scanning electron micrograph of a sagittally transected 10 days aged p.c. mouse embryo (heart removed). Pharyngeal pouches are indicated (↑). b_1 = first branchial arch; f = forebrain; rp = Rathke's pouch; os = optic stalk.

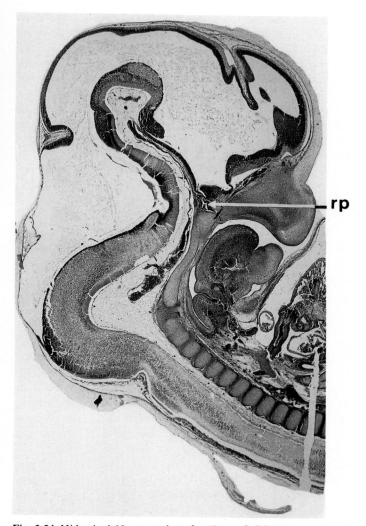

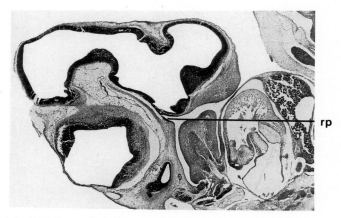

Fig. 3.33 Parasagittal 10-μm section of a 10-mm C–RL human embryo. rp = Rathke's pouch.

Fig. 3.34 Midsagittal 10-μm section of a 17-mm C–RL human embryo. The cranial base has developed. rp = Rathke's pouch.

cord, the organ of Chievitz, remains after the occurrence of cell degeneration and interruption of the basement membranes in this plate (17 mm C–RL). In front of this organ, between the same swellings, another epithelial plate develops, the first anlage of the parotid gland (17 mm C–RL). These outgrowing processes into the primitive oral cavity result in a reduction in the size of the cavity itself and of the primitive mouth opening. After these transformations the primitive mouth opening has its definitive proportions and can be called the permanent mouth opening.

The late development of the face and skull (⩾17 mm C–RL)

In the previous developmental period the neural walls had fused. Subsequently the swellings in the embryonic face fused superficially with each other and also those in the neck. At the end of this period the different facial swellings are still visible, indicated by grooves (Fig. 3.31). The face is flat and the two nasal elements are separated by the internasal groove. In the mesodermal compartment of all these swellings and around the brain cell condensations are recognizable. Among them are parts of the desmocranium, for example the precartilage of the otic and nasal capsules, the percartilage of Meckel (first branchial arch) and of Reichert (second branchial arch), the prospective bone centres, and the premuscular blastema of the facial muscles. The latter develop in connection with their innervating nerves. Microscopically the first differentiations are seen about the 17 mm C–RL stage, except for the otic capsule and some other parts of the chondrocranium, which starts slightly earlier (13–17 mm C–RL, O'Rahilly 1983, Vermeij-Keers 1967).

In general, it can be concluded that differentiation of the mesenchyme into cartilage, bone centres and musculature takes place after transformation of the respective swellings in the head–neck area.

DEVELOPMENT OF THE PERMANENT FACE

In the period of 17–27 mm C–RL the outgrowth and differentiation of the nasal septum (part of the nasal capsule) in a frontocaudal direction leads to the disappearance of the internasal and interorbital grooves. This process can be described as merging, because of the fact that no epithelial plate is ever observed at the site of these grooves (Fig. 3.2). Additionally, the distance between the eyes decreases relatively. At this time the proportions in the face resemble practically the adult situation, in which the two nasal structures are forming the nose. The swellings of the upper and lower eyelids, already present in the previous developmental period, are growing out in stages of about 17 mm up to 34 mm C–RL. They adhere and a narrow epithelial plate is formed. Cell degeneration in this

plate is never observed and the plate opens again in late fetal life. The lower eyelid is composed of the lateral nasal and maxillary processes, and the upper one of a swelling of the forehead (Fig. 3.31).

DEVELOPMENT OF THE PERMANENT ORAL AND NASAL CAVITIES

From 17 mm C–RL onwards epithelial plates in the upper and lower jaws, the dental laminae and the labial grooves, preliminary stages of the teeth and the lips, respectively, develop. The lower teeth and lip originate from the mandibular processes and the upper from the medial nasal and maxillary processes (Fig. 3.3l). The upper lip and jaw grow out in a caudal direction, and so the distance between the external nostrils, bounded by the medial and lateral nasal processes, and the mouth opening increases (Fig. 3.31). As a consequence the primitive palate formed by all the three facial swellings is transformed into the primary

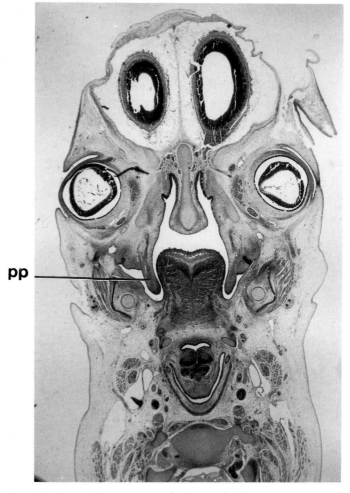

Fig. 3.35 Frontal 10-μm section of a 26-mm C–RL human embryo. The palatine processes (pp) in vertical position.

palate, consisting of only the medial nasal and maxillary processes.

At the same time, at the 17 mm C–RL stage, the first indication of the palatine processes, swellings of the maxillary processes are visible. At either side they grow out into the primitive oral cavity next to the tongue, which reaches in these developmental stages up to the nasal septum (Fig. 3.35). In embryos of about 27 mm C–RL the palatine processes are shifted from a vertical to a horizontal position, now above the tongue. Simultaneously the mandible takes a more frontal position (Vermeij-Keers 1967, Schade 1973). These palatine processes adhere to the primary palate occipitally, in other words just in front of the frontal border of the primitive choana. Furthermore they make contact with each other and with the nasal septum, consisting of both medial nasal processes (Fig. 3.36). This contact takes place in a fronto-occipital direction and is completed in embryos of 34 mm C–RL (Vermeij-Keers 1967). At the contact places epithelial plates develop (Vermeij-Keers 1967) which disappear locally by cell degeneration (Ferguson 1981, Pratt et al 1984, Vermeij-Keers et al 1983a), and fusion of the palatine processes with each other and with the nasal septum is the result, i.e. the secondary palate (Fig. 3.37).

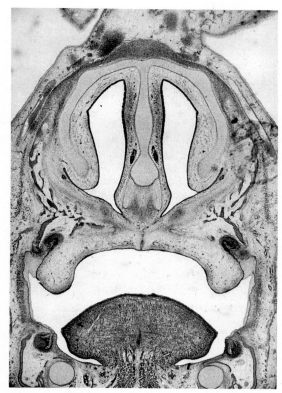

Fig. 3.37 Frontal 10-μm section of a 35-mm C–RL human embryo. The epithelial plates have disappeared locally by cell degeneration.

Owing to the development of the secondary palate the primitive oral cavity is divided horizontally into two parts. The inferior part becomes the permanent oral cavity. The superior part is subdivided vertically by the nasal septum. Now the permanent nasal cavities are formed, consisting of frontally the primitive nasal cavities plus occipitally the superior part of the primitive oral cavity. As a consequence the internal openings of the permanent nasal cavities into the pharynx are the permanent choanae.

DEVELOPMENT OF THE FACIAL MUSCLES

In the literature the premuscular blastema of the facial musculature is said to migrate from the second branchial arch into the face (e.g. Futamura 1906, Gasser 1967). This process is considered to take place in a very short time and to manifest itself independent of the stage of development of the skull and the face. Careful examination of the development of the deep and superficial facial muscles indicate, however, that these muscles develop locally by an interaction between the nerve branches and the mesenchyme (Vermeij-Keers 1967). The differentiation into premuscular blastema starts after the transformations in a special area (e.g. the m. orbicularis oculi develops in the eyelids after they have closed (34 mm C–RL), and the m. orbicularis oris does not arise until the vestibulum oris has

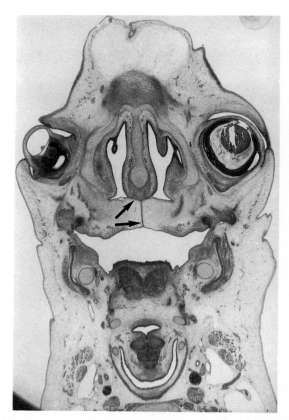

Fig. 3.36 Frontal 10-μm section of a 33-mm C–RL human embryo. Epithelial plates are present between both palatine processes and the nasal septum ($\uparrow$).

developed (27 mm C–RL)). Generally the differentiation of the facial muscles is preceded by the development of the bone centres of the facial skeleton.

DEVELOPMENT OF THE SKULL (17–155 mm C–RL, 7–20 weeks)

The osteocranium develops from the chondrocranium, forming chiefly the base of the skull, and from the membrane bones. The preliminary stage of both is the desmocranium. The anlage of the chondrocranium starts in the midline during the transformation of Rathke's pouch (14–15 mm C–RL). When this pouch is closed off and only connected with the oral epithelium via an epithelial stalk, the definite position of the base of the skull in continuity with the developing nasal septum, part of the nasal capsule, is a fact (17 mm C–RL, Vermeij-Keers 1967) (Fig. 3.34). The first bone centres arise in the membrane bones (17–50 mm C–RL) followed by those in the different parts of the chondrocranium (30–140 mm C–RL, Starck 1955).

In the literature the developmental stages (given by mm C–RL) in which the onset of the ossification starts, are described at different times of the development of the embryo. These discrepancies are most probably freaks of nature and are in fact not very important. Most important, however, is the number of bone centres within one bone, and the outgrowth of the bone centres towards each other followed by fusion or suture formation between bone centres. Various opinions concerning the number of bone centres within one bone also exist in the literature (e.g. O'Rahilly & Gardner 1972). These variations, however, are easy to explain when adult normal skulls are examined (Vermeij-Keers et al 1983b, and this chapter). In these skulls extra sutures are present within membrane bones developing normally from a single bone centre, for example the bipartite zygomatic bone.

The number of bone centres developing in membrane bones and the embryonic stage in which the bone centres arise are summarized in Table 3.1.

Initially the upper jaw is formed from separate elements: the premaxillae and the maxillae. Each premaxilla differentiated from the mesenchyme of the medial nasal process, has two bone centres and bears two incisor teeth. These bone centres grow out and fuse with each other and with the single centre of the maxilla. Each parietal bone develops from two fusing centres. The maxilla, and the palatine, zygomatic, nasal and lacrimal bones each develop mainly from a single centre, whereas the mandible, the frontal, the vomer and the interparietal bones are formed by paired centres. The bone centres of the vomer and interparietal fuse immediately, those of the mandible form initially the symphysis of the mandible, whereas the frontal bone centres form the frontal suture. Both the symphysis

Table 3.1 Ossification of membrane bones of the skull

Bone	C–RL (mm)	Number of bone centres
Maxilla	17	1
Mandible	17	1 L, 1 R
Palatine	23	1
Premaxilla	23	
	50	2
Zygomatic	24–25	1
Pars squamosa	25*	1
Frontal	26	1 L, 1 R
Pterygoid	30*	1
Parietal	31	
	40	2
Vomer	32	1 L, 1 R
Pars tympanica	32–34*	1
Interparietal	32–34*	1 L, 1 R
Nasal	34	1
Lacrimal	40	1

* After Starck (1955).

of the mandible and the frontal suture ossify in the first and second year after birth, respectively.

Ossification of the chondrocranium begins at the 30 mm C–RL stage, when the majority of the membrane bone centres are already present.

The number of bone centres developing in the various bones of the chondrocranium and the developmental stage in which the centres arise are given in Table 3.2.

The occipital, sphenoid and temporal bones are of intramembranous and cartilage origin, whereas the ethmoid bone consists initially of cartilage only (see Tables 3.1 and 3.2). In the cartilage of the occipital bone four bone centres appear around the foramen magnum. The ventral centre corresponds to the basioccipital, both lateral centres which bear the condyles are indicated as exoccipitals and the dorsal one as supraoccipital. The interparietal, of intramembranous origin, develops from two paired centres and joins the supraoccipital to the occipital squama (Figs.

Table 3.2 Ossification of the chondrocranium

Bone	C–RL (mm)	Number of bone centres
Supraoccipital	30 mm*	1
Exoccipital	37 mm*†	1
Alisphenoid	37 mm†	1
Basioccipital	51 mm*	1
Orbitosphenoid	60 mm*†	
Basisphenoid	65 mm*	1 L, 1 R
Presphenoid	90 mm*	1 L, 1 R
Petrosum	110–130 mm*	>3
Incus	110 mm*†	
Malleus	117 mm*	
Inferior nasal concha	130 mm*	
Ossicula Bertini	130 mm*	
Ethmoid	130 mm*	
Stapes	140 mm*	

* After Starck (1955).
† After De Beer (1937).

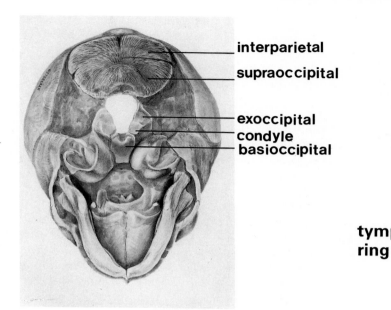

interparietal
supraoccipital

exoccipital
condyle
basioccipital

Fig. 3.38 Base of a fetal skull, in caudal view (total length of fetus 17.5 cm, at 4 months). Interparietal, supraoccipital, exoccipital, condyles and basioccipital parts at the occipital bone.

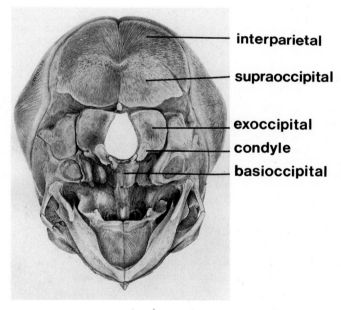

interparietal

supraoccipital

exoccipital

condyle

basioccipital

Fig. 3.39 Base of a fetal skull, in caudal view, at 6½ months.

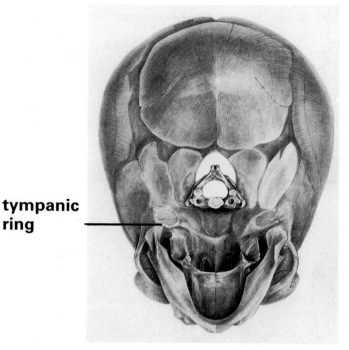

tympanic ring

Fig. 3.40 Base of the neonatal skull, in caudal view, with cervical vertebrae.

3.38–3.42). The total number of bone centres that arises in the cartilage of the future sphenoid bone is controversial. Arey (1965) speaks of 10 principal centres and Lemire (1986) describes that there are at least 14 separate ossification centres plus several others in the ossicula Bertini, parts of the dorsal extension of the nasal capsule, which fuse with the presphenoid postnatally. In addition Arey (1965) mentions that intramembranous bone enters the composition of this bone, one centre forming the orbital and temporal portion of each ala magna and another centre forming the mesial lamina of each pterygoid process. Starck (1955) indicates only the latter. The temporal bone develops out of four different portions, i.e. the petrous, the squamosal and tympanic portions and the styloid process. The latter originates from cartilage of the dorsal end of the second branchial arch. The squamosal and tympanic portions are both of intramembranous origin and their bone centres differentiate in embryos of 25 and 32–34 mm C–RL, respectively (Table 3.1). Within the cartilage of the petrous portion over three principal centres of ossification develop, producing a bony capsule about the inner ear (Starck 1955). The mastoid process bulges out of the petrous bone after birth (Arey 1965) (Figs. 3.38–3.42).

The ossification of the nasal capsule cartilage concerns the ethmoid bone, the inferior concha and the ossicula Bertini (Table 3.2). In the literature the inferior concha is also indicated as maxilloturbinal, suggesting its origin in the maxillary process. However, as described earlier the inferior concha is part of the lateral nasal process and therefore the term maxilloturbinal must be avoided. Data concerning the pattern of ossification of the nasal capsule are scarce. According to Starck (1955) the ossification starts in the medial concha, whereas the cribriform plate, the crista galli and perpendicular plate ossify latest. The

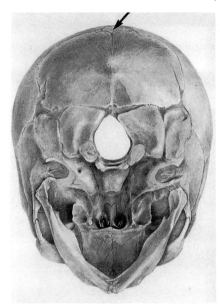

Fig. 3.41 Base of a skull, in caudal view, in the first year of life. Note the os inca (↑).

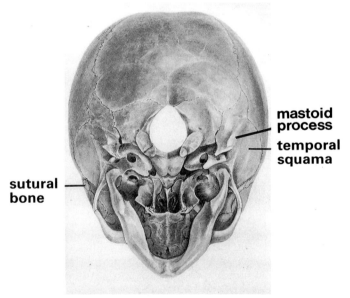

mastoid process

temporal squama

sutural bone

Fig. 3.42 Base of the skull, in caudal view, of a child of 2 years old. Note the difference in bony structure during the development of the bones and the final suture formation (Figs. 3.38–3.42).

number of ossification centres is not available. The inferior concha and the ossicula of Bertini develop as independent bones, of which the ossicula fuse with the sphenoid bone.

It is obvious that bones of such a complicated shape, developing during a long period of intrauterine life and studied via different techniques, should cause discrepancies concerning the number of bone centres; and in the case of the ethmoid the number is even lacking. As already mentioned, the exact number of bone centres seems not very important. More important is the extent of outgrowth of the bone centres within the cartilage, which shape is delimited during the formation of the chondrocranium; for example the cranial base angle was found to remain unchanged at approximately 128° (Diewert 1983, 1985). The spatial proportions of the chondrocranium are defined after the transformations of the neural groove and tube, Rathke's pouch, the branchial arch system and the sense organs. Furthermore the development and outgrowth of the intramembranous bone centres take place with respect to the chondrocranium.

Bone centres within the cartilage of the chondrocranium and those of membranous origin grow out towards each other and fuse directly or form synchondroses and sutures (Figs. 3.38–3.42). The synchondroses cranii develop within the chondrocranium as cartilaginous junctions between bone centres. These can be located within or between future bones. The intersphenoidal synchondrosis extends between the two halves of the body of the sphenoid bone. The anterior and posterior intraoccipital synchondroses are located between the basi- and exoccipital and the posterior between the ex- and supraoccipitals, all parts of the future occipital bone (Figs. 3.38–3.42). Between future bones the petro-occipital, the spheno-occipital and sphenopetrosal synchondroses are formed. Disappearance of the synchondroses within bones by fusion of the bone centres involved takes place postnatally (Lemire 1986).

Suture formation at places of synchondroses between future bones also starts postnatally. Prenatally sutures are narrow mesenchymal connections between the respective bones (Figs. 3.38, 3.39). The formation of sutures of the membrane bones of the skull starts in embryos of 25 mm C–RL, i.e. with the symphysis of the mandible, whereas almost all sutures are present in specimens of 7.5 cm C–RL, 14 weeks of development (Vermeij-Keers et al 1983a).

The question why some bone centres can fuse directly and others form sutures with or without a cartilaginous intermediate stage remains unanswered. In the case of suture formation the mesenchymal or cartilaginous area between bone centres must be different from that of fusing bone centres. Perhaps this difference dissolves in the normal situation when an existing suture ossifies during ageing, in the pre- or postnatal or in the adult situation. Probably the occurrence of programmed cell degeneration within a suture is responsible for the existence of that suture. Consequently lack of programmed cell degeneration causes ossification of a suture. Further investigations concerning this subject are necessary.

MACROSCOPIC OBSERVATIONS IN HUMAN SKULLS

About 2400 human skulls, representing an unselected

collection with respect to craniofacial defects, were used to assess the occurrence of agenesis of bones, the absence of sutures, the presence of persistent and extra sutures and fusion defects within bones.

Agenesis of bones was seen only for the nasal bones, in six of the 2400 skulls (Fig. 3.43).

With absence of sutures is expressed the normal situation in which ossification of sutures occurs during ageing, and the abnormal situations of premature synostosis and non-formation of sutures, i.e. a bony cleft between bones. The last was observed in four cases. In one, a neonatal skull, the frontal suture was missing, caused by arrested growth of both frontal bone centres (Fig. 3.44) In another the zygomatic arch showed a break at the site of the temporozygomatic suture. Both the temporal process of the zygomatic and the zygomatic process of the temporal bone were shortened and rounded (Vermeij-Keers et al 1983a). In the third case (fetus Eb148) several sutures were not formed, e.g. the frontozygomatic suture, the spheno-frontal, sphenomaxillary and sphenoparietal sutures (Fig. 3.45). And in the last case the interparietal suture shows a defect.

Persistent sutures, e.g. the frontal suture then indicated as metopic suture and the incisive suture, and remnants of sutures such as in the symphysis of the mandible, were observed frequently.

An extra suture can be defined as a suture within a bone that normally develops from a single bone centre or from multiple fusing centres. This phenomenon was seen four

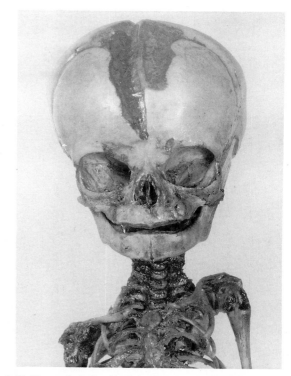

Fig. 3.44 Neonatal skull with defective outgrowth of the paired frontal bone centres, i.e. defective formation of the frontal suture.

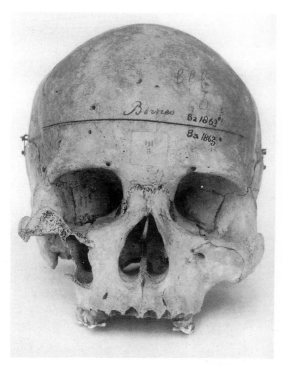

Fig. 3.43 An adult skull in frontal view. Both nasal bones are missing.

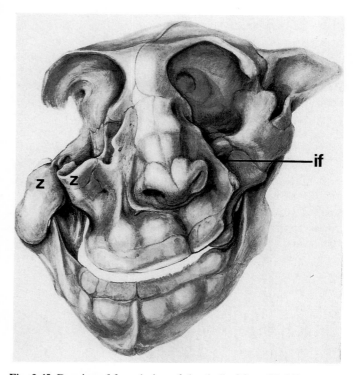

Fig. 3.45 Drawing of frontal view of the skull of fetus Eb 148. Schistasis of the corpus maxillae medial to the infraorbital foramen (if) (left side) and schistasis of the zygoma. Both parts of the zygoma are indicated with z. There were gaps in place of sutures and the lateral wall of the right orbit was not closed.

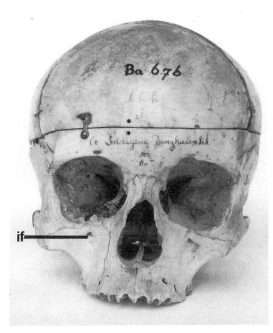

Fig. 3.46 Frontal view of an adult skull with an extra suture of the right maxilla medially to the infraorbital foramen (if).

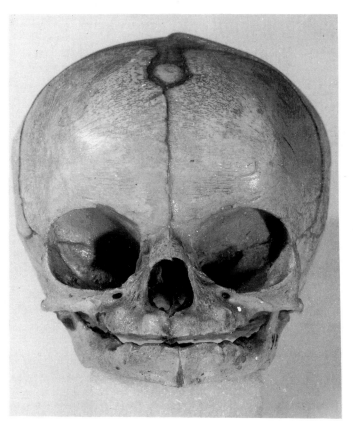

Fig. 3.47 Frontal view of a neonatal skull with a sutural bone.

times unilaterally in the maxilla, not always on the same side or same location (Fig. 3.46). Two of these extra sutures were present in the body of the maxilla (one lateral and the other medial to the infraorbital foramen) and two in the frontal process of the maxilla. The bipartite or tripartite nasal bone was present in six skulls and the bipartite zygomatic in 13 skulls. Furthermore the inca bones were found frequently (Fig. 3.41), as well as the different ossa suturarum (Figs. 3.42, 3.47). A fusion defect within a bone is caused by deficient outgrowth of one bone centre or more if that bone develops from multiple bone centres. The result is a bony cleft within it. In nine skulls this type of defect was observed. Five of them show a cleft in the primary palate uni- or bilaterally, i.e. between the premaxilla and maxilla, all with palatoschisis. Another example demonstrates a defect between the premaxilla and maxilla without palatoschisis (Fig. 3.48). Foetus Eb148 shows, apart from the missing sutures, a schistasis of the right zygoma and a schistasis of the left maxillary corpus medial to the infraorbital foramen (Fig. 3.45). Finally, two cases have a bony defect in the midline of the occipital squama.

ABNORMAL CRANIOFACIAL DEVELOPMENT

Knowledge of the normal morphogenetic and differentiation processes in the human brain, face and cranium is necessary to understand the derailments that occur during abnormal development. In the literature some of the

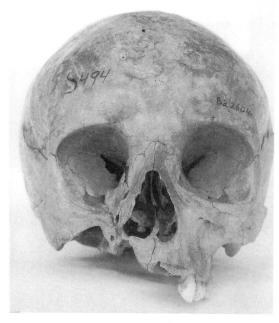

Fig. 3.48 Frontal view of an adult skull with a fusion defect between the premaxilla and maxilla (right side).

malformations are explained as embryological, in terms of fusion (His 1892), and merging (Patten 1961) theories of the facial swellings; others — the rare craniofacial clefts — do not fit into these schemes (Kawamoto 1976). For the last category other explanations are proposed such as amniotic bands and adhesions, splitting off parts of the facial swellings (e.g. Morian 1887). Ploner (1957), however, questioned the importance of the amniotic bands and considered, imitating Politzer (1937), followed by Pfeifer (1967), the atypical clefts as the results of ruptures of the embryonic face caused by external damage. According to Johnston (1975), for example, defects in neural crest cell migration should lead to the most extreme malformations in man, such as cyclopia and hypertelorism.

There are differences of opinion not only about the abnormal development of the brain, face and cranium, but also about the classification and nomenclature of these malformations. Pure topographically oriented classifications are published by, for example, Tessier (1976) and Kawamoto (1976), using a cleft-numbering system. Pfeifer (1967, 1974) and Mazzola (1976) took some embryological considerations into account in an otherwise topographically subdivided face. They all use the term cleft erroneously.

According to *Dorland's Medical Dictionary* (1981) a cleft is defined as 'a fissure or elongated opening, especially one occurring in the embryo or derived from a failure of parts to fuse during embryonic development'. Vermeij-Keers et al (1983a,b, and this chapter) and Van der Meulen et al (1983) (Ch. 9) use the term cleft in that sense. In addition a new nomenclature is proposed using the general term dysplasia, i.e. abnormality in development, instead of the term 'cleft', and introducing a new classification based only on the embryological development of the brain, face and cranium.

From the present knowledge it may be concluded, without involving the theory of neural crest cell migration, that derailments in the basic developmental processes occurring in the cephalic region (cell proliferation, degeneration and differentiation) can lead to the various malformations observed in man. Three different groups of malformations can be distinguished:

cerebrocranial dysplasias — malformations of the brain and cranium;
cerebro-craniofacial dysplasias — facial defects involving the brain and/or the eyes and cranium;
craniofacial dysplasias — defects of the face and cranium only.

All three groups can be subdivided into early or primary and late or secondary developmental defects. Examples are taken from the teratological collection of the Department of Anatomy and Embryology of Leiden University.

Cerebrocranial dysplasias

The early or primary defects develop during the transformation of the neural plate via the neural groove into the neural tube. The outgrowth of the headfolds and/or neural walls is deficient along the longitudinal axis of the embryo, resulting in craniorachischisis, or is partly deficient in cases of cranium bifidum apertum and spina bifida aperta. The term cranium bifidum apertum is introduced as analogous to spina bifida aperta. The 66 cases available of cranium bifidum apertum can be subdivided into anencephaly totalis, i.e. holoanencephaly (30 cases), anencephaly partialis, i.e. meroanencephaly (14), and exencephaly (22 cases). In all cases of cranium bifidum apertum the eyes, the diencephalic part of the prosencephalon, are normally developed. The anterior neuropore which separates the two nasal fields is closed. In cases of anencephaly the deficiency of outgrowth can be caused by insufficient proliferation of the neuroectoderm and of the mesectoderm in the telencephalic part of the prosencephalon, the mesencephalon and the rhombencephalon. The exencephaly is another example of insufficient outgrowth of the headfolds and/or the neural walls. In this case the proliferation of the neuroectoderm seems sufficient, but the formation and/or proliferation of the mesectoderm is unsatisfactory. Primary defects can also be caused by insufficient cell death at the place of contact between the otherwise normally proliferated neural walls. Discontinuity of the basement membranes does not occur (see description of the cleft lip) and fusion of the walls does not take place. The plate opens again and forms a groove (compare the development of the inferior nasal meatus), resulting in a complete cleft. This mechanism explains the reopening of the neural tube, described by Gardner (1964, 1966, 1980) and Padget (1970, 1972). They, however, indicate that this is caused by too high a pressure of the liquor cerebrospinalis or by neuroschisis and bleb formation of the skin by the leaking of liquor cerebrospinalis, respectively. Under experimental conditions a raised pressure of the cerebrospinal fluid of rat embryos cultured in vitro has never caused a schisis of the neuroectoderm of the neural tube, but the neural tube is dilated (Smits-van Prooije, unpublished data).

All primary clefts show an ectodermal defect along the extension of the affected epithelial plate, i.e. the plate between the opposed neural walls. After fusion of the neural walls mesectoderm will separate the surface ectoderm from the neuroectoderm of the neural tube in the fusion zone. The neural tube then grows out and differentiates into tel-, di-, mes-, met- and myelencephalon. In the mesodermal compartment around the developing human brain the desmocranium will be outlined as a mass of dense mesenchyme in which the chondrocranium and membrane bones of the osteocranium will differentiate in developmental stages around 17 mm C–RL. In general, the development of the human brain coincides with that of the human cranium. If the outgrowth of the brain is insufficient, such as is the case in microencephaly, the neurocranium is microcephalic. Both are secondary defects or dysplasias.

Skull formation can be explained as outgrowing bone centres, intramembranous or endochondral, making contact with each other. At the places of contact fusions of bone centres occur, or sutures develop. Secondary bony defects arise during formation of the neurocranium due to absence of: (1) anlage of bone centres, e.g. absence of a frontal bone centre with dilatation of the underlying half of the telencephalon; (2) outgrowth of bone centres between two adjacent membrane or endochondral bones or between a combination of both; these are bony defects situated between two bones at sites of sutures; e.g. between the two frontal bone centres the frontal suture is missing. Another example concerns a bony defect at the place of the interparietal suture. Fetus Eb148 (Fig. 3.45) shows bony defects between several membrane bones and an endochondral bone, the sphenoid bone; (3) outgrowth of one or more bone centres in bones (membrane and/or endochondral) having multiple bone centres; these are bony defects within a bone, e.g. the two cases with a bony defect in the midline of the occipital squama.

These secondary defects are indicated as cranium bifidum occultum. When these malformations are associated with protrusion of meninges and/or brain tissue through the defect and are covered with ectoderm the term cranium bifidum cysticum (meningocele or meningoencephalocele) can be used (see also Ch. 9).

Cerebrocraniofacial dysplasias

EARLY OR PRIMARY DEFECTS (≤17 mm C–RL)

To this group belong cases of cyclopia (a single eye or closely approximated eyes, with all integrades, synophthalmus and synorbitism, in a single orbit), with or without proboscis and cases of hypotelorism. In a 6.5 mm human embryo with a single nasal placode localized in front of two eye-cups, and in 12 human fetal cases, and in two fetal skulls, the midfacial region was more or less deficient (Vermeij-Keers et al 1987). In the embryo the area between the nasal placodes — the interplacodal area — was missing, resulting in a single undulated nasal placode, as if formed from two fused nasal placodes, (Fig. 3.49). In normal embryos both medial nasal processes, with the internasal groove in between, will develop within the interplacodal area (Figs. 3.8, 3.11). In the two fetal cyclopic skulls this missing area is indicated by the agenesis of, for example, the two premaxillae, the nasal septum, the nasal and lacrimal bones and the

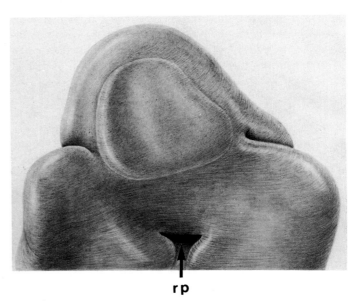

Fig. 3.49 Artist's impression of a caudofrontal view of a reconstruction of a human embryo (6.5 mm C–RL). The superficial contours with a single undulated nasal placode are indicated. rp = Rathke's pouch.

ethmoid. The maxillae had fused in the midline and the narrow flat palate, consisting of maxillae and palatine bones, was closed. The deformed vomer, composed of two triangular pieces of bone, was situated perpendicular to the occipital side of the palate and sutured the pterygoid processes. One of the cyclopic skulls had no proboscis and a single frontal bone developed from one midline bone centre; the other had a bony proboscis constructed of three bone centres.

Of the 12 human fetuses one had cyclopia (single eye in a single orbit), arhinia without proboscis and otocephaly (agnathus with astomus), four had synophthalmus (fused eyes in a single orbit), three of them had arhinia without and one had arhinia with proboscis; there were two cases of synorbitism (two eyes in a single orbit) and arhinia with proboscis; one of these two had otocephaly (Fig. 3.50) and in a further five cases hypotelorism was present. One of these fetuses showed otocephaly and extreme hypotelorism (but the orbits were separated), and arhinia with a septate proboscis, i.e. ethmocephaly (type II of De Myer et al 1964; and Ch. 9). The four other examples had flat noses, a cleft palate and agenesis of the premaxillae, the median part of the upper lip and of the nasal septum, corresponding to type IV of de Myer et al (1964). Externally, all the 12 fetuses exhibited fusion of the right and left eye related to the associated organs, and they lacked the premaxillae and nasal septum. In normal embryos this corresponds to the interplacodal area. In type V of De Myer et al (1964), showing hypotelorism with premaxilla anlage, the interplacodal area is present but too narrow (Vermeij-Keers et al 1983a, 1987). All specimens described above were microcephalic, and according to De Myer et

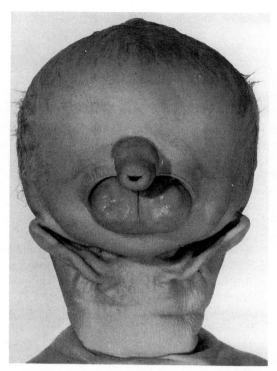

Fig. 3.50 Frontal view of a fetal face showing otocephaly, synorbitism and arhinia with proboscis.

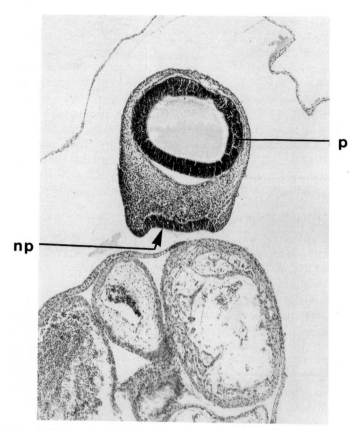

Fig. 3.51 Horizontal 10-μm section of the single undulated nasal placode (np) of a human embryo (6.5 mm C–RL; Fig. 3.49). Note the narrow holoprosencephalon (p). No amniotic bands are present.

al (1964) and Mieden (1982) they are holoprosencephalic. In the literature several theories are proposed for pathogenesis of cyclopia and hypotelorism, such as amniotic band adhesions (Jones 1975), lack of closure of the anterior neuropore (Tessier 1976), and the abnormal positioning of the notochord (Cohen et al 1971). But in the 6.5 mm embryo the neural tube was closed, no amniotic bands were present and the position of the notochord was normal. The forebrain, however, was too narrow, and the interplacodal area, i.e. the medial nasal processes, was missing (Fig. 3.51). It might be concluded that both the neuroectoderm and mesoderm were already affected at an early stage of development. According to experiments carried out in mammals (Smits-van Prooije 1986), the mesoderm of the preliminary midface consists of mesectodermal cells, originating from the neural crest and surface ectoderm placodes of the headfolds present in the preneural plate, in the presomite stages. From the 4-somite stage onwards only the neural crest of the prosencephalon and the optic neural crest active in the 13- to 20-somite stage deposit mesectodermal cells in the mesodermal compartment of that part of the head region. Therefore it can be concluded that in cases of cyclopia and hypotelorism the outgrowth of the neuroectoderm and the formation of mesectoderm are deficient (Vermeij-Keers et al 1987).

In the literature two hypotheses concerning the normal development of the eyes are discussed: whether the eyes

derive from a single median eye primordium or from paired lateral primordia (De Myer 1977). According to Smits-van Prooije et al (1985; murine embryos) and Müller & O'Rahilly (1985; human embryos) one eye primordium develops in each prosencephalic part of the neuroectoderm of the headfolds. The same can be concluded from all microscopically studied cyclopia cases, as one eye in one orbit showed signs of fusion of two eye primordia, e.g. a bifurcated optic nerve (Smith & Boulgakow 1927 and Vermeij-Keers et al 1987). Therefore cyclopses, with or without proboscis, and hypotelorismic cases must have the same abnormal stages in early embryological development of the prosencephalon in relation to the eyes. In cyclopses and hypotelorismic specimens with proboscis the dislocation of the nasal placode(s) in the nasal field(s) outside the range of the maxillary processes would lead to the malformation. Both malformations are frequently accompanied by otocephaly, which can be explained by the persistence of the buccopharyngeal membrane.

Because of the localization of the eye primordia in the prosencephalic neural walls, the eyeballs, except for the lens, form part of the brain. Therefore the malformations of the neural elements of the eyeballs are grouped with the cerebro-craniofacial dysplasias. The lens develops as an ectodermal placode in front of the optic vesicle and in continuity with the nasal fields. The influence of the lens on the size of the eyeball is very important. For example primary congenital aphakia (e.g. Mann 1958, Manschot 1963, 1966, 1969) occurring as a part of the rubella syndrome (Vermeij-Keers 1975b) causes anophthalmia or microphthalmia, microorbitism and hypoplasia of the faciocranium on the affected side. The term faciocranium is introduced to replace the term viscerocranium, the latter implying that part of the skull which is derived from the branchial arches. Since the maxillary processes form no part of the first branchial arch. the term viscerocranium is misplaced.

During the normal development of the mammalian eyeball (Silver & Hughes 1973) and lens (Schook 1980) cell degeneration occurs. In 1974 Silver & Hughes postulated that lack of cell degeneration in the early stage of eye development inhibits the invagination of the optic vesicle and subsequently leads to anophthalmia or microphthalmia. In addition the optic fissure will not be formed. Abnormal formation of the optic fissure (Silver & Hughes 1973) and improper closure of the fissure (Arey 1965) cause congenital colobomata of the iris, ciliary body, retina and/or choroid tunic. The fissure closes normally without cell degeneration (Silver & Hughes 1974) and with fusion of its basement membranes, i.e. basal intraepithelial fusion (Vermeij-Keers et al 1983a).

LATE OR SECONDARY DEFECTS (⩾17 mm C–RL)

After closure of the neural tube transformations of the neuroectoderm take place owing to outgrowth of the neuroectoderm into the lumen of the primitive tubular brain and into superficial directions. Symmetrical outgrowth into the lumen causes apical fusion of the neuroectoderm, and outgrowth into superficial directions causes basal fusion of the basement membranes of the neuroectoderm, i.e. the final shape of the cavities of the brain and formation of the commissures, respectively. In cases of extreme hypertelorism the corpus callosum, a telencephalic commissure originating at the 54 mm C–RL stage (Hochstetter 1919), is often missing. Other examples of failures of appearance of parts of the brain in combination with craniofacial defects are arhinencephalia with arhinia, with or without probiscis, and arhinencephalia with trigonocephalia. In the latter synostosis of the metopic suture has taken place or the frontal bone has originated from a single bone centre. The external nose can be normal (Warkany 1975). For hypotheses of the development of arhinia, see pages 52, 53, 55.

Craniofacial dysplasias

EARLY OR PRIMARY DEFECTS (⩽17 mm C–RL)

Under normal conditions the transformations occurring in the embryonic face take place after closure of the anterior neuropore, lying in the midline of that face between the two nasal fields. This localization is found in mouse embryos (Smits-van Prooije 1986, Vermeij-Keers et al 1983a) as well as in human examples (O'Rahilly 1967, O'Rahilly & Gardner 1971). Disturbances of the closing mechanism at the final point of closure can explain dermoid (midline) cysts and midline fistulas (Vermeij-Keers et al 1983a), which are generally indicated as separate entities (e.g. Mazzola 1976). In both cases 'inclusion' of ectoderm exists as a result of insufficient cell degeneration of neuro- and/or surface ectodermal cells of the anterior neuropore. The presence of neural crest activity at that place can explain the development of the dermoid cyst. The ultimate position of these defects on the back of the nose can be explained by the development of that organ. The nasal placodes evolve within the nasal fields, separated by the interplacodal area. Around both nasal placodes, three swellings grow out with respect to the prosencephalon and transform the placodes, via the nasal grooves, into the nasal tubes. During this transformation the two medial nasal processes grow from the interplacodal area, with the internasal groove in between. The internasal groove, initially the closing place of the anterior neuropore, still present at the 17-mm stage, becomes the back of the nose in later stages (Fig. 3.31) by a process indicated as merging. As a consequence the dermoid cyst and midline fistulas are indicated as internasal dysplasias (Ch. 9). Patten (1961) postulated that the above-described deformities are merging defects, and therefore develop after 17 mm C–RL.

All the other primary defects are based on derailments of the development of the nasal placodes and/or of the transformations of the facial swellings. As already indicated the nose develops out of two separated elements. Therefore when there is one nasal element present the term nasal aplasia can be used instead of 'half-nose', and when both elements are lacking arhinia can replace 'agenesis of the nose' (Vermeij-Keers et al 1983a; Van der Meulen et al 1983). Following the normal events of development of the nose, nasal aplasia and arhinia can be explained in the first place by lack of evolution of the nasal fields and/or the nasal placodes. This situation can be demonstrated in an abnormal human embryo of 9.5 mm C–RL with the prosencenphalon not closed; neither the optic sulci nor the nasal fields and placodes are present. Under normal conditions the prospective medial and lateral nasal and maxillary processes are situated around the nasal placode (6.0–6.5 mm). In the absence of the placode(s) these processes will not grow out and, for instance, the nasolacrimal duct(s) will not develop. The result is a non-transformed mesenchymal block in which subsequently bone tissue differentiates. A second possibility in the genesis of nasal aplasia and arhinia can be found in the persistence of the bucconasal membrane(s). In a 20-mm C–RL embryo this bilateral phenomenon is accompanied by undeveloped nasolacrimal ducts, under-developed nasal lumina, which means, for example, that the inferior conchae failed to form. There are no primitive choanae and the mesenchyme of the primary palate is in continuity with that of the future base of the skull (e.g. the sphenoid bone), thus forming a block of mesenchyme in which bone will differentiate. Normally, the bucconasal membrane breaks and disappears by cell degeneration at the 17-mm stage, causing the primitive choana. In specimens with nasal aplasia or arhinia, cell degeneration has probably failed to occur.

An abnormal localization within the nasal field out of the range of the maxillary processes can explain nasal aplasia or arhinia with proboscis (see under cerebrocraniofacial dysplasias). Furthermore, Kirchmayer (1906) and McLaren (1955) described patients with a practically normally developed nose in combination with proboscis, and other primary dysplasias such as cleft lip and palate. It is postulated that the combination of a normal nose with proboscis can be the result of differentiation of a double nasal placode within one nasal field (Vermeij-Keers et al 1983a). The same explanation can be used for nasal and rhinal duplication. In these cases the duplication is present in one or in both nasal fields, respectively. In diprosopia, for example — nasal duplication with an extra orbit (Mazzola 1976) — the possibility of conjoined twins should be considered.

Fusion processes taking place between the facial swellings during the early embryonic development of the face, and between the palatine processes during secondary palate formation, can explain primary or true clefts. These clefts can be caused by derailments during the different phases of the fusion process. In the first phase, owing to insufficient outgrowth of the facial swellings, i.e. insufficient cell proliferation and/or extracellular matrix formation, the processes do not come into contact with each other and the epithelial plates cannot develop (mouse embryos, Trasler and Leong 1982). In the adhesion phase some cells have the capacity to make cell contacts and to establish an epithelial plate. When this phenomenon is lacking the epithelial plate will not be properly formed. The third phase is characterized by cell death in a normally developed epithelial plate. Absence of cell degeneration in the ectoderm of the epithelial plates results in the existence of the basement membranes and the plate itself. The plate opens again and forms a groove (cf. the development of the inferior nasal meatus and the adhesion and opening of the eyelids). This situation can be demonstrated in a 22 mm C–RL human embryo (Heidelberg collection) with a cleft on the left side of the upper lip. The facial swellings on the right side are normally fused and the epithelial plate of Hochstetter has disappeared completely owing to cell degeneration. The epithelial plate on the left side, which shows neither cell degeneration nor cell proliferation and has uninterrupted basement membranes, is still present (Fig. 3.52).

Incomplete clefts, i.e. tissue bridges, can be caused by incomplete disappearance of the epithelial plate. The remnants of the epithelial plate open again and form a groove. Derailments in all the three phases of the fusion process can play a part, alone or in combination, in the development of such deformities.

The primary or true clefts all coincide with the localization of an epithelial plate (Fig. 3.31):

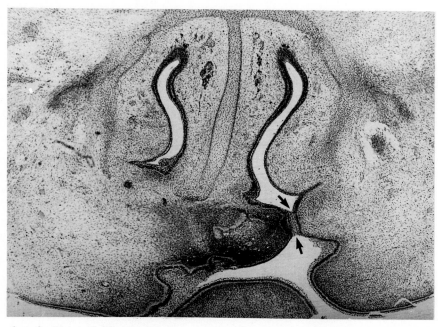

Fig. 3.52 Frontal 10-μm section of a 22-mm C–RL human embryo with a unilateral cleft lip (Heidelberg collection). The persistent epithelial plate on the left side showed no signs of cell degeneration (↑).

1. between the lateral nasal and maxillary processes on the lateral side and the medial nasal process on the medial one;
2. between the lateral nasal and maxillary processes;
3. between the maxillary and mandibular processes;
4. between the palatine processes.

In all these primary or true clefts an ectodermal defect exists along the extension of the affected epithelial plate. In other words the ectoderm above the affected epithelial plates has not fused. The epithelial plate of Hochstetter coincides with the localization described in (1) above and corresponds to the common cleft lip: cheiloschisis or cheilognathoschisis. The nasolacrimal groove indicates the cleft in (2) above and is often combined with a common cleft lip. This defect running from the mouth through the nose to the swelling of the lower eyelid lateral to its inner canthus corresponds to the oro-naso-ocular cleft, i.e. Morian I (1887). In this type of cleft the nasolacrimal duct is absent, or patent in less severe cases. Type (3) above describes the maxillomandibular dysplasia or macrostomia corresponding to the ectodermal part of Tessier's 'no. 7 cleft' (1976). The parotid gland and duct, normally coming from the epithelial plate between the maxillary and mandibular processes, may be absent. The localization in (4) above marks the cleft palate: the hard and/or the soft cleft palate. The defects of the bones and musculature involved are the result of the non-fusion of the swellings. In the literature (e.g. Patten 1953) two fusing mandibular swellings are described. But in mouse, rat and human embryos an epithelial plate between these swellings was never observed (Vermeij-Keers et al 1983a). Therefore schisis of the mandible must have another explanation (see below).

LATE OR SECONDARY DEFECTS (≥17 mm C–RL)

The fusion processes of the face are completed around the 17-mm C–RL stage. In that stage the ectoderm of the face has closed, the mesenchymal cores of the swellings have fused, and the differentiation of the mesenchyme into bone centres, cartilage and facial muscles begins. During the late development of the face the number of the bone centres and their degree of outgrowth are most important. Defective differentiation and outgrowth cause the secondary defects or dysplasias. They can arise through:

1. The absence of anlage of bone centres, such as the absence of the malar bone in the Treacher Collins syndrome, absence of one frontal bone (see Ch. 9, frontal dysplasia) and agenesis of the nasal bones.
2. The absence of outgrowth of bone centres between two adjacent future bones, cartilaginous or membranous. These bony defects are situated at sites of sutures: for example, sphenofrontal, maxillozygomatic, zygofrontal,

intermaxillary dysplasia (between both premaxillae), intermaxillopalatinal dysplasia (submucous cleft palate) and intermandibular dysplasia (Ch. 9); in this chapter (see above), fetus Eb148 in which several sutures were not formed (Fig. 3.45) and a neonatal skull lacking the frontal suture (Fig. 3.44).

3. The absence of outgrowth of one or more bone centres in future bones having multiple bone centres. The bony defects are located within the affected bones. This category can be subdivided into:
   (a) Bony defects localized at sites where normally bone centres fuse, for example between the premaxilla and maxilla (see Fig. 3.48), and in the midline of the occipital squama.
   (b) Bony defects with a highly variable localization within a membrane bone, according to the localizations of the extra sutures of, for example, the zygoma and maxilla (see Tessier 1976, nos 10 and 11, 4 and 5; i.e. Morian II and III and their variations (1887); see Ch. 9, medial and lateral maxillary dysplasias, and fetus Eb148). Fetus Eb148 shows a secondary defect of the left corpus maxillae medially with regard to the infraorbital foramen, i.e. Morian II, and medial maxillary dysplasia (Ch. 9). The nose and both nasolacrimal ducts are not involved. But when a secondary defect concerns the frontal process of the maxilla instead of its corpus, then the nasolacrimal duct (at the 15-mm C–RL stage already present as a solid epithelial cord still separated from the nasal lumen) will be affected or damaged during the development of the facial skeleton, ≥17 mm C–RL. In such a case the duct or remnants of the duct will be found. According to Ask & van der Hoeven (1921) many variations in the outgrowth of the lacrimal ducts under normal and abnormal conditions are possible. The lateral maxillary dysplasia corresponds to Morian III and its localization is lateral with regard to the infraorbital foramen. It is obvious that direction and localization of these dysplasias vary widely.
4. Hypoplasia of bone(s) or parts of bone(s) after normal development and outgrowth of the bone centres, for example, hypoplasia of the maxilla or mandible. This defect is often combined with other malformations.

   All the various defects coinciding with points (1)–(4) can be classified under the term dysostosis.
5. Premature synostosis between bones of the faciocranium and/or neurocranium. The formation of sutures starts in the faciocranium in embryos of about 25 mm C–RL and in the neurocranium at the 55-mm C–RL stage. In fetuses of 14 weeks gestation, i.e. about 7.5 cm C–RL, practically all the sutures are formed. Up to now it is not known what causes premature synostosis. It is postulated here that instead of the normal suture formation fusion of bone centres takes

place. This can be demonstrated in a 16-week-old fetus with a cloverleaf skull. This subclass of dysplasias develops quite early during the period of differentiation of the mesenchyme into bone centres. In addition Diewert (1983, 1985) has indicated that after 7 weeks of development the cranial base angle of the chondrocranium remains unchanged at approximately 128°. Therefore abnormal angles of the chondrocranium, indicating some synostotic syndromes, can be developed before the 17-mm stage. The nomenclature of these synostotic sutures should be, for example, sagittal dysplasia, metopic dysplasia and sagittocoronal dysplasia (Bertelsen 1958, Van der Meulen et al 1983, Ch. 9).

Apart from the differentiation into bone centres within the mesenchyme, differentiation into cartilage and musculature takes place (about the 17-mm C–RL stage). In these embryos the nose is composed of two nasal elements separated by the internasal groove. These embryos show physiologically a flat nose and hypertelorism. During the late development of the face the internasal groove disappears owing to the outgrowth and differentiation of the nasal septum (cartilage) in the frontocaudal direction, i.e. in a process called 'merging'. Simultaneously (17–27 cm C-RL) the distance between the eyes decreases relatively, because of a relative lag in transverse growth. So orbital hypertelorism or teleorbitism can be explained by insufficient relative decrease of the midfacial part (Fig. 3.31). In that case the interorbital as well as the outerorbital distances are increased, and the angle between the lateral walls of the orbits is increased (see Ch. 9; Vermeij-Keers et al 1984). Interorbital hypertelorism must be distinguished from orbital hypertelorism (Van der Meulen & Vaandrager 1983, Vermeij-Keers et al 1984). In interorbital hypertelorism only the interorbital (bony) distance is increased, and the angulation between the lateral walls is normal. This situation is seen in cases of craniosynostosis, encephaloceles, pneumatoceles and craniotubular dysplasia, and is based on differentiation defects of bone centres, e.g. absence of nasal bones and schistasis (failure to form sutures) between two different bones, i.e. cranium bifidum occultum. In pseudohypertelorism (Converse et al 1970) the intercanthal distance is increased and both bony orbital distances are normal. Interorbital as well as orbital hypertelorism can be grouped as bony defects under frontonasoethmoidal dysplasias (Ch. 9). Pseudohypertelorism is only an abnormality of the soft tissues.

Orbital hypertelorism and some minor defects are the result of insufficient outgrowth and merging of the internasal groove, for example the subtle bifidity of the nasal tip (Ch. 9). In the literature these defects, located in the midline of the face, are classified under various terms, such as medial cleft face syndrome (De Myer 1967), frontonasal dysraphia (Mazzola 1976), frontonasal dysplasia (Sedano et al 1970) and cleft no. 0 and 14 according to Tessier

(1976) and Kawamoto (1976). In addition, different malformations are grouped under the same syndrome. The most extreme example concerns the holoprosencephaly series reckoned among Tessier's cleft no. 0 and 14 (Tessier 1976, and Kawamoto 1976). Furthermore De Myer (1967) places the median cleft palate in the median cleft face syndrome.

From an embryological point of view the holoprosencephaly series belongs to the early or primary defects of the cerebro-craniofacial group, and the median cleft palates to the subclass of primary clefts of the craniofacial group. All these examples exclude the median cleft face syndrome. The major anomalies of De Myer (1967) — orbital hypertelorism, cranium bifidum occultum, median cleft nose (bifid nose and Doggennase), median cleft prolabium and median cleft premaxilla — are all late or secondary defects. Cranium bifidum occultum, whether or not combined with encephaloceles, and median cleft premaxilla are explained by insufficient outgrowth of the paired frontal bone centres and of the bone centres of both premaxillae, respectively. The median cleft nose and median cleft prolabium can be explained by the persistence of the internasal groove (cf. the real lip and nose of rodents and among them the hare). Therefore they can be classified under internasal dysplasia. The cartilage of the nasal septum — in extreme cases a duplication forming a Y — and the soft tissues are deficient.

Another defect in differentiation of cartilage and soft tissues concerns a cleft or notch of the nostril, i.e. no. 1 cleft of Tessier (1976) or a paramedian anomaly according to Mazzola (1976), and nasoschisis (Ch. 9). In this case the early development of the nose has been normally completed, with both external nostrils present (≤17 mm C–RL). During the later development of the nose (≥17 mm) the outgrowth and differentiation of the mesenchyme into cartilages of the ala are defective. The suggested failure of fusion between the medial and lateral nasal processes that would cause nasoschisis (e.g. Mazzola 1976) has not been observed. The bony and cartilaginous defects in secondary dysplasias include imperfect development of facial muscles, connective tissues and tissue of ectodermal origin. Defects characterized by interrupted skin (ectoderm) can be classified as secondary clefts (fetus Eb148). In these cases the influence of amniotic bands was proposed, but in all the examples under study interference of development by amniotic bands or external damage was not found (Vermeij-Keers et al 1983b).

Many secondary dysplasias are accompanied by defects of the eyelids, for example colobomata, cryptophthalmia (complete fusion of the eyelids) and microblepharon. Normally the eyelids grow out after the 17-mm stage and adhere in embryos of 34 mm C–RL. In the case of cryptophthalmia the eyelids have fused instead of adhering and have failed to open again during late fetal life. The development of colobomata and complete absence of the lid (ablepharon) must have taken place during the outgrowth of the swellings of the eyelids. Defects of the m. orbicularis oculi are present. It is obvious that the development of the eye and the orbit influence the development of the eyelids. This is, for example, the case in microblepharon.

Secondary dysplasias in the corner of the temporal and zygomatic bones and the mandible are frequently coupled with defects of the external and middle ear and, rarely, of the internal ear (see Ch. 9, zygo-auromandibular, temporo-aural and temporo-auromandibular dysplasias). Both the external and middle ear are derivatives of the first and second branchial arches and their transformations take place exactly in the same developmental period, and derailments occur at both places. The fistulas, sinuses, cysts and tags are all remnants of the branchial system transformations, and are primary or early defects. Microtia and anotia referred to under atretic ears in Ch. 9 could be explained as early defects in cases of anotia and microtia with a blind or absent external auditory meatus. In that case the tympanic membrane is not formed. In examples with a meatus and rudiments or a reduction of the auricle or pinna the developmental arrest is later ($\geqslant$17 mm C–RL). The same holds for prominent, adherent and constricted ears (see Ch. 9). Combinations of early and late defects belonging to the cerebrocranial, the cerebrocraniofacial and craniofacial groups are possible.

All the deformations mentioned can be associated with anomalies in other regions of the body. It depends on the developmental stage of the different parts of the embryo and the asymmetry in development which regions are affected.

ACKNOWLEDGEMENTS

The author wishes to express her gratitude to Mr H. G. Wetselaar for the preparation of drawings, Mr C. J. van der Sijp and Mr J. H. Lens for photography, and Dr R. E. Poelmann who provided the scanning micrographs. The manuscript was corrected by Drs H. E. Whitehead-van Prooije, and typed by Mrs E. A. H. Bruyn and Mrs E. Hopman-Witte.

REFERENCES

Adelmann H B 1925 The development of the neural folds and cranial ganglia in the rat. Journal of Comparative Neurology 39: 19–171

Adelmann H B 1936 The problem of cyclopia. Quarterly Review of Biology II: 161–304

Arey J B 1965 Developmental anatomy, 7th edn. Saunders, Philadelphia

Ask F, and van der Hoeven J 1921 Beiträge zur Kenntnis der Entwicklung der Tränenröhrchen unter normalen und abnormen Verhältnissen, letzteres an Fällen von offener schräger Gesichtsspalte. Albrecht von Graefes Archiv fur Klinische und Experimentelle Ophthalmologie 105: 1157–1196

Bartelmez G W, Blount M P 1954 The formation of neural crest from the primary optic vesicle in man. Contributions to Embryology of the Carnegie Institution 35: 55–91

Batten E H 1958 The origin of the acoustic ganglion in the sheep. Journal of Embryology and Experimental Morphology 6: 597–615

Bertelsen T I 1958 The premature synostosis of the cranial sutures. Acta Ophthalmologica Suppl. 51: 24–34

Cohen M M Jr, Jirasek J E, Guzman R T, Gorlin R J, Peterson M Q, 1971 Holoprosencephaly and facial dysmorphia: nosology, etiology and pathogenesis. Birth Defects, Original Article Series 7: 125–135

Converse J M, Ransohoff J, Mathews E S, Smith B, Molenaar A 1970 Ocular hypertelorism and pseudohypertelorism. Journal of Plastic and Reconstructive Surgery 45: 1–13

De Beer G R 1937 The development of the vertebrate skull. Clarendon Press, Oxford. pp 354–373

De Myer W 1967 The median cleft face syndrome. Differential diagnosis of cranium bifidum occultum, hypertelorism, and median cleft nose, lip and palate. Neurology 17: 961–971

De Myer W 1977 Holoprosencephaly (cyclopia–arhinencephaly). In Vinken P J, Bruyn G W (eds) Handbook of clinical neurology, vol. 30, part I. Congenital malformations of the brain and skull. North Holland, Amsterdam. pp 431–478

De Myer W, Zeman W, Palmer C G 1964 The face predicts the brain: diagnostic significance of median facial anomalies for holoprosencephaly (arhinencephaly). Pediatrics 34: 256–263

Diewert V M 1983 A morphometric analysis of craniofacial growth showing changes in spatial relations during secondary palatal development in human embryos and fetuses. American Journal of Anatomy 167: 495–522

Diewert V M 1985 Development of human craniofacial morphology during the late embryonic and early fetal periods. American Journal of Orthodontics 88: 64–76

Erickson C A, Weston J A 1983 A SEM analysis of neural crest migration in the mouse. Journal of Embryology and Experimental Morphology 74: 97–118

Ferguson M W J 1981 Developmental mechanism in normal and abnormal palate formation with particular reference to the aetiology, pathogenesis and prevention of cleft palate. British Journal of Orthodontics 8: 115–137

Futamura R 1906 Ueber die Entwicklung der Facialmuskulatur des Menschen. Anatomische Hefte 30: 433–516

Gaare J D, Langman J 1980 Fusion of nasal swellings in the mouse embryo. DNA synthesis and histological features. Anatomy and Embryology 159: 85–99

Gardner W J 1964 Diastomyelia and the Klipper–Feil syndrome. Cleveland Clinic Quarterly 31: 19–44

Gardner W J 1966 Embryologic origin of spinal malformations. Acta Radiologica Diagnosis 5: 1013–1023

Gardner W J 1980 Hypothesis: overdistension of the neural tube may cause anomalies of non-neural organs. Teratology 22: 229–238

Gasser R F 1967 The development of the facial muscles in man. American Journal of Anatomy 120: 357–376

Gasser R F 1979 Evidence that sclerotomal cells do not migrate medially during normal embryonic development of the rat. American Journal of Anatomy 154: 509–524

Geelen J A G 1980 The teratogenic effects of hypervitaminosis A on the formation of the neural tube. Thesis, Nijmegen.

Geelen J A G, Langman J 1977 Closure of the neural tube in the cephalic region of the mouse embryo. Anatomical Record 189: 625–640

Geelen J A G, Langman J 1979 Ultrastructural observations on closure of the neural tube in the mouse. Anatomy and Embryology 156: 73–88

Glücksmann A 1951 Cell deaths in normal vertebrate ontogeny. Biological Reviews 26: 59–86

Hinrichsen K 1985 The early development of morphology and patterns of the face in the human embryo. Advances in Anatomy, Embryology and Cell Biology 98: 1–79

His W 1892 Die Entwicklung der menschlichen und thierischer Physiognomien. Archiv für Anatomie und Physiologie Anatomischer Abteilung: 384–424

Hochstetter F 1891 Ueber die Bildung der inneren Nasengänge oder primitiven Choanen. Verh Anat Ges (Anatomischer Anzeiger Suppl) 6: 145–151

Hochstetter F 1919 Beiträge zur Entwicklungsgeschichte des menschlichen Gehirns. I. Deuticke, Vienna

Hochstetter F 1950 Ueber die Beteiligung der Gesichtsfortsätze an der Bildung des primitiven Gaumens. Anatomischer Anzeiger 97: 217–224

Hörstadius S 1950 The neural crest. Oxford University Press, Oxford

Johnston M C 1966 A radioautographic study of migration and fate of the cranial neural crest cells in chick embryo. Anatomical Record 156: 143–155

Johnston M C 1975 The neural crest in abnormalities of the face and brain. In: Bergsma D (ed) Morphogenesis and malformations of face and brain. Liss, New York pp 1–18

Jones K L 1975 Aberrant tissue bands in the face and brain defects. In: Bergsma D (ed) Morphogenesis and malformations of face and brain. Liss, New York. pp 205–206

Karnovsky M J 1965 A formaldehyde-glutaraldehyde fixative of high osmolarity for use in electron microscopy. Journal of Cell Biology 27: 137A

Kawamoto H K 1976 The kaleidoscopic world of rare craniofacial clefts: order out of chaos (Tessier classification). Clinics in Plastic Surgery 3: 529–572

Kirchmayr L 1906 Ein Beitrag zu den Gesichtsmissbildungen. Zeitschrift fur Chirurgie 81: 71–81

Kosaka K, Hama K, Eto K 1985 Light and electron microscopic study of fusion of facial prominences. A distinctive type of superficial cells at the contact sites. Anatomy and Embryology 173: 187–201

Le Douarin N M 1975 The neural crest in the neck and other parts of the body. In: Bergsma D (ed) Morphogenesis and malformations of face and brain. Liss, New York. pp 19–50

Le Douarin, N M 1982 The neural crest. Cambridge University Press, Cambridge

Lemire R J 1986 Embryology of the skull. In: Cohen M M Jr (ed) Craniosynostosis: diagnosis, evaluation and management. Raven Press, New York. pp 105–129

McLaren L R 1955 A case of cleft lip and palate with polypoid nasal tubercle. British Journal of Plastic Surgery 8: 57–59

Mann I C 1958 Developmental abnormalities of the eye, 2nd edn. British Medical Association, London

Manschot W A 1963 Primary congenital aphakia. Archives of Ophthalmology 69: 571

Manschot W A 1966 L'aphakie congénitale primaire et la trisomie 13–15. In: Travaux d'ophthalmologie moderne. Masson et Cie, Paris. p 243

Manschot W A 1969 Die kongenitale primäre Aphakie in genetischer Sicht. Klinische Monatsblatter fur Augenheilkunde 154: 1

Mazzola R F 1976 Congenital malformations in the frontonasal area: their pathogenesis and classification. Clinics in Plastic Surgery 3: 573–609

Mieden G D 1982 An anatomical study of three cases of alobar holoprosencephaly. Teratology 26: 123–133

Minkoff R 1980 Regional variation of cell proliferation within the processes of the chick embryo: a study of the role of 'merging' during development. Journal of Embryology and Experimental Morphology 57: 37–49

Moore K L 1982 The developing human. Clinically oriented embryology, 3rd edn. Saunders, Philadelphia.

Morian R 1887 Ueber die schräge Gesichtsspalte. Archiv fur Klinische Chirurgie Chir 35: 245–288

Morriss G M, Thorogood P V 1978 An approach to cranial neural crest cell migration and differentiation in mammalian embryos. In: Johnston M H (ed) Development of mammals, vol. 3. North Holland, Amsterdam. pp 363–412

Müller F, O'Rahilly R 1983 The first appearance of the major divisions of the human brain at stage 9. Anatomy and Embryology 168: 419–432

Müller F, O'Rahilly R 1985 The first appearance of the neural tube and optic primordium in the human embryo at stage 10. Anatomy and Embryology 172: 157–169

Noden D M 1975 An analysis of the migratory behavior of avian cephalic neural crest cells. Developmental Biology 42: 106–130

O'Rahilly R 1966 The early development of the eye in staged human embryos. Contributions to Embryology 38: 1–42

O'Rahilly R 1967 The early development of the nasal pit in staged human embryos. Anatomical Record 157: 380

O'Rahilly R 1973 Developmental stages in human embryos. Part A: embryos of the first three weeks (stages 1 to 9). Carnegie Institution of Washington Publication 631.

O'Rahilly R 1983 The timing and sequence of events in the development of the human eye and ear during the embryonic period proper. Anatomy and Embryology 168: 87–99

O'Rahilly R, Gardner E 1971 The timing and sequence of events in the development of the human nervous system during the embryonic period proper. Z Anat Entwickl Gesch 134: 1–12

O'Rahilly R, Gardner E 1972 The initial appearance of ossification in staged human embryos. American Journal of Anatomy 134: 291–308

O'Rahilly R, Gardner E 1979 The initial development of the human brain. Acta Anatomica 104: 123–133

O'Rahilly R, Müller F 1981 The first appearance of the human nervous system at stage 8. Anatomy and Embryology 163: 1–13

Padget D H 1970 Neuroschisis and human embryonic maldevelopment. New evidence on anencephaly, spina bifida and diverse mammalian defects. Journal of Neuropathology and Experimental Neurology 29: 192–216

Padget D H 1972 Development of so-called dysraphism, with embryologic evidence of clinical Arnold–Chiari and Dandy–Walker malformations. Johns Hopkins Medical Journal 130: 127–165

Patten B M 1953 Human embryology, 2nd edn. Churchill, London

Patten B M 1961 The normal development of the facial region. In: Pruzansky S (ed) Congenital anomalies of the face and associated structures. Thomas, Springfield, Ill.

Peter K 1950 Nochmals über die Beteiligung der Geischtsfortsätze an der Bildung des primitiven Gaumens. Anatomischer Anzeiger 97: 225

Pfeifer G 1967 Die Entwicklungsstörungen des Gesichtsschädels als Klassifikationsproblem. Zahn-, Mund-, und Kieferheilkunde 48: 22–40

Pfeifer G 1974 Systematik und Morphologie der kraniofazialen Anomalien. Forkschritte der Kiefer- und Gesichts-Chirurgie 18: 1–14

Ploner L 1957 Die schräge Gesichtsspalte. Fortschritte der Kiefer- und Gesichts-Chirurgie 3: 334–340

Poelmann R E 1980 Differential mitosis and degeneration patterns in relation to alterations in shape of the embryonic ectoderm of early postimplantation mouse embryos. Journal of Embryology and Experimental Morphology 55: 33–51

Poelmann R E, Verbout A J 1985 3-D reconstructions in anatomy using a semi-automatic device. Verhandlungen Anatomischen Gesellschaft 79: 155–156

Poelmann R E, Vermeij-Keers Chr 1976 Cell degeneration in the mouse embryo: a prerequisite for normal development. In: Müller-Bérat N et al (eds) Progress in differentiation research. North-Holland, Amsterdam

Poelmann R E, Dubois S V, Hermsen C, Smits-van Prooije A E, Vermeij-Keers Chr 1985 Cell degeneration and mitosis in the buccopharyngeal and branchial membranes in the mouse embryo. Anatomy and Embryology 171: 187–192

Politzer G 1937 Neue Untersuchungen über die Entstehung der Gesichtsspalten. Monatsschrift fur Ohrenheilkunde und Laryngo-Rhinologie 71: 63–73

Pratt R M, Dencker L, Diewert V M 1984 2,3,7,8-Tetrachlorodibenzo-p-dioxin-induced cleft palate in the mouse: evidence for alterations in palatal shelf fusion. Teratogenesis, Carcinogenesis, and Mutagenesis 4: 427–436

Raven C P 1937 Experiments on the origin of the sheath cells and sympathetic neuroblasts in Amphibia. Journal of Comparative Neurology 67: 221–241

Schade G J 1973 De embryonale schedel-ontwikkeling bij opwekking van een gespleten verhemelte. Thesis, Amsterdam.

Schook P 1980 A spatial analysis of the localization of cell division and cell death in relationship with morphogenesis of the chick optic cup. Acta Morphologica Neerlando-Scandinavica 18: 213–229

Sedano H O, Cohen M M Jr, Jirasek J, Gorlin R J 1970 Frontonasal dysplasia. Journal of Pediatrics 76: 906–913

Silver J, Hughes A F W 1973 The role of cell death during morphogenesis of the mammalian eye. Journal of Morphology 140: 159–170

Silver J, Hughes A F W 1974 The relationship between morphogenetic cell death and the development of congenital anophthalmia. Journal of Comparative Neurology 157: 281–302

Smith S, Boulgakow B 1927 A case of cyclopia. Journal of Anatomy 61: 105–111

Smits-van Prooije A E 1986 Processes involved in normal and abnormal fusion of the neural walls in murine embryos. Thesis, Leiden.

Smits-van Prooije A E, Vermeij-Keers Chr, Poelmann R E, Mentink M M T, Dubbeldam J A 1985 The neural crest in presomite to 40-somite murine embryos. Acta Morphologica Neerlando-Scandinavica 23: 99–114

Smits-van Prooije A E, Poelmann R E, Mentink M M T, Dubbeldam J A, Vermeij-Keers Chr 1986 WGA-Au as a novel marker for mesoderm formation in mouse embryos, cultured in vitro. Stain Technology 61: 97–106

Smits-van Prooije A E, Vermeij-Keers Chr, Dubbeldam J A, Mentink M M T, Poelmann R E 1987 The formation of mesoderm and mesectoderm in presomite rat embryos cultured in vitro, using WGA-Au as a marker. Anatomy and Embryology 176: 71–77

Starck D 1955 Embryologie. Georg Thieme Verlag, Stuttgart.

Sulik K K, Lauder J M, Dehart D B 1984 Brain malformations in prenatal mice following acute maternal ethanol administration. International Journal of Developmental Neuroscience 2: 203–214

Tessier, P 1976 Anatomical classification of facial, craniofacial and laterofacial clefts. Journal of Maxillofacial Surgery 4: 69–92

Theiler K 1972 The house mouse. Development and normal stages from fertilization to 4 weeks of age. Springer Verlag, Berlin

Töndury G 1950 Zur Entwicklung des menschlichen Gesichtes und zur Hasenschartengenese. Schweizerische Medizinische Wochenschrift 80: 10–12

Töndury G 1964 Embryology of clefts. In: Hotz R (ed) Early treatment of cleft lip and palate. Huber, Stuttgart. pp 17–24

Trasler D G, Leong S 1982 Mitotic index in mouse embryos with 6-aminonicotin- amide-induced and inherited cleft lip. Teratology 25: 259–265

Van der Meulen J C, Vaandrager J M 1983 Surgery related to the correction of hypertelorism. Journal of Plastic and Reconstructional Surgery 71: 6–17

Van der Meulen J C, Mazzola R F, Vermeij-Keers Chr, Stricker M, Raphael B 1983 A morphogenetical classification of craniofacial malformations. Journal of Plastic and Reconstructional Surgery 71: 560–572

Vermeij-Keers Chr 1967 De facialis musculatuur en transformaties in het kopgebied. Thesis, Leiden

Vermeij-Keers Chr 1972a Transformations in the facial region of the human embryo. Advances in Anatomy, Embryology and Cell Biology 46: 1–30

Vermeij-Keers Chr 1972b Degeneration in the epithelial plate of Hochstetter in the mouse: a light and electron microscopic study. Acta Morphologica Neerlando-Scandinavica 9: 386–387

Vermeij-Keers Chr 1975a The development of the nose, with the naso-lacrimal duct of the human embryo. Acta Morphologica Neerlando-Scandinavica 13: 126–127

Vermeij-Keers Chr 1975b Primary congenital aphakia and the rubella syndrome. Teratology 11: 257–265

Vermeij-Keers, Chr, Koppenberg J 1985 The oro-ocular clefts and the amniotic band theory. Teratology 32: 36A

Vermeij-Keers Chr, and Poelmann R E 1980 The neural crest: a study on cell degeneration and the improbability of cell migration in mouse embryo. Netherlands Journal of Zoology 30: 74–81

Vermeij-Keers Chr, Mazzola, R F, Van der Meulen. J C, Stricker M, Raphael B 1983a Cerebro-craniofacial and craniofacial malformations: an embryological analysis. Cleft Palate Journal 20: 128–145

Vermeij-Keers Chr, Koppenberg J, Maat G J R 1983b The oro-ocular clefts, an embryological subdivision. Orbit 2: 111–120

Vermeij-Keers Chr, Poelmann, R E, Smits-van Prooije A E, Van der Meulen J C 1984 Hypertelorism and the median cleft face syndrome. An embryological analysis. Ophthalmic Paediatrics and Genetics 4: 97–105

Vermeij-Keers Chr, Poelmann R E, Smits-van Prooije A E 1987 6.5 mm human embryo with a single nasal placode: cyclopia or hypotelorism? Teratology 36:1–6

Verwoerd C D A, Van Oostrom C G 1979 Cephalic neural crest and placodes. Advances in Anatomy, Embryology and Cell Biology 58: 1–75

Warkany J 1975 Congenital malformations. Year Book Medical Publishers, Chicago

Wen I C 1928 The anatomy of human embryos with seventeen to twenty-three pairs of somites. Journal of Comparative Neurology 45: 301–376

Weston J A 1963 A radioautographic analysis of the migration and localization of trunk neural crest cells in the chick. Developmental Biology 6: 279–310

Weston J A 1981 The regulation of normal and abnormal neural crest cell development. Advances in Neurology 29: 77–95

4. Craniofacial development and growth

M. Stricker, B. Raphael, J. Van der Meulen, R. Mazzola

INTRODUCTION

'The great mystery of life has until now been the problem of growth' (Gley, quoted in Dieulafe, p. 127). According to Dieulafe (1933), growth is the result of an individual process connected with the earliest periods of life: with the period of enlargement in the quaternary system of Beaugrand (in the Dechambre dictionary); with the first three seasons in the weekly system of Littré brought to light from the *Treatise of Weeks* and based upon the cabbalistic metaphysics of the number 7.

The term 'growth' is ambiguous. The layman understands it to be the process which continues until adulthood is reached. In an effort to make the understanding of normal growth simpler a scheme has been devised which divides the growth process into three stages:

organization
ossification
adaptation

Because of the overlap in interest between the embryologist and the clinician, this chapter will arbitrarily begin with ossification.

It is, however, necessary to emphasize that there is a discordance in time and in space between organogenesis and morphogenesis (Fig. 4.1), which accounts for the fact that the topographical boundaries of a bone are not strictly the same as those of the facial processes.

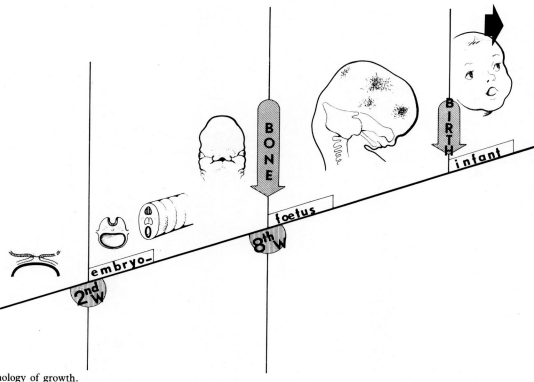

Fig. 4.1 Chronology of growth.

The mesenchymal tissues develop into processes at the core of which ossification centres appear and expand. These osseous parts will be subject to forces generated by different functions, of which muscle is the most representative element.

Craniofacial growth is a dynamic process balancing form and function. This precarious equilibrium is easily disturbed at various levels by passive or active alteration of one of the mechanisms involved. Growth is studied at its osseous component because bone can be measured.

OSSIFICATION

The formation of the bony structures by mesenchymal differentiation is the result of the selection of collagen fibres capable of becoming calcified. According to Grasse (1967) that selection occurs in vertebrates. Ossification starts before and continues after birth in accordance with two modalities:

1. direct, membranous;
2. indirect, endochondral, through cartilage.

It conforms to a topographical and chronological scheme and the sites of appearance, named ossification centres, are clearly related to nerve territories, while growth of the bony part is regulated by dynamic factors in which the muscles have a major role.

'The brain plays an important role in the morphology of the bones of the skull.' Le Double (1903) in his *Traité des Variations des Os de la Face* was already conscious of the pre-eminent importance of the brain and its sensory expansions — the placodes and the cranial nerves — in determining the formation of bony structures. One may therefore postulate that in each bone there is a primary neural part and a secondary muscular part. The initial neural structure is in the form of a square and it is striking to note that the organization of the facial skeleton involves a succession of such right-angled formations.

The distribution of the ossification sites appears to be determined by the sites of neural emergence and ossification occurs in the presence of a nerve — sensory or of special sense (Figs. 4.2, 4.3). The term neuromatricial axis was therefore coined by Laude et al (1978), in relation to the mandible. These neuromatricial axes defined by the emergence of a nerve at the origin of the initial neural square exist for each bony unit, as we shall see. Formation of the bony skeleton either by direct ossification in the mesenchyme or following the intermediate deposition of cartilage proceeds in directions which are determined by the brain or its sensorial or sensitive extensions. The facial expansions of the cartilaginous skull bear witness to this.

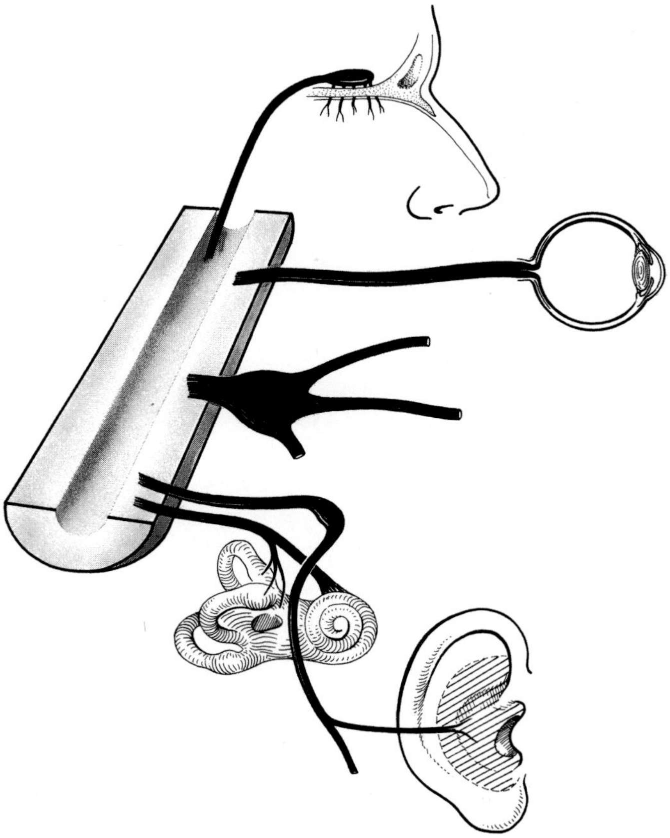

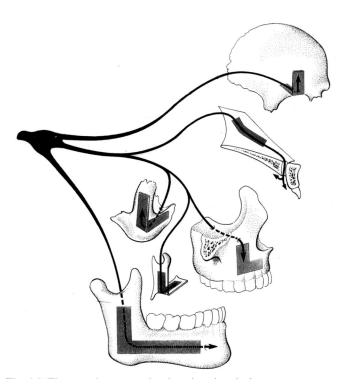

Fig. 4.2 The sensory encephalic antennae.

Fig. 4.3 The neural squares related to the trigeminal nerve.

The mandibular model (Fig. 4.4)

Arbitrarily the mandible is discussed first because the term 'neuromatricial axis' was applied to this model. The chondrocranial expansion (Meckel's cartilage) is a primary cartilage with autonomous proliferation, surrounded by mesenchymal tissue which has a neuraxial orientation (Laude et al 1978, Delachapelle 1981).

Ossification starts at the site of nerve bifurcation, the mental foramen. The mesenchyme is anterior and external

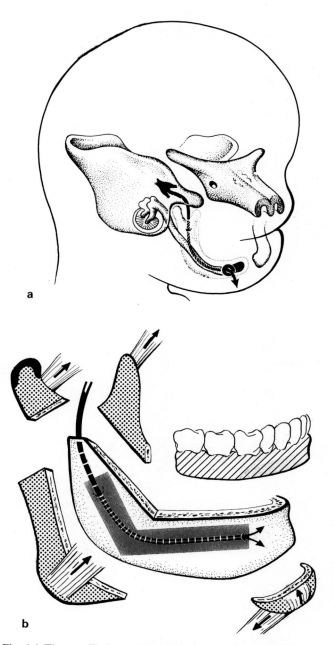

b

Fig. 4.4 The mandibular model: (a) Meckel's cartilage and the mandibular 'externation'; (b) the muscular and dentoalveolar complements.

to the cartilage, so that the anterior part only of Meckel's cartilage is intraosseous. Because of this and analogous to the formation of the cranium one may speak of mandibular externation (Sakka 1980). The bony mandible, in fact, covers the cartilaginous model. Apophyseal areas under muscular control are then deposited on this mandibular mesenchyme by secondary chondrification. These include the coronoid process, gonion, chin apophysis, etc.

APOPHYSIS OF THE MANDIBULAR CONDYLE

This part is the only one to persist in the form of cartilage, because of its articulation with the squamous bone (Fig. 4.5). It is formed by prechondroblasts which are subject to mechanical influences, generated by the activity of the masticatory muscles, in particular the external pterygoid. The fact that the embryo already opens its mouth in the 8th week is proof of this.

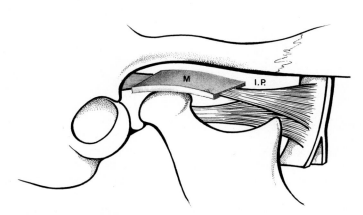

Fig. 4.5 The pterygo-meniscocondylar complex (Dubecq–Petrovic). M = meniscus; i.p. = internal pterygoid muscle.

Maxilla (Fig. 4.6)

The initial neural structure organizes itself around the ossification centre situated at the point where the infraorbital nerve emerges. This is the only centre recognized as such by Scott, who observed an L-shaped development, with frontal and palatine processes connected by an external frontal wall. In contrast Dixon (1953) described two centres, each responsible for one branch of the square: an infraorbital ossification centre and another, anterior premaxillary or incisive centre, situated at the bifurcation of the anterior and superior dental nerve.

The structure is completed by a muscular apophysis at the insertion of the masseter. The definitive shape is determined by the combination of pneumatization, posterior muscle pressure and dental growth. The role of a fat pad in the transmission of pressure must be stressed in this respect (Latham 1976).

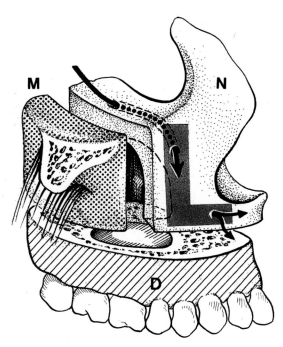

Fig. 4.6 Ossification of the maxilla. N = neural medially; M = muscular laterally; D = dentoalveolar inferiorly.

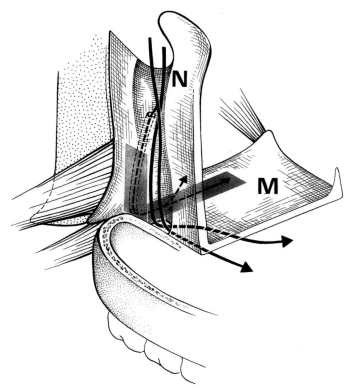

Fig. 4.7 Ossification of the palatine. N = predominantly vertical; M = predominantly horizontal.

Premaxilla

The premaxilla or intermaxillary bone has long been a matter for controversy. It forms the anterior corner of the maxillary arch, sealing its top and consisting of an independent bone.

Its ossification, related to that of the vomer, with which it constitutes a functional strut, is determined in part by the emergence of the internal sphenopalatine nerves in the palatine canal and completed by the internal frontal bone under the control of the rhinencephalon. The clinical manifestation of a defect, a hyporhinencephaly, provides an excellent example. The discussion about the premaxilla concerns the relationship of the maxillopremaxillary suture (incisor–canine) to the site of the alveolar defect in clefts. The concordance is illusory and the premaxilla is an example of the topographical discordance between the territories of the facial processes and the distribution of the bony elements.

Palatine bone (Fig. 4.7)

The right-angled structure starts with the ossification centre situated at the point of emergence of the palatine nerves, where the two laminae unite. The horizontal part develops as a result of the muscle activity in the velopharyngeal sling, as demonstrated by the absence of the horizontal plate in rare cases of agenesis of a hemipalate.

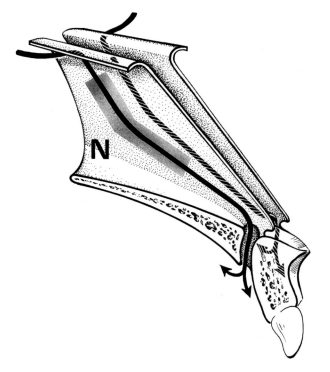

Fig. 4.8 Ossification of the vomer. N = only neural.

Vomer (Fig. 4.8)

This structure originally has a double origin arising from two ossification centres in contact with the nasal capsule. A groove is formed, concave surface upward, in the vicinity of the internal sphenopalatine nerves.

Basi-presphenoid (Fig. 4.9)

Related to the facial mass, this structure controls its situation through the pterygoidal apophyses. The origin of the latter is uncertain, being purely mesenchymal in the view of Kier and Dollander (1973) but of dual origin for most authors: a mesenchymal external wing and a cartilaginous internal wing. The double neural square is determined by contact with the nerve of the pterygoid canal, later joined to the muscular outer wing and through this to the alisphenoid, in this case the greater wing. The alisphenoid combines the lesser and greater wings — the former cartilaginous, the latter mesenchymal — under the influence of the temporalis muscle. The lesser wings arise from the optic expansions of the chondrocranium.

Ethmoidal bone (Fig. 4.10)

Arising entirely from the nasal capsule, and initially divided by two grooves, this structure develops into a central mesethmoid (Grasse 1967) and two lateral masses or ectethmoids. The most anterior part of the mesethmoid becomes permanently cartilaginous, forming the axis of the olfactory neuromatrix, which also has a coordinating role related to respiration.

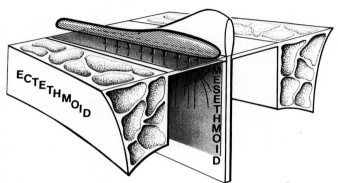

Fig. 4.10 The square of the mesethmoid.

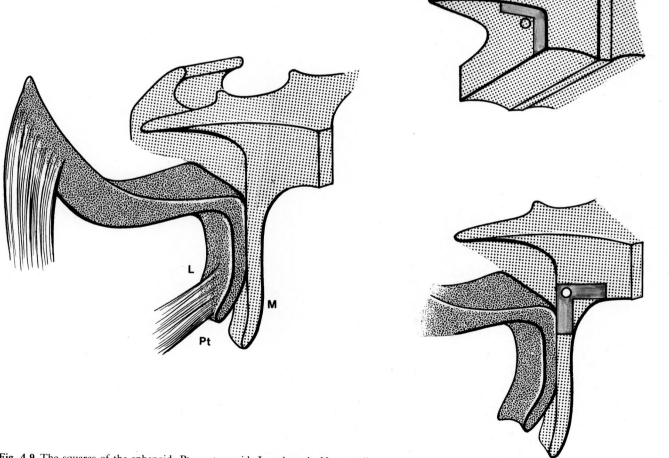

Fig. 4.9 The squares of the sphenoid. Pt = pterygoid; L = lateral; M = median.

Malar bone (Fig. 4.11)

Classically, this is formed by the confluence of three ossification centres: superior or postzygomatic (Albrecht, anterior or prezygomatic, and posteroinferior or hypozygomatic, with the zygomatic canal within (Toldt 1912, Le Double 1903, Rambaud & Renault).

The ossification centre is at the site of emergence of the temporozygomatic branch of the orbital nerve, itself a branch of the maxillary nerve. The bone is completed through muscles of mastication and its double origin is confirmed by the findings at operation in patients with mandibulofacial dysostosis.

Frontal bone (Fig. 4.12)

The fronto-orbital structure develops around the frontal nerve, a branch of the ophthalmic nerve. It has an internal orbital portion and an external frontal part (Cuvier 1805) due to division of the nerve into internal orbital and supraorbital branches. The internal branch protects the eye and in lower species it fulfils that purpose. In man its protective function has become adapted with the development of the brain: with its corresponding contralateral companion it forms a specific structure, the forehead, adorned with a median apophysis, the anterior superior nasal spine, which is of cartilaginous origin. Two

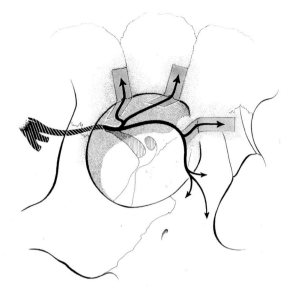

Fig. 4.12 Ossification of the frontal bone; the three squares.

secondary ossification centres, located high up, help to shape the forehead.

Temporal bone (Fig. 4.13)

The larger sensorial part, which is primitive and cartilaginous, is organized around the otic placode as the periotic

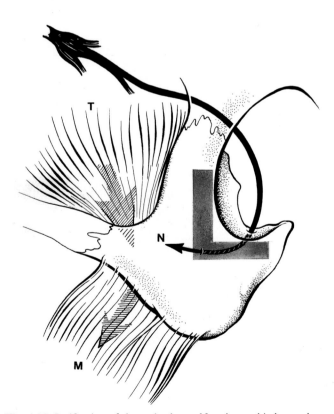

Fig. 4.11 Ossification of the malar bone. N = juxtaorbital neural square; M = masseter muscle.

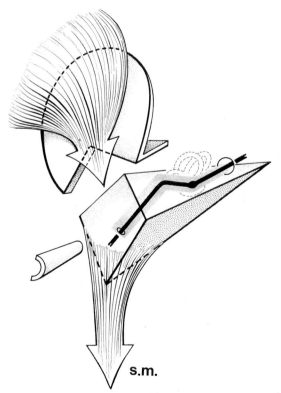

Fig. 4.13 Ossification of the temporal bone. s.m. = sternomastoid muscle.

capsule. It forms the petrosal pyramid, with an expansion towards the cervical region (Reichert's cartilage), in indirect relationship to the hyoid bone.

The squamous portion is fibrous and its growth depends on the balance between the brain and the temporalis muscle. The ossification centre of the zygomatic bone and the apophysis of the condyle of the mandible appear at the same time (dynamic relationship).

Occipital bone (Fig. 4.14)

Anteriorly, the basioccipital is cartilaginous, a satellite of the basi-postsphenoid with which it forms the clivus of Blumenbach, although separated by the spheno-occipital synchondrosis. It is a mixed structure independent of the neuraxis, combining the parachordal cartilages with the sclerotomes of the occipital somites. Posteriorly, the membranous portion, tilted backwards, is part of the cervical muscular system.

THE MECHANISMS OF GROWTH

Two contradictory entities stand out in the midst of apparent great complexity — the cartilage and the periosteum — each corresponding to a particular type of ossification with specific dynamics.

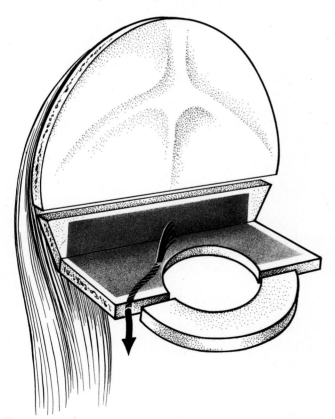

Fig. 4.14 Ossification of the occipital bone.

The cartilaginous system constitutes a primary area of growth — *active*, because it is stimulated by intrinsic dynamic forces, at least where primary cartilage is concerned.

The periosteal system, in contrast, is an area of *passive* secondary growth, influenced by forces upon it. This system is composed of three structures: the sutures, simple intermediary periosteum (to use Lebourg's (1948) phrase) and named expanding joints with automatic adaptation (Delaire 1974); the periosteum, influenced by muscular insertions which are responsible for apposition and resorption, according to the theory held by Enlow 1968; and the alveolodental ligament, a specific site for transitional periosteum, the tooth-bone organ (Ten Cate).

The cartilaginous system

This forms the basilar groove, site of active primary growth, and is analogous to the epiphyses of the long bones. The condylar cartilage is an exception, being a site of secondary passive growth dependent on the forces acting upon it, in particular the external pterygoidal muscle.

THE CHONDROCRANIUM (Fig. 4.15)

The paraxial mesoblastic layer on the inferior aspect of the neural tube becomes condensed at the 11-mm stage to form a gutter, concave above and posteriorly. It produces a continuous cuff around the sensory buds — the sensory capsules — with projections on both sides towards the branchial arches. Three elements may be distinguished.

The basal pedestal

This structure supports the brain and consists of two portions:

a posterior portion — parachordal — which, with the assistance of the sclerotome of the occipital somites, forms the basioccipital bone, the future clivus and the posterior branch of the basal field;

an anterior portion — prechordal. This is the presellar branch of the basal field, consisting of hypophyseal and prehypophyseal trabeculae. It is a precursor of the basisphenoid.

The sensorial projections

Posteriorly, these consist of the optic capsules, which are situated in front of the occipital bone. Anteriorly, they are formed by the chondroethmoid.

The chondroethmoid (Fig. 4.16) is the key anterior structure in the craniofacial borders.

Laterally it generates two optic processes: one temporal, one orbital. The temporal process corresponds to the root of the greater wing, and the orbital to the lesser or

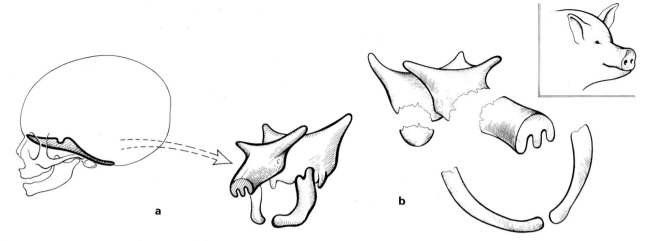

Fig. 4.15 (a) The chondrocranium; (b) the different components; nasal capsule, optic capsule and facial expressions.

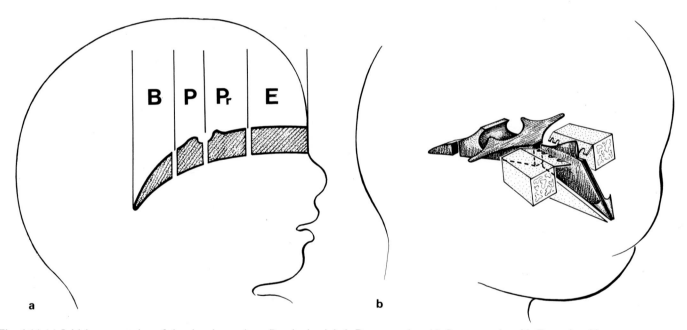

Fig. 4.16 (a) Initial segmentation of the chondrocranium. B = basioccipital; P = postsphenoid; Pr = presphenoid; E = ethmoid; (b) the chondroethmoid.

orbitosphenoidal wing of some writers. According to Dollander (1973) the orbitosphenoid is distinct from the chondroethmoid and later becomes attached to the chondrosphenoid.

Anteriorly, it possesses a snout-like projection, the nasal capsule, which consists of a sagittal plate or mesethmoid, extending from the sphenoid to the caudal edge of the septum, and two lateral masses or ectethmoids connected by the lamina cribrosa. The anterior part of the lateral borders of the nasal capsule will form the cartilaginous roof of the nasal pyramid.

Scott (1955) has stressed the duality within the chondroethmoid of the cranial, mesethmoid, the facial ecteth-

moid, and the connection of the cribriform plates. This notion is reflected in human clinical practice by some interorbital malformations.

Visceral expansions

The otic or auditory capsules have two ventral extensions, which are unequal in length.

The first is Meckel's cartilage, described in 1859 by Serres. This is the cartilaginous basis for the first arch and has a dual destination: a dorsal tympanic and a transitional ventral mandibular.

The second extension is Reichert's cartilage, which is a kind of miniature replica of Meckel's cartilage, situated behind and below this structure and stretching from the temporal region to the hyoid bone. It forms the styloid process, the stylohyoid ligament, which is sometimes ossified, and the lesser horn of the hyoid. It provides the basis for the second or hyoid arch.

The chondrocranium becomes ossified but its growth is an active process, involving the proliferation and the division of chondroblasts. This cellular activity takes place at two sites, as follows.

The synchondroses (Fig. 4.17)

These are areas of growth cartilage which separate the zones of ossification in the cartilage of the base, analogous to the epiphyseal cartilage of the long bones, but organized as a dual-action epiphysis, to use Scott's (1955) expression. This specific activity has been confirmed in tissue cultures made by Charlier & Petrovic (1967). The synchondroses, which are primary growth centres, are very vulnerable to insults; their excision arrests the growth of the base of the skull (Moss 1969).

The mesethmoid

The growth of the sagittal strut of the mesethmoid, more commonly called the cartilaginous septum is a subject on which there is some disagreement. Various authors, including Moss et al (1968), after studies of partial excision in the dog, have stated that it has no intrinsic growth but only acts passively by the transmission of pressure. Others, in fact a majority of authors, following Sarnat (1963) and then Petrovic (1970), have demonstrated intrinsic growth by cell division in the upper part of the cartilaginous sagittal plate.

Thus the mesethmoidal part exerts a sagittal pressure upon the anterior mesenchymal structures, through a dual mechanism: indirectly by transmitting the activity of the spheno-occipital synchondrosis through the sphenoid; and directly by contributing through its own activity, which paradoxically appears not to fade towards the age of 10 years, when the perpendicular plate ossifies. It continues

through the cartilaginous septum, as shown by the clinical example of nasal kyphosis and by its age of onset (prepubertal).

This chondroethmoidal activity is not limited to a sagittally directed thrust. Its action is also distributed fanwise by the wedging effect of the lateral masses upon the interorbital area, and more anteriorly of the nasal cartilaginous roof. It should be stressed that at birth the ethmoid bone is still tripartite — mesethmoid, ectethmoid and lamina cribrosa — but already pneumatized, anteriorly as well as posteriorly (Shapiro 1954).

It can readily be seen that premature fusion (synostosis) of the ethmoidal and sphenoidal components, separately or together, results in distortion of the sagittal thrust, so that the lateral distribution becomes preponderant. The lesser wings suffer the direct effect and grow vertically.

The basal synchondroses (Fig. 4.17) generally close at about the time of birth, with the following exceptions: the spheno-occipital synchondrosis, which remains open until adolescence; and the periethmoidal systems, which close when the lamina cribrosa ossifies (at the age of 3 years, according to Scott). In fact, there are many examples of joints between a cartilaginous part and a fibrous part, which strictly speaking are neither synchondroses nor sutures, but a sort of compromise: synchondrosutures.

Synchondrosutures (Fig. 4.18)

These are heterogeneous structures, consisting of an active cartilaginous side, a primary site; and a passive fibrous

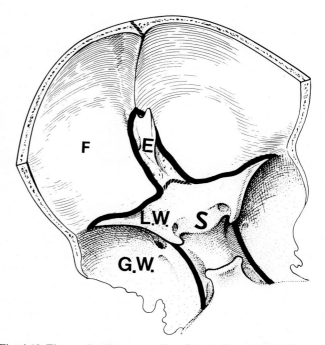

Fig. 4.18 The synchondrosutures. F = frontal; E = ethmoid; S = sphenoid: L.W. = lesser wing, G.W. = greater wing.

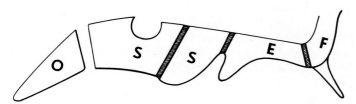

Fig. 4.17 The synchondroses. O = spheno-occipital; S = intersphenoidal; E = sphenoethmoidal; F = ethmoidofrontal.

side, an adaptive site, which is dynamically a real hemi-synchondrosis. They are distributed in the periphery of the basal pedestal and consist of:

The Budin synchondrosuture, situated at the junction of basiocciput and exo-occiput.
The sphenoalar synchondrosutures, between the body of the sphenoid and the greater wings of that bone.
The sphenofrontal synchondrosutures, between the frontal bone and the lesser wing of the spenoid.
The ethmoidofrontal synchondrosutures:
    mesethmoidofrontal, anteriorly and unpaired;
    ectethmoidofrontal, laterally and paired.

THE CONDYLAR CARTILAGE

The condylar cartilage is the only example of secondary cartilage in practice. The prechondroblasts of secondary cartilages are young cells. They have not undergone differentiation and are very sensitive to mechanical pressures. The persistence of the condyle is explained by the movements at the temporomandibular joint.

The conditions of action of this condylar cartilage have been fully elucidated by Petrovic et al (1968). The lateral pterygoid muscle provides the motor stimulus and the condyle behaves in an adaptive manner which is very similar to that of a suture site.

The interpretation of clinical facts is distorted by the simultaneous alteration of joint motility and muscle action. The responsibility lies not with the condyle but with its 'activators'.

The periosteal system (Fig. 4.19)

'The periosteum forms bone' (Duhamel). As long ago as 1867, Ollier stated two fundamental facts:

Periosteum, separated from its bone and from its natural connections, can produce bone.
Bone without periosteum remains viable.

The behaviour of this omnipresent tissue varies with the topographical situation.

LINING PERIOSTEUM

The periosteum is a fibrous membrane which covers the skeleton externally. In contrast to older views that it is produced by bone tissue, we now know that 'periosteum produces bone' through its inner, deep, osteogenic layer, while also determining its shape. Its vascular contribution predominates. It puts the finishing touch to the shape of the bone, being engaged in bone resorption or apposition, depending upon the forces which act upon it.

There is no doubt about the fact that periosteum is

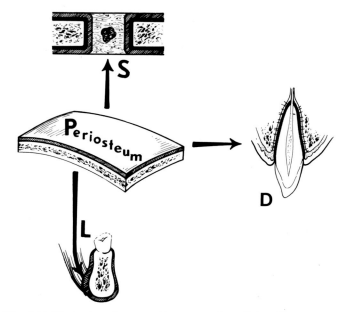

Fig. 4.19 The periosteal system. S = suture; L = lining; D = dentoalveolar ligament.

osteogenic, but it acts indirectly. Thus, a fragment of periosteum produces bone only under favourable conditions. The periosteal sheath demonstrates a particular mode of behaviour of the mesenchymal fibrous tissue when in contact with bone. Benninghof (1931) postulated the existence of a periosteal matrix specific for each bony structure.

In fact, periosteum forms, limits and models a structure, providing it with an appearance and an activity which varies from time to time and from place to place. The bony unit is defined by the periosteum.

The potential of periosteum for bone formation wanes with time, its capacity for regeneration following the same course. Its activity oscillates between apposition and resorption, depending upon the location. Enlow (1982) stressed this and his conclusion appears to be corroborated by the experimental studies by Atherton (1974) in the pig. This author reversed the anatomical situations of the nasal and palatine mucosae, and obtained bone resorption in the palate after transposition of the nasal mucosa. Finally, the productivity of periosteum depends essentially upon the state of pressure.

The lining periosteum, common to the whole system of the individual, has a specific appearance in two locations: at the suture site, which is an arrangement characteristic of the craniofacial region, but differing in the face and the cranial vault owing to the presence of a dural sac within the latter and in the alveolodental ligament.

THE SUTURES

Lebourg (1948) considered the suture to be intermediary

periosteum analogous to growth cartilage. He and Seydel were the first, in 1931 and 1932, to study the nature and the role of the facial and cranial sutures, originally considered to be simple ligamentous connections. Their histology was examined in detail by Pritchard et al (1956), in animals and in man. Enlow (1968) and Ten Cate resumed the idea of Lebourg (1931), that periosteum, suture and periodontium are identical. The technique of organotypical culture (Petrovic et al 1968) shows the functional significance.

Presutural stage

The approximation of 'bony territories' within the mesenchymal tissue takes place in ways, which differ in the face and in the vault of the skull. The concept of 'bony territory' developed by Pritchard et al (1956) fully agrees with our own view of the periosteal matrix (described by Benninghof 1925), which combines the bony part and its periosteal lining, subdivided into an inner productive layer and an external limiting layer. When the bony territories come into contact, the mesenchyme ensures that each of the bones keeps its own identity, as a result of the formation of a limiting fibrous border in front of each extremity. However, an intermediate zone persists. Lying between the two layers, it represents the nucleus of the suture which guarantees its mobility and thus its effectiveness, because of its immunity with respect to ossification. This immunity probably results from the vascular characteristics of the suture.

Sutural organization (Fig. 4.20)

According to Pritchard et al (1956), the suture is organized into five different layers. Scott (1955) distinguishes only between three:

1. The fibrous peripheral layer of periosteum, both internal as well as external, splits at the edge of the bone into a linking membrane, which bridges the suture and a limiting membrane lining the border of

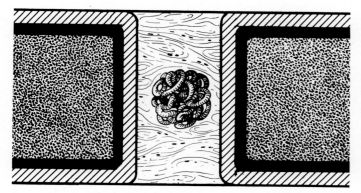

Fig. 4.20 Sutural organization.

each piece of bone. It is formed by osteogenic fibres, which give rise to the Sharpey fibres.
2. The transitional layer, between the limiting membrane and the bone, loose and very cellular. This is an osteogenic zone which resembles in every way the intermediate zone of the peridontal membrane (Enlow 1982).
3. The intermediate layer: the nucleus, consisting of highly vascular very loose tissue.

Sutural types

The structure of the suture, described above, differs in the cranium and in the face. In fact, the approximation of bones in the face occurs within loose mesenchymal tissue devoid of a guiding structure, whereas in contrast the dura mater represents a rail for the spatial expansion of the vault (Moss 1978).

The presence of the dura mater characterizes the skull, providing moulding influence and a guiding structure for the developing bone. But it also constitutes a permanent threat to the patency of the suture because of the very high osteogenic property of the periosteal layer. The facial suture is less endangered as it is delimited by less productive periosteum. The morphology of the suture is reminiscent of that of a diarthodial joint (Haines 1947, Pugeaut 1968) and histology may reveal areas of cartilage within the suture, either after fusion or after trauma (Moss 1978). The bony margins may relate to each other in two ways (Scott 1955): edge to edge or in an overlapping manner, with bevelled surfaces.

Each arrangement relates to one type of growth. Bone deposition in the edge to edge suture takes place within the suture site itself, either in one of the two bony margins or in both of them. These arrangements lead to a displacement of the suture on the non-appositional side (as Girgis & Pritchard 1956 have shown by partial destruction of one side). In the overlapping suture, bone deposition takes place on one of the aspects of the bones, resulting in displacement by apposition and resorption, as stated by Enlow (1982).

Sutural evolution and functional significance

There are three successive stages in the life of the suture, as defined by Lebourg & Seydel (1932a):

initial stage, young suture — synfibrosis;
adult stage, arrested suture — synarthrosis;
terminal stage, old suture — synostosis.

Classically, bone fusion starts in the inner table (Hanotte 1898). In fact, it involves both tables from the outset (Sitsen 1933, Todd 1971) but the advance is more rapid in the inner table. The histology has been studied in detail by Laitinen (1956).

The periosteum of the capsule and the basal membrane fuses at the level of the osseous borders. The intermediate layers show poor vascular supply and fatty degeneration. The Sharpey fibres increase in number and in area of distribution. The linking layers thicken. Bone trabeculae penetrate the suture to form bridges. The synostosis starts when brain growth ceases and when the intracranial pressure falls (Loesh & Windhold 1922). The central nucleus is then compressed, resulting in ischaemia and fibrosis. However, the external parts remain open because they are subject to mechanical influences, specifically those of mastication. According to some anthropologists (Firu 1957) there is a correlation between lack of teeth and the obliteration of sutures. The facial suture differs a little from its cranial counterpart. It has a longer programme of growth, related to the absence of an equivalent of the dura mater on its inner aspect.

Sutural systems (Scott 1955)

Each suture is part of a system. According to Scott, the sutures of the vault and the facial skeleton are organized into five different systems.

1. The facial circum-maxillary system (Fig. 4.21), separating the maxilla from the adjacent structures, the malar, palatine, nasal, lacrimal and ethmoidal bone.
2. The craniofacial system (Fig. 4.22), separating the maxilla from the frontal bone and the other facial bones from the cranial base: the frontal bone, the ethmoidal bone and the sphenoid.
3. The coronal system (Fig. 4.23), between the anterior cranial fossa (frontal bone, ethmoidal bone and sphenoid) and the middle cranial fossa (temporal and parietal bones). At the level of the pterion the system bifurcates around the greater wing into the spheno-parietal suture posteriorly and the sphenofrontal suture anteriorly. The temporozygomatic suture is an important element. At the level of the cranial base, and more particularly in the pterygopalatine fossa, the coronal system is closely related to the perimaxillary and craniofacial systems.
4. The sagittal system (Fig. 4.24): complete at birth it divides the vault in two halves. The system begins with the interparietal suture and continues in the metopic, internasal and intermaxillary sutures. It includes the mandibular symphysis and the mediopalatine suture.
5. The lambdoidal system (Fig. 4.25). Situated between the occipital bone and the middle cranial segment it becomes connected to the spheno-occipital synchondrosis in the same way as the posterior root of the coronal system.

Function of the sutures

Lebourg & Seydel (1932b) were the first to insist on the

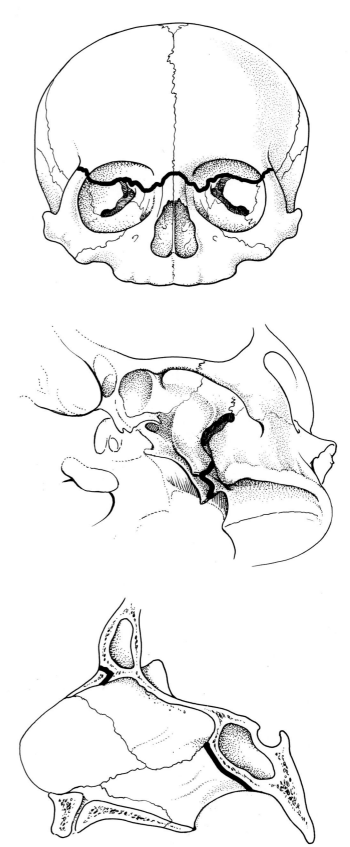

Fig. 4.21 The craniofacial system.

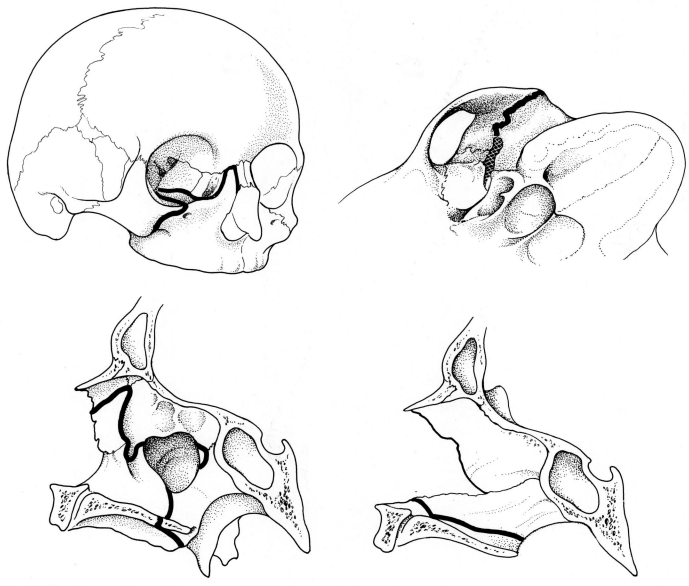

Fig. 4.22 The circum-maxillary system.

role played by the sutures in cranial and facial growth, comparing them to 'intermediary periosteum'. Earlier in 1851 Virchow made a comparison with growth cartilage. In contrast to the synchondroses, however, the sutures are only the site of secondary growth, passive and adaptive (Scott 1967).

After excision of a suture and following osseous regeneration, a new suture appears at the same site provided the dura mater is intact (Troitzky 1932). Excision of a suture does not interfere with cranial growth (Moss 1962). A suture isolated in an organotypic culture does not show any proliferative potential; Charlier & Petrovic (1967) have demonstrated this in rats, showing that the development of bone was due to the division of young conjunctival cells and thus confirming the observations of Selma and Sarnat

(1957) in their studies of the frontonasal suture of the rabbit and the results of transplantation of the zygomaticomalar suture recorded by Koski in 1968.

The suture, cranial as well as facial, therefore behaves as an 'expanding joint' with automatic correction through adaptative conjunctival proliferation and marginal ossification (Delaire 1978).

The predetermination of the sutural site

Von Gudden (1874) held the opinion that the site of the suture was determined by the arrangement of the bony parts. The experiments of Pritchard et al (1956) have confirmed this view.

Prior to the meeting of the bones there is no histological

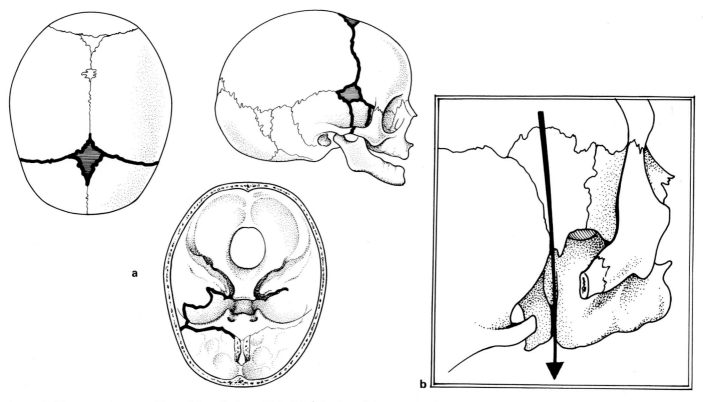

Fig. 4.23 The coronal system: (a) cranial projections; (b) facial projection of the coronal axis.

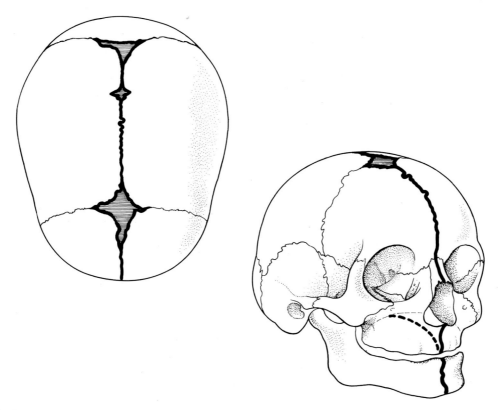

Fig. 4.24 The sagittal system.

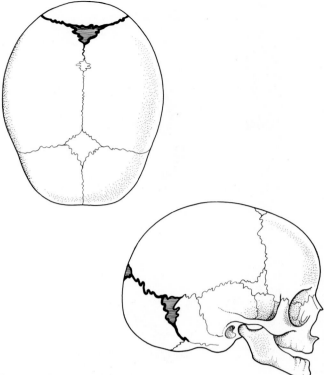

Fig. 4.25 The lambdoid system.

specialization of a suture. Is it then justified to conclude that the suture site is not predetermined? Certainly not. Shillito noticed the appearance of a neosuture at the site of a craniectomy and one of our observations points in a similar direction. Regeneration of the lambda was seen by van der Werf after partial loss of the vault.

The topographic distribution of the suture sites seems to be determined at the genetic organization level. According to Moss the suture exists in a 'predetermined form' in the cranial mesenchyme shortly before the meeting of the osseous edges — which to us seems obvious.

The mechanical characteristics of the suture

Elasticity alone as suggested by Bolk & Thoma is an inadequate characteristic. The suture is in a state of permanent conflict between: (1) the formation of bone at the osseous edges by subperiosteal apposition as shown in the experiments of Scalori (displacement of trans-sutural clips), of Laitinen (1956), and of Giblin & Alley (1944) (visualization of coloured layers with alizarin); (2) the protection of a central hydrostatic cushion, responsible for the patency of the suture and its potential for growth in reply to the encephalic thrust and is this sense a veritable regulating mechanism; (3) the preservation of osseous alignment by the division of the periosteum in uniting and capsular membranes.

The sutural space, subject to the mechanical stimulus of encephalic thrust and undulation caused by differential growth, assures thus the connection of the osseous segments. The presence of cartilaginous deposits within the nucleus gives evidence of microtraumas exerted on the suture. In addition to its corrective role the suture can adapt the production of bone to external mechanical constraint (intentional deformities).

Ryoppy in 1965 transplanted a suture of the vault to a site of epiphyseal growth, showing that the form of the suture was strictly dependent on mechanical activity. In contrast a suture transplanted to the abdominal wall (Watanabe et al 1957) is quickly replaced by fibrous tissue.

Experimental synostosis

Experimental fusion of a suture may be obtained: (1) by trans-sutural clipping, as demonstrated by Laitinen in cats; (2) by excision or destruction of the sutural periosteum according to Moss (1960), although cauterization of the suture, performed in 118 rat skulls in utero by Girgis & Pritchard (1958), did alter the suture but not the shape of the cranium; and (3) by an osseous graft, transversely blocking the suture; (Giblin & Alley 1944 inserted a parietal graft across the coronal suture).

It therefore appears that immobilization of any part of the sutural space will result in the fusion of that part followed by an extension of that fusion along the suture. This concept is supported by the study of physiological synostosis, which begins when encephalic expansion has come to a stop, and by the experiments of Moss carried out in rats. Sectioning of the falx in this animal prevents fusion of the frontal suture posteriorly. Fusion begins again following cicatrization of the falx.

The adaptive sutural system appears to preserve its patency only when subject to mechanical stimuli essentially of an internal nature — the cephalic thrust, which is transmitted directly or orientated by the sutural sac. This guarantee of patency provided by mobility does not explain the origin of premature synostosis during which course the sutural system fails to react to the cephalic thrust.

The fused suture has lost its faculty for adaptation and proliferation. The reasons for this we intend to discuss later on.

ALVEOLODENTAL LIGAMENT

This ligament or periodontal membrane consists of bundles of collagen fibres placed between the cement and the alveolar bone. It changes in shape and in structure during the development of the tooth and its evolution. It stabilizes the root of the dental organ during the period of reciprocal changes in the alveolar bone and in the erupting tooth. There are three layers of collagen fibres:

(1) internal, adjacent to the root, anchored to the cement, structurally very stable;

(2) external, juxta-alveolar, where there are frequent reorganizations of the bundles of fibres;

(3) intermediate, unstable, consisting of precollagen fibres which penetrate between the first two layers.

The model tooth–parodontium ligament is an example of an apposition–resorption mechanism. Thus the activity of the outer layer may be resorptive or appositional, depending upon the direction of pressure exerted upon the system. Because of this, the movement of the tooth through the alveolar bone stems from simultaneous anterior resorption and posterior apposition.

THE ACTIVATORS OF GROWTH

Cellular proliferation, cerebral thrust and function play an important role in the activation of growth.

Cellular proliferation

Cellular proliferation, essentially cartilaginous in the transformation of prechondroblasts into chondroblasts, has been discussed in the section on the cartilaginous system, under synchondroses.

Cerebral thrust (neurocranial adaptation of Rabischong 1960) (Fig. 4.26)

The nervous system not only induces the material of its protective envelope but it also regulates its development by repressing the conjunctival cover, the expansion of which is determined by this internal thrust, during cerebral growth.

The cranial box, first membranous and cartilaginous, later osseous, reacts to telencephalic expansion in a variety of ways. It channels and distributes the forces produced by the internal pressure. It pushes the cortex backward by elevation of the anterior branch of the basal compas and it remodels the cortex by opposing its expansion through the formation of an orbitofrontal square and a resistant ossified cap, thus forcing the brain to spread out posteriorly and laterally and to form folds and fissures.

This encephalic action is canalized by the dural sac, which like a floating tent finds support partly in basal attachments provided by the lesser wings of the sphenoid and the superior borders of the petrous bones, and partly also in the supple median partition, the cerebral falx.

Relation between function and growth

Moss in 1952 presented his theory of the functional matrices, basing it on the ideas put forward by Van der Klaauw in 1945. These structural entities are bound by

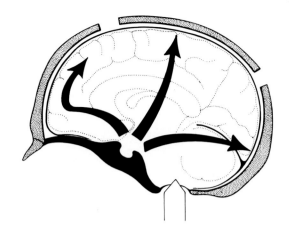

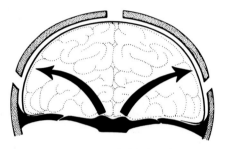

Fig. 4.26 Neurocranial adaptation (Rabischong).

one or several functions, each corresponding to a skeletal unit as a biomechanical support of its function. The dynamics result either from the variation of pressures within the cavities or from muscular activity.

The speculations of Moss have been contradicted by the facts (Dambrain 1986); however, the effect of function on growth is real.

Respiration does not play a preponderant morphogenetic role and mastication is only of minor importance (the osseous bases are virtually normal in anodontia).

The facial skeleton contains various cavities which also participate in the activation of growth.

THE EMPTY (AIR FILLED) CAVITIES

These pneumatic cavities act like caissons. The nasal fossae and their adnexa provide the best examples of this type.

THE FULL (SENSORIAL) CAVITIES

These are represented by the orbital cavity, which is expanded by the globe and its muscles, and the buccal cavity, which is surrounded by a muscular sling and filled by the tongue.

It appears that the expansion of the empty cavities is a result of muscle function, the fat pads serving to transmit pressure to the osseous walls (Latham & Scott 1970). Muscle forms therefore the predominant element in this stimulating and modelling activity, by the mechanism of apposition–resorption (Fig. 4.16).

Enlow (1982) demonstrated the displacement of an osseous lamina by deposition of bone on one site and resorption on the opposite site. This mechanism, initially described by Lacoste in his thesis on 'la decourbure des os du crane chez le mouton' at the level of the vault is essential in facial growth, more particularly in the maxillary area, 'movement is indispensable for harmonious growth'.

THE REGULATION OF GROWTH

Van Limborg (1982) has divided the regulating factors into three groups: genetic, epigenetic, and environmental. This division allows a correlation with the cybernetic model proposed by Petrovic (1970).

Genetic or intrinsic factors

The impact of these concerns above all the chondrocranium, the size and form of which are determined by DNA transcription. Koski (1968) held the opinion that the cranial base could be influenced by mechanical factors, but other experimental studies do not support this view. On the other hand, the size and form of the bony complex are mainly determined by the genetic programme which also defines the type of growth (Fig. 4.27), the latter constituting a familial characteristic.

Genetic information plays an important role at the skeletal level, but it also affects the muscles through the medium of muscular tonus responsible for posture (Bell et al 1980).

Epigenetic factors

Congenital unilateral anophthalmia constitutes an excellent clinical model of the role played by these factors within a functional complex.

Environmental factors

The origin of these factors may be of a local nature when due to a disturbance of one or more functions causing apraxias. It may be of a general nature when endocrine and nutritional disorders are involved. The hormonal impact is also important. Dimensional sexual variations demonstrate the role of sex hormones.

Somatotropic hormone plays an essential role in cartilaginous cell division and in the prepubertal growth spurt of the mandible. Pituitary adenomas causing acromegaly provide a typical clinical example of this type of disturbance.

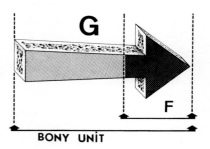

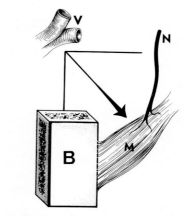

Fig. 4.27 Development of a bony unit: (a) the role of genetic programme and function on the growth of a bony unit. F = function; G = genetic programme; (b) different structures influencing the growth of the bony unit (B). M = muscle; N = nerve; V = vessel.

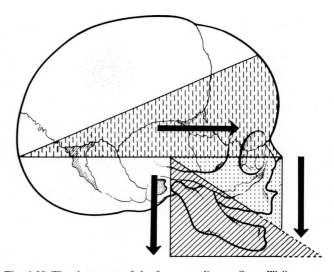

Fig. 4.28 The three ages of the face according to Greer-Walker.

THE PROGRESSION OF GROWTH

Synthesis

Craniofacial growth fluctuates from one region and one period to another and corresponds to the primordial concept of a timetable. Its progression is determined by a schedule, the main features of which have been envisaged by Greer-Walker (1961) in his definition of the three ages of the face (Fig. 4.28). The present authors, in their initial and fragmental approach, have modified this conception and distinguish between three periods, each with a different topography. In fact, the error lies in the deliberate wish to superimpose space and time (Fig. 4.29a,b).

The formation of the skull and face involves three successive and interconnected mechanisms. The first of these, the sagittal thrust has only the frontal plane as a reference and is accomplished with the help of directional squares. The second and third have a 3-dimensional reference. Multi-directional expansion is provided, medially, by bipartite bands (Fig. 4.30a) and laterally, by directional squares. The three mechanisms together finally achieve an equilibrium.

THE SAGITTAL THRUST (Fig. 4.30b)

This is the initial force related to the axis of symmetry common to all living creatures. Its action is distributed along a basocranial strut which starts at the spheno-occipital synchondrosis. The sphenoid, with its vomeropremaxillary projection, is the activator. This strut glides through the stirrup which has been formed by the two pterygo-palatomaxillary squares. The brain plays a capital role but only temporarily.

TRANSVERSE DISTRIBUTION (Fig. 4.30c)

The sagittal thrust acts on a series of superimposed transverse bands: a frontal band, a nasomaxillary band and a mandibular band, all of which have a clear functional objective. Each band is interrupted in the middle, a disposition which favours the formation of harmonious curves.

LATERAL COMPENSATION (Fig. 4.30c)

This mechanism is directed by the sphenoid under the dual control of the greater wing and the pterygoid. The position of the greater wing determines the site of the insertion of the temporal, which models the coronoid process. The relation between the pterygoid bone and the ramus is affected by the pterygoid muscles.

FINAL EQUILIBRIUM (Fig. 4.31)

Craniofacial balance is completed by occlusion, which testifies to the maxillomandibular relation and is a meeting point of genetic heritage and functional habits.

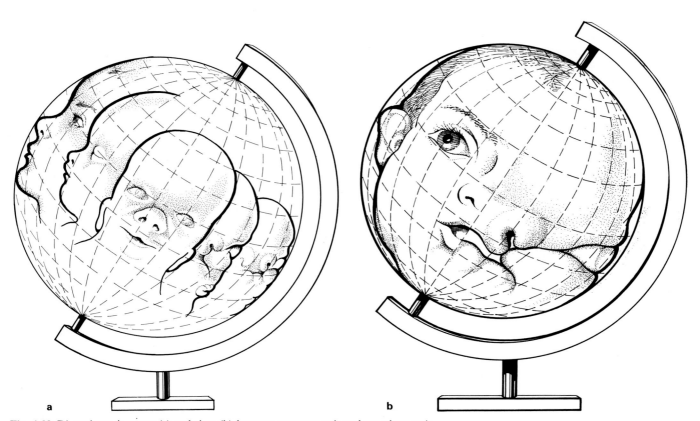

a   b

Fig. 4.29 Discordance in space (a) and time (b) between organogenesis and morphogenesis.

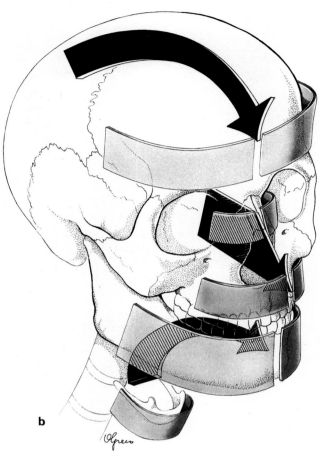

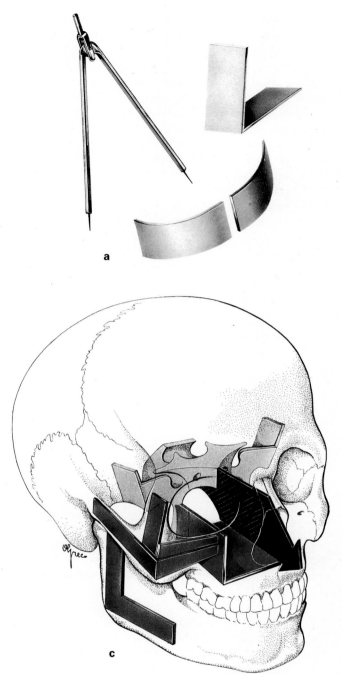

Fig. 4.30 The progression of growth: (a) the architectural symbols — compass, square and interrupted bands; (b) the sagittal thrust, its different components and the transverse distribution by means of bipartite bands; (c) transverse distribution and lateral compensation.

Conclusion: the helix (Fig. 4.32).

Development takes place along a helix which starts at the cranium, simultaneously at the base and at the vault, and then courses to the midline through the chondroethmoid, where a first anterior curve is made in conjunction with the sagittal thrust.

The helix continues over the maxillary band laterally and posteriorly towards the temporal bone, where a second curve turns medially and anteriorly over the mandibular band. The helix is a simplified representation of craniofacial development and it represents a symbol of evolution. It is striking to note that this construction encompasses both morphogenesis and pathology as well as a classification of the malformations.

THE RHYTHM OF GROWTH

Growth is a continuous phenomenon but it takes place with varying speed and in separate locations. Adult dimensions are reached at different ages, depending on the regions involved. A classic example is the discrepancy between growth of the cranium, which continues until the age of 3 years and that of the face, which is affected by growth spurts differing in direction, location and time.

The relation between the cranium and the face changes with time. The ratio is 8:1 at birth, becomes 4:1 in childhood at the age of 5 years to diminish to 2:1 in the

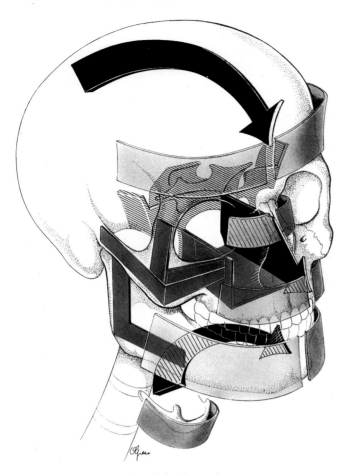

Fig. 4.31 The synthesis of craniofacial growth.

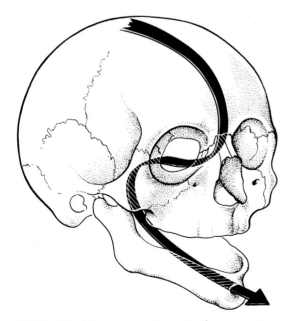

Fig. 4.32 The helix of growth; beginning in the cranium it courses through the maxillofacial complex and ends at the mandible.

adult. Facial dimensions at the age of 3 months are equivalent to 40% of those of the adult, to 70% at the age of 2 years and to 80% at the age of 5 years. The rhythm follows that of statural growth, although with a slight delay as Björk (1955a) has demonstrated by making comparative curves of sutural, condylar and statural growth. Sutural growth stops 2 years before the termination of statural growth. In addition the speed of growth decreases after 5 years of age until the arrival of puberty. This period is associated with an acceleration of growth of a hormonal origin and followed by rapid retardation, to stop at the age of 17 years.

The time of sutural obliteration may reflect the rhythm of growth, although an arrest of sutural activity, difficult to determine at times, does not necessarily mean that there is a synostosis. Nevertheless, it seems useful to report the observations of Firu (1971) on the obliteration of facial sutures in a study of 194 infant skulls and 600 adult skulls (see Table 4.1)

Table 4.1 Patent sutures

	Age (years)	Per cent patent
Interincisivo canines	2	96
	4	45
	8	14
Maxillo palatine	2	100
	6	100
	18	75
Zygotemporal	70	84
Maxillomalar	25	92
	70	40

Growth proceeds in accordance with a predictable rhythm, the appreciation of which makes it possible to decide upon the proper moment for the surgical correction of a malformation. Thus:

The initial period of cranial growth in a lateral direction affects the face until the completion of the sphenoid.

The sagittal thrust predominates in the first year of life, more particularly in the first 6 months.

The vertical growth will correspond to the evolution of the ocular globes until the age of 3 years, and thereafter to that of the teeth.

Mandibular growth will finally be regulated by prepubertal hormonal stimulation (hypophysis).

Thus, the balance of a normal face, and even more of a malformed or operated face, is threatened by critical periods in which disturbance may occur, the two most important periods being the transition between deciduous and adult dentition, and puberty with the spurt of mandibular growth.

THE SECTORS OF GROWTH

The craniofacial complex is subdivided into sectors, each with an independent and characteristic evolution, related to the different rates of growth in different regions. This lack of synchrony later diminishes because of the total interdependence of the sectors. In the end there is global harmony. Asynchronous morphogenetic development is particularly striking when it concerns the skull and the face.

Growth of the skull is an example of continuous development in the short term. It is unifactorial, directed by a single activator, the 'brain', with the quasi-exclusive 'suture' mechanism. In contrast the face shows discontinuous growth in the long term. It is multifactorial, with successive mechanisms such as synchondroses, sutures and apposition–resorption.

The encephalic sector (0–2 years) (Fig. 4.33)

This sector is characterized by the encephalic thrust, the only factor able to expand the vault. For as long as the patency of the cranial sutures permits this, the thrust is exerted in all directions, finding support in the fixed structures of the base, particularly the clivus, supported by the vertebral column. It positions the elements which make up the vault, pushing the occipital bone backward, the parietal and squamous temporal bone outward and the fronto-orbital structure forward and upward.

This frontal square has a nasal extension which is comparable to the central protection of the Greek helmet and is formed by the time the period of encephalic expansion is completed. The favoured intermediary between the brain and the mesenchymal envelope is the dural sac. The inner partitions of this sac are attached to the bone and help to shape the skull. One of these, the falx cerebri, is inserted into both the frontal bone and the mesethmoid, and induces a slight restraining effect on the length of the median axis.

The position of the frontonasal band will determine the high position of the maxillary bone. The hypothesis of maxillary forward swing postulated by Delaire is in our opinion incorrect. The encephalic sector shows a preponderant development in the first 2 years of life, waning in the third year. The brain indeed doubles its volume in the first 6 months and triples it at the end of the first year. It is easy to see that even the smallest obstacle to this thrust will affect the morphological features. Patency of the sutures is a 'sine qua non' condition for an effective cephalic dynamic. Growth assessment is made by measuring the skull circumference and by calculating the indices from the diameter. This clinical craniometry has as its corollary a volumetric craniometry which is essentially radiological (table of skull circumference measurements and changes in cranial indices).

The initial bipartite character of the forehead allows for a very harmonious distribution of the fan-like expansion over the bony contour. The frontal band has an aperture in its middle part which permits the ethmoid to protrude.

The sagittal thrust of the brain is based on the sphenoid, the only completed bone present at birth, which allows lateral expansion by means of its greater wings.

The median-sagittal sector (centrofacial complex) (Fig. 4.34)

This can roughly be likened to a sagittal strut. It is exceedingly complex in the orientation and heterogeneity of its structures. Extending from the spheno-occipital synchondrosis to the premaxilla and supported by the base of the skull and the facial mass, the sector consists in fact of two distinct portions with differing morphogenesis: the spheno-ethmoidonasal portion, which is chondrocranial and highly placed; and the vomeropremaxillary and pterygo-palatomaxillary portions, which are of mesenchymal origin and situated in the inferior and anterior part. The first is sabre-shaped gliding on the second.

SPHENO-ETHMOIDONASAL PORTION

At the centre this contains the mesethmoid, based upon the sphenoid, which transmits the activity of the spheno-occipital synchondrosis. Anteriorly it terminates in the nasal septum and the lateral cartilaginous expansions.

The mesethmoid is flanked by the ectethmoid or lateral masses, which direct the position of the ethmoidonasal band by their expansion and ossify in the fourth month of intrauterine life (in the fifth month according to Scott 1967). Their connection to the mesethmoid, the lamina cribrosa, ossifies towards the end of the third year.

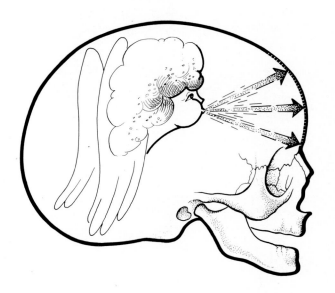

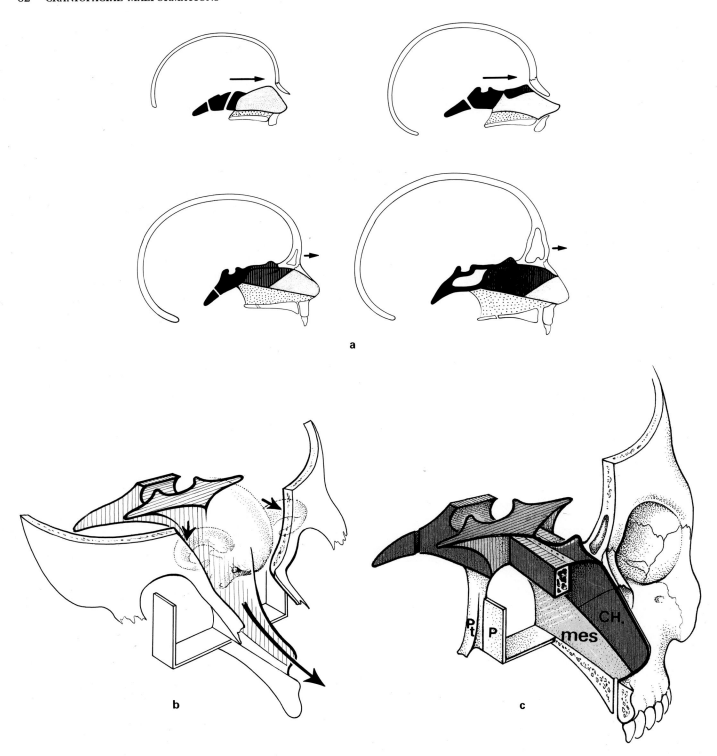

Fig. 4.34 The medial sagittal sector: (a) evolution of the chondrocranium according to Baume; (b) the sphenoethmoidal ram; (c) the dual character of the medial strut — superiorly chondroid (CH) (spheno-ethmoidonasal sector), inferiorly mesenchymal (mes); vomeropremaxillary lamina; pterygomaxillary stirrup (Pt–P).

The interorbital position is defined by the union of the mesethmoid and of the ethmoid so far achieved. The mesethmoid ossifies from back to front from the end of the first year but union with the vomer occurs only towards the age of 10 years. Until that time the nasal septal strut remains bipartite.

Vomeropremaxillary portion

The vomer, buttressed by the body of the sphenoid, propels the maxilla through a fan-like suture, early, rapidly and powerfully, as shown in total bilateral cleft palate by the extreme forward position of a premaxilla, which is not restrained by muscle. The role of the cartilaginous septum and of the so-called ligament of Latham (1970) has virtually no effect in determining the shape or the position of the premaxilla.

Battered children without a septum and an anterior nasal spine following post-traumatic resorption have an almost normal premaxilla.

Pterygo-palatomaxillary portion

The pterygoid process, a rigid strut placed perpendicular to the body of the sphenoid, controls the position of the middle face. Anteriorly, it supports the square of the palatine bone, which forms a transition with the maxillary bone. This square constitutes a stirrup as a result of their midline contact, through which courses the sagittal plate of the vomeropremaxillary plate.

Thus, at birth, the cartilaginous skull forms a complex which is interrupted only by the spheno-occipital synchondrosis, the sphenomesethmoidal synchondrosis and the mesethmoidofrontal synchondrosis (Ford 1958). The mesethmoid is a single bone and the frontal bone becomes one. Thus at the age of 1 year, a rigid frontosphenoidal bridge is formed between the orbits, at a time when growth of the eyeball is important.

A central opening allows the passage of the tripartite ethmoidal plate above, lying on the sphenoid with the sabre-like vomeropremaxillary plate, also lying on the sphenoid and pointing towards the palatomaxillary stirrup. This synopsis, highlighting the fundamental role of the sphenoid, is an old concept, already supported by Topinard (1875): not only does this 'central point' directly control the superior sectors and the middle fossa through the greater wings, connected to the petrous pyramids, but it also exerts its influence on the middle third of the face — first upon the position of the maxillary bone, and later upon the lateral compensatory movement through the pterygoid processes and by muscle action: the pterygoid processes — semi-mobile directional pillars with varying lateral obliquity — regulate the transverse dimension of the maxillary through the palatine stirrup and through the action of the pterygoid muscles which act upon the tuber-

osity; the muscle action of the pterygoids, attached to the middle fossa, determine the lateral drift of the mandible. It can thus be seen that each sector, once it has become ossified, gives support to muscles whose activity will play a part in the development of the subsequent segment.

The lateral sector (spheno-temporomandibular complex) (Fig. 4.35)

This sector, the spatial situation of which is determined by the greater wing of the sphenoid, is not only subject to the muscular influence of the temporal muscle but also to that of the pterygoidal muscles, which are attached to the lower pillar of the sphenoid, the pterygoid. In addition, greater wing and temporal bone together determine the forward projection of the external orbit, namely the fronto-zygomaticomalar subcomplex. Finally, the mandible appears to be clearly dependent only on the base of the skull in a direct or indirect manner, justifying Laude's terminology of 'craniomandibular field' (1978).

SPHENO-TEMPORAL PORTION

This forms an osteomuscular buttress whose bony supports consist of the greater wing of the sphenoid, lying on the

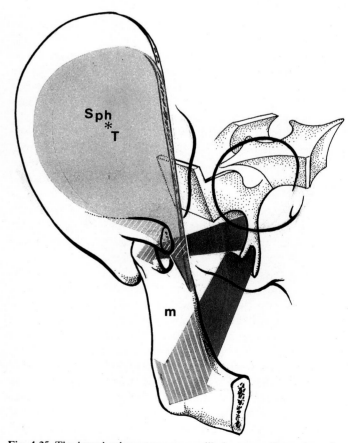

Fig. 4.35 The lateral spheno-temporomandibular sector. It consists of two parts: sphenotemporal (Sph–T) and pterygomandibular (Pt–m).

squamous temporal with a limited contact with the petrous temporal bone. It is situated in a strategic region, with the inferior divergences of the coronal sphenoparietal system behind and the sphenofrontal anteriorly. The zygomatic bone is supported by the sphenozygomatic suture, whose patency ensures effective propulsion of the zygomatic ring by the temporalis muscle.

PTERYGOMANDIBULAR PORTION

This portion consists of two short and thick muscles which arise from the pterygoid processes and diverge towards the extremities of the ramus, whose drift they in part control. The upper or lateral pterygoid muscle runs to the temperomandibular joint, which is a mobile transition between the petrous temporal and the mandible.

The inferior or medial pterygoid muscle reaches the gonion, connected with the zygomaticomalar subcomplex by the masseter muscle mass, with which it forms the pterygomasseter propulsion band.

Two points should be stressed: the pre-eminent role of the greater wing and the dependence of the mandible upon the skull.

Linguo-mandibulo-hyovertebral sector (Fig. 4.36)

This sector marks the transition between the neural and visceral parts of the craniofacial complex. Here muscle predominates over bone; function is pre-eminent in determining growth, but especially in the completion of the structures; the mandible horseshoe, a superficial skeletal element, demarcates the floor of the mouth, within which the lingual muscle mass develops.

The anterior segment of the mandible regulates the position of the tongue, but only in a very relative fashion. Thus the lingual muscle lying on the hyoid is suspended, on the one hand from the base of the skull and on the other hand from the pharyngeal musculature. The hyoid bone, a structure ossified within muscle — a true link between the mandible anteriorly and the skull posteriorly — ensures that the larynx and the air-channels are supported.

It is a transitional bone without a true function and seems to play a role in achieving vertical reorientation of the muscle supports. A miniature of the mandible, a cage suspended from the body of the mandible, its position is directly related to the growth of the vertebral axis. The work of Bench (1963) suggests that the hyoid bone migrates downward, from the level C3–C4, at the age of 3 years to the level of C4 in adulthood. Initiallly, the distance between the spine and the hyoid bone remains constant up to the age of puberty, but in the prepubertal growth spurt the chin carries the hyoid apparatus forward.

The spine forms the fixed posterior point of reference

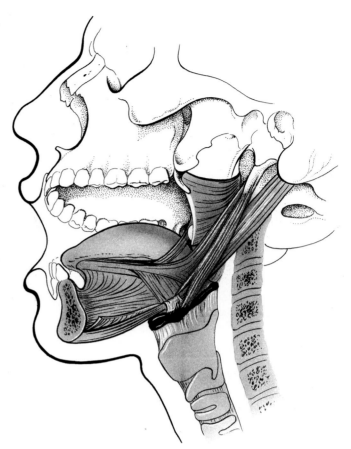

Fig. 4.36 The linguo-mandibulo-hyovertebral sector.

in indirect relation to the lingual mass through the pharynx and the constrictor muscles. With the tongue it defines the respiratory channel, whose functional role is obvious.

The tongue is a muscular visceral organ, located at the centre of oral functions. It acts not only as a single muscle but also as a proprioceptive receptor. Perceived sensations condition functional habits (Weiffenbach 1972). The lingual muscle and its environment (the lingual box) are closely related. The configuration of the palatal roof is extremely important. The tongue takes part in different functions — suction, deglutition, phonation — and it must conform to their modifications. With this adaptive capacity the tongue is one of the key elements in the rehabilitation of oral dyspraxias.

The dentoalveolar sector

As a finishing touch to facial harmony the dentoalveolar sector develops within the neuromuscular corridor, in which there is no pressure. The dentoalveolar arches are in constant search of occlusal balance, protecting the teeth from vertical pressure (Fig. 4.37) which is perpendicular to their long axis.

CONCLUSION

Harmonious craniofacial growth answers to three imperatives: neurosensory induction (neural inductor); growth potential (mesenchymal effector); and muscular balance (muscular activity).

The bony unit provides a typical example of the interaction between the major impact of the genetic programme and the minor influence of functional habits. In this exciting game, form, as a result of growth, needs a partner — force — produced by dynamic activity dependent on proprioceptive information. The craniofacial complex is entirely innervated by the trigeminal nerve and frontal symmetry is organized along a sagittal plane.

Craniofacial form produced by growth is a compromise between the innate and the acquired, although their contribution is unequally divided.

The influence of postural and functional habits is restricted to the inferior part of the face, which is of visceral origin and symbolized by the tongue at the junction of the neural and visceral parts of the craniofacial complex.

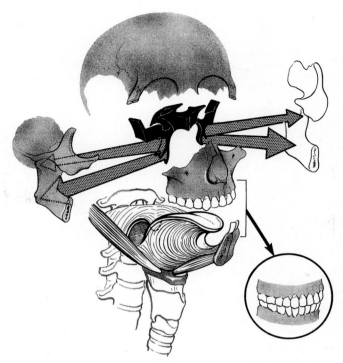

Fig. 4.37 Sectors of morphogenesis and growth: (1) Cranioencephalic; (2) Medial-sagittal; (3) Latero-craniofacial (spheno-temporomandibular); (4) Linguo-hyomandibulo-vertebral; (5) Dentoalveolar.

REFERENCES

Adolph E F 1964 Perspectives of adaptation in some general properties. In: Dill D B, Adolph E F Wilber C G (eds) Handbook of physiology, section 4. American Physiological Society, Washington, DC pp 27–36

Alhopuro S 1978 Premature fusion of facial sutures with free periosteal grafts. Scandinavian Journal of Plastic and Reconstructive Surgery (suppl 17): 1–68

Alhopuro S, Ranta R, Ritsila 1973 Growth of the facial skeleton in guinea pigs after experimental fusion of the premaxillo-maxillary suture. Proceedings of the Finnish Dental Society 69: 263–265

Andersen H, Mathiessen M 1967 Histochemistry of the early development of the human central face and nasal cavity with a special reference to the movement and fusion of the palatine processes. Acta Anatomica 68: 473–508

Appleton A B 1934 Postural deformities and bone growth. Lancet 1: 451–454

Arey L B 1965 Developmental anatomy. Saunders, London

Atherton J D 1974 The growth of the bony palate of the pig consequent to transpositioning the oral and nasal mucoperiosteum. Cleft Palate Journal 11: 429–438

Babler W J, Persing J A 1982 Experimental alteration of cranial suture growth: effects on the neurocranium, basicranium and midface. In: Dixon A D, Sarnat B G (eds) The international conference on factors and mechanisms influencing bone growth Liss, New York

Babula W J, Smiley G R, Dixon A D 1970 The role of the cartilaginous nasal septum in midfacial growth. American Journal of Orthodontics 58: 250–263

Badoux D M 1966 Framed structures in the mammalian skull. Acta Morphologica Neerlando-Scandinavica 5: 347–360

Baer J G 1965 Cours d'anatomie comparée des vertèbres. du Griffon, Neuchatel

Baer M J, Ackerman J L 1966 A longitudinal vital staining method for the study of apposition in bone. In: Evans F G (ed) Studies on the anatomy and function of bone and joints. Springer-Verlag, New York

Barrett R H, Hanson M L 1974 Oral myofunctional Disorders. Mosby, St Louis

Bassett C A L 1965 Biophysical principles affecting bone structure. In: Bourne G H (ed) The biochemistry and physiology of bone, vol. III. Academic Press, New York

Bassett C A 1972 A biophysical approach to craniofacial morphogenesis. Cranio-facial Conference, Nimegue

Baume L J 1961 The postnatal growth activity of the nasal cartilage septum. Helvetica Odontologica 5: 9–13

Baume L J 1968 Patterns of cephalofacial growth and development. A comparative study of the basicranial growth centers in rat and man. International Dental Journal 18: 489–513

Behrents R G 1975 The influence of the trigeminal nerve on facial growth and development. MS thesis, Case Western Reserve University

Bell W H, Proffit W R, White R P 1980 Surgical correction of dentofacial deformities. Sanders, London

Bench R W 1963 Growth of the cervical vertebrae as related to tongue, face and denture behaviour. American Journal of Orthodontics 49: 183–214

Benninghoff A 1925 Form und Bau der Gelenk Knorpel in Ihren Beziehungen zur Function. Zeitschrift fur Zellforschung 2: 783–862

Benninghoff A 1931 Uber die Entstehung funktioneller Strukturen. Verhandlungen der Anatomischen Gesellschaft 39: 62–70

Bercher J, Psaume J 1953 Les geno-neuro-dystrophies faciales. Dystrophies de la region du sphenoide. Presse Medicale 61: 1190–1193

Bergland O 1974 The role of the nasal septum in mid facial growth in man elucidated by the maxillary development in certain types of facial clefts. Scandinavian Journal of Plastic and Reconstructive Surgery 8: 42–48

Bergsma D (ed) 1975 Morphogenesis and malformations of face and brain. Liss, New York

Bernard R, Giraud F, Spriet A, Mattei J F 1974 Le rapport craniofacial, ses applications a la pathologie malformative. Journal de Genetique Humaine 22: 205–209

Bertelsen T I 1958 The premature synostosis of the cranial sutures. Acta Opthalmologica (suppl 51): 1–176

Björk A 1955a Facial growth in man; studies with the aid of metallic implants. Acta Odontologica Scandinavica 13: 9–34

Björk A 1955b Cranial base development. A follow-up x-ray study of the individual variation in growth occurring between the age of 12 and 20 years and its relation to brain case and face development. American Journal of Orthodontics 41: 198–225

Björk A 1968 The use of metallic implants in the study of facial growth in children: method and application. American Journal of Physical Anthropology 29: 243–254

Björk A 1969 Prediction of mandibular growth rotation. American Journal of Orthodontics 55: 209–233

Björk A 1972 The role of genetic and local environmental factors in normal and abnormal morphogenesis. Proceedings of the Craniofacial Conference Swets & Zeitlinger, Nijmegen. pp 67–80

Björk A, Skieller V 1976 Postnatal growth and development of the maxillary complex. In: McNamara J A Jr (ed) Factors affecting the growth of the midface. Monograph 6, Craniofacial Growth Series, Center for Human Growth and Development. University of Michigan, Ann Arbor

Blechschmidt E 1961 The stages of human development before birth — an introduction to human Embryology. Saunders, Philadelphia

Blechschmidt M 1976 The biokinetics of the basicranium. In: Bosma J F (ed) Symposium on development of the basicranium. DHEW Pub No (NIH) 76–989, Bethesda

Blumenbach J F 1795 On the natural variety of mankind, 3rd Ed. Dietrich Gottingen

Bolk L 1915 On the premature obliteration of sutures in the human skull. American Journal of Anatomy 17: 495–523

Bosma J F 1967a Symposium on oral sensation and perception. In: Bosma J F (ed) Oral sensation and perception. Thomas, Springfield, Ill.

Bosma J F 1967b Second symposium on oral sensation and perception. In: Bosma J F (ed) oral sensation and perception. Thomas, Springfield, Ill.

Bosma J F 1975 Form and function in the mouth and pharynx of the human Infant. In: McNamara J A Jr (ed) Control mechanisms in craniofacial growth. Monograph 3, Craniofacial Growth Series. Center for Human Growth and Development, University of Michigan, Ann Arbor

Brachet A 1956 Traité d'embryologie des vertèbres. Masson, Paris

Brash J C 1929 The growth of jaws and palate. In: The growth of the jaws, normal and abnormal, in health and disease. Dental Board, London

Brodie A G 1941 On the growth pattern of the human head from the 3rd month to the 8th year of life. American Journal of Anatomy 68: 209

Buffon L Comte de 1775–1776 In: Kendrick W, Murdock J (eds) A natural history. London

Burston W R, Hamilton W J, Walker D G 1964 Symposium: malformation of the face. British Dental Journal 116: 285

Carlson D S, Poznanski A 1982 Experimental models of surgical intervention in the growing face: histochemical analysis of neuromuscular adaptation to altered muscle length. In: McNamara J A Jr, Carlson D S, Ribbens K A (eds) The effect of surgical intervention on craniofacial growth. Monograph No 12, Craniofacial Growth Series, Center for Human Growth and Development. University of Michigan, Ann Arbor

Carlson D S, McNamara J A Jr, Graber L W, Hoffman D L 1980. Experimental studies of growth and adaptation of the temporomandibular joint. In: Irby W B (ed) Volume III. Current concepts in oral surgery. Mosby, St Louis

Chaconas F J, Caputo A A, Davis J C 1976 The effect of orthopedic forces on the cranio-facial complex utilizing cervical and headgear appliances. American Journal of Orthodontics 69: 527–539

Charlier J P, Petrovic A 1967 Recherches sur la mandibule de rat en culture d'organes: le cartilage condylien a-t-il un potentiel de croissance independant? Orthodontie Française: 38: 165–175

Chierici G 1977 Experiments on the influence oriented stress on bone formation replacing bone grafts. Cleft Palate Journal 14: 114–123

Chierici G, Harvold E P, Vargervik K 1973 Morphogenetic experiments in facial asymmetry: the nasal cavity. American Journal of Physical Anthropology 38: 191–300

Cleall J F 1972 Circumstances limiting the development and verification of a comprehensive theory of craniofacial morphogenesis. Acta Morphologica Neerlando-Scandinavica 10: 115–126

Coleman W 1977 Biology in the nineteenth century. Problems and form, function and transformation. Cambridge University Press, Cambridge

Cox N H, van der Linden F P G M 1971 Facial harmony. American Journal of Orthodontics 60: 175

Cox R L 1970 Muscular development and maturation of the dentofacial complex: normal and abnormal. American Speech and Hearing Association Report 5: 20–32

Creekmore T D 1967 Inhibition or stimulation of the vertical growth of the facial complex, its significance to treatment. Angle Orthodontist 37: 285–297

Cuvier G 1805 Leçons d'anatomie comparée. Paris

Dahlberg A A, Graber T M (eds) 1977 Orofacial growth and development. Mouton, The Hague

Daniels G H Kremenak C R Jr 1971 Median structures of the midface and their role in growth control systems. Journal of Dental Research 50 (Suppl): 1498

De Beer G R 1937a The vertebrate skull. Oxford University Press, Oxford

De Beer G R 1937b The development of the chondrocranium of homo sapiens. In: The development of the vertebrate skull. New York: Oxford Press. p 355

Dechambre A 1857 Dictionnaire usuel des Sciences médicales, 3rd edn. Paris, Masson

Delachapelle C L 1981 La mandibule. Deux ou trois choses que je sais d'elle. Contribution a un abord structural. These pour le Doctorat d'Etat en Biologie Humaine. Amiens

Delaire J 1972 La croissance maxillaire: deductions therapeutiques. Transactions of the European Orthodontic Society 81–102

Delaire J 1974 Considerations sur l'accroissement du premaxillaire chez l'homme. Revue de Stomatologie et de Chirurgie Maxillo-Faciale 75: 951–970

Delaire J 1975 Les mechanismes de la croissance du squelette facial. In: Orthopedie dento-faciale bases fondamentales. Prelat, Paris. pp 72–124

Delaire J 1978 The potential role of facial muscles in monitoring maxillary growth and morphogenesis. In: Carlson D S, McNamara J A Jr (eds) Muscle adaptation in the craniofacial region. Monograph 8, Craniofacial Growth Series. Center for Human Growth and Development, University of Michigan, Ann Arbor

Diamond M 1946 Posterior growth of the maxilla. American Journal of Orthodontics and Oral Surgery 32: 359–364

Dieulafe, Dieulafe R 1933 L'enfant. Paris, Bailliere et fils

Diewert V M 1982a A comparative study of craniofacial growth during secondary palate development in four strains of mice. Journal of Craniofacial Genetics and Developmental Biology 2: 247–263

Diewert V M 1982b Contributions of differential growth of cartilages to change in craniofacial morphology. Progress in Clinical and Biological Research 101: 229–242

Dixon A D 1953 The early development of the maxilla. Dental Practitioner 9: 10

Dollander A 1973 Elements d'embryologie. Embryologie generale (1). Flammarion, Paris

Droschl H 1975 The effect of heavy orthopedic forces on the sutures of the facial bones. Angle Orthodontist 45: 26–35

Dureux J B 1955 Le probleme des malformations associees des genopathies et embriopathies neuro-ophtalmiques. Leur incidence au cours des malformations du squelette cranio-facial. These Med, No 72, Nancy

Duterloo H S, Bierman M W J 1977 Morphological changes in alveolar bone during development of the dentition in man. In: McNamara

J A Jr (ed) The biology of occlusal development. Monograph 7, Craniofacial Growth Series. Center for Human Growth and Development, University of Michigan, Ann Arbor

Enlow D H 1968 The human face. Harper & Row, New York

Enlow D H 1982 Handbook of facial growth. Saunders, Philadelphia

Epker B N, Schendel S A, Washburn M 1982 Effects of early superior repositioning of the maxilla on subsequent growth: III. Biomechanical considerations. In: McNamara J A Jr, Carlson D S, Ribbens K A (eds) The effects of surgical intervention on craniofacial growth. Monograph No 12, Craniofacial Growth Series. Center for Human Growth and Development, University of Michigan, Ann Arbor

Eschler J 1970 L'influence des muscles masseter et ptérygoidien sur le développement et la croissance de la mandibule. Actualités Odonto-Stomatologie 89: 7–28

Faulkner J F, Maxwell L C, White T P 1978 Adaptations in skeletal muscle. In: Carlson D S, McNamara J A Jr (eds) Muscle adaptation in the craniofacial region. Craniofacial Growth Series, Monograph No 8. Center for Human Growth and Development, University of Michigan, Ann Arbor

Firu P 1971a Le developpement du massif facial: 1. Ontogénèse de la région cranio-faciale. Revue Belge Med Dent 26: 105–130

Firu P 1971b Le developpement du massif facial 2. Croissance et sutures cranio-faciales. Revue Belge Med Dent 26: 283–298

Firu P, Neagu V, Georgescu 1957 Contribution a l'etude des sutures craniennes. In: Problemes d'anthropologie. Bucarest

Ford E H R 1958 Growth of the human cranial base. American Journal of Orthodontics 44: 498–506

Freng A 1978 Growth in width of the dental arches after partial extirpation of the midpalatal suture in man. Scandinavian Journal of Plastic and Reconstructional Surgery 12: 267–272

Frost H M 1963 Bone remodelling dynamics. Thomas, Springfield, Ill

Frost H M 1964 The laws of bone structure. Thomas, Springfield, Ill

Frost H M 1973 Orthopaedic biomechanics. Thomas, Springfield, Ill

Gans C 1974 Biomechanics: an approach to vertebrate biology. Lippencott, Philadelphia

Gasser R F 1967 The development of the facial muscles in man. American Journal of Anatomy 120: 357–376

Gasson N, Petrovic A 1972 Mecanismes et regulation de la croissance antero-posterieure du maxillaire superieur. Recherches experimentales, chez le jeune rat, sur le role de l'hormone somototrope et de la cloison nasale. Orthodontie Française 43: 255–270

Giblin N, Alley A 1944 Studies on skull growth: coronal suture fixation. Anatomical Record 88: 143–153

Gillespie J A 1954 The nature of the bone changes associated with nerve injuries and disuse. Journal of Bone and Joint Surgery 36: 464–474

Girgis F, Pritchard J J 1956 Experimental alteration of cranial suture patterns. Journal of Anatomy 9: 573

Girgis F G, Pritchard J J 1958 Effects of the skull damage on the development of sutural patterns in the rat. Journal of Anatomy 92: 39–51

Gisel A 1974 Influence of the environment on the growth and formation of the human skull. Wiener Medizinische Wochenschrift 124: 353–357

Goss R J 1972 Theories of growth regulation. In: Goss R J (ed) Regulations of organ and tissue growth. Academic Press, New York. pp 1–11

Graber T M, Swain B F 1969 Current orthodontic concepts and techniques. Saunders, Philadelphia

Grasse P P 1967 Traite de zoologie. Mammiferes: tegument et squelette 16, 1. Masson, Paris

Greer Walker D 1961 Malformations of the face. Livingstone, Edinburgh

Gregory W K 1929 Our face from fish to man. Putman, New York

Haines R W 1947 The development of joints. Journal of Anatomy 81: 33–55

Hall B K 1982 Tissue interactions controlling the differentiations of bone in the craniofacial skeleton. In: Dixon A D, Sarnat B G (eds) The international conference on factors and mechanisms influencing bone growth. Liss, New York

Ham A W, Harris W R 1971 Repair and transplantation of bone. In: Bourne G H (ed) The biochemistry and physiology of bone, vol. III. Academic Press, New York

Hanotte M 1898 Anatomie pathologique de. l'oxycephalie. These Med, Paris

Hartshorn D F 1970 Facial growth effects of nasal septal cartilage resection in beagle pups. Thesis, Department of Otolaryngology and Maxillogacial Surgery, University of Iowa, Iowa City

Harvold E P 1979 Neuromuscular and morphological adaptations in experimentally induced oral respiration. In: McNamara J A Jr (ed) Naso-respiratory function and craniofacial growth. Monograph 9, Craniofacial Growth Series. Center for Human Growth and Development, University of Michigan, Ann Arbor

Heft J 1960 The growth of the periosteum and bone marrow in long bones. Experimental study on the tibia of the rabbit. Ceskoslovenska Morphologie 8: 238–250

Henry H L 1976 An experimental study of external force application to the maxillary complex. In: McNamara J A (ed) Factors affecting the growth of the midface. Monograph 6, Craniofacial Growth Series. Center for Human Growth and Development, University of Michigan, Ann Arbor

Hirschfield W J, Moyers R E 1971 Prediction of craniofacial growth: the state of the art. American Journal of Orthodontics 60: 435

Horowitz S L, Osborne R 1971 The genetic aspects of cranio-facial growth. In: Moyers R E, Krogman W M (eds) Craniofacial growth in man. Pergamon Press, Oxford. pp 183–191

Houpt M I 1970 Growth of the craniofacial complex of the human fetus. American Journal of Orthodontics 58: 373

Howells W W 1957 The cranial vault: factors of size and shape. American Journal of Anthropology 15: 19–48

Hoyte D A N 1966 Experimental investigations of skull morphology and growth. International Review of General and Experimental Zoology 2: 345–407

Hoyte D A N 1971 The modes of growth of the neurocranium: the growth of the sphenoid bone in animals. In: Moyers R E, Krogman W M (eds) Cranial facial growth in Man. Pergamon Press, Oxford. p 77

Hoyte D A N, Enlow D H 1966 Wolff's law and the problem of muscle attachment on resorptive surfaces of bone. American Journal of Physical Anthropology 24: 205–214

Humphrey T 1969 Reflex activity in the oral and facial area of the human fetus. In: Bosma J F (ed) Oral sensation and perception, 2nd symposium. Thomas Springfield, Ill. pp 195–233

Humphrey T 1971a Human prenatal activity sequences in the facial region and their relationship to postnatal development. American Speech and Hearing Association Report 6: 19–37

Humphrey, T 1971b Development of oral and facial motor mechanisms in human fetuses and their relation to craniofacial growth. Journal of Dental Research 50: 1428–1441

Ingervall B, Thilander B (1972) The human spheno-occipital synchondroses. I. The time of closure appraised macroscopically. Acta Odontologica Scandinavica 30: 349–356

Isaacson R J, Erdman A G, Hultgren B W 1981 Facial and dental effects of mandibular rotation. In: Carlson D S (ed) Craniofacial biology. Monograph 10, Craniofacial Growth Series, Center for Human Growth and Development. University of Michigan, Ann Arbor

Johnson L C 1966 The kinetics of skeletal remodeling. A further consideration of the theoretical biology of bone. Birth Defects Original Article Series 2: 66–142

Johnston M C 1975 Morphogenesis and malformation of face and brain. Birth Defect, 11: 1

Kemble J V H 1973 The importance of the nasal septum in facial development. Journal of Laryngology and Otology 87: 379–386

Kissel P, Dureux J B, Tridon P 1959 Incidence des malformations du systeme nerveux au cours des malformations du squelette cranio-facial. Collection Internationale sur les Malformations Congénitales Encéphaliques 159: 204

Knese K H 1956 Die periostale Osteogenese und Bildung der Knochenstruktur bis zum Sauglingsalter. Zeitschrift fur Zellforschung 44: 585–643

Koski K 1968 Cranial growth centers: facts or fallacies? American Journal of Orthodontics 54: 566–583

Koski K 1971 Some characteristics of cranio-facial growth cartilages. In: Moyers R E, Krogman W M (eds) Cranio-facial growth in man. Pergamon Press, Oxford

Koski K 1977 The role of the craniofacial cartilages in the postnatal growth of the cranio-facial skeleton. In: Dahlberg A A, Graber T M (eds) Orofacial growth and development. Mouton, Hague

Koski K, Ronning O 1969 Growth potential of subcutaneously transplanted cranial base synchondroses of the rat. Acta Odontologica Scandinavica 27: 343–357

Kreiborg S, Pruzansky S 1971 craniofacial growth in patients with premature craniosynotoses. Transaction of conference on craniofacial anomalies, New York

Kremenak C R Jr 1972 Circumstances limiting the development and verification of a complete explanation of craniofacial growth. Acta Morphologica Neerlando-Scandinavica 10: 127–140

Kremenak C R Jr, Searls J C 1971 Experimental manipulation of midfacial growth: a synthesis of five years of research at the University of Iowa Maxillofacial Growth Laboratory. Journal of Dental Research 50: 1488–1491

Kremenak C R, Hartshorn D F, Demjen S E 1969 The role of the cartilaginous nasal septum in maxillofacial growth: experimental septum removal in beagle pups. Journal of Dental Research 48: abstract 32

Kremenak C R Jr, Huffman W C, Olin W H 1971 Maxillary growth inhibition by mucoperiosteal denudation of palatal shelf bone in non cleft beagles. Cleft Palate Journal 7: 817–825

Krogman W M 1976 craniofacial growth and development: an appraisal. Yearbook of Physical Anthropology (1974) 18: 31–64

Kvinnsland S 1971 The sagittal growth of the foetal cranial base. Acta Odontologica Scandinavica 29: 699

Kvinnsland S 1973 Growth potential of autografts of cartilage from the nasal septum in the rat. Plastic and Reconstructional Surgery 52: 557–561

Kvinnsland S 1974 Partial resection of the cartilaginous nasal septum in rats: its influence on growth. Angle Orthondontist 4: 135

Kvinnsland S, Breistein L 1973 Regeneration of the cartilaginous nasal septum in the rat, after resection: its influence on facial growth. Plastic and Reconstructional Surgery 51: 190–195

Lacroix P 1951 The organization of bones. Churchill, London

Laitinen L 1956 Craniosynostosis. Thesis. Annals Paediatric Fenn 2 (Suppl. 6): 18

Latham R A 1968 A new concept of the early maxillary growth mechanism. Transactions of the European Orthodontics Society: 53–63

Latham R A 1970 Maxillary development and growth: the septo-premaxillary ligament. Journal of Anatomy 107: 471–478

Latham R A 1976 An appraisal of early maxillary growth mechanisms. In: McNamara J A Jr (ed) Factors affecting the growth of the midface. Monograph 6, Craniofacial Growth and Development. University of Michigan, Ann Arbor

Latham R A, Scott J H 1970 A newly postulated factor in the early growth of the human middle face and the theory of multiple assurance. Archives of Oral Biology 15: 1097–1100

Latham R, Deaton T, Galabrase C 1975 A question of the role of the vomer in the growth of the premaxillary segment. Cleft Palate 12: 351–355

Latham R A, Hoffman H, Munro L I 1977 Structure of cranial sutures in craniosynostosis. Third international congress on cleft palate and related craniofacial anomalies, Toronto

Laude M, Thilloy G, Delachapelle C et al 1978 Introduction a l'analyse cranio-mandibulaire (Rapport au 51e Congres de la SFODF). Orthodontie Française 49: 1–120

Lebourg L 1931 La dysarthrose cranio-faciale. These Med, Paris

Lebourg L 1948 Significations des sutures osseuses céphaliques. Revue de Stomatologie 49: 331–335

Lebourg L, Seydel S 1932a Sur quelques points du developpement postnatal de la boite cranienne Annales d'Anapathologie et Medico-Chirurgie Paris

Lebourg L, Seydel S 1932b Nature evolution et role des articulations de la face: leur importance physiopathologique. Revue de Stomatologie 34: 193–210

Le Double A F 1903 Traité des variations des os du crane de l'homme. Vigot, Paris

Limborg J 1970 A new view on the control of the morphogenesis of the skull. Acta Morphologica Neerlando-Scandinavica 8: 143–160

Limborgh J 1972 The role of genetic and local environmental factors in the control of post natal craniofacial morphogenesis. Acta Morphological Neerlando-Scandinavica 10: 37

Linder-Aronson S 1979 Naso-respiratory function and craniofacial growth. In: Naso-respiratory function and cranofacial growth series. Center for Human Growth and Development, University of Michigan, Ann Arbor

Linge L 1973 Tissue changes in facial sutures: incident or mechanical influences. Thesis, University of Oslo

MacKeown M 1975a The influence of environment on the growth of the craniofacial complex. A study on demonstration. Angle Orthodontist 45: 137–140

MacKeown M 1975b The allometric growth of the skull. General mode and prediction of facial growth. American Journal of Orthodontics 67: 412–422

McNamara J A Jr 1972 Neuromuscular and skeletal adaptations to altered orofacial function. Monograph no 1, Craniofacial Growth Series. Center for Human Growth and Development, University of Michigan, Ann Arbor

McNamara J A Jr (ed) 1975a The role of muscle and bone interaction in craniofacial growth. In: Control mechanisms in craniofacial growth. Monograph 3, Craniofacial Growth Series. Center for Human Growth and Development, University of Michigan, Ann Arbor

McNamara J A Jr (ed) 1975b Control mechanisms in craniofacial growth. Monograph 3, Craniofacial Growth Series. Center for Human Growth and Development, University of Michigan, Ann Arbor

McNamara J A Jr (ed) 1976 Factors affecting the growth of the midface. Monograph 6, Craniofacial Growth Series. Center for Human Growth and Development, University of Michigan, Ann Arbor

McNamara J A Jr (ed) 1979 Naso-respiratory function and craniofacial growth. Monograph 9, Craniofacial Growth Series. Center for Human Growth and Development, University of Michigan, Ann Arbor

Melsen A 1972 The morphogenesis of the human head. Acta Morphologica Neerlando-Scandinavica 1: 3–9

Melsen B 1974 The cranial base. Acta Odontologica Scandinavica 32: 1–126

Mew J R C 1981 Factors influencing maxillary growth. Proceedings of Symposium Anatomischam Institute, Rostock

Miroue M A, Rosenberg L 1975 The human facial sutures: a morphologic and histologic study of the age changes from 20 to 95 years. Master's thesis, University of Washington, Seattle

Moffett B C 1969 Remodeling changes of the facial sutures, periodontal and temporomandibular joints produced by orthodontic forces in rhesus monkeys. Bulletin of the Pacific Coast Society of Orthodontics 44: 46–49

Moffett B C 1972 A research perspective on craniofacial morphogenesis. Proceedings of the Craniofacial Conference. Swets & Zeitlinger, Nijmegen. pp 122–141

Moffett B C 1973 Remodeling of the craniofacial skeleton produced by orthodontic forces. Symposium of the IVth International Congress of Primatology Vol 3. Craniofacial biology of primates. pp 180–190

Moore R N 1979 Morphology, growth and maturation. In: Saunders B (ed) Pediatric oral and maxillofacial surgery. Mosby, St Louis

Morin J, Hill J, Anderson J, Grainger R 1963 A study of growth in the interorbital region. American Journal of Ophthalmology 56: 895–901

Moss M L 1962 The functional matrix. In: Kraus B S, Riedel R A (eds) Vistas in orthodontics. Lea & Febiger, Philadelphia

Moss M L 1969 A theoretical analysis of the functional matrix. Acta Biotheoretica 18: 195–202

Moss M L 1972a The regulation of skeletal growth. In: Goss R J (ed) Regulation of organ and tissue growth. Academic Press, New York

Moss M L 1972b Functional cranial analysis and the functional matrix. In: Schumacher G H (ed) Morphology of the maxillo-mandibular apparatus. Thieme, Leipzig

Moss M L 1974 Neurotrophic regulation of craniofacial growth.

Presentation at lst annual symposium of control mechanisms in craniofacial growth, The University of Michigan, Ann Arbor

Moss M L 1975 Neurotrophic regulation of craniofacial growth. In: McNamara J A Jr (ed) Determinants of Craniofacial Form and Growth. Ann Arbor, University of Michigan

Moss M L 1976 The role of the nasal septal cartilage in midfacial growth. In: McNamara J A Jr (ed) Factors affecting the growth of the midface. Monograph 6, Craniofacial Growth Series. Center for Human Growth and Development, University of Michigan, Ann Arbor

Moss M L 1978 The design of bones. In: Owen R, Goodfellow J W, Bullough P G (eds) Scientific foundations of orthopaedics and the Surgery of trauma. Heinemann, London

Moss M L 1983 Entwicklungsmechanik: the functional matrix hypothesis and epigenetics. In: Graber T M (ed) The physiologic basis of functional appliances. Mosby, St Louis

Moss M L, Moss-Salentijn L 1978 The muscle–bone interface; an analysis of a morphological boundary. In: Carlson D S, McNamara J A Jr (eds) Muscle adaptation in the craniofacial region. Monograph 8, Craniofacial Growth Series. Center for Human Growth and Development, University of Michigan, Ann Arbor

Moss M L, Bromberg B E, Song I C, Eisenman G E 1968 The passive role of nasal septal cartilage in mid-facial growth. Plastics and Reconstructional Surgery 41: 536–542

Moyers R E, Krogman W M 1971 Craniofacial growth in man. Pergamon, Oxford

Nairn R I 1956 The circumoral musculature: structure and function. British Dental Journal 138: 49–56

Ohyama K 1969 Experimental study on growth and development of dento-facial complex after resection of cartilaginous nasal septum. Bulletin of the Tokyo Medical and Dental University 16: 157–176

Ollier L 1867 Traité experimental et clinique de la regeneration des os et de la production artificielle des tissus osseux. Masson & Cie, Paris

Ollier L 1885 Traité des resections et des operations conservatrices qu'on peut pratiquer sur le systeme osseux. Masson & Cie, Paris

O'Rahilly R, Gardner E 1973 The initial appearance of ossification in staged human embryos. American Journal of Anatomy 134: 291–308

Oudet C 1979 Rythmes nycthemeral et saisonnier de la vitesse de croissance du squelette et de la susceptibilitè du cartilage condylien de la mandibule a l'egard des dispositifs orthopediques. Thèse de Doctorat en Biologie Humaine, Universite Louis Pasteur, Strasbourg

Persson M 1973 Structure and growth of facial suture. Odontology Review 24: 146

Persson K M, Roy W A, Persing J A, Rodeheaver G T, Winn H R, 1979 Craniofacial growth following experimental craniosynostosis and craniectomy in rabbits. Journal of Neurosurgery 50: 187–197

Petrovic A 1970 Recherches sur les mechanismes histophysiologiques de la croissance osseuse craniofaciale. Annals of Biology 9: 303

Petrovic A, Charlier S P 1967 La synchondrose spheno-occipitale de jeune rat en culture d'organes: mise en evidence d'un potentiel de croissance independant. Comptes Rendus de l'Academie de Science 265: 1511–1513

Petrovic A, Charlier S P, Herrmann G 1968 Les mecanismes de la croissance de la face. Recherches sur le cartilage de la cloison nasale et sur les sutures craniennes et faciales de jeunes rats en culture d'organes. Comptes Rendus de l'Association Anatomique 53: 1376–1382

Poswillo D E 1975 Causal mechanisms of craniofacial deformity. British Medical Bulletin 31: 101–106

Powell T V, Brodie A G 1964 Closure of the spheno-occipital synchondrosis. Anatomical Record 147: 15–23

Prahl B 1968 Sutural growth. Investigation on the growth mechanism of the coronal suture and its relation to cranial growth in the rat. Doctoral thesis, University of Nijmegen

Pritchard J J, Scott J H, Girgis F G 1956 The structure and development of cranial and facial sutures. Journal of Anatomy 90: 73–86

Pruzansky S 1961 Congenital anomalies of the face and associated structures. Thomas, Springfield, Ill

Pugeaut R 1968 Le probleme neuro-chirurgical des craniostenoses. Cahier de Médecine Lyonnais 44: 3343–3357

Rabischong P 1960 Étude des variations morphologiques du crane et de la main. Leurs relations avec les encephalopathies de l'enfance. Thèse médicale, no 57 Nancy

Ranley D M 1980 A synopsis of craniofacial growth. Appleton-Century-Crofts, New York

Ryoppy S 1965 Transplantation of epiphyseal cartilage and cranial suture. Acta Orthopaedica Scandinavica (supll 82) 1–106

Sakka M 1980 Morphologie evolutive, Table Ronde du CNRS, Paris

Sarnat B G 1963a Postnatal growth of the face: some experimental considerations. International congress of Plastic Surgery, Washington 3: 66, 423–424

Sarnat B G 1963b Postnatal growth of the upper face: some experimental considerations. Angle Ortodontist 33: 139–161

Sarnat B G 1968 Growth of bones as revealed by implant markers in animals. American Journal of Physical Anthropology 29: 255–286

Sarnat B G 1971 Clinical and experimental considerations in facial bone biology: growth, remodeling and repair. Journal of the American Dental Association 82: 876–889

Sarnat B G 1976 The postnatal maxillary–nasal–orbital complex: some considerations in experimental surgery. In: McNamara J A Jr (ed) Factors affecting the growth of the midface. Monograph 6, Craniofacial Growth Series. Center for Human Growth and Development, University of Michigan, Ann Arbor

Sarnat, B G, Engel M B 1951 A serial study of mandibular growth after removal of the condyle in the macaca rhesus monkey. Plastic and Reconstructional Surgery 7: 364

Sarnat B G, Wexler M R 1966 Growth of the face and jaws after resection of the septal cartilage in the rabbit. American Journal of Anatomy 118: 755–767

Schowing J 1959a Influence de l'excision du rhombencephale et du mesencephale sur la morphogenese du crane chez l'embryon de poulet. Comptes Rendus de l'Académie de Science 248: 2391–2393

Schowing J 1959b Influence de l'excision de mesencephale et du prosencephale sur la morphogenese du crane chez l'embryon de poulet. Comptes Rendus de l'Académie de Science 249: 170–172

Scott J H 1967 Dento-facial development and growth. Pergamon Press, London

Selman A J, Sarnat B G 1957 Growth of the rabbit snout after extirpation of the frontonasal suture: a gross and serial roentgenographic study by means of metallic implants. American Journal of Anatomy 101: 273–293

Selye H, Bajusz E 1958 Effect of denervation on experimentally induced changes in the growth of bone and muscle. American Journal of Physiology 192: 297–301

Shapiro H H 1954 Maxillo-facial anatomy with practical applications. London, Lippincott

Sicher E L 1980 Oral anatomy, 7th edn. Mosby, St Louis

Siegel M I 1976 Mechanisms of early maxillary growth — implications for surgery. Journal of Oral Surgery 34: 106–112

Sitsen A E 1933 Zur Entwicklung der Nahte des Schadeldaches. Zeitschrift fur Anatomie und Entwicklingsgesch 101: 121–152

Slavkin H C 1979 Development of craniofacial biology. Lea & Febiger, Philadelphia

Solow B, Tallgren A Head posture and craniofacial morphology. American Journal of Physical Anthropology 44: 417–436

Sperber G H 1981 Craniofacial embryology, 3rd edn. Wright, Bristol

Stamrud L 1959 External and internal cranial base. A cross sectional study of growth and association in form. Acta Odontologica Scandinavica 17: 239–244

Stark R B 1973 Development of the face. Surgery, Gynecology and Obstetrics 137: 403

Stenstrom S J, Thilander B L 1967 Facial skeleton growth after bone grafting to surgically created premaxillary suture defects: an experimental study on the guinea pig. Plastics and Reconstructional Surgery 40: 1–12

Stenstrom S J Thilander B J 1970 Effects of nasal septal cartilage resections on young guinea pigs. Plastic and Reconstructional Surgery 45: 160–170

Storey E 1972 Growth and remodeling of bone and bones. American Journal of Orthodontics 62: 142–165

Stutzmann J, Petrovic A 1976 Experimental analysis of general and local extrinsic mechanisms controlling upper jaw growth. In: McNamara J A Jr (ed) Factors affecting the growth of the midface.

Monograph 6, Craniofacial Growth Series. Center for Human Growth and Development, University of Michigan, Ann Arbor

Takagi Y 1964 Human postnatal growth of vomer in relation to base of cranium. Annals of Otology, Rhinology and Laryngology 73: 238–247

Tessier P, Delaire J, Billet J, Landais H 1965 Considerations sur le developpement de l'orbite. Ses incidences sur la croissance faciale. Revue de Stomatologie 63: 27–38

Theunissen J J W 1973 Het fibreuze periosteum. Doctoral thesis, University of Nijmegen

Thilander B, Ingervall B 1973 I. The human spheno-occipital synchondroses. II. A histological and microradiographic study of its growth. Acta Odontologica Scandinavica 31: 323–334

Thompson D 1968 On growth and form. Cambridge University Press, Cambridge

Toldt C 1912 Atlas d'anatomie humaine. Adaptation française par Lucien M. Paris, Editions Scientifique et Medical

Topinard P 1876 L'anthropologie. Reinwald, Paris

Tridon P 1958 Les dysraphies cranioencephaliques. Thèse medicale Nancy

Troitsky V 1932 Zur Frage der Formbildung des Schadeldaches (Experimentelle Untersuchung der Schaedeldachnhate und der damit verbundenen Erscheinungen). Zeitschrift fur Morphologie und Anthropologie 30: 504–534

Trowell O A, Chir B, Willmer E N 1938 Studies on the growth of tissues in vitro. VI. The effects of some tissue extracts on the growth of periosteal fibroblasts. Journal of Experimental Biology 16: 60–70

Vallois N V 1954 La capacite cranienne chez les Primates superieurs et le Rubicon cerebral. Comptes Rendus de l'Académie de Science 238: 1349–1351

Van der Klaauw C J 1945 Cerebral skull and facial skull. A contribution to the knowledge of skull structure. Arch. Neerl. Zool. 7: 16–37

Van der Klaauw C J 1948 Size and position of the functional components of the skull. Arch. Neerl. Zool. 9: 1–559

Van Limborgh J 1970 A new view on the control of the morphogenesis of the skull. Acta Morphologica Neerlando-Scandinavica 8: 143–160

Van Limborgh J 1982 Factors controlling skeletal morphogenesis. In: Dixon A D, Sarnat B G (eds) The international conference on factors and mechanisms influencing bone growth. Liss, New York

Van Limborgh J 1983 Morphogenic control of craniofacial growth. In: McNamara J A Jr, Ribbens K A, Howe R P (eds) In: The clinical alteration of the growing face. Monograph 14, Craniofacial Growth Series. Center for Human Growth and Development, University of Michigan, Ann Arbor

Verwoerd, C D A, Urbanus N A M, Verwoerd-Verhoef 1979 Growth mechanisms in skulls with facial clefts. Acta Otolaryngology 87: 335–339

Von Gudden B 1876 Recherche experimentale sur la croissance du crane. Delahaye, Paris

Watanabe M, Laskin D, Brodie A G 1957 The effect of autotransplantation on growth of the zygomato-maxillary suture. American Journal of Anatomy 100: 319–329

Weiffenbach J M 1972 Discrete elicited notions of the newborn's tongue. In: Bosma J F (ed) Third Symposium on Oral Sensation and Perception

Weinmann J P Sicher H 1955 Bone and bones, 2nd edn. Mosby, St Louis

Wieslander L 1974 The effect of force on cranio-facial development. American Journal of Orthodontics 65: 531–538

5. Comparative anatomy

M. Stricker, B. Raphael, C. Mentre, J. Van der Meulen, R. Mazzola

'Comparative anatomy is the fixed and permanent state of organogenesis in man' (Serres 1859).

THE ANIMAL SKULL

'For man, it is a humiliating truth that he must include himself in the class of Animals' (Buffon 1749).

A skull structure is first seen in the cyclostome fishes, which have no jaws. It becomes tripartitional in reptiles and achieves its tubular form in mammals.

The cephalic extremity of animals is divided into a neural and visceral cranium and directed forward in the horizontal plane, to aid in the search for food. Basically it is a jaw supported by the temporal bones. This jaw is alerted and indirectly activated by the sense of smell, by sight, and by hearing. It is guided by the brain, oriented by the vestibulocerebellar system. The visceral portion or dental cranium of the anthropologists is clearly predominant.

This malleable skull is subject to internal encephalic and external muscular and postural forces. The exocranial forces are influenced by the cervical and masticatory musculature and by cephalic posture. The evolution of the animal skull into the human skull proceeds through three transforming phases:

1. Vertebralization — the formation of a vertebral column is made possible by the selection of collagen fibres destined to produce a matrix for ossification.
2. Primatization — the progressive acquisition of an erect posture sets the forelimbs free.
3. Humanization — the modification of neurosensory priorities and of encephalic organization, leading to the acquisition of facial and above all of verbal expressions; culminating in the development of language.

Development of the primate starts with anthropogenesis, and hominization becomes engraved in the cerebral cortex, with motor functions within the precentral gyrus, and sensory functions within the postcentral gyrus.

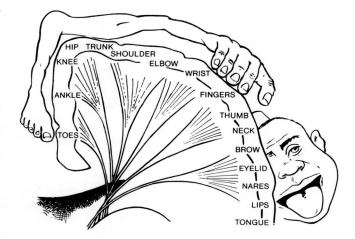

Fig. 5.1 The homunculus of Penfield.

The homunculus (Fig. 5.1) demonstrates the great importance of the orofacial structures, which represent one-third of its surface equal to that of the hand and that of the remaining part of the body. This rapid orofacial differentiation is probably related to the need for communication, brought about by social life.

MEANS OF STUDY

The comparative study of skulls requires reliable, definitive references. Previous anthropologists, such as Huxley (1868), based their study on the basilar plane, the nasion–basion, but progressive angulation of the base in vertebral evolution made this criterion unreliable.

The Vestibular plane linking the lateral semicircular canals is, however, a suitable plane of reference (Girard 1929) (Fig. 5.2). In fact, the vestibule orientates the cephalic extremity and stabilizes it in the three planes of space, thus enabling coordinated movements.

The studies performed by the Lille school have shown that the orientation of the vestibular plane on the face is

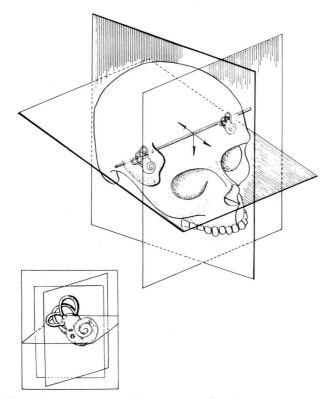

Fig. 5.2 The vestibular axis of Girard, Perez and Delattre.

constant. In addition to this criterion, the palatine plane and the posterior facial plane have also proved useful. These planes intersect angles which are essential anthropometric criteria in measurement and comparison:

1. the angle created by the intersection of vestibular and palatine planes measuring 15°;
2. the angle created by the intersection of the palatine and posterior facial planes measuring 150°;
3. the planum–clival angle or sphenoidal angle, which measures the opening of the basal compass (Fig. 5.3);

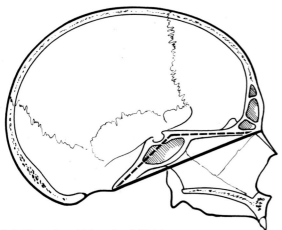

Fig. 5.3 The sphenoidal angle of Welcker.

4. the planum–pterygoid angle, which measures the orientation of the midface;
5. the palatobasilar angle of Escat, described in his inaugural thesis in 1894. It measures 20° in the neonate and 50–70° in the adult, and is considered to reflect facial projection.

HUMANIZATION OF THE SKULL

The mammalian and the human skull are composed of the same elements but differ greatly in shape. Aristotle considered the human characteristics to be the erect posture and the cephalization index, i.e. the ratio between the volume of the brain and body weight. The lower limit of cerebral volume is 800 ml (the cerebral Rubicon of Vallois 1954).

Morphological evolution divides the skull into morphofunctional entities (Sakka 1980) in which the composing elements develop in a manner dissociated in time and space.

The two tables of the cranial vault evolve in a different manner (Figs. 5.4 and 5.5). The outer table is under the influence of muscular factors, while the internal table is modified by neural factors. This is the reason why external and internal landmarks do not correspond and the value of external craniometry is questionable.

Humanization of the skull (Fig. 5.6) is the result of complex remodelling; the factors influencing this change are:

1. the alteration in postural forces from horizontal to vertical, and the influence of gravity;
2. the modification of the neurosensory hierarchy, in which vision takes precedence over olfaction;
3. the transformation of feeding patterns affecting the dental system and mastication;
4. the sophistication of facial and particularly of oral expression, by the acquisition of language, which is associated with the development of nasal respiration and the apparition of a larynx.

These changes take place simultaneously in the different sectors but will be considered separately here for the sake of convenience.

The brain

The modelling of the brain is the result of the moulding of the cerebral vesicles around the hypothalamus. The neopallium covers the archipallium, which corresponds to the regressing olfactory brain. This movement of the brain is organized around the vestibular axis and the vestibular plane, and proceeds in concordance with craniofacial evolution.

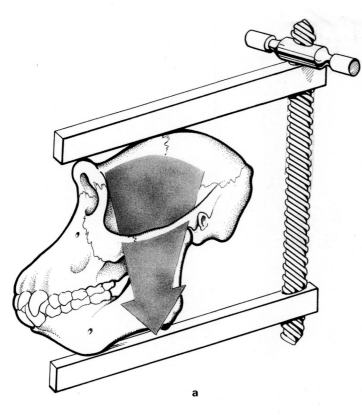

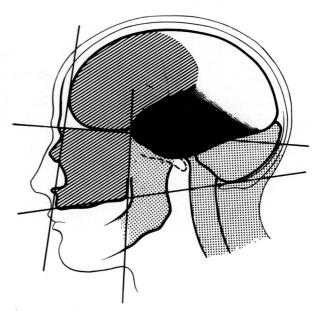

Fig. 5.5 Relationship between the territories of the brain and the skull.

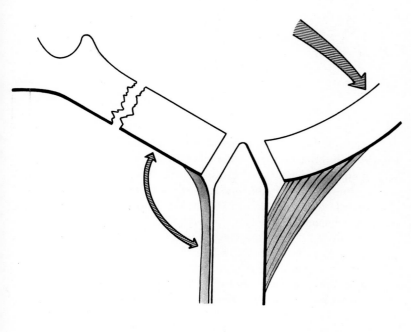

b

Fig. 5.4 Muscular influence on the outer table of the skull: (a) masticatory vice; (b) posture and gravity.

The alterations in the craniofacial relationship

In the animal the posterior part of the skull opens directly into the vertebral canal. Straightening of the trunk and curvature of the cervical spine, which are related to erect posture (Sakka 1980), lead to a posterior modification in the skull shape posteriorly. The skull basculates and the nape of the neck appears. The occipital funnel tilts backward and inferiorly and this movement causes the foramen magnum to assume a horizontal plane at the base of the skull. In addition the clivus moves upwards, together with the petrous parts of both temporal bones. As a result, the clivus–planum angle is reduced and the sphenoidal prominence penetrates into the skull (Fig. 5.7).

Laterally, the squamous parts of the temporal bone are displaced backwards. The tentorium cerebelli raises itself, together with the veins of the superior petrosal and lateral sinuses. This displacement opens a breach in the vault of the skull above the cartilaginous basiocciput, leaving a space (Fig. 5.8) for the complementary bones of Le Double (1903, 1906) which originate from the mesenchyme between the obelion and the inion. On the external aspect of the skull, the zygomatic arches, which resemble shafts, are secured to the vestibular axis.

Posteriorly, the insertion of the muscular masses marks the division between the posterior fossa, which is attached to the cervical spine, and the anterior part of the skull, which is in direct relation to the midface.

The displacement of the posterior skull affects the anterior arm of the basal compass, the planum. The basilar axis (planum–clivus) bends at its weakest point, the sella turcica. The planum elevates in a posterior direction and the clivus descends somewhat more in an anterior

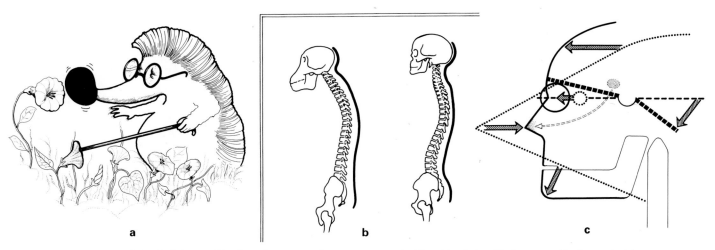

Fig. 5.6 Humanization of the skull by modification of posture and neurosensory priorities: (a) relationship between olfaction and vision; (b) change in posture; (c) scheme of craniofacial evolution.

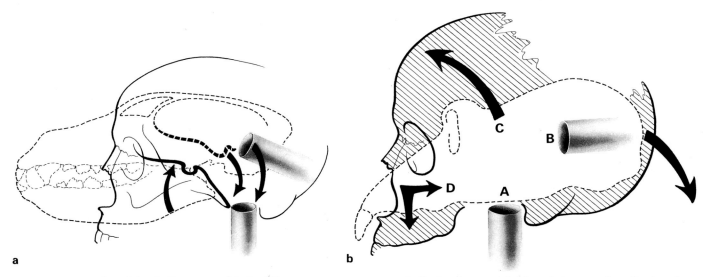

Fig. 5.7 Humanization of the skull represented in its different components. a = verticalization; b = occipital basculation; c = frontalization; d = facial retrusion.

direction, thus reducing the sphenoidal angle. This phenomenon is associated with shortening of the basilar axis.

According to Topinard (1891): 'the sphenoid is the only stationary bone of the skull and the centre around which all development takes place. Together with the pterygoids it forms a true flying buttress for the midface.'

The position of the (so-called) main facial block is dictated by the planum–pterygoid angle, and vertical elongation of the pterygoids produces an increase in the height of the nasal respiratory passage, especially behind in the choanal region.

The face, drawn towards the skull by the rise of the planum, is roofed anteriorly by the cribriform plate and by the horizontal part of the frontal bone. Posteriorly it is bordered by two vertical rami, the pterygoids, and laterally by the horizontal rami, the zygomas.

Because of the modifications due to the alimentary and sensory conditioning mentioned above, a regression occurs that opens the facial angle (Camper 1791) (Fig. 5.9). The snout thus becomes the mouth. This regression also involves the teeth, which are reduced in number from 40 to 32 and become changed in shape and in size.

The reduced size of the face, which is made lighter by pneumatization, releases the masticatory vice and frees the supraorbital region from its constraint, thus permitting verticalization of the eyes and frontalization of the orbit by elevation of the visual axis (Fig. 5.10). The orbit becomes vertical and separates from the temporal fossa at the anthropoid stage. The frontal bone moves forwards and downwards as telencephalization of the brain takes place. The frontal thrust over the nasal capsule determines the shape of the nose and also draws the temporal bones

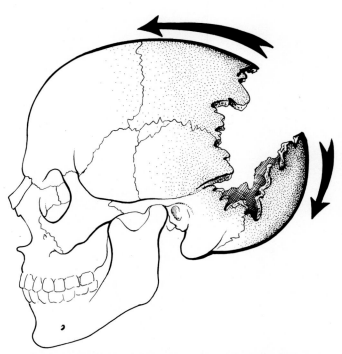

Fig. 5.8 Occipital basculation opens the breach filled by the parietal bones (the complementary bones of Le Double).

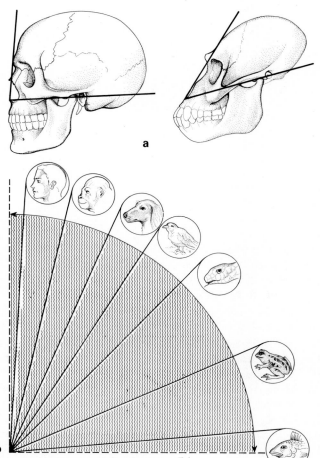

Fig. 5.9 The facial angle of Camper.

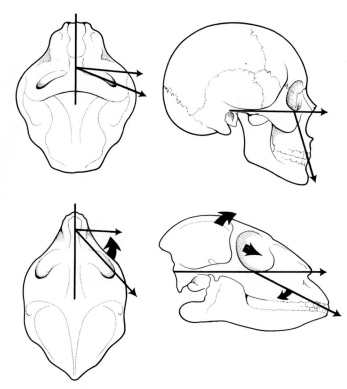

Fig. 5.10 Autonomization and verticalization of the orbital axis.

forwards, pushing the zygomas outwards to give shape to the cheek.

In the centre of the face, the sensory organs are no longer concentrated around the jaw but lie near the brain, where they are protected by the skull. The splanchnocranium gives way to the neurocranium, so that the cephalic extremity is no longer a jaw but a brain (Fig. 5.11).

In mammals a nasal respiratory part becomes apparent between the neural and visceral cranium. The turbinates and sinuses develop, completing the nasal fossa which appeared in reptiles by the formation of a palatal vault.

In the lateral region, evolution proceeds in a similar manner by condensation of bony elements and their integration in the skull.

The primitive reptilian joint between the square and the articular bones gives way to a mammalian articulation between the dental and squamous bones (Fig. 5.12). After a transitory stage of coexistence, only the dental/squamous joint remains, situated in the centre of a masticatory muscular complex. This is innervated entirely by the trigeminal nerve. The articular remnants which are incorporated into the skull as the petrous part of the temporal bones develop and the clivus is displaced, contributing to the formation of the middle ear.

A mechanical concept which is too strict must be avoided. The role of the brain is precocious and primordial,

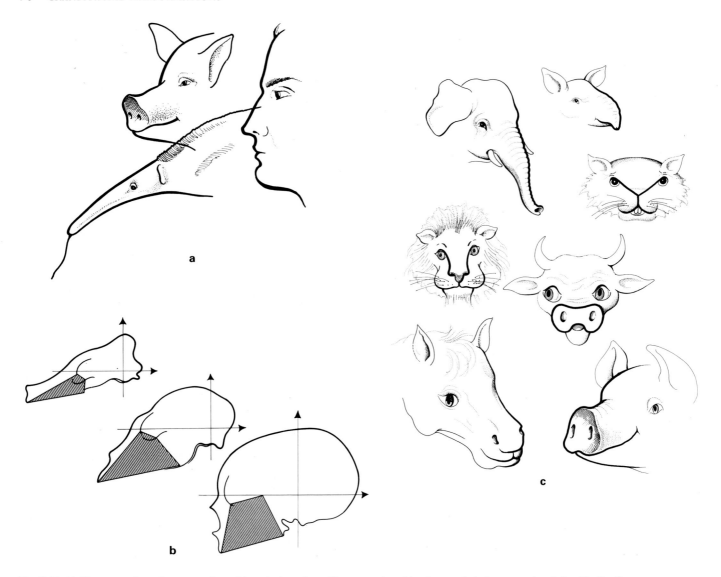

Fig. 5.11 (a) From muzzle and snout to face; (b) evolution of maxillary complex; (c) a humouristic interpretation (after Taullard).

as the studies of Schowing (1968) have demonstrated. The collection of phenomena which affect the craniofacial complex, including osseous expansion, muscular retraction, sensorial incorporation and perfection of facial proportions, was given the name 'cranial externation' by Sakka (1980). The skull expands, incorporating the adjacent structures under the influence of the brain.

MIMIC EXPRESSION AND LANGUAGE

Emotional mimic expression and communication with the outside world by verbal language have reached a high degree of development in the human species. Mimic expression is made possible by the action of the mimic muscles innervated by the facial nerve and the sensibility provided by the trigeminal nerve (Fig. 5.13). Individualization is due to typical morphological characteristics.

The mimic musculature has its origin in the sphincter colli of vertebrates. The elevation of the head devides the sphincter in two portions which develop in opposite directions. The vertebral portion forms the platysma, a continuous layer which extends from the clavicle to the mandible and the labial commissures, to which it gives off the risorius muscle. The dorsal portion is directed towards the superior region and divides itself in two layers: an occipital layer behind the ear, and a temporo-orbital layer in front of the ear.

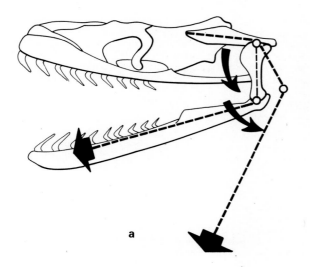

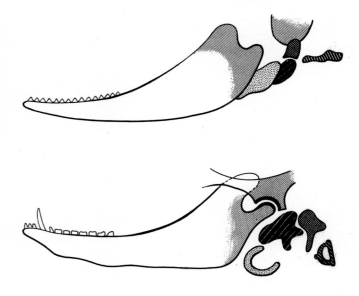

Fig. 5.12 Temporomandibular evolution from reptile to man:
(a) double articulation of the reptile; (b) progressive simplification with
cranial externation.

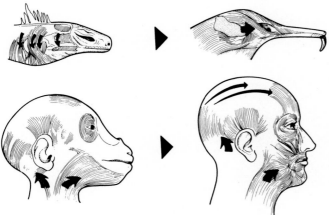

Fig. 5.13 Phylogenesis of mimic muscles.

Development and sophistication of the mask of mimic
muscles is dictated by the facial nerve, which augments its
distribution.

The laryngeal sphincter, originally a simple constriction
within the horizontal respiratory axis, evolves into a
sophisticated protective sphincter when vertical orientation
of the axis occurs and its muscular suspension to the
mandible is perfected.

The anterior portion of the mandibular bone seems to
correspond to the development of a phonatory instrument.
The formation of a mental projection proceeds simultaneously but its significance is controversial.

REFERENCES

Anthony J 1952 L'influence des facteurs encéphaliques sur la brisure
  de la base du crane chez les primates. Annales de Paléontologie
  38: 69–79
Baer J G 1958 Anatomie comparée des vertébrés. Masson, Paris
Baer J G 1965 Cours d'anatomie comparée des vertébrés. du Griffon,
  Neuchatel
Brachet A 1956 Traité d'embryologie des vertébrés. Masson, Paris

Buffon 1749 Histoire naturelle générale et particulière avec description
  du cabinet du Roy. Imprimerie Royale, Paris
Camper P 1791 Verhandeling over het natuurlijk verschil der
  wezenstrekken in menschen van onderscheiden landaart en
  ouderdom. Wild & Altheer, Utrecht
Cayotte J L 1970 Les grands chemins de l'homme. Discours de
  réception à l'Academie de Stanislas, Nancy

De Beer G R 1971 The development of the vertebrate skull. Clarendon Press, Oxford

Delattre A 1951 Du crane animal au crane humain. Masson, Paris

Delattre A, Fenart R 1960 L'hominisation du crâne étudiée par la méthode vestibulaire. Editions CNRS, Paris

Escat J M E 1894 Evolution et transformations anatomiques de la cavité naso-pharyngienne. Thèse médecine, Paris

Girard L 1929 L'attitude normale de la tête determinée par le labyrinthe de l'oreille. Bulletin Société Anthropologie de Paris 10: 79–99

Grasse P P 1967 Les mammifères. Traité de Zoologie, T16, Masson, Paris

Gregory W K 1929 Our face from fish to man. Putman, New York

Huxley J 1942 Evolution of the modern synthesis. Allen & Unwin, London

Huxley Th H 1868 De la place de l'homme dans la nature. Traduction Dally, Paris

Le Double A F 1903 Traité des variations des os du crane de l'homme et de leur signification au point de vue de l'anthropologie zoologique. Vigot, Paris

Le Double A F 1906 Traité des variations des os de la face de l'homme et de leur signification au point de vue de l'anthropologie zoologique. Vigot, Paris

Mentre C, Friot J M 1976 Aspect phylogénétique de la pyramide nasale. Société. Anatomique de Paris, 26 novembre

Perez F 1922 Craniologie vestibienne, ethnique et zoologique. Bulletin Société Anthropologie de Paris 3: 16–32

Piedelievre R, Clavin P, Derobert L 1948 La régression faciale au point de vue phylogénétique. Annales de Médecine Légale 29: 210–212

Rabischong P 1960 Etude des variations morphologiques du crane et de la main. Thèse médecine, Nancy

Rouviere H 1949 De l'animal à l'homme. Masson, Paris

Sakka M 1980 Morphologie évolutive, morphogénèse du crane et origine de l'homme. Table ronde CRNS, 24–27 juin, Paris

Schowing J 1968 Mise en évidence du role inducteur de l'encéphale dans l'ostéogénèse du crane embryonnaire des poulets. Journal of Embryology and Experimental Morphology 19: 83

Serres E R A 1859 Anatomie comparée transcendante. Principes d'embryogenie, de zoogenie et de teratogenie. Firmin Didot, Paris

Topinard P 1891 Transformation du crane animal en crane humain. Anthropologie 11: 659

Vallois N V 1954 La capacité cranienne chez les primates supérieurs et le Rubicon cérébral. Comptes Rendus de l'Academie des Sciences 12: 1349–1351

6. Craniofacial anatomy (surgical and functional)

M. Stricker, B. Raphael, J. Van der Meulen, R. Mazzola

'Every craftsman must be familiar with the material on which he works' (Henri de Mondeville, 1260–1320).

Once the remodelling processes of morphogenesis are completed we can divide the 'finished skull' into five anatomical sectors, corresponding to the morphogenic areas. One should bear in mind that the different skeletal components tend to adapt themselves to their assigned function, albeit with some architectural reshaping.

These anatomical sectors will be considered from a strictly surgical and functional point of view. In fact the great majority of craniofacial surgical procedures require access to the 'craniofacial frontiers', more commonly called the 'deep regions of the face' in standard texts on topographic anatomy.

Confidence in the performance of such an operation comes from precise acquaintance with the anatomy. From a surgical point of view, the cephalic extremity can also be subdivided arbitrarily into five sectors (Fig. 6.1) which correspond to the morphogenetic areas of growth:

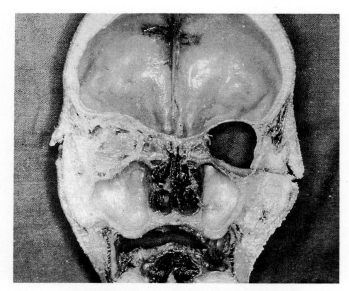

b

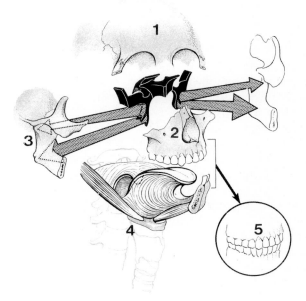

a

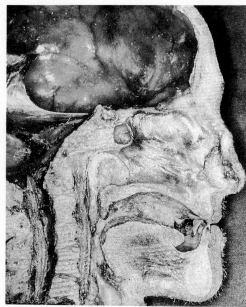

c

Fig. 6.1 The craniofacial section: (a) spatial impression of the different sectors; (b) coronal and (c) sagittal sections, showing the different sectors and the orbit, as zone of transition between the cranium and the face.

99

1. the cranium, corresponding to the encephalic areas;
2. the median sagittal area;
3. the spheno-temporo-zygomandibular area;
4. the linguo-mandibulo-hyovertebral area;
5. the alveolodental area, a regional feature specific to the face.

These regions do not constitute independent areas; their relations are always closely interdependent, particularly at certain connecting zones: craniomaxillary, craniomandibular and maxillomandibular. In addition, a complementary equilibrium is involved, which is related to the vertical position of the head on the vertebral column, the craniovertebral and vertebromandibular relationship.

The cephalic extremity consists of two structures, as dissimilar as they are inseparable: the cranium and the face.

THE CRANIUM

The term derives from the Greek word *cranios* (above). This ovoid structure, with its large posterior end, precariously balanced on the spine and occasionally referred to as the cranial box, is composed of two parts: the vault, a thin continuous cap serving as a protecting structure; and the base, a thick discontinuous pedestal, pierced by afferent blood vessels and efferent nerves, the true hilum of the brain.

The vault is formed by several bones which are not very thick: the frontal bone, single and median, the two parietals and the upper part of the occipital bone. On the lateral aspect there are two depressions: the two temporal fossae.

THE CRANIUM OF THE NEWBORN

The cephalic extremity, disproportionately large in comparison with the rest of the body, associates a voluminous cranium with protruding frontal and parietal eminences and a face which has only $\frac{1}{8}$ of the volume of the cranium. This will be $\frac{1}{16}$ at the age of 2 years and $\frac{1}{2}$ in adulthood. The skeletal parts, small in number, are separated from each other by bands of connective tissue — the sutures — or by cartilaginous zones — the synchondroses.

The sutures and the fontanelles (Fig. 6.2)

The skeletal parts do not yet reinforce the connective envelope in its totality. They are separated by membranous spaces named sutures when they divide two bones. The word fontanelle indicates a site of suture junction between three or four bones.

Anterior fontanelle. This is lozenge-shaped, measuring 4–5 cm in anteroposterior diameter and 3 cm in transverse

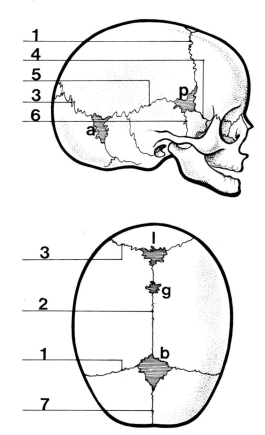

Fig. 6.2 Sutures: (1) coronal, (2) sagittal, (3) lambdoid, (4) sphenofrontal, (5) parietosquamous, (6) sphenotemporal, (7) metopic; frontanelles: b = bregmatic, l = lambdoid, p = pteric, a = asteric, g = Gerdy's.

diameter, and is placed at the junction of the sagittal and coronal suture. It closes at approximately 1 year of age, although some controversy still exists about this time.

Posterior fontanelle. Triangular in form, this is situated at the intersection of the sagittal and parieto-occipital sutures. It closes at 2 months of age.

Anterolateral fontanelle (of Gasser). This is rectangular and placed at the junction of the coronal and sphenoparietal sutures; closure takes place between the third and sixth month of life.

Posterolateral fontanelle. This is also rectangular and situated at the intersection of the parietomastoidal, parieto-occipital and occipitomastoidal sutures. Obliteration occurs during the first year.

These four fontanelles are placed at the four corners of the parietal bone. Other fontanelles, called accessory, may be observed: the sagittal fontanelle of Gerdy, lozenge-shaped, situated halfway between the anterior and posterior fontanelle, may be confused with the first of these two; the orbital fontanelle, on the inner side of the orbit between the frontal bone, the os planum and the smaller wing of the sphenoid, disappears commonly at the eighth month of fetal life; the nasofrontal fontanelle is located between the two frontal bones.

Remodelling of the cranium occurs during its passage through the pelvic canal by superposition of bones at suture levels.

Sutures of the vault. The sutures are 1–10 mm wide at birth and become obliterated progressively by a process of physiological synostosis. One can distinguish:

1. the coronal suture which separates the frontal and parietal bone. According to Richard (1957), synostosis of the coronal suture progresses rapidly until the sixth month and from then on more slowly up to the 18th month. Fusion of the inner tables is completed at 3 years of age;
2. the sagittal suture between the parietal bones. Fusion of the inner tables takes place at 2 years of age;
3. the metopic suture between the two frontal bones. It closes before birth and disappears towards the 15th month of life;
4. the lambdoidal sutures between the parietal bones and the occipital bone;
5. the parietosquamous sutures, separating the parietal bones from the squamous parts of the temporal bones;
6. the sphenofrontal and sphenoparietal sutures, normally of minor importance. Their role becomes significant in cranio-faciostenosis.

Sutures of the face. These are similar to those of the cranial vault. They unite the bones of the facial complex and the latter to the vault and the cranial base.

THE CRANIUM OF THE CHILD

The study by Sysak (1960) and that of Olivier (1965) on 38 skulls showed no characteristics typical for an infantile skull. The frontal eminences are more pronounced than the parietal. As a result, the maximum length of the skull must not be measured at the glabella but more superiorly, at the ophryon.

The metopic suture remains open in its lower part. The external occipital eminence is practically absent and does not appear until the age of 6 years, according to Augier (1931). The younger the bone the less relief is visible.

THE CRANIUM OF THE ADULT

The vault

This consists, first, of a hairy part: the scalp, i.e. the vertex and its surroundings. The differentiated cranial part of the skin has a number of characteristics (Fig. 6.3) besides its hairiness: an avascular plane between the galea (epicranial aponeurosis) and the pericranium, which is

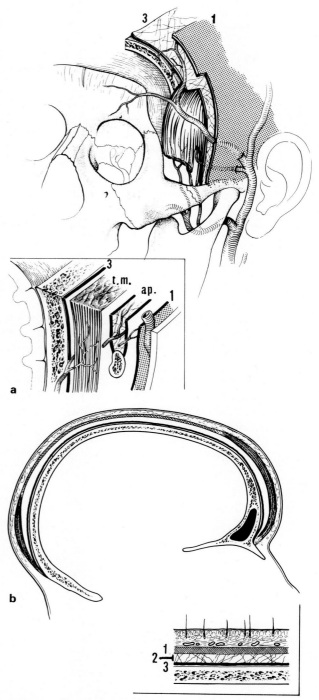

Fig. 6.3 The vault and the scalp: (a) vascular distribution over the lateral part of the vault and osteomuscular relationship; (b) fascial distribution (osteomuscular) within the scalp: (1) epicranium (epicranial aponeurosis or galea), (2) avascular plane of Merkel, (3) pericranium (or periosteum). t.m. = temporalis muscle; ap. = aponeurosis.

easily dissectable; a generous blood supply; a scarcity of nerve endings; and a well-vascularized pericranium — the outer layer of the cranial periosteum, the inner being the dura mater. The vault, a protective cap for the brain, is modelled by it, and therefore receives its vascular and nervous supply from two sources: anteriorly and posteriorly.

The second component of the vault is a hairless part, the forehead, whose morphological role is of cardinal importance. Some consider the forehead as the upper third of the face. From a strictly anatomical point of view the frontal bone and its orbital and nasal reflection are common to both the vault and the facial complex. However, ontogenical arguments attribute not only the forehead to the vault but also the shared lower part, the orbito-nasofrontal square.

The anatomical relationships of the vault are few and do not constitute chief hazards for the surgeon except along the midline. The relationships of importance (Fig. 6.4) are:

1. the dura mater, which is loose except at patent suture sites when physiological synostosis has not yet, taken place;
2. the vascular elements, particularly the superior longitudinal sinus with the torcular posteriorly, the transverse sinus and branches of the middle meningeal artery;
3. the frontal sinus. According to Poirier, the frontal sinus appears towards the end of the second year, reaches the size of a pea during the seventh year and attains its full development between 15 and 20 years.

The orbito-nasofrontal transitional zone constitutes the superior orbital contour, marked by the hairy eyebrows and the nasofrontal angle. The latter is formed by the skeletal nasal roof, a process of the frontal bone equivalent to the nasal protector of helmeted knights.

Laterally the break in the fronto temporal slope produces a contour, the gradation of which should be scrupulously preserved. Anteriorly, the vault supports the frontomalar and fronto-maxillonasal buttresses, which transmit the masticatory forces.

The base (Fig. 6.5)

The pedestal of the skull, or basal compass, is formed by a small number of bony elements whose characteristic solidity and stability are interrupted anteriorly. It constitutes a stairway with three unequal steps — the posterior, middle and anterior fossae — reproducing the tribasilar bone of Virchow (basiocciput, basisphenoid and presphenoid). The three bony elements, of which the anterior presphenoid or ethmoid forms the weak point, are disposed in two regions radiologically — anterior and posterior — sketching the arms of a compass whose centre is the sella turcica.

The anterior fossa. This space is of particular interest to the surgeon. It is a transitional structure which snakes along the whole length of the craniofacial territory, to which it provides the natural route of access. This territory can be divided into three portions: an unpaired midline area, or median sagittal sector, leading to the nasopharynx, immediately below; two paired lateral areas, the orbital

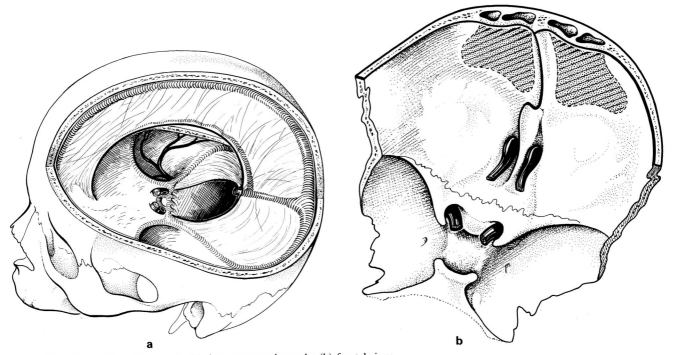

a   **b**

Fig. 6.4 The relationships of the vault: (a) dura mater and vessels; (b) frontal sinus.

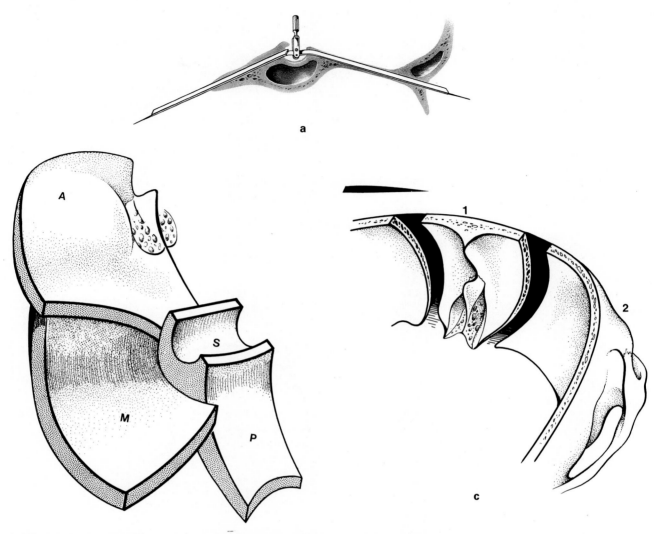

Fig. 6.5 The cranial base: (a) basal compass; (b) the three steps of Virchow: A = anterior, M = middle, P = posterior, S = sella turcica; (c) the areas of the anterior borderline: (1) medial (naso-maxilloethmoidal), (2) lateral (orbito-zygotemporal).

regions, where the morphogenetic sectors meet and which are therefore mandatory routes for the surgeon.

The anterior fossa, the main part of the presellar arm of the basal compass, is supported by the body of the sphenoid which extends laterally as the lesser wings, articulating with the frontal bone.

The cribriform plate lies sheltered at its centre. This area is identical to the olfactory grooves, as these support the olfactory bulbs and allow passage to their branches. This olfactory organ lying on the roof of the nose represents the main source of danger but laterally the optic canals are very close and anteriorly the frontal bone harbours the contaminated sinus.

The dura mater, which is free over three-quarters of its circumference, is firmly attached to the apophysis of the crista galli and to the foramen caecum, an important surgical landmark. Laterally, the orbital roofs, often convex and sometimes marked by spicules, terminate at the lateral root of the lesser wing.

The middle fossa. This extends from the posterior border of the lesser wings of the sphenoid to the upper border of the petrous pyramids. The endocranial portion, related to the temporal lobes, is only indirectly involved in surgical procedures. However, osteotomies carried laterally or distally in the anterior fossa must respect the integrity of the dura in the middle fossa. The central region is to be avoided because of the increasing risk encountered here.

The base forms the neurovascular hilum of the skull and the foramina are situated mainly in the middle fossa, pointing in the following directions to the orbit: through the optic foramen and the sphenoidal fissure; to the face, through the foramina rotundum, ovale and spinosum; and to the neck, through the carotid canal and the foramen lacerum. The middle meningeal artery and its branches run in bony grooves, starting in the lateral part of the middle fossa.

The posterior cerebellar fossa. This is an area of no interest for the craniofacial surgeon.

THE FACE

The centrofacial complex (Fig. 6.6)

This has the shape of a pyramid with a wide base and constitutes the central part of the face, extending backwards to the nasopharynx. It corresponds to the sagittal medial morphogenetic sector.

This middle third, a maxillo-ethmoidonasal complex, is framed by the two maxillary segments, buttressed between by their horizontal plate (the palatal vault), and firmly secured by the premaxillary projection anteriorly.

The maxillae are suspended from the middle part of the frontal bone and covered by the bony bridge of the nose, which rests on three thin sagittal plates: the medial walls; an orbitoethmoid mosaic of translucent bone; and the osteocartilaginous nasal septum.

The tip of the nose crowns the whole, modelled by its cartilages. Deep inside, the centrofacial complex supports the velum or rather the palatopharyngeal muscle slings (Chancholle 1980) (Fig. 6.7).

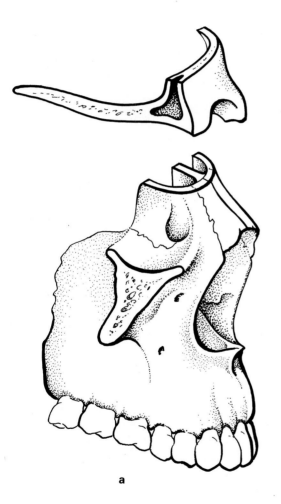

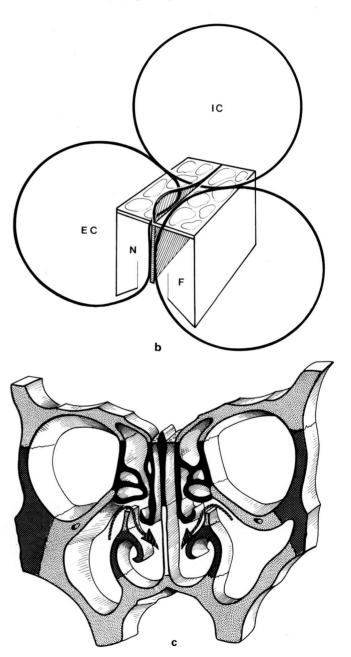

Fig. 6.6 The centrofacial pyramid: (a) the nasal maxillo-ethoidonasal unit; (b) nasal fossae (NF): the vascular meeting point between the external (EC) and internal (IC) carotid systems; (c) pneumatization.

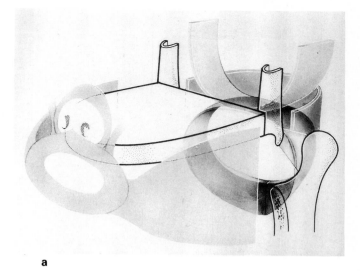

a

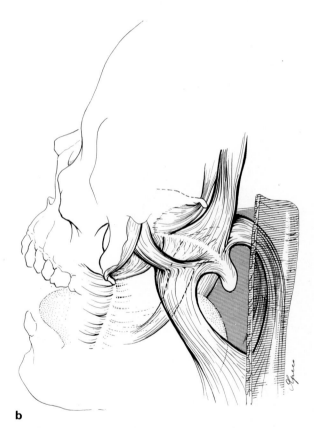

b

Fig. 6.7 The muscular slings: (a) the anterior facial sling of Chancholle; (b) the posterior facial sling or velopharyngeal sphincter.

Sensation is provided by the infraorbital nerves, originating from the maxillary branch of the trigeminal nerve (V2).

The blood supply is from the facial artery, superficial and deep (internal) maxillary arteries, and it must be stressed that this territory forms a transitional zone between the internal and external carotid systems.

The characteristic fragility of the complex stems not only from the translucent bony mosaic described above but also from the presence of air cavities — the nasal fossae and their accessory sinuses — which are very prone to infection.

The orbitonasal junction contains the ducts of the lacrimal system.

THE LATERAL SPHENO-TEMPORO-ZYGOMANDIBULAR SECTORS

These are the corridors (Fig. 6.8) from the vault of the skull to the mandible, the oral cavity and the pharynx. Their meaning is essentially dynamic, by reason of the presence of the temporalis muscle, the predominant element of the craniomandibular relationship.

These lateral corridors widen towards the skull base and communicate freely with the pterygoid regions, which contain the second component in the dynamics of the mandible i.e. the pterygoid muscles. Their shape is that of an incomplete bony funnel with a skin covering, circumscribed by the greater wing of the sphenoid superiorly and medially and by the squamous part of the temporal bone medially and posteriorly. The external hemi-circumference consists for nine-tenths of its extent of the temporal arch.

This funnel leads inferiorly to the ramus, the third component in movements of the mandible, situated anterior to the external auditory meatus.

The junction inferiorly is with the mandibular sector by means of the masseter, a muscular offshoot of the temporalis, and laterally it is with the cervical corridor, the zone through which the vessels course. The profusion of important structures must be noted: they involve the vascular axes, the deep facial and superficial temporal arteries and the third division of the trigeminal nerve.

The pterygoid and the tuberosity constitute the anterior internal wall. The bony auditory canal, placed on the mastoid, represents the posterior wall. The inner slope of the funnel forms a thick, resistant sphenomalar beam, which extends from the pterion.

The outer part, purely cutaneous above as far as the zygoma, ends below in the parotid compartment. The facial nerve emerges here as its superior temporofacial branch and constitutes the chief hazard in surgical approaches.

THE ORBIT

This transitional bony cavity between the skull and the face is one-third ethmoidal, one-third sphenoidal and one-third maxillonasal. Classically it has the form of a pyramid with a quadrangular base, but according to Winkler (1964) it is more often triangular. The funnel of the orbit is approximately 30 mm in size in the adult, with a depth of

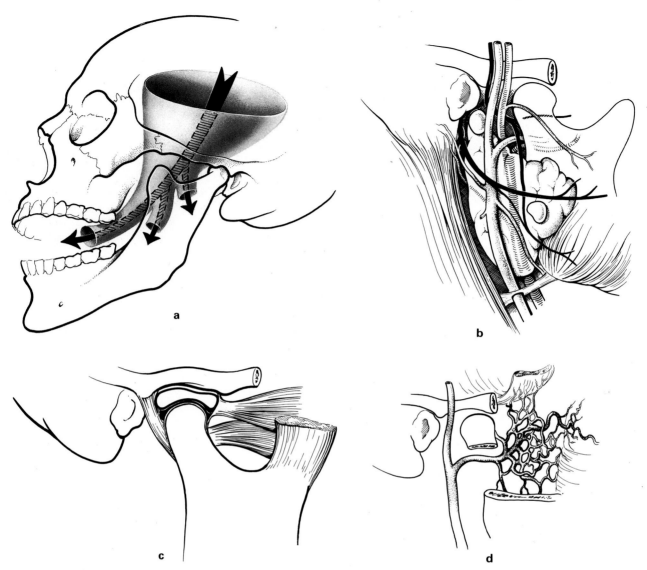

Fig. 6.8 The lateral sector: (a) the temporal funnel; (b) the vascular axis and facial nerve; (c) the temperomandibular joint; (d) deep vascular axis of the face and its venous plexus.

45 mm. The anterior orifice has a height of 35 mm and a width of 40 mm; the main orbital axis runs obliquely forward and outward.

The orbit consists of two parts: the fragile orbital cone and the anterior orbital ring — thick and resistant, the true surgical orbit (Fig. 6.9).

The eyeball, its motor apparatus and the fatty tissue are held within the periosteal sac of the periorbit, which forms an anatomical and surgical plane allowing for easy dissection from the bony walls. At the rim this sac passes into the fibroelastic tissue of the eyelids and is continuous with the septum.

The eyeball, a sphere 24 mm in diameter and 6.5 ml in volume, lies well forward in the cavity, protected by the movable anterior wall of the eyelid and lodged in the cavity formed by Tenon's capsule.

The orbital fat contained within the septum forms the fatty pad of Charpy, organized into several compartments and vulnerable to injuries.

The anterior wall (Fig. 6.10), a movable partition, is formed by the two eyelids, attached to the periphery by the palpebral ligaments and suspended at the edges from the septum radiating over the eyelids. The lids are lined by the conjunctival mucosa and glide over the eyeball, especially the upper lid. They protect the globe and spread the film of tears, later drained to the nasal cavity by a system of ducts.

Each eyelid has a central ocular and a peripheral orbital

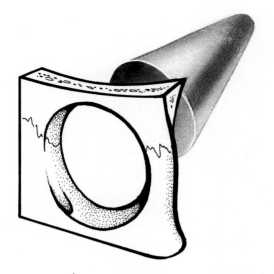

Fig. 6.9 The two parts of the orbit: the posterior cone and the anterior ring or movable orbit.

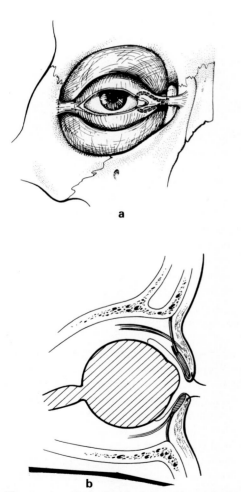

Fig. 6.10 The anterior palpebral wall of the orbit: (a) frontal view; (b) sagittal view.

part. Seen from in front, one distinguishes between the ciliated lateral temporal zone and the medial nasolacrimal zone.

THE LINGUO-HYOMANDIBULO-VERTEBRAL SECTOR (Fig. 6.11)

Extending on either side and fused medially, this sector forms the cephalic floor. It has the shape of a horseshoe, open above and behind. It comprises a mobile bony mandibular framework and a muscular suspension mechanism for static and dynamic balance of the tongue and laryngotracheal apparatus (Fig. 6.12). In front it circumscribes the oral cavity, while behind it has close and complex relations with the muscles of the pharynx, namely the superior constrictor, which provides support from the midline cranially. Thus we can speak of the dynamic pharyngo-linguo-hyomandibular complex (muscle sling of Chancholle).

THE ALVEOLODENTAL SECTOR

The alveolus lives and dies with the tooth (Fig. 6.13), the dental organ conditioning its bony and fibromucous environment, the 'periodontium'. This alveolodental entity is important in all areas of medicine, from physiology to the treatment of disease.

Teeth often characterize the pathology of the face,

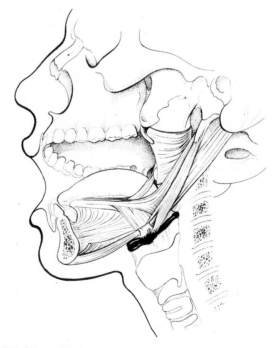

Fig. 6.11 Linguo-hyomandibulo-vertebral sector.

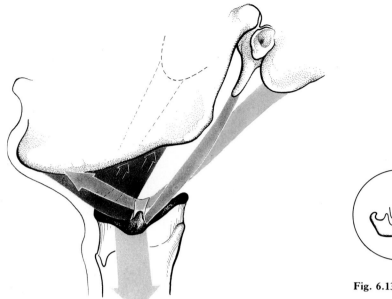

Fig. 6.12 Suspension of the visceral axis by means of the hyoid bone.

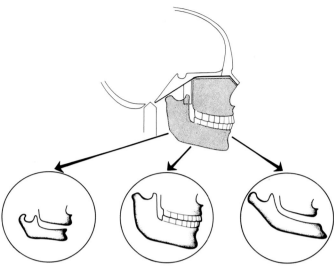

Fig. 6.13 The three ages of the alveolodental sector.

malformations not excepted; they suffer the direct or indirect impact of the malformation.

The relationship between the dental arches defines what is conventionally called 'occlusion', i.e. maximum inter-cuspidation between the arches, sanctioning the cranio-maxillomandibular relation. It is established only at the time of the second dentition.

In the edentulous baby, where swallowing is primarily labial during suckling, a relation exists between the gum margins. In the child with deciduous or mixed dentition, the occlusion changes as the teeth erupt and the prepub-ertal increase of hormonal secretion occurs. In the adolescent and the adult, a specific type of occlusion is established. Normally its stability is definitive. However, the alveolodental sector also has an adaptive character to be stressed, emanating from its compensatory potential. In fact, orthodontic correction involves this region in 90% of cases.

ORAL CAVITY (Fig. 6.14)

This compartment has four walls and two orifices, whose movements are involved in respiratory and digestive physiology.

The walls consist of:

1. a bipartite roof, formed anteriorly by the rigid bony palate, which is fixed and bears the alveolar ridge; and posteriorly by the soft palate which is mobile and can move backwards and upwards;
2. a pliant floor, supported by a muscular hammock from the hyoid bone and itself supporting the tongue, which emerges from it in the midst of the linguohyomandi-bular complex;
3. two side-walls, the cheeks, whose elasticity and contrac-tility produced by the buccinator slings permit great variations in the size of the cavity.

The orifices are two in number:

1. the anterior orifice, a simple structure with sphincteric activity, animated by the orbicularis oris and its connec-tions with the musculocutaneous mask of the face;
2. the posterior orifice, or 'isthmus of the gullet', both a sphincter and an anti-reflex valve.

This structural complexity is characterized by a close inter-action between the different components, both at rest as well as in the performance of the main oral functions (respiratory, phonatory, alimentary). These various visceral functions are not all automatic and stereotyped;

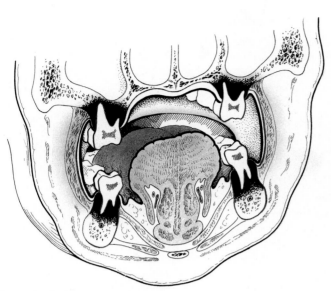 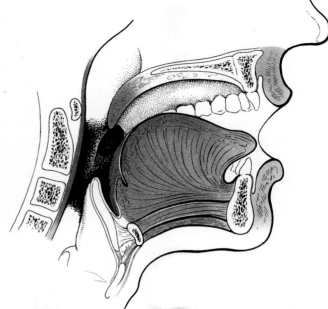

Fig. 6.14 The oral cavity.

they are integrated into the specific orofacial comportment of the individual, a mixture of the innate and the acquired, conferring an intrinsic dynamic behaviour.

At the heart of this dynamic interchange the antagonism between tongue and lips is dominant, and the resultant effect represents the primordial element in positioning of the teeth and thus in the equilibrium of occlusion.

CRANIOMETRY

Many craniometric studies have attempted to determine whether the development of the skull is dependent on the growth of the brain. Of course, this does not apply to the craniosynostoses. We shall here consider successively the clinical and then the radiographic methods of craniometry, particularly techniques permitting assessment of malformation rather than mere volume.

Clinical or external craniometry

Clinical measurements are subject to error, as the bony skull is surrounded by a fatty and muscular skin envelope which varies considerably in thickness from place to place. Nevertheless, clinical craniometry remains of great practical interest.

SKULL CIRCUMFERENCE

This is measured with a soft tape and refers to the greatest circumference of the vault, comprising the frontal and parietal eminences and the most prominent part of the occiput.

In the particular case of cranial pathology, this parameter is insufficient as it does not give information on the shape of a skull whose growth is not uniform in all directions. For this reason, different diameters must be measured.

THE DIAMETERS

As the skull is not spherical in shape, two diameters have to be considered.

The anteroposterior diameter is measured by calipers or a compass with curved arms between the extreme points of the sagittal plane, and joins the glabella to the most distant part of the occipital vault.

The biparietal diameter, or maximum width, is the greatest distance between the two parietal eminences, just above the external auditory meati. To these two fundamental measurements may be added measurement of the minimum frontal diameter. This diameter must be determined using a compass with curved arms, whose tips must be placed behind the external orbital apophyses of the frontal bone. This diameter gives the width of the anterior part of the skull.

Radiographic measurements

Radiography affords the clinician greater precision in his judgements, because the thickness of the bone and skin coverings can be excluded from the measurements and, in some cases, the features of the skull base can be taken into consideration. However, the standard anteroposterior and lateral views require correction for the radiographic magnification, unless teleradiography is used. Like many authors, we prefer the radiographic measurements for assessing the longitudinal, transverse and vertical diameters. The last, of course, is clinically inaccessible.

THE DIAMETERS

Measured on anteroposterior views, the biparietal diameter or maximum endocranial width is the distance between the most widely separated points of the parietal eminences. The anteroposterior diameter or maximum endocranial length is the distance between the nasion and the inion.

The vertical diameter is defined sometimes as the distance between the vertex and the pyramid of the petrous bone and sometimes as the projection of the vertex on the nasio-basion line (Bertelsen 1958). This method does not prejudge the position of the vertex and eliminates the impression of undue elevation of the vault in certain craniostenoses with a marked anteriorly situated vertex. In addition, basilar impression as a source of error is also reduced.

CEPHALIC INDICES

The cephalic indices are ratios of two diameters. They provide a quantitative picture of the morphological appearance of the skull, in both horizontal (horizontal cephalic index) and sagittal (vertical cephalic index) planes.

Horizontal cephalic index (HCI, Retzius index):

HCI = maximum width/maximum × 100

The normal range is between 76 and 80, the limits of mesocephaly (Pugeaut 1968, Rabischong 1960). Outside that range we can refer to dolichocephaly and to brachycephaly. The index can change with age; the child aged 7 years is thus more brachycephalic than the newborn.

Vertical cephalic index (VCI):

VCI = height of skull/length of skull × 100

The normal range is between 58 and 63, but the figure is of little practical value.

BASE OF SKULL

The complexity of the contours of the base of the skull and

its dual allegiance to both the face and the cranium make it difficult not only to take measurements but also to assess the results. The angle of Welcker is the only measurement made at all frequently, its magnitude being sometimes useful in pathology. Many authors consider this to be the only quantitative value for the base of the skull.

The sphenoidal angle, or angle of Welcker, is defined as the obtuse angle lying between the horizontal plane which joins the centre of the sella and the nasion and the plane of the quadrilateral plate. Its normal values range between 115° and 120° in the adult and between 130° and 140° in the newborn (Lefebre 1955). According to Bertelsen 1958, the mean is 117° before the age of 20 years and 116° thereafter.

The basal angle of Bogaert (between the nasion–tubercle and sella–basion lines) has substantially the same values as the angle of Welcker.

The foramino-clival angle is determined by the plane of the clivus and the line joining the basion and the opisthion. The normal value is 125° ± 2.5° after the age of 4 years.

The facial angle of Cloquet lies between the line joining the nasion to the alveolar tip and that running from the latter to the basion. Its normal value is 62°.

The intercanthal interval or distance between the medial walls of the orbits is measured on teleradiography in the anteroposterior view. This interval gives the distance between the orbits and is complementary to clinical measurements and to the interpupillary and intercaruncular intervals.

CRONQVIST INDEX (Fig. 6.15)

This index relates the cranial measurements to measurements of the face. It is defined by the following formula:

$$I = \frac{\text{height} + \text{length} + \text{width}}{\text{intercondylomandibular distance}} \times 10$$

According to Lacamp 1973 this index is normal both in the craniostenoses and in microcephaly.

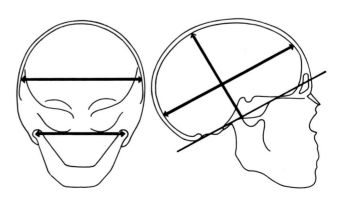

Fig. 6.15 The Cronqvist index.

Direct planimetry: extension to cranial volumetry

Some authors, recently including Frerebeau & Jourdan (1975) in Montpellier, have used the Kent planimeter, a polar planimeter, capable of determining the plane surfaces of complex geometric figures. A wheel within this instrument rotates and measures the cranial surfaces as seen in anteroposterior and lateral films of the skull.

Volumetry rests on the assumption that the cavity of the skull resembles that of an ellipsoid. Jouve et al (1973) have developed a formula which assesses the volume of the skull from craniometry and a single linear measurement.

The measurements obtained provide an objective assessment, as a percentage, of the increase in cranial areas and volumes following corrective operations.

Many other very complex formulae have been suggested. Of these, the formula of Rabischong yields fairly precise results, the values obtained being close to those revealed by a cast.

MORPHOLOGY

One may distinguish two territories characterized by their type of covering: the hairy scalp — cranial; and the hairless skin — facial — marked by hairy zones at typical sites — the eyebrows, the moustache and the beard, varying with the sex.

The visible surface of the face therefore extends from the hairline (trichion) to the superior cervical crease. Three superposed levels may be differentiated (Fig. 6.16a): the upper frontal level, belonging to the cranium and located between the hairline and the upper orbital ridge; the middle maxillary level, situated between the upper orbital ridge and the occlusal plane; and the inferior mandibular level, located between the occlusal plane and the upper cervical fold.

The proportions have long been established. Initially artists and sculptors recognized a balance between these levels according to the rule of thirds (Leonardo da Vinci).

The facial skin is lined by the mimic muscles (Fig. 6.16b), which are innervated by the facial nerve. In addition, the face possesses and shelters sensory organs open to the outside by fissures and orifices with varying or no mobility. The mobile orifices are the palpebral fissures and the buccal cleft. The semimobile orifices are the nostrils and the immobile orifices are the external auditory meatis.

ORGANIZATION

Architecture

The relations between the cranium, the maxilla and the mandible have been discussed above.

CRANIOMAXILLARY RELATIONSHIP

The skull and the facial mass form a fixed relationship (Fig. 6.17), not only of contiguity but also of continuity and interdependence. Wedged beneath the base of the skull, the facial mass is connected to the pterygoid process through the intermediate palatine bones, and to the body of the sphenoid through the septonasal strut. It is fixed laterally by the zygomatic arch and suspended from the frontal bone by the apophyses of the malar bones and of the maxillae.

It is organized in three sagittal plates: two laterally solid and thick, and extending from the pterions; and one medially, the septovomerian strut, which is placed on the intermaxillary zone and is responsible for projection of the premaxillary through the vomeropremaxillary suture in a fan-shaped manner.

The palatine bone, a small oddly shaped piece of bone, is in our view the key to the architecture of the face. It leans against the pterygoid process, takes part in the formation of the orbit, frames the vomer and gives way to the deep vessels of the facial complex. Its role is crucial in determining malformations due to synostosis (retromaxillary) and to palatal clefting (Latham 1976).

The bony architecture is conditioned by the nature and orientation of the forces acting on the skeleton. The facial region is subject to the vertical constraints of mastication and therefore arranges its osseous trabeculae vertically in areas of strength, the pillars of Weinmann & Sicher (1955). These pillars are separated by zones of weakness.

The pillars (Fig. 6.18) are composed of a vertical part and horizontal reinforcements and their structure has been well described by Benninghoff (1931), Ombredanne, (1909), Felizet (1895), Weinmann & Sicher (1955).

The zones of weakness are often caisson-type air cavities, the role of which is important in the transmission of forces.

The facial complex is weakened by the presence of two kinds of cavities: air cavities, accessory to the nasal fossae — these are the so called sinuses of the face, whose extent determines the degree of pneumatization; and receptor cavities — these are the orbits, for the peripheral receptors of vision.

CRANIOMANDIBULAR RELATION

The relationship between the mobile mandible and the skull is variable in a dual way: directly through the temporo-mandibulodental joint of Frey, the position of the glenoid conditioning that of the condyle; and indirectly through the shrouds of the temporalis and the pterygoid muscles.

The mandible consists of four parts: the bony basilar arch or body, the alveolodental arch, and the two ascending rami. The bony architecture is organized in

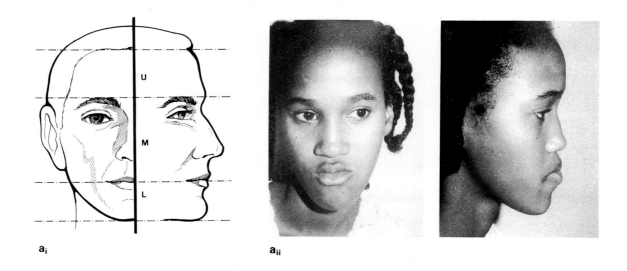

a_i

a_ii

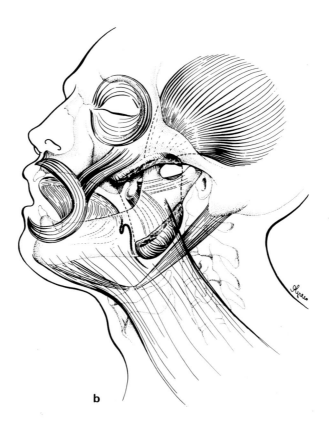

b

Fig. 6.16 (ai,aii), (b)

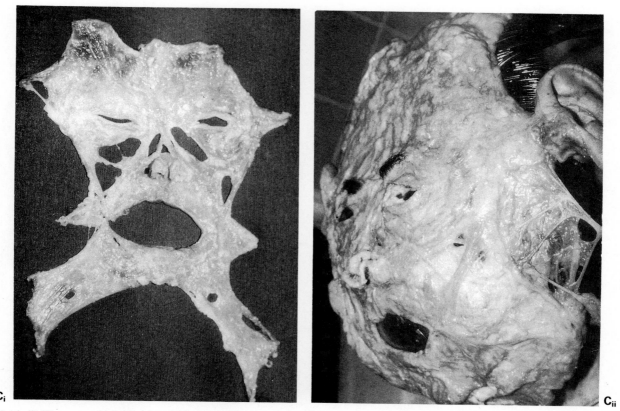

C_i   C_{ii}

Fig. 6.16 (ai,aii) The upper third (U), the middle third (M), and the lower third (L) of the face; (b) the mimic muscles; (c) dissection in adult and infant.

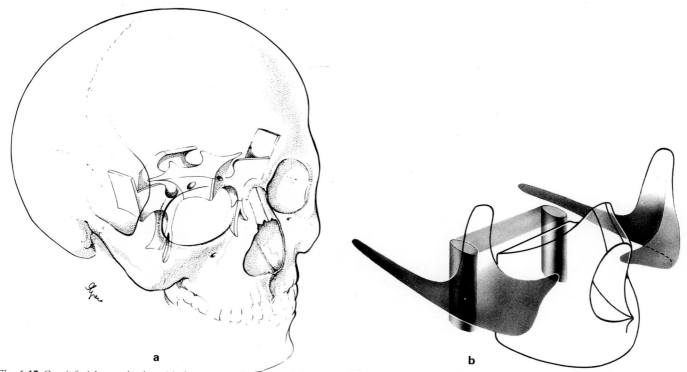

a   b

Fig. 6.17 Craniofacial organization: (a) the commanding post of the sphenoid; (b) the face framed by the zygomatic arch and the pterygoids.

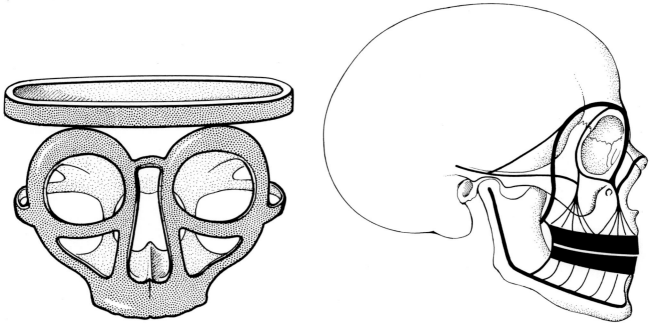

Fig. 6.18 The facial architecture: the pillars according to Weimann–Sicher–Benninghoff.

trabeculae arranged in the axis of the bone and demonstrable by Indian ink impregnation (Vanneville 1971).

MAXILLOMANDIBULAR RELATIONS

These are both direct and indirect: direct, through the masseter and pterygoid muscles; and indirect, via the temporo-mandibulodental joint. The maxilla and mandible are separated by the buccal cavity, which contains one of the elements essential to this relationship — the lingual muscle or tongue — attached to the mandible but orientating its action in all directions. The mandible supports the lingual musculature and also the hyoid bone which holds the apparatus of the larynx.

Dynamics

In man, an erect mammal, the head is balanced on the vertebral axis between two main muscle masses: laterovertebral posteriorly; and masticatory and mandibulohyoid anteriorly (Brodie's schema) (Fig. 6.19).

The muscles are arranged in slings which are interdependent. A failure of balance affecting one sling leads to disturbed equilibrium in adjacent slings. This forms part of a chain reaction.

The adipose compartments in the temporal (buccal fat pad of Bichat) and pterygomaxillary region fulfil an undisputable mechanical role. As Latham (1970) emphasized, they transmit the pressure exerted by the muscles to the skeleton.

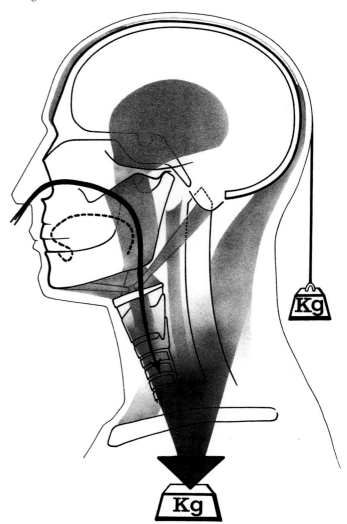

Fig. 6.19 The modified Brodie scheme.

REFERENCES AND BIBLIOGRAPHY

Augier M 1931 Squelette céphalique. In: Poirier, Charpy (eds) Traité d'Anatomie Humaine, Tome 1, Fasc 1. Masson, Paris

Bernard R, Jouve P, Pinsard N et al 1973 La radio-planimétrie cranio-faciale, méthode d'estimation du dévelopement cérébral. Son application à la détermination des microcéphales. Journal de Radiologie, Electrologie et Médecine Nuclèaire 54: 285–290

Bertelsen T I 1958 The premature synostosis of the cranial sutures. Thèse médecine, Copenhagen

Chancholle A R 1980 Les boucles musculo-apóneurologiques velo-pharyngofaciales. Etude fonctionnelle. Annales de Chirurgie Plastique 25: 135–146

Lacamp B 1973 Evaluation des dimensions du crâne de l'enfant normal de 0 à 7 ans. Application à la pathologie cranienne. Thèse médecine, Toulouse

Latham R A 1976 An appraisal of early maxillary growth mechanisms. In: McNamara J A (ed) Factors affecting the growth of the midface. University of Michigan, Ann Arbor

Lefebvre J, Faure C, Metzger J 1955 Action du cerveau sur le crâne au cours des premières années de la vie. Journal de Radiologie, Electrologie 36: 297–307

Olivier G 1965 Anatomie anthropologique. Vigot. 488pp

Ombredanne L 1909 Maladies des machoirnes. Baillière, Paris

Pugeaut R 1968 Le problème neurochirurgical des craniosténoses Cahiers Médicaux Lyonnais 44: 31

Rabischong P 1960 Etude des variations morphologiques du crâne et de la main. Thèse médecine, Nancy

Richard J 1957 Contribution à l'étude radiologique des sutures craniennes chez l'enfant normal dans la microcéphalie et dans la maladie de Minkowski–Chauffard. Thèse médecine, Paris

Sysak N S 1960 The age morphology of the human cranium. Anatomischer Anzeiger 108: 1–19

Weinmann J R, Sicher H 1955 Bone and bones: fundamentals of bone biology, 2nd edn, Kimeton, London

Winckler G 1964 Manuel d'anatomie topographique et fonctionnelle. Masson, Paris. 524pp

7. Microanatomy and pathology of craniofacial structures

R. Dambrain

INTRODUCTION

The development and growth of the skull and face is the result of a precise programme in time and space. This programme, in turn, is dependent upon the activity of bipolar cartilage and the bony sutures as well as the apposition–resorption mechanism which takes place at the surface of the skeleton.

The first part of this chapter is devoted to the study of this programme; the second is reserved for the craniofacial anomalies which are caused by disturbances of this process.

In the first part, histological and microradiographic observations on the normal growing child and adult craniofacial structures provide suitable material to study the manifold activities taking place at the level of the cranial base.

This research will enable us to understand the conditions necessary for a balance to be maintained between the skull and its developing cerebral contents and the growing dental material in the maxillary complex.

The second part is a study of craniofacial abnormalities. These will be divided into different sections: the first concerns the premature and localized closure of the sutural gaps in craniosynostosis and faciostenosis and the second will be devoted to various important dysmorphic syndromes which are called (cerebro-) craniofacial dysplasias.

MATERIAL AND METHODS

The skulls of ten human fetuses, from 15 to 20 weeks old, were thoroughly examined. Control samples of the skull from newborn children, or from children under 1 year old, were difficult to obtain. Indeed, the majority of the skulls available came from children of the same age as the abnormal subjects. These had died from cardiac or renal diseases, and there was indirect or direct associated skeletal pathology. That is why suture specimens from a little girl who died suddenly at 9 months, as the result of a thymoma, have been used as control segments. To this exceptional case should be added 18 fragments, comprising sutures belonging to normal sagittal and coronal systems, taken at the time of a neurosurgical operation. These specimens were available to the pathologists when the skull was being remodelled in the treatment of skull dysmorphies, particularly craniostenosis. Their interest is due to the fact that in faciostenosis surgery bony tissues cannot be removed. This is the reason why, until now, we obtained a collection of specimens mainly belonging to the vault.

Thirty-two cases of craniosynostosis were examined: 15 trigonocephalies, 10 scaphocephalies, 3 brachycephalies and 4 plagiocephalies.

Seventeen craniofacial dysostoses were also examined, 5 of which were subject to postmortem examination: there were 5 oxycephalies, 2 Apert's syndromes, 4 cloverleaf skulls (3 died), 2 Pfeiffer's syndrome, and 1 partial 16 trisomic (who died). In addition, we also examined 3 congenital calcified chondrodystrophies (2 died).

Classical histological methods were used in the study of the fetuses. The specimens were dissected, divided into different samples, fixed in formaldehyde neutralized by sodium carbonate and decalcified in a solution consisting of equal parts of formic acid 8N and sodium formate 1N. They were embedded in paraffin, cut using microtome (American Optical, Spencer 820) into 7-μm thick sections, oriented in the three planes and stained by Masson's trichrome methanol.

For older fetuses over 23 weeks, for newborn babies, for older children and for adults, we preferred more appropriate methods for the calcified tissue. Those, used in the Human Anatomy Laboratory, have been previously described (Dhem 1967).

The specimens were embedded in methyl methacrylate, without preliminary decalcification. They were then cut into transverse slices using an automatic saw (type 32, Safag, Bienne, Switzerland). The sections were reduced to a uniform thickness of 80μm by manual grinding on a ground glass plate under methanol. The sections were

118 CRANIOFACIAL MALFORMATIONS

microradiographed (Baltograph*BF-50/20, Balteau, Liège) and stained using methylene blue.

RESULTS

The histological observations of the ossification process of the fetuses and children enabled us to define important differences in connection with the skeletal pieces of the skull, and led to a study of the disorders met with among dysmorphias.

Fetus and normal child

The bony framework of the skull proceeds according to the membranous and endochondral modality. The description of the growth of the bones of membranous origin is based on new concepts, which enables the explanation of the appearance of malformed skulls. Reference will be made to the special case of the mandible.

MEMBRANOUS OSSIFICATION

The complexity of the membranous skeleton varies according to the areas observed and the rapidity of its growth necessitates the presence of specialized tissue: chondroid tissue.

The areas observed

The membranous bones form the dome of the skull and most of the facial bones. They appear, in precise places, on supports of mesenchymal origin which develop into intensely vascularized connective tissue delineated by a fibrillar layer. Transformations of the ground substance and of the connective cells lead to the deposit of mineral salts and set osteogenesis in motion. This process begins about the 70th day and progresses from anterior to posterior. Before acquiring their own rigidity, these structures develop on surfaces of cartilaginous origin (chondrocranium) or within the envelope of the nervous system (the ectomeninx).

In the first case, the development of the growing bones usually overlaps the limits of the cartilaginous base in one of two ways, as shown in Figure 7.1. These ways differ according to the observed cranial or facial area, the complexity of the form and functions of these being quite different.

At the skull level, the vault will develop at the core of the most external envelope of the brain in order to protect it (Fig. 7.2). The ossifying mesenchymal tissue, formed

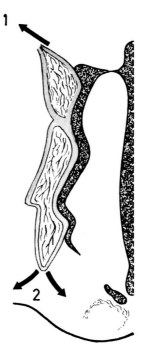

Fig. 7.1 Diagram of a coronal section cut in a 15-week-old fetus, crossing the internal orbital process, frontal process and alveolar bone of premaxilla. The osteogenesis advancement into the cranial area (1) and its invasion in the facial area (2).

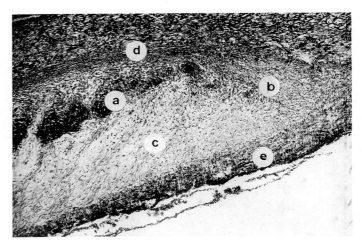

Fig. 7.2 The temporal edge of the temporoparietal suture shows the osseous flat (a), the cambium (b), the fibrillar layer (c), the pericranial membranous (d) and the dura mater (e) (×53).

within the ectomeninx, divides the latter into two membranes; the external or pericranium and the internal or dura mater. The bone grows towards the neighbouring skeletal piece (Fig. 7.3) and together they determine the boundaries or sutures which are concordant or bevelled. The ectomeninx as well as the cartilages of the base can be used as a matrix in the fabrication of flat bones.

At face level, the ossification process corresponds to the

* Gift of the Fonds National de la Recherche Nationale (FNRS), Brussels, Belgium.

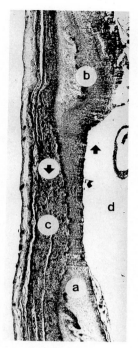

Fig. 7.3 Temporal bone (a) and parietal bone (b) are converging in the ectomeninx. Temporal muscle (c) and the brain (d) exert opposite pressure (arrows) (×9).

complex forms of the cartilaginous models and its development enables it to adapt to more diverse conditions (Fig. 7.4).

The osteogenic process of the maxilla takes place by the superposition of sagittal planes. The two osseous lamellae grow along two fronts. They extend bilaterally in a centrifugal direction to envelop the dental germs, and also advance medially, skirting the cartilaginous model towards

the vomer. This supplies the principal elements of the midfacial skeleton: the premaxilla and postmaxilla, on the one hand, and the postmaxilla and palatine bone which are separated by square-shaped spaces on the other hand (Fig. 7.5). These spaces are filled with connective tissue of a dense fibrous type. Development so far prepares the face for the action of the 'ethmoidal ram'. The ethmoidal cartilaginous septum, with the vomer to which it is closely related, influences the spatial disposition of the different constituents of the face. In addition the three-dimensional form of the face or the borders of the skeleton will become adorned with gutters and crests to guide and protect the rich vasculonervous network of the face, to provide sites of insertion for the muscles and to facilitate their arrangement at the base of the skull.

Flat junctional bones are also added: these comprise the thick zygomatic bones, the thin nasal bones, the lacrimal bones and the inferior turbinates. The sutures which divide these bones look like the sutures of the vault but the Scott scheme is applied differently with regard to the position of the fibrillar layers and membranes (Pritchard et al 1956).

The chondroid tissue

Membranous ossification does not take place immediately. The increase in the size of the brain and its accessory structures is such a rapid phenomenon that the rate of the fibrous bone deposit would not be sufficient to build a sufficiently extended calcified skeleton. The skeletal formation therefore has to undergo an intermediary stage during which tissue rich in calcium is formed. This tissue is similar to woven bone, but deposition occurs more rapidly. Formerly it was incorrectly called chondroid bone

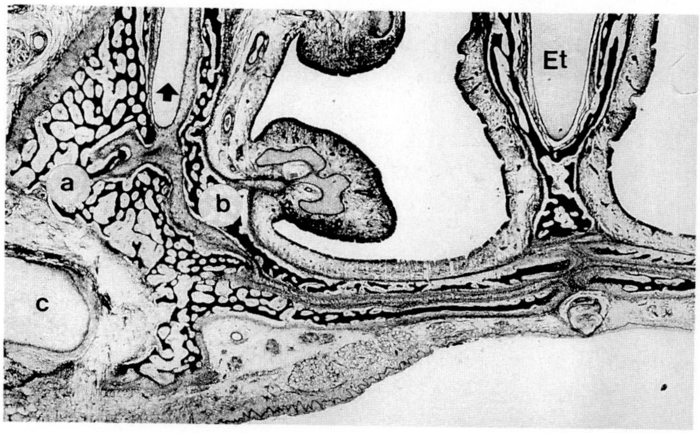

Fig. 7.4 Coronal section cut in a 15-week-old fetus crossing (a) the premaxilla and (b) postmaxilla, which are disposed at right-angled planes, allowing for their sliding into the sagittal plane. Centrifugal progression of the ossification to envelop the dental germs (c). Cartilaginous model (arrow). Et = ethmoidal septum (×4).

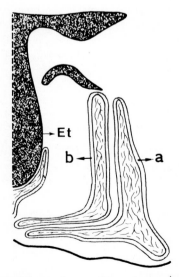

Fig. 7.5 Diagram of the section cut 20 mm back from the one illustrated in Fig. 7.1. The postmaxillar (a) and palatine bone (b) are disposed in right-angled planes.

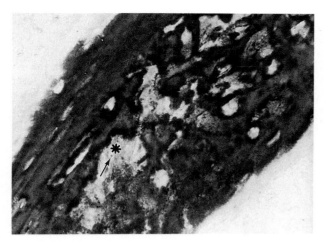

Fig. 7.6 Morphological characteristics of the chondroid tissue. Methylene blue staining. Cell lacuna (arrow), unmineralized matrix (×312).

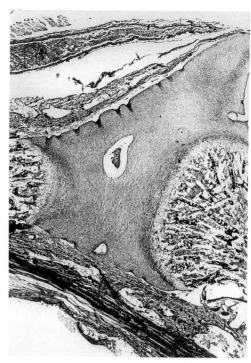

Fig. 7.7 Sagittal section in spheno-occipital synchondrosis (×6).

(Schaffer 1888), or chondroid tissue (Grohe 1899). Its morphological characteristics, which are different from those of the osseous and cartilaginous tissue, were studied in the symphyseal region of the growing human mandible (Goret-Nicaise 1981 a,b,c, 1982, Goret-Nicaise & Dhem 1982).

Chondroid tissue can be found in the whole of the viscerocranium. Microscopic examination of thick non-demineralized sections demonstrates two centric lacunae around every cell (Fig. 7.6). The first one — round, smooth and close to the cell — resembles a chondrocytic lacuna; the second one lies outside the first and has an irregular edge. This uneven border is due to small granular aggregations of mineralized material and corresponds to the limit of visible calcification on microradiography. The weak affinity of chondroid tissue to methylene blue and the calcification process prohibits its absorption by the cartilage. Examination of the microradiographs shows numerous, large, irregular and sometimes confluent lacunae and a fundamental substance with a very high degree of calcification.

ENDOCHONDRAL OSSIFICATION

The base of the skull is formed from the transformation of a cartilaginous matrix by endochondral ossification. In different places this elaborately profiled cartilage undergoes an ossification process which is largely completed during the first few years of life. Between the ossifying areas, bipolar fertile spaces persist and these are the synchondroses (Fig. 7.7). Most of those centres disappear completely by ossification during the first year (e.g. the intrasphenoidal suture) or change into a fissure (e.g. fissure between the petrous part of the temporal bone and the sphenoid bone). The spheno-occipital synchondrosis is an exception. It persists for many years and enables sagittal growth to occur.

Another site of cartilaginous growth is the ethmoidal septum. It acts on the maxillary constituents by the intermediary of the vomer (Fig. 7.4).

The cartilaginous growth centres associated with mastication and breathing functions influence in turn the adaptive growth centres of the sutures and the midfacial planes.

THE GROWTH OF MEMBRANOUS BONE

The sutures which determine viscerocranial growth become apparent from the 17th week but microradiographic examination of calcified specimens is only possible five weeks later. We distinguish sutures of the vault, of the face, and the sutures at the limit between the membranous and endochondral skull.

The sutures of the vault

The sagittal system of the vault has been chosen as an example of the evolution of these adaptable centres. Figure 7.8 indicates four different stages in the fetus and the newborn.

At 23 weeks (Fig. 7.8a) the calcified pieces were formed exclusively by chondroid tissue lamellae, separated by parallel spaces. These lamellae were stretched here and there by a wide non-calcified band. At 28 weeks (Fig.

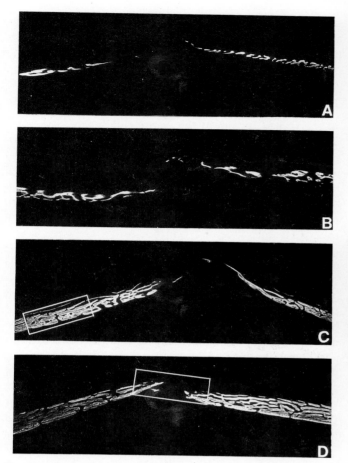

Fig. 7.8 Microradiograph of the sagittal suture (a) at 23 weeks, (b) at 28 weeks, (c) at 33 weeks, and (d) at birth (×2.6).

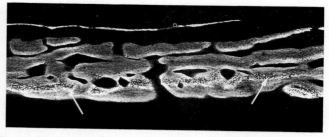

Fig. 7.9 Enlargement (×45) of the frame in Fig. 7.8(c). A fragment of parietal bone of a 33-week-old fetus indicates that chondroid tissue (arrows) constitutes the support for woven bone deposit, mainly on its external side.

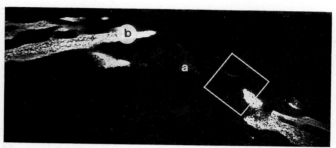

Fig. 7.10 Enlargement (×22.4) of the frame in Fig. 7.8(d). The sagittal suture at birth is only filled by chondroid tissue with two different layers of mineral contents. In (a) none are visible, while (b) shows saturation. The framed area corresponds to the region reproduced in Fig. 7.11.

7.8b) the first lamellae of chondroid tissue join other lamellae progressively and form a support for the deposit of narrow lamellae on the external side. In Figure 7.8(c) at 33 weeks, and in Figure 7.8(d) in the newborn, the documents demonstrate the mixed modality of calcification which is both osseous and chondroid. The difference between both stages is quantitative.

One specimen shows that the chondroid tissue forms a continuous framework. On both sides of this frame, but especially on the external surface, osseous tissue is deposited. In the perisutural areas, however, calcified tissue is only represented by chondroid tissue.

An enlargement enables the dynamics around the sutural area (Fig. 7.9) to be seen. Radiography in the 33 week fetus confirms that the chondroid tissue is the frame of the skeletal piece, adapted to strong internal pressure. It also emphasizes the rapid ossification on the external side of the hypercalcified plate (Fig. 7.9). This phenomenon differs from that in the growing long bones where, on the contrary, the deposit affects both sides of the plate (Ponlot 1960). In the perisutural region calcified tissue is uniquely represented by chondroid tissue (Fig. 7.10)

which reacts to the strong cerebral pressure from within. Indeed, mineralization of the most advanced position is microscopically visible, but is not seen on a photograph. So, to observe the movement of this extremity toward its homologues, we must examine the stained section (Fig. 7.11).

The sutural edges are united by mixed fibrillar bundles and separation of these edges as a result of tension is

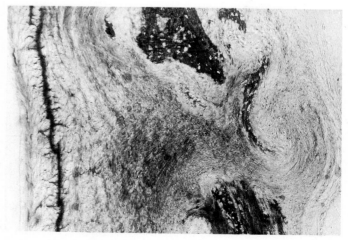

Fig. 7.11 Relations between the fibre bundles and recently deposited chondroid tissue, stained with methylene blue (×60).

immediately followed by the apposition of chondroid tissue.

In the second 6 months, a differentiation in the skeletal piece appears which results in the formation of two lamellae, an internal and an external intercepting the diplöe. The expanding external layer consists of woven bone. The internal one is more compact and made of lamellar bone which is deposited slowly.

The appearance of the parietal bone during the whole of the cephalic growth is illustrated in Figure 7.12(a), and its sutural edges, formed by chondroid tissue, in Figure 7.12(b).

In adulthood ossification progressively seals the sutural

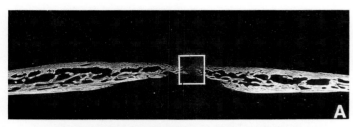

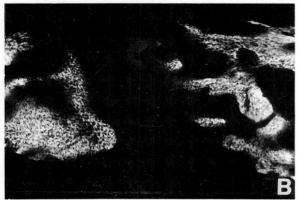

Fig. 7.12 (a) Differentiation of parietal bones in a 2½-year-old child (×2); (b) enlargement of the frame shown in (a) (×72). The growth is exclusively represented by chondroid tissue deposit.

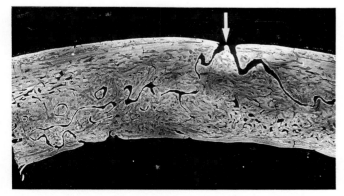

Fig. 7.13 Microradiograph of an adult sagittal suture. The arrow indicates the confluence between coronal and sagittal sutures (×8).

fissure (Fig. 7.13). Having become narrow, discontinuous and undulating it runs in compact osseous tissue in which important remodelling is present.

The sutures of the face

In the frontal section of the young child's face, the right-angled space separating the pre- and postmaxilla disappears (Fig. 7.14a). By contrast, the postmaxilla and palatal area maintain their own individuality and remain separated by a narrow non-mineralized band, the right-angled form of which is obvious (Fig. 7.14b). Transversely, the relations between the facial pieces are realized through rounded bands, oriented ventrodorsally. They emphasize the curved form between the postmaxilla and palatine bone and the premaxilla and vomer (Fig. 7.14c). The maxilla will rapidly expand in an anterolateral direction by means of a forefront of chondroid tissue. The premaxilla is pulled forward by the vomerine plate. This movement is achieved by its continuity with the ethmoidal septum, which transmits the activity of the spheno-occipital synchondrosis.

The role of these spaces during growth is that of sliding planes, able to respond to the developing forces. They allow a very speedy development in the newborn by an active movement in a sagittal direction. The maintenance of the posterior space will be useful in dentofacial development throughout childhood and adolescence.

In addition to the sliding planes, the face presents sutures, similar to those described in the vault, which retain their permeability for a long time. When growth is completed, the sutures do not ossify but develop a resilience which provides protection from shocks. From this point of view, the maxillo-vomerine suture is an excellent example of how the vomer is able to slide on the maxillary rail (Fig. 7.15).

Between cartilaginous and membranous bone, there is a strip of connective tissue. Once the ossification process is induced in the cartilage, the aspect of the two sides, of membranous and endochondral origin, is similar to an ordinary suture (Fig. 7.16). This region could be called a 'synchrondro-membrano-suture' to evoke its double origin.

New concepts clearly emerge from the analyses:

1. The adaptive growth centres of the skull are of two different kinds. The first is sutural and responds to the progressive growth, exerted by the brain, and the ocular globes. The second is sliding and contributes to the 'dental skull', allowing sufficient space for the teeth and the accomplishment of the facial functions.
2. The osseous parts of the viscerocranium are systematically preceded by the deposit of chondroid tissue. The constant presence of this tissue on the sutural edges in fetuses and young children, as in the peripheral areas of the future maxilla, attest to its essential role during

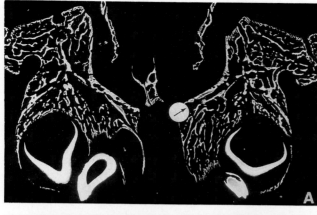

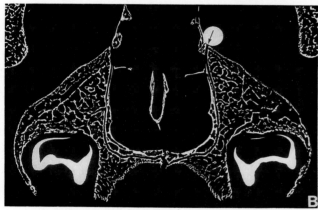

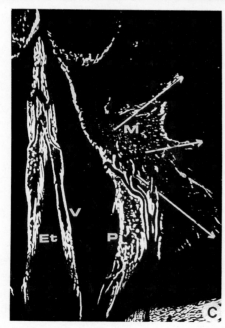

Fig. 7.14 Microradiograph of the space separating the 'dental skull' pieces. In the frontal plane, the pre-/postmaxillary area (a), and the postmaxilla/palate (b), are arrowed. The sliding plane is observed transversely in (c). Et = ethmoidal septum; V = vomer; P = palatine bone. Arrows indicate centrifugal growth of the maxillary bone, M.

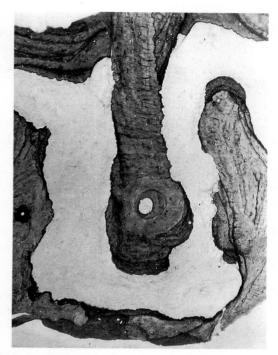

Fig. 7.15 Maxillo-vomerine of a 30-year-old woman.

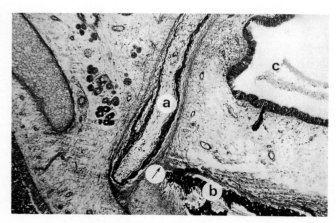

Fig. 7.16 At the limit of endochondral (a) and membranous (b) skull, the 'chondro-suture' is shown (arrow). Specimen from the face near the maxillary sinus (c) (×64).

the periods when membranous ossification is greatly to the fore.

3. The potentialities for rapid deposit of the chondroid tissue permit the sutural space to be reduced and thus protect the brain. By not completely filling the sutural space, the chondroid tissue leaves the skull free to develop.

The regular curvilinear osseous pieces develop by conjoint activity of the sutural and periosteal elements. The sutures are stimulated by the tension on and the separation of their edges by adaptable connective proliferation and by marginal ossification through the intermediary of chondroid tissue deposition. Chondroid tissue similarly permits the mineralization of the skeletal pieces at an accelerated rate.

THE MANDIBLE

The most recent and complete growth scheme of the mandible (Goret-Nicaise 1986) permits this bone to be considered a harmonious group of three modules, the ontogenesis of which is fundamentally different. As a group they form the basis of a fourth alveolar unit, the presence and the development of which is closely linked to the development of dental germs (Fig. 7.17).

The initial unit, consisting of woven bone and located dorsally in connection with the foramen mentale, is the unique mandibular ossification nucleus. Its length is fixed at the 14th week.

The ventral unit, situated between the foramen mentale and the midline, results successively from the lengthening of Meckel's cartilage and, after the 20th week, exclusively from the symphyseal sutural growth.

Sutural mesenchyme takes part in the growth because of its differentiation into cartilage or chondroid tissue. This tissue separates the two half-mandibles by the production of fibrous tissue, by the increase in the size of the chondriola symphysea, and by formation of the chin bones.

The dorsal units form the base for the mandibular body and ramus. Its growth centres — condylar and coronoid — contribute to the dorsoventral lengthening of the mandible and assure the increase in height of the ramus.

Until the postnatal period, the alveolar unit is formed by woven bone, cartilage and chondroid tissue. The

initial module

ventral module

dorsal module

alveolar module

subperiosteal osteogenesis

R → resorption

→ direction of the growth

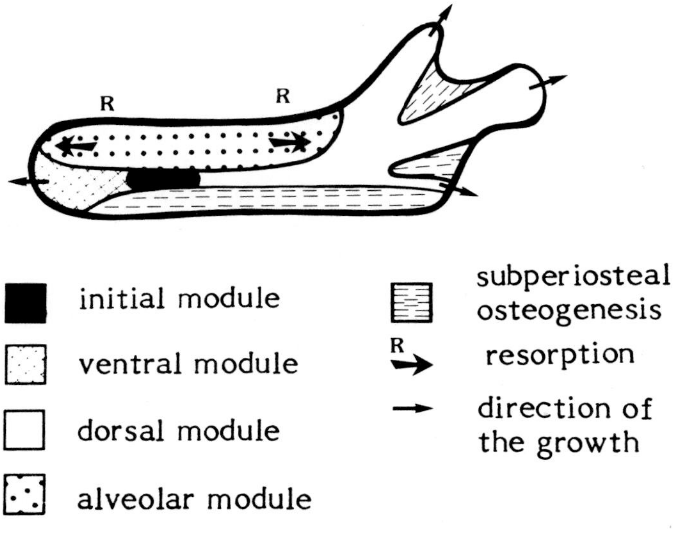

Fig. 7.17 Diagram of human mandibular ontogenesis according to Goret-Nicaise (courtesy of the author).

growth of dental germs provokes a ventral and dorsal lengthening of this unit by resorption of the medial wall of the central incisor tooth and of the ventral area of the dorsal unit.

The detailed observations of the evolution of the symphysis towards synostosis resemble those made at the sutural level.

The chondroid tissue persists in the symphyseal edges in the form of large areas, intercepted by vascular cell spaces. There appears to be a resorption of chondroid tissue by multinucleated cells and an apposition of lamellar bone. This substitution continues until synostosis formation.

There seem to be two determining agents: the first is the differentiation of ectomesenchymal cells in calcified tissue, eventually associated with a reduction of mitotic activity, and the second is the medial progress of chondroid tissue resorption and substitution by lamellar bone.

Osteogenesis in craniofacial abnormalities

The programme governing craniogenesis can be altered by a premature ossification of the sutural centres and/or the degeneration of cartilaginous centres. The disturbance of this programme leads to craniofacial abnormalities, which are classified in Table 7.1.

Table 7.1

Membranous skull
Craniosynostosis
    Premature ossification situated in one or two sutures is the main characteristic
Craniofacial dysostoses
    Premature ossification concerns several sutures and the failure of osseous tissue in one or more skeletal pieces. It is often associated with extra cranial anomalies, whose chromosomal origin and neurological mechanism are sometimes detailed

Endochondral skull
Chondrodystrophia
    The degeneration of growing centres in the cranial base is associated with synostosis in several cranial sutures

CRANIOSYNOSTOSIS

The example is a trigonocephaly affecting a 12-month-old child and characterized by the closure of the metopic suture. The presumed sutural area is recognizable by the sharp arching of the internal wall. This results in a thickening of the suture, which is eight times the normal size (Koskinen-Moffett 1982). The orientation of some rare osseous lamellae, perpendicular to the skeletal pieces, is another sign of craniosynostosis (Fig. 7.18). The evolution of the closure indicates that ossification began near the base and on the internal side of the sutural area (Fig. 7.19) (Dhem et al 1983).

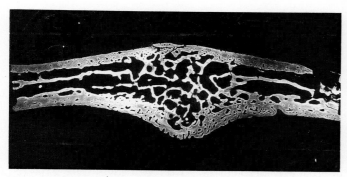

Fig. 7.18 Microradiograph of frontal synostosis (×15).

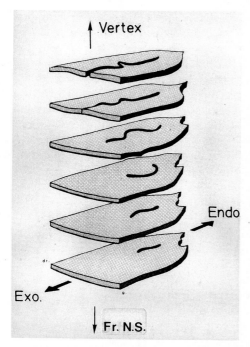

Fig. 7.19 Diagram illustrating the evolution in space of the premature ossification of the frontal suture. Endocranial (Endo.), exocranial (Exo.) sides, frontonasal suture (Fr.N.S.).

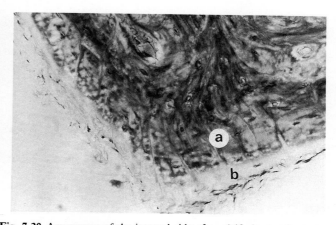

Fig. 7.20 Appearance of the internal side of a calcified sutural space: the interdependence between osseous deposit and dura mater fibre. The orientation of dura mater fibres (a) is perpendicular to the osteoblast axis and preosseous border (b) (×105).

Contrary to most current theories (Moss 1954), the dura mater is not responsible for the pathological ossification. Indeed, osteogenesis is visible on the internal side of the bone as a preosseous border of pale colouring. The direction of the dura mater fibres (Fig. 7.20) is perpendicular to that of the osteoblasts, which are arranged along the preosseous border. There, as Dhem & Vincent (1965) demonstrated, with regard to the incorporation of the patellar ligament in the tibial tuberosity of a growing dog, when osteogenesis is guided by soft tissue bone deposition is parallel to the included fibres.

CRANIOFACIAL DYSOSTOSES

Craniofacial dysostoses are hereditary diseases whose genetic transmission often takes place according to the dominant modality.

The clinical aspect of the head which is typical of some syndromes illustrates serious osteogenesis programming defects. Those defects affect the whole sutural system (e.g. Crouzon's syndrome) or are predominant in a localization of the vault involving skull development in height (excluding partial 16 trisomy, cloverleaf skull and Pfeiffer's syndrome).

Crouzon's disease and oxycephaly

In Crouzon's disease, at any level of slicing the appearance of sutures under the microscope does not differ (Fig. 7.21). The external surface is the seat of regular apposition, whereas on the internal face an osteoclastic resorption of variable degree takes place. This unusual resorption explains the formation of crests and pillars whose appearance does not differ from the bone tissue that was recently deposited on the surface (Dambrain & Dhem 1984).

The failure of the osteoclastic mechanism and the absence of bone differentiation of the primary bone are accompanied by the fusion of all the sutures. This fusion changes the vault into an inextensible envelope.

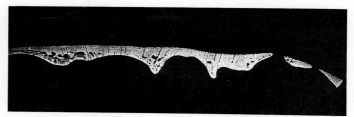

Fig. 7.21 Microradiograph of a section cut from a skull affected by Crouzon's disease (×2.4).

This illness is marked by an anomaly in the erection of the desmocranium which opposes cerebral expansion. The anomaly affects the mechanism of bone resorption, without which it would not be possible to affirm whether the abnormality is at the level of recently ossified tissue or of the osteoclasts.

The findings of a surgical operation accord with this point of view since the exeresis of bone fragments can re-establish the usual profile of a flat bone.

In this illness, there is no relation to the usual type of craniosynostosis. It is a craniofacial dysostosis and, as the general aspect of the vault suggests, oxycephaly seems to be an anomaly related to Crouzon's syndrome.

Partial 16 trisomy

Observations of the case of a baby girl, who died when only 4 months old, showed a very early closure of the frontal and coronal sutures, followed by a sagittal suture synostosis. The cessation of the functions resulted in at least three features. It influenced the disposition of the basal skeletal pieces but without causing the disappearance of the synchondrosis. It led to an absence of transversal expansion (hypotelorism, ogival palate), and it also provoked a turricephaly as compensation.

Detailed observations, which will be published later, are summarized as follows and indicate that the forehead, by the disappearance of the sutures, was reduced to a unique angular part at the summit (Fig. 7.22a). It was about four times thicker than the part observed in the specimen skull

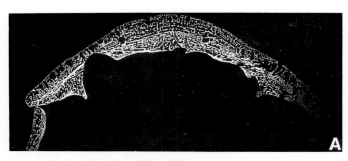

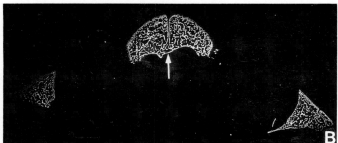

Fig. 7.22 Microradiograph of two coronal sections from a partial 16 trisomy: (a) in the forehead area there is frontal and coronal synostosis; (b) the parietal area where the suture is only closed at its internal extremity (arrow) is shown; the presence of digital markings and the perforation of the parietal bones (×2.3) are seen.

and consisted of two clearly distinctive layers. The internal layer, uneven on the cerebral side, was composed of bone trabeculae tangential to the skull, except in three areas corresponding to sutural gaps.

The external layer was formed of thinner osteochondroid trabeculae, located without any definite orientation. It enclosed no structures similar to a sutural area. In the section dealing with the two parietal bones (Fig. 7.22b), the skull consisted of only one layer divided by a deep fissure. This latter represents the sagittal suture with the internal extremity closed. Two broad edges were so jagged as to cause perforations of the parietal bones, far from the sutural areas.

Microradiographic and histological analysis of thick non-demineralized sections brought to light little-known phenomena which enabled us to understand, at least partially, the causes of the disorders of the cranial skeleton. This investigation demonstrated that, as in simple craniosynostosis, the laws governing the growth of the membranous bone were not applicable, because of the abnormal behaviour of the sutural mechanism and the disorders introduced in the 'apposition–resorption' process. The global volume of the cranium and the X-rays were normal, which showed that the brain and the growing centres of the skull base cannot be held responsible.

The anomaly, doubtless of chromosomal origin, itself caused by an unknown mechanism (Cohen 1977), seems to have begun early in the gestation period by a premature closure of the coronal and sagittal sutures. This stenosis was responsible for the formation of a rigid limit of the anterior cranial wall.

In spite of the cerebral pressure, osteoclastic resorption was not produced at the level of the diseased areas and the brain had been diverted towards the syncciput, where the vascular growth seemed to restrain the closing process of the suture.

Going further afield from the forehead, the antagonism between the influence related to the merging of the sutural banks and the influence resulting from the forces of cerebral expansion is of advantage to the brain, as seen in the progressive depth of the digital-shaped pattern.

This observation can only be explained by the refractory character of dystopic osseous tissue to osteoclasis. In other words, the calcified tissue constitutes a breach in the harmonious development of the brain and obliges the latter to obtain sufficient size for its expansion at a distance from the stenosis.

Cloverleaf skull and Pfeiffer's syndrome

Cloverleaf skull and Pfeiffer's syndrome constitute in varying degrees the constitutive signs of the association of craniosynostosis and hydrocephaly.

At the level of the base, the synchondroses are porous. But in the vault craniosynostosis begins by the closure of

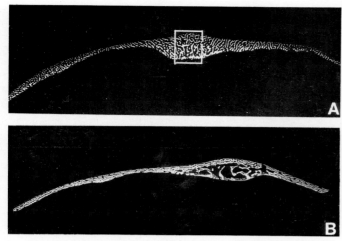

Fig. 7.23 Microradiograph of the vault (a) in cloverleaf skull (32-week fetus) mainly formed by chondroid tissue, and (b) in Pfeiffer syndrome (6 months old), characterized by a woven bone deposit.

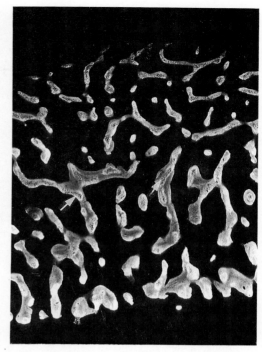

Fig. 7.24 Enlargement of the frame of the coronal suture in the cloverleaf skull of Fig. 7.23(a). Arrows indicate the chondroid tissue (×47).

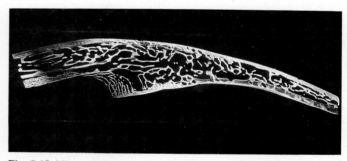

Fig. 7.25 Microradiograph of a coronal suture synostosis. The internal side shows an irregularity, which at first sight appears to be an alteration of the implantation (×3.8) of the dura mater fibres.

the temporoparietal suture, which is the first obstruction to the expansion of the brain and to cephalorachidian liquid expansion. The stenosis then extends in the coronal system, reaching eventually the lambdoidal suture and finally the sagittal suture. This evolution in time and space explains either the tricuspid form of the cloverleaf skull or the globular aspect in Pfeiffer's syndrome.

X-ray examination classically demonstrates the existence of prominent digital markings. In a more pronounced degree, the whole of the vault which has been prematurely submitted to internal pressure is uniformly thin, except for the very thick skull of the occipital bone (Fig. 7.23).

The microradiographic appearance of the summit of the vault is of a thin lamella in both diseases. The parietal and frontal bones are united by an ossified and thick sutural area. In the cloverleaf skull, brain expansion is so rapid that the continuity of the vault requires a deposit of chondroid tissue on its external surface (Fig. 7.24) (Dambrain et al 1987).

In the most severe forms of cloverleaf skull, the characteristics of this tissue are seen to be inadequate and the squamal part of the temporal bone is reduced to a fibrous envelope. These two diseases demonstrate in a positive way that the excessive pressure, caused by hydrocephaly, is inoperative on the synostosis.

Once again, the osseous tissue filling the suture is refractory to osteoclasis.

CHONDRODYSTROPHIA

A case of unilateral acrocephalosyndactyly

Synchondrosis degeneration associated with a prematurely closed neighbouring suture is an example. Since the osseous tissue organization at the level of the vault presents

a pagetoid aspect (Fig. 7.25), a viral infection must be retained.

Direct examination of the skull base taken from a 2½-year-old child indicated a clear hypodevelopment on the right side. It was the result of the ossification of the sphenotemporal synchondrosis on the same side (Dambrain 1977). This abnormality spread at the level of the vault in the coronal sutural system.

The irregularity of the internal face shows that fusion took place by a procedure which differs from those we have already described in simple craniosynostosis (Fig. 7.26). At first sight, this aspect suggested that the serious upset which took place at the level of the skull base

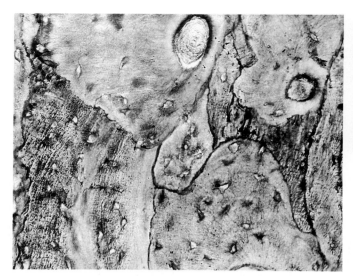

Fig. 7.26 Pagetoid aspect of osseous tissue organization, perhaps due to a viral infection. Methylene blue staining (×58).

automatically influenced the building of the vault. The fusion of the two edges, which had slid together, seems to be an argument in favour of a retraction of the ectomeninx.

Congenital calcifying chondrodystrophia

This is another example of disease where the growing centres of the base are affected by a calcifying necrosis, resulting in a globular form of the vault and retromaxillism. The lesion is located in the hyaline cartilage (Fig. 7.27) which initially undergoes a calcification caused by

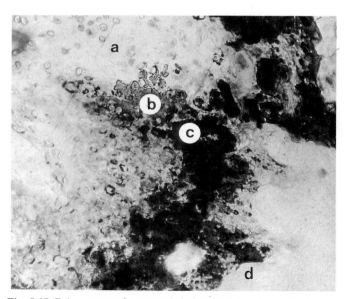

Fig. 7.27 Enlargement of a congenital chondrodystrophic calcifying area (methylene blue staining). The skull base is altered in the hyaline cartilage area (a) by mineralization in intracellular spaces (b) and cellular lacunae (c), ending in cystic degeneration (d) (×105).

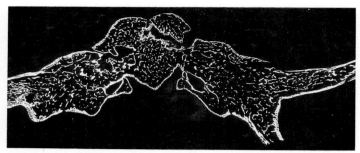

Fig. 7.28 Microradiograph of a coronal section in the congenital chondrodystrophic calcifying area, with an asymmetry of the base (×5).

vascular disturbance. The microradiographic aspect of a coronal section of the skull base illustrates the consecutive asymmetry (Fig. 7.28) (Dambrain 1983).

GENERAL CONCLUSIONS

The bone formation of the skull involves endochondral and intramembranous tissues. Intramembranous ossification is preceded by the deposition of chondroid tissue, which is very speedily elaborated in accordance with the need of the brain envelope.

Development of the membranous skull proceeds in two different ways. At the level of the vault and lateral face, the centrifugal pressure of the brain and occular globes, as well as the influence exerted by the muscles, results in tension on the sutures.

At the level of the 'dental skull' expansion of the brain and the cranial base and the numerous orofacial functions exert forces in ventrodorsal and lateral directions through the ethmoid bone on particular structures: the sliding planes. One of these planes between post- and premaxilla is transient, while the other between the postmaxilla and palatine bone is operational, at least during the body's growth: the spaces separating the skeletal pieces are adaptive growing centres (sutures) which become the site of resistance (fissure), and later disappear by an ossification process, exactly programmed in time and space.

The programme can be altered pathologically by early ossification. Abnormal deposits of osseous tissue on the internal side of the suture cannot be the result of the dura mater activity. The passive modality of the insertion of this latter in the bone tissue and the absence of a systemic relation between the ossification of the vault and the base will stimulate further research into the etiopathology of craniostenosis.

The hypothesis of an intrauterine pressure skull (Graham and Smith 1980, Higginbottom et al 1980) seems unfounded, since no experience shows that joining the suture edges by compression only has ever caused craniosynostosis.

The histochemical study of sutures seems more advisable. Some factors, important in the maintenance of sutural permeability, would be absent and would permit an ossification refractory to ostealasia. This hypothesis would explain calcification of stenotic skulls, which contrasts with the digital markings.

REFERENCES

Cohen M M Jr 1977 Genetic perspectives on craniosynostosis and syndromes with craniosynostosis. Journal of Neurosurgery 47: 886

Dambrain R 1977 Aspects anatomo-pathologique des crâniosténoses. In: Montaut J, Stricker M (eds) Dysmorphies crânio-faciales. Les synostosee prématurées (crâniosténoses et faciosténoses). Rapport du XXVII Congrès Annuel de la Société de Neuro-Chirurgie de langue francaise. Masson, Paris, pp. 60–72

Dambrain R, Frijns J P 1983 La chondrodystrophie calcifiante congénitale. In: Delaire J (ed) Thérapeutiques médicales et chirurgicales des syndromes malformatifs. Ve Congres francais de stomatologie et chirurgie maxillo-faciale. Paris, Masson, pp 287–297

Dambrain R, Dhem A 1984 Histological and microradiographical study of Crouzon's disease. International Journal of Tissue Reactions 6: 275–280

Dambrain R, Freund M, Verellen G, Pellerin P, Francke J P, Dhem A 1987 Considerations about the cloverleaf skull. Journal of Craniofacial Genetics and Developmental Biology 7: 387–401

Dhem A 1967 Le remaniement de l'os adulte. Thesis, University of Leuven

Dhem A, Vincent A 1965 Analyse microradiographique du squelette. Recipe, 10: 515–536

Dhem A, Dambrain R, Thauvay C, Stricker M 1983 Contribution to the histological and microradiographic study of the craniostenosis. Acta Neurochirurgie 69: 259–272

Graham J M, Smith D W 1980 Metopic craniosynostosis as a consequence of fetal head constraint; two interesting experiments of nature. Pediatrics 65: 1000–1002

Goret-Nicaise M 1981a I. Ueber das Wachstum des Unterkiefers beim Menschen. Fortschritte der Kieferorthopadie 42: 405–427

Goret-Nicaise M 1981b II. Tierexperimentelle Vergleichsuntersuchung mittels zweier extraoraler mandibulärer Kräfte. Fortschritte der Kieferorthopadie 42: 429–440

Goret-Nicaise M 1981c Influence des insertions des muscles masticateurs sur la structure mandibulaire du nouveau-né. Bulletin de l'Association des Anatomistes 65: 287–296

Goret-Nicaise M 1982 La symphyse mandibulaire du nouveau-né. Etude histologique et microradiographique. Revue de Stomatologie et de Chirurgie Maxillo-faciale 83: 266–272

Goret-Nicaise M 1986 La croissance de la mandibule humaine: conception actuelle. Thesis, University of Leuven

Goret-Nicaise M, Dhem A 1982 Presence of chondroid tissue in the symphyseal region of the growing human mandible. Acta Anatomica 113: 189–195

Grohe B 1899 Die Vita propria der Zellen des Periosts. Virchows Archiv (Pathologische Anatomie), 155: 428–464

Higginbottom M C, Jones K L, James H E 1980 Intrauterine constraint and craniosynostosis. Neurosurgery 6: 39–44

Koskinen-Moffett L K, Moffett B C Jr, Graham J M Jr 1982 Cranial synostosis of human sutures. Progress in Clinical and Biological Research 101: 365–378

Moss M L 1954 Growth of the calvaria in the rat. The determination of osseous morphology. American Journal of Anatomy 94: 333–359

Ponlot R 1960 Le radiocalcium dans l'étude des os. Thesis University of Leuven

Pritchard J J, Scott J H, Girgis F G 1956 The structure and development of cranial and facial sutures. Journal of Anatomy 90: 73–86

Schaffer J 1888 Die Verknöcherung des Unterkiefers und die Metaplasiefrage. Ein Beitrag zur Lehre von der Osteogenese. Archiv fur Mikro-Anatomie 32: 266–377

Genetics

8. Genetics of craniofacial malformations

M. F. Niermeyer, J. Van der Meulen

INTRODUCTION

Craniofacial malformations highlight some perspectives of the function of the plastic surgeon at the crossroads of modern medical care, with emphasis on reconstructive surgery of congenital malformations in a multidisciplinary team.

During this process, which usually involves a long period of close contact between the surgeon and his or her team with the patient and his or her parents, the latter will have many questions about the nature and origin of the malformation, and about options for treatment, and risks of recurrence in future children and grandchildren. This need for genetic counselling has stimulated many centres for plastic and reconstructive surgery to establish close working relations with centres for genetic counselling. The fascinating development of craniofacial surgery and the rapidly accumulating insights into causes of birth defects and genetic disorders, all mainly derived from original work during the last few decades, solved many questions; however, one should consider that the number of 'unknowns' still largely exceeds the solved problems.

At the same time, the perspective for parents of a child with a congenital malformation became essentially different: full genetic counselling has replaced the former assumption that 'lightning doesn't strike twice', as an answer to the question about the risk of recurrence.

Genetic counselling is the process of informing consultees about the nature, therapeutic modalities, implications and risks of recurrence and options for prevention of a disorder or handicap either occurring in him/herself or in a relative (Ad Hoc Committee on Genetic Counselling 1975). The counselling process is based upon the precise identification of the nature and — if possible — the (genetic) cause of a malformation or a syndrome.

CAUSES OF CONGENITAL MALFORMATIONS OR HANDICAPS

The incidence of congenital physical and/or mental handicaps in newborns is estimated as ±5%. The main causes are summarized in Table 8.1.

Table 8.1 Causes of congenital malformations

	Estimated incidence (%)
Genetic factors	
Chromosal disorders	0.5
Single-gene disorders	1
Multifactorial disorders (polygenetic and environmental)	
at birth	2
disorders of later life	5
Non-genetic factors	
Maternal infections	
Maternal metabolic derangements and genetic diseases (diabetes, hypertension, thyroid disorders, PKU)	
Maternal use of medicines or toxic substances	
Maternal exposure to radiation	
Disturbances of embryonic differentiation and fetal growth	

Genetic factors

CHROMOSOMAL DISORDERS

The human karyotype consists of 46 chromosomes: 22 pairs of autosomes (non-sex chromosomes) and one pair of sexchromosomes — XX in the female and XY in the male.

About 50% of fertilizations lead to a spontaneous abortion, largely because of a chromosomal imbalance in the sperm or egg. The incidence of chromosomal disorders at birth is 0.5% and most of these are numerical aberrations caused by non-disjunction at gametogenesis in either parent. Trisomy 21 (Down's syndrome) is the most frequent anomaly (±1 in 700 newborns), with a specific combination of facial features, cardiac and other malformations and mental retardation.

The risk of recurrence is ±1% in subsequent children. In a minority of cases of Down's syndrome, the additional material of chromosome 21 is translocated (attached to) another chromosome, e.g. chromosome 14. One of the parents may be a carrier of this translocation (in balanced form), with a risk of 5–20% of having a child with Down's syndrome.

Trisomies of the other autosomes are less frequent, e.g. trisomy 13 (±1 in 10 000), trisomy 18 (±1 in 7000). Numerical aberrations of the sex chromosomes have lesser effects on the phenotype, and generally cause infertility and lack of secondary sexual characteristics. Turner's syndrome (45,X0) has an incidence in newborns of 1 in 8000, Klinefelter's syndrome (47,XXY) of ± 1 in 1000, and the XYY syndrome also ±1 in 1000.

Structural chromosomal abnormalities may be translocations, inversions, deletions, etc. The phenotype of the patient will be dependent upon the presence of supernumerary and/or loss of chromosomal segments and in most cases there is a pattern of multiple malformations (often in multiple areas or organs) with mental retardation. The pattern of malformations in the different chromosomal syndromes is extensively reviewed in Schinzel (1984).

Diagnosis of a chromosomal disorder in a patient is important not only for the clinical management but also for counselling the parents about the risks of recurrence (especially if a structural chromosomal aberration is inherited) and about the options for prenatal diagnosis after chorionic villus sampling (CVS) in the 10th week or amniocentesis in the 16th week in a future pregnancy.

SINGLE-GENE DISORDERS

Since every chromosome contains several hundreds of thousands of genes, a mutation (invisible at chromosome analysis) may cause a variety of abnormalities. About 1% of newborns has a (combination of) mental and/or physical handicap because of the presence of a single or a double dose of a mutant gene. There is a wide variety of some 3000 syndromes or malformations, involving all (combinations of) organ systems (see McKusick 1988) and new syndromes are being described in the specialized journals at an increasing rate. The main features of the inheritance of single-gene determined disorders are subsequently described for autosomal dominant, autosomal recessive, X-linked recessive and X-linked dominant disorders.

Autosomal dominant inheritance

The presence of a mutant gene in a patient causes symptoms, irrespective of the presence of a normal gene at the same gene locus. Since all autosomal genes are present in duplicate, one inherited from each parent on an autosome (= a non-sex chromosome), a mutation (change) in one of the genes of a single pair of genes may have either no effect on the phenotype (and only when present in double dose are they associated with autosomal recessive disorders), or cause abnormalities in the phenotype of an individual. Disorders with autosomal dominant inheritance are clinically manifesting in heterozygotes. A heterozygote is the person carrying two different genes at a single gene locus: one normal and one mutant. A homozygote is a person who carries two identical normal or mutant genes.

Autosomal dominant inheritance is seemingly a straightforward and simple genetic mechanism. Disorders with autosomal dominant inheritance are clinically manifesting in heterozygotes, i.e. the presence of a mutant gene causes symptoms irrespective of the presence of a normal gene at the same gene locus on the homologous chromosome.

In the classical situation one may observe (Fig. 8.1):

1. A carrier of the abnormal gene transmits this gene (and the disorder) to 50% of his or her offspring, with an equal risk to sons and daughters.
2. The disorder is transmitted from one generation to the next by affected male and female individuals, without 'skipping' a generation.
3. Unaffected individuals from such a pedigree do not carry the gene and accordingly their offspring will not transmit the disorder to their children.
4. 'First cases in a family' may be caused by a (relatively rare) spontaneous mutation and can transmit the disorder to their offspring.

These observations will only be made when the gene shows full penetrance, i.e. causes symptoms detectable in all gene carriers. Achondroplasia is an example of such a disorder and a classical pedigree might show the pattern of Figure 8.1.

In rare situations a person may be homozygous (carrying two identical mutant genes) for an autosomal dominant disorder, which will usually cause a very severe expression as compared to the heterozygous form, e.g. homozygous (lethal) achondroplasia.

In practice, autosomal dominant inheritance provides a number of special problems in analysis and counselling, because variation of expression (variation in the number and/or degree of symptoms in a carrier of the gene) frequently occurs.

Penetrance is the percentage of gene carriers who are identifiable as such by showing symptoms. It is a statistical term. Non-penetrance accordingly indicates the percentage of individuals carrying a gene without showing any detectable symptoms (for discussion, see McKusick 1972). The clinician is mostly concerned about variability of expression of a mutant gene.

Real causes of this variability are largely conjectural, but one general principle is the unpredictability of the interaction between the normal gene (and/or its gene product, like an enzyme or protein) and the mutant gene. Variation

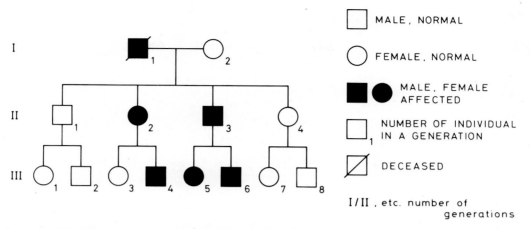

☐	MALE, NORMAL
○	FEMALE, NORMAL
■ ●	MALE, FEMALE AFFECTED
☐₁	NUMBER OF INDIVIDUAL IN A GENERATION
⊘	DECEASED

I/II , etc. number of generations

Fig. 8.1 Pedigree in autosomal dominant inheritance with full penetrance of the gene.

in expression shows two aspects: age-dependent variation and non-age-dependent variation.

Age-dependent variation in expression. The onset of symptoms in an individual carrier of a mutant gene may occur at varying age, often only in adult or later life. Polycystic kidney disease (adult type) and Huntington's chorea are classical examples. In myotonic dystrophy there may be an extreme variation within families in age of onset of the symptoms. In the absence of a precise test for presymptomatic carrier detection, the counselling of apparently healthy relatives from these families is sometimes difficult. Certain growth patterns of craniofacial structures may cause a contrasting pattern, since in some craniostenosis syndromes an apparently normal appearance of the skull at adult age may obfuscate the aberrant form in the early years of life.

Variation in expression, independent of age. Only a few autosomal dominant disorders are fully penetrant with little variation in expression (e.g. achondroplasia) and the majority shows a large degree of variation in symptoms (Fig. 8.2). It is wise never to assume a relative of a patient with such a disorder is unaffected without careful examination (Harper 1981) and special tests may be required before counselling of such a relative becomes possible, as in neurofibromatosis or tuberous sclerosis. Modifying influences, like sex of the affected parent, have been described for a limited number of these conditions, like myotonic dystrophy, in which the intrauterine milieu of an affected mother definitely increases the risk of an affected child developing the early (neonatal) severe form of the disorder. The awareness of variation of expression may help in the analysis of an apparent sporadic case of a dominantly inherited disorder. The importance of establishing this accurately is shown for example in Apert's disease (most cases are new mutations). For siblings of a patient with a new mutation the risk is no greater than for the general population in the absence of germinal mosaicism in a parent; if either parent is shown to be affected, this risk is 50%!

Table 8.2 lists some craniofacial disorders with an

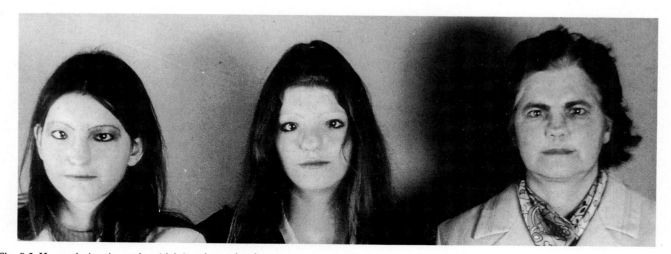

Fig. 8.2 Hypertelorism in mother (right) and two daughters.

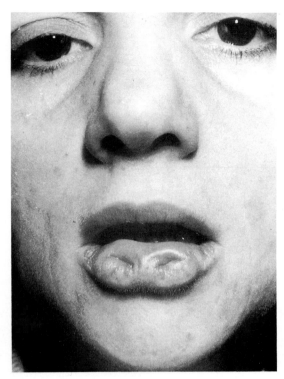

Fig. 8.3 Van der Woude's syndrome.

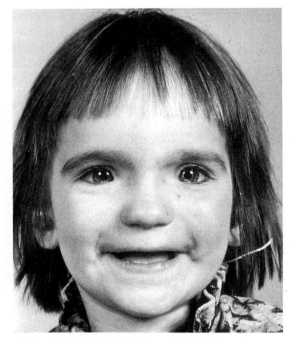

Fig. 8.4 Waardenburg's syndrome.

autosomal dominant type of inheritance. Such a listing, of course, does not attempt completeness and reference should be made to standard texts in this field (Gorlin & Pindburg 1976, Cohen 1978, Goodman et al 1977,

Table 8.2 Some craniofacial malformation syndromes with autosomal dominant inheritance

Blepharophimosis syndrome
Waardenburg's syndrome (Fig. 8.3)
Treacher Collins syndrome
Van der Woude's syndrome (Fig. 8.4)
Popliteal pterygium syndrome
Oculodentodigital syndrome
EEC syndrome
  (Ectrodactyly, ectodermal dysplasia, clefting)
Craniostenosis syndromes
  Crouzon's syndrome
  Saethre–Chotzen syndrome
  Pfeiffer's syndrome
  Apert's syndrome

McKusick 1986). The presence of genetic heterogeneity in many of these syndromes (i.e. the occurrence of apparently identical or similar clinical entities caused by different mutations, sometimes with different modes of inheritance) may be another factor to be considered in the analysis of every individual patient. With small family sizes (as in Western countries) this is a typical problem in isolated cases.

In autosomal recessive inheritance, the parents of the affected patient are healthy, but are heterozygous (carriers) for a normal gene A and a mutant gene a. Every one of their children, irrespective of its sex, has a risk of 1 in 4 of being affected (homozygous aa, for the mutant gene) (Fig. 8.5).

Their unaffected offspring each has a 2 in 3 chance of being a carrier, which will generally neither be a problem to their health nor to their offspring. If they marry a non-consanguineous partner who has generally a chance of 1 in 50 to 1 in 200 of being a carrier for the same disorder, they will have a risk of 1 in 200 to 1 in 800 for affected offspring. Similarly, an affected patient has a risk of 1 in 100 to 1 in 400 for affected offspring.

Table 8.3 Some craniofacial syndromes with recessive inheritance

Cryptophthalmus syndrome
Orofacial digital syndrome type II
Robert's syndrome
Carpenter's syndrome

Table 8.3 is a summary of autosomal recessive disorders with predominant craniofacial abnormalities. The recognition of this type of inheritance, especially in present-day small families with one affected case, is difficult. The clear delineation of the symptoms may be helpful in a number of cases. Detection of parental consanguinity can be an important indication but is no prerequisite for autosomal recessiveness (with many ASR syndromes having heterozygote frequencies of 1 in 50 to 1 in 200). In the rarer ASR syndromes the likelihood of consanguinity is increased.

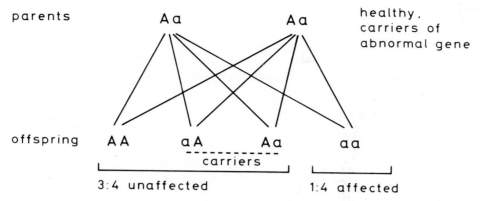

Fig. 8.5 Autosomal recessive inheritance.

Genetic heterogeneity may complicate the differentiation from a new dominant mutation. A family history, search for consanguinity, study of parents and family photographs may be helpful in these situations.

X-linked inheritance

Genes located on the female sex chromosome (the X chromosome) are present in a double dose in a female and in a single dose in a male individual. However, most genes on the X chromosome are inactivated shortly after conception at the time of implantation of the female embryo. This inactivation is irreversible for the cell and its descendants.

If a female is heterozygous for a mutation of a gene on one of her X chromosomes, the consequences for her phenotype are unpredictable and dependent upon the type of cooperation (or correction) between cells expressing the normal and the mutant gene, respectively. In X-linked recessive inheritance, the general rule is that the heterozygous female does not show expression of the trait; however, partial expression in some syndromes has been described and may be useful in heterozygote dectection, for instance in Aarskog's syndrome (e.g. hypertelorism),

Lowe's syndrome (cataracts in females), the otopalatodigital syndrome, etc.

The consequences of this type of transmission (Fig. 8.6) for carriers follow from the X chromosomal location of the mutant gene and in a mating with a normal male the chances are as follows. Sons have a 50% chance of being unaffected and a 50% chance of being affected (the genetic information on the Y chromosome is different from that on the X chromosome and unable to compensate the effects of the mutant gene). Daughters will be unaffected; they have a 50% chance of being non-carriers and a 50% chance of being carriers. With some exceptions (e.g. as indicated above) most carriers will be free of symptoms.

The pedigree will show the occurrence of the condition in males in every subsequent generation, transmitted by unaffected females to half of their male offspring, and male to male transmission does not occur. Affected males (when able to reproduce) will have unaffected sons and all their daughters will be obligate heterozygotes.

In X-linked dominant inheritance, there is clear expression of the gene mutation in a heterozygous female, whereas affected males may be more severely affected, as in Albright's hereditary osteodystrophy and the Coffin Lowry syndrome.

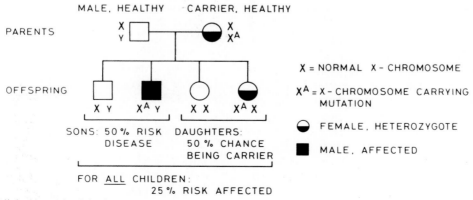

Fig. 8.6 Pedigree in X-linked recessive inheritance.

In contrast to X-linked recessive inheritance, affected females may have both affected daughters (50%) and affected sons (50%) (the latter more severely). Affected males (if able to reproduce) will transmit the condition to *all* their daughters and none of their sons. The extreme of this type of inheritance, as observed in the Goltz syndrome (focal dermal hypoplasia), incontinentia pigmenti, etc., is lethality in males, which gives the typical observation of female-to-female transmission, often with an increased rate of spontaneous abortions.

X-linked mutations may either be transmitted in families, or occur as de novo mutations. In X-linked recessive diseases with no reproduction in affected males, one-third of cases is estimated as being caused by new mutations (either having arisen in the maternal oocyte, or obtained by the mother from one of her parents). Some X-linked dominant disorders with very severe manifestations are observed only sporadically in female patients and are believed to represent new X-linked dominant mutations, lethal in males, e.g. one form of agenesis of the corpus callosum (Aicardi's syndrome). Table 8.4 lists some X-linked disorders (out of a total of ±200) showing craniofacial symptoms.

Table 8.4 Some craniofacial syndromes with X-linked inheritance

Albinism–deafness syndrome
Amelogenesis imperfecta (two types)
Coffin–Lowry syndrome
Aarskog's syndrome
Focal dermal hypoplasia
X-linked hydrocephaly
Lowe's syndrome
Mucopolysaccharidosis II (Hunter)
Oro-facio-digital syndrome (type I)
Oto-palato-digital syndrome (Taybi)

MULTIFACTORIAL INHERITANCE

A number of malformations or diseases are caused by the combination of multiple genetic factors (polygenic), with or without environmental contributions. The genetic risks in this model do not follow the simple Mendelian ratios.

Individuals having a combination of additive genetic factors together with possible external risks will show a particular malformation when the combination of these factors surpasses the developmental threshold for the process involved, e.g. closure of the lip and/or palate, to proceed normally. This liability shows a normal distribution in the general population, with only a small number of individuals exceeding the threshold and showing the malformation (Fig. 8.7a). First-degree relatives (sharing half of their genes with the index case, e.g. sibs and parents) have a liability intermediate between that for the general population and that for the index cases (Fig. 8.7b) and their risk of developing the malformation will be higher than in the general population.

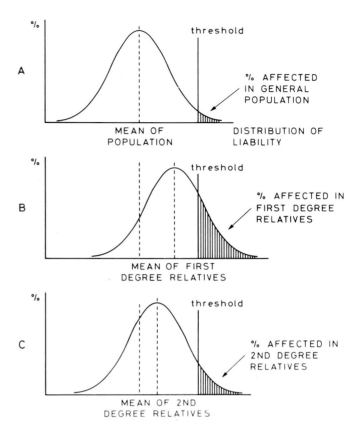

Fig. 8.7 Risks (liability) of multifactorial disorders.

In second-degree relatives, there will be a drop-off of the risk as compared to the first-degree relatives (Fig. 8.7c).

The difference in risk between the general population and first-degree relatives of affected probands may be mathematically derived and is influenced by the population incidence of the disorder, being approximately the square root of the incidence of the malformation in the particular population. This implies that the more common the type of malformation, the higher is the recurrence risk in first-degree relatives. Differences between populations are to be considered in using empirical data obtained in various countries, e.g. the incidence of neural tube defects shows important differences between countries, regions and populations.

The following factors are relevant in the analysis and estimation of genetic risks in multifactorial disorders (see Harper 1981, Fraser & Nora 1986):

1. The risk is greatest among first-degree relatives and decreases with distance of relationship (Fig. 8.7a–c). This is different from the classical Mendelian risk. The magnitude of the risk is usually in the order of 3–10% for first-degree relatives and will be nearly equal to the population risk for third-degree relatives.

2. The risk to first- and second-degree relatives will be dependent on the population incidence of the specific malformation or disease. In practice, the latter data are not generally available and empirical data (obtained in studying larger series of patients and their relatives) are being used. These should, ideally, be obtained from the population of the index cases.

3. The risks for first-degree relatives, being sibs or children of patients, are comparable, which is at variance with classical Mendelian inheritance. This is confirmed for neural tube defects and cleft lip or palate (Bonaiti-Pellie & Smith 1974).

4. Sex differences in liability may influence the recurrence risk. If a malformation has a higher frequency in boys, this implies that the threshold for a girl will be more to the right (Fig. 8.7a) and accordingly more 'risk factors' are required for a girl to develop the malformation. First-degree relatives of an affected girl will have a higher recurrence risk than of an affected boy. A number of malformations show these deviations from the sex ratio (Table 8.5), e.g. pyloric stenosis (more frequent in boys), congenital dislocation of the hip (more frequent in girls), and this affects the risks to future brothers or sisters of index cases.

5. The more severe forms of a certain malformation tend to have greater risks of recurrence, reflecting the greater liability, or the presence of more additive genes in the index case. Hirschsprung's disease shows this effect,

with increased recurrence risk in the long segment type (Bodian & Carter 1963).

6. If multiple family members are affected, this will increase the number of additive risk genes in that particular family and, accordingly, the recurrence risks with close (first-degree) relatives contributing more to the risk than more distant relatives. Two siblings with cleft lip and palate (CLP) will increase the risk for the next to ±10%. Risk tables for several malformations have been developed for these situations (Spence et al 1976, Bonaiti et al 1982).

The application of this model in cases of common congenital malformations is only justified when the malformation occurs as a single abnormality in an otherwise normal patient, which may be the situation in the majority of cases. However, since all 'common' and less common single malformations may be part of either a chromosomal disorder, a non-genetic syndrome or a single-gene disorder, a full clinical evaluation of the patient and evaluation of the family history is essential, before counselling is given along the lines of the multifactorial principle. Whereas most cases of cleft lip (and palate) may be single malformations, there are some 150 syndromic associations known (Table 8.6) (for review, see Cohen 1978). The same heterogeneity may be found in craniostenosis, etc. (Cohen 1986). In studying the family history, the pattern of irregular occurrence of a malformation may suggest multifactorial inheritance, when no specific Mendelian pattern is observed. However, autosomal dominant disorders with variable expression (which may show reduced penetrance) may mimic this situation.

This is not only of theoretical interest, but will stimulate clinicians and geneticists to study relatives of patients before arriving at conclusions on the mode of inheritance.

Numerous malformations and syndromes belong to the possible multifactorial or polygenic group, and Table 8.7 is a summary of syndromes listed under these headings in Goodman's (1977) atlas.

Non-genetic and unknown genesis malformations

Table 8.7 indicates a multitude of malformations or syndromes, in which concepts on aetiology are conjectural. Malformations or syndromes observed as sporadic in offspring of normal non-consanguineous parents that cannot be categorized into a well-known syndrome or a chromosomal disorder may be classified as a 'single case'. They can be explained by different mechanisms and incur extremely varying risk to siblings, as listed in Table 8.8.

The clinical statement 'sporadic case in child of healthy, unrelated parents' has less reassuring implications than usually assumed. Evaluation of the history of the pregnancy, clinical appearance of the child (and its parents) and scrutiny of the family history may help in classifying

Table 8.5 Common single congenital malformations of multifactorial origin**

Type	Sex ratio (Male : Female)	Recurrence risk to sibling (parents normal) (%)		
		All sibs	Male sibs	Female sibs
Cleft lip ± cleft palate	2 : 1	4–5		
Cleft lip and palate	1 : 1.3	2–6		
Clubfoot	2 : 1	2–8		
Cardiac defects (most types)		3–4		
Neural type defects				
Spina bifida	1 : 1.5			
Anencephaly	1 : 3	3–5		
Pyloric stenosis	5 : 1	3		
Male index case*			4	2.7
Female index case			9	3.8
Congenital dislocation of hip	1 : 5			
Male index case			3.6	7.1
Female index case			1	5.1
Hirschsprung's disease	3 : 1	3–15		
Short aganglionic segment	5 : 1			
Male index case			4	0.6
Female index case			8	2.9
Long aganglionic segment	2 : 1			
Male index case			7	11.1
Female index case			18.2	9.1

* Index case = first affected patient with disorder or malformation in family.
** Data summarized in Smith 1976, Harper 1981.

Table 8.6   Malformations as part of heterogeneous syndromes

	Chromosomal	Single-gene disorders	Unknown, non-genetic	Syndromic associations with N associations
Cleft lip and/or palate	+	+	+	154
Craniostenosis	+	+	+	57
Hypertelorism	+	+	+	
Robin complex	+	+	+	18
Neural tube defects	+	+	+	

Table 8.7   Multifactorial* (MFR): genetic or non-genetic syndromes with craniofacial symptoms

	Possible mode
Sturge–Weber syndrome	Non-genetic?
Möbius' syndrome	MFR–non-genetic
Frontonasal dysplasia syndrome	MFR–heterogeneous
Goldenhar's syndrome (oculo-auriculovertebral dysplasia)	MFR–non-genetic
Aglossia–adactylia syndrome	MFR–non-genetic
Amniotic band syndrome	Non-genetic
Cleft lip ± cleft palate (as single malformation)	MFR
Cleft palate	MFR
Craniosynostosis (non-syndromic)	?
Sagittal craniosynostosis (some forms)	MFR

* Compare Tables 8.3–8.8; some syndromic associations of known genesis show malformations that may be multifactorial if occurring as a single malformation.

Table 8.8   'Sporadic case' in a family — possible risks of recurrence:

Possible causes of malformations in a child with normal karyotype and normal parents

Cause	Risk of recurrence to siblings of index case
New mutation for an autosomal dominant disorder	Nil
Autosomal recessive disorder	25%
X-linked disorder	
New mutation in index case	Nil
Mother carrier of X-linked recessive disorder	50% to males
Mother carrier of X-linked dominant disorder	50% to males 50% to females
Multifactorial disorder	3–5%
Largely non-genetic or known non-genetic	Slight to nil

a number of these situations, but some unsolved cases will remain. The following environmental or non-genetic factors may then be considered.

MATERNAL INFECTIONS IN PREGNANCY

Some viral (rubeola, herpes, cytomegaly), parasitic (toxoplasmosis) and bacterial (lues) infections are well-known causes of mostly combinations of multiple organ maldevelopments. Single malformations are less frequent (or noticed). Maternal hyperthermia per se of an infection has

been suggested as a causative factor but this is not firmly established (Shiota 1987). There is no general agreement on the effect of hyperthermia as a single factor (Saxen et al 1982).

MATERNAL METABOLIC DERANGEMENTS

Inherited or acquired metabolic derangements are expected to jeopardize embryonic differentiation, and juvenile diabetes mellitus (insulin-dependent diabetes mellitus) is the most studied situation, where the fetus has a two- to threefold elevated risk of a (complex) malformation like cardiac defects, neural tube defects, skeletal absence-deformities of the axial skeleton (sacral agenesis), etc.

Microcephaly and/or cardiac defects and/or mental retardation are well-known risks to infants of mothers with phenylketonuria, especially when a dietary phenylalanine restriction has not been reinstituted from before pregnancy (Levy et al 1983).

The maternal milieu may be influencing the expression of certain genetic disorders, as has been demonstrated in myotonic dystrophy; when the mother is affected, her child has not only a 50% chance of being affected with this autosomal dominant disorder but, if so, the child is likely to show the severe, neonatal form of the disorder with striking hypotonia, whereas affected children of affected fathers show a later onset of the disease (Harper 1979).

Vitamin deficiencies and caloric deficiencies in pregnancy have long been suspected as causes of malformations; however, no precise data of this are available (Schardein 1985). The preconceptional and early pregnancy supplementation of folic acid and multivitamin to reduce the recurrence risk of neural tube defects (as observed in the UK by Smithells) is to be confirmed in other countries (Schardein 1985).

MATERNAL USE OF MEDICATIONS AND SUBSTANCES OF USE AND ABUSE

A multitude of drugs, when used in pregnancy, have been associated with fetal malformations. Many of these associations are weak and the data from the Collaborative Perinatal Study in the USA (Heinonen et al 1977) give long listings of drugs used in pregnancy, with relative risk factors of 1.2–2.5 for a variety of malformations. Stronger associations are known for a number of drugs (Schardein 1985).

The anticancer drugs (by acting as antimitotic agents, as antimetabolites or as mutagens) may by one or several mechanisms cause malformations.

The anticonvulsants (especially diphantoin) probably carry an elevated risk. However, it was observed (Heinonen et al 1977) that maternal epilepsy per se (in the absence of maternal use of antiepileptics) may increase the risk of cardiac defects and facial clefts in the fetus. Maternal valproate use in pregnancy has been shown to give a risk of 1–2% for a fetal neural tube defect (Robert & Guibaud 1982, Lindhout & Meinardi 1984).

Vitamin A and its potent analogue retinoic acid have been recognized as very potent animal and human teratogens, possibly by their interference with the development of cranial neural crest cells (Webster et al 1986) or other cellular functions. Retinoic acid, by its potency and storage in fatty tissues during extremely long periods, makes this substance very dangerous for women of reproductive age. Exposure (during or even when discontinued several months before pregnancy) has been associated with spontaneous abortion, craniofacial malformations (microtia, anotia, maldevelopment of facial bones and calvaria, cleft secondary palate), cardiac defects (conotruncal or branchial arch mesenchymal tissue defects), thymic abnormalities, hydrocephaly and other central nervous system structural defects (neuronal migration disturbances, cerebellar hypoplasia, etc.) (Lammer et al 1985). Discontinuation of the isoltretinoin derivative (with a shorter half-life) before pregnancy probably has no later adverse effects.

Megadoses of vitamin A (25 000 IU daily), as recommended by some for general health reasons, are in the range associated with fetal defects (Shepard et al 1986).

The susceptibility for drug-induced malformations might be related to maternal or fetal genetic factors, leading to the production of toxic substances in certain mothers or fetuses who have a specific pharmacogenetic trait. Recognition of these susceptibilities by testing for enzyme polymorphisms, etc., awaits further research.

Exposure to toxic and mutagenic substances in the environment is a well-known problem nowadays. As an example, organic solvents have been related to facial clefting in a Finnish study (Holmberg et al 1982). The analysis of many compounds used in industry or in agriculture (pesticides, etc.) has been greatly facilitated by the bacterial mutagenesis test as developed by Ames. However, the extrapolation of these data to human exposure during pregnancy remains speculative (Barlow & Sullivan 1982).

Despite the established in vitro potential for mutagenic and teratogenic effects of dioxin (TCDD) it has been difficult to demonstrate increased incidence of chromosomal aberrations or congenital defects in the offspring of exposed men and woman (Tenchini et al 1983, Friedman 1984). Careful collection of exposure data is, however, very important in all 'ill-understood' cases.

The maternal ingestion of high amounts of alcohol, especially in early pregnancy, has recently been shown to be associated with the fetal alcohol syndrome: a combination of mild mental retardation, mild microcephaly, short palpebral fissures, absence of philtrum, thin upper lip, elevated risk of cardiac defects and facial clefting. This pattern of malformation might be one of more frequent (estimated incidence 1 in 1000 births in the Western world) environmentally induced complexes of birth defects (for review see Rosett & Weiner 1984).

EXPOSURE TO RADIATION

Radiation influences cell division and the integrity of the DNA of the genetic code. Exposure during pregnancy only carries a teratogenic risk when administered at relatively high dosages, as in therapeutic irradiation (Otake & Schull 1984). There are relatively few well-proven associations of low-level maternal radiation and fetal malformations (Brent 1979, Mossman & Hill 1982). Protective measures, of course, are indicated whenever possible. The problem in the analysis is that radiation-induced mutations will only be noticed if dominant; recessive mutations are very difficult to recognize (Brent 1979).

Other sources of radiation include microwaves (shortwave electromagnetic radiation) (Roberts & Michaelson 1985). There is no evidence for a teratogenic potential. This also applies to diagnostic ultrasound. This has been proven to be unharmful to mother and fetus, whereas most experimental evidence indicates that at the frequencies and intensities used in diagnosis no detrimental effect on DNA is to be expected (Williams 1983).

DISTURBANCES OF EMBRYONIC DIFFERENTIATION AND FETAL GROWTH

The extensive knowledge of human embryology and fetal development both at the microscopic and macroscopic level is slowly becoming supplemented with new concepts on the intricate relationship between cellular differentiation, histogenesis and morphogenesis and prospects for the understanding of basic teratological mechanisms.

Vascular disruption causing focal haemorrage has been produced in experiments with a linoleic acid deficient diet (Martinet 1958), maternal injection (Jost 1961) with adrenalin and vasopressin and uterine ischaemia (Franklin & Brent 1964) caused by clamping of its vasculature. Poswillo (1966) has demonstrated in animal models that anomalies such as hemifacial microsomia, Goldenhar's syndrome and mandibulofacial dysostosis may result from the selective destruction of differentiating normal tissues by an expanding haematoma.

Amniotic disruption has been held responsible for the development of craniofacial clefting and amniotic bands, together with visceral and extremity defects. The incidence of this syndrome has been reported to vary from 1 in 5000 to 1 in 15 000 (Torpin 1968, Baker & Rudolph 1971). Familial incidence has not been reported, and the fact that facial clefts have been observed in one or two monozygotic twins (Velasco 1980) clearly demonstrates that non-genetic factors may be involved in their production. Torpin (1968) has stressed the role of maternal trauma and premature amnion rupture in the production of the syndrome, and his observations are consistent with those made in experiments.

Amnion rupture or experimental amniocentesis (Trasler et al 1956, Poswillo 1966, Kendrick 1967, DeMyer & Baird 1969, Singh et al 1974, Kino 1975, Kennedy & Persaud 1977), is known to produce compression-related malformations, some of which are due to restricted mobility, leading to mechanical postural deformations. Others, however, are caused by ischaemia, resulting in focal haemorrhage and necrosis of previously normal tissues affecting the craniofacial complex (encephaloceles, hydrocephalus, palatal clefts), the vertebrae (spina bifida), and the limbs (constriction ring anomalies, acrosyndactyly, etc.) The spectrum of abnormalities produced by these experiments only rarely includes oblique facial clefts, but despite this the possibility should be considered that oblique facial clefts and other anomalies also have their origin in compression-related focal fetal dysplasia (Miller et al 1981, Graham et al 1980). Oblique facial clefts (Van der Meulen 1985) and constriction ring defects of the extremities are frequently observed (Wilson et al 1972, Boo-Chai 1970, Gunther 1963, Dey 1973, Mayou & Fenton 1981) in the amnion rupture syndrome, together with amniotic bands. The origin of these bands may, however, be readily explained by the healing of fetal defects with adhesion formation. Differences in the nature and incidence of the several defects can be explained by a variation in susceptibility of the developing area and by the timing and severity of the causative insult.

While some teratological mechanisms, potentially involved in the production of a variety of craniofacial dysostoses, can thus be explained, those at the origin of dyschondroses such as achondroplasia and some chondrodystrophies which will affect facial development by their effect on the growth of the chondrocranium are far from being understood.

In a number of disorders, the absence or deficient structure of molecules with important function in histogenesis and morphogenesis facilitates the understanding of pathophysiology of a syndrome, as in the Ehlers–Danlos syndrome (collagen defects of various types) and in some of the enamel hypoplasias.

Future developments will come not only from analysis of the human genome by analysis of the DNA at the level of the gene, using restriction enzyme analysis, but also from analysis of the consequences of genetic defects at the level of molecular organization. The defect of the dynein arms of cilia in Kartagener's syndrome is a relevant example since cilia may be important in morphogenetic movement (as shown by the association of situs inversus with this syndrome) (Afzelius 1985).

Another line of future research is the influence of immunogenetic factors (like the HLA complex) on human development. In mice, certain strains show an association between certain H2 (histocompatibility system) loci and clefting susceptibility, which association remains to be studied in humans.

GENETICS OF SOME SELECTED CRANIOFACIAL MALFORMATIONS

The scope of this chapter does not allow discussion of specific syndromes, nor the synopsis of the wide field of craniofacial malformations. There are several excellent recent sources available, which are essential in the analysis of specific questions (Gorlin et al 1976, Stewart & Prescott 1976, Cohen 1978). Because of their frequency in the practice of a plastic surgeon, facial clefting, craniostenosis and hypertelorism and their associations will be briefly discussed.

Cleft lip with or without cleft palate (CL/P)

This malformation may occur either as a single malformation, or in a complex of a syndromal association with clefting. In some of these, the associated defects will point to the diagnosis, as in the chromosomal trisomies. In others, the associated defects may be absent (as in the cleft lip with lip-pits syndrome) and only study of relatives may lead to the correct diagnosis. For counselling, the exclusion of one of the many syndromic associations is of importance (for an excellent review, see Cohen 1978). If syndromal occurrence of CL/P is estimated to represent only ±3% of cases, the number of syndromal associations doubled between 1971 and 1978; 154 of these were known in 1978 (Table 8.9).

Table 8.9 Causal analysis by cleft type (Sphrintzen et al 1985)

Cause	Cleft lip only (%)	Cleft lip and palate (%)	Cleft palate Overt (%)	Cleft palate Submucous (%)
Multifactorial	67	54	41	34
Monogenic	0	13	20	21
Teratogenic	4	3	5	3
Chromosomal	4	3	1	3
Disruption/deformation	4	5	9	0
Unknown	21	22	24	40

Cleft palate (CP), occurring as an isolated, non-syndromic malformation, is thought to be aetiologically heterogeneous. The multifactorial threshold model will apply to most cases.

Occasional families may show a Mendelian type of inheritance. Autosomal dominant and X-linked recessive inheritance has been observed for CP, with variable manifestations of CP, submucous CP and bifid/absent uvula (Rollnick & Kaye 1986). A full family history is apparently essential before counselling can be given to parents of 'isolated' cases of CP.

Associated anomalies were reported in the older literature in 3–7% of the children with cleft lip and/or palate, with the highest incidence with clefting only of the secondary palate and the lowest with cleft lip alone. In a more completely studied population of 1000 patients with CL, CP or CLP, Shprintzen et al (1985) found associated anomalies in 63.4%. Half of these latter patients have recognized syndromes, sequences or associations, while the other half has unique syndromes (Cohen 1981).

Among significant findings were the presence of small stature in 27% of the patients, microcephaly in 25% and mental retardation in 28%. Main diagnostic categories were isolated clefts in 47%, clefts as part of a syndrome (22%) or sequence (8%) or association (1%) or provisionally unique syndrome (22%).

Frequent diagnosis included the velo-cardiofacial syndrome (5%), van der Woude's syndrome (cleft lip ± lip-pits) (Fig. 8.3) (4–5%), Stickler's syndrome (hereditary arthro-ophthalmopathy) (3.8%), isolated Robin sequence (3.5%), fetal alcohol syndrome (3%), Goldenhar's syndrome (facio-auriculovertebral syndrome) (2.4%), Treacher Collins syndrome (2.2%). The referring diagnosis was correct in only 43% of cases, often because of underestimation of the disorder.

Such a complete evaluation of causes by a team of different specialists, and including full dysmorphology evaluation, karyotyping (when indicated) and family study, revealed the distribution of causes as indicated in Table 8.9.

The implications for genetic counselling of parents and patients and their relatives is obvious. The use of risk tables (Bonnait-Pellie et al 1974) for counselling for CL/P cases is possible, when it is sufficiently clear that a multifactorial origin is most probable. This will help in estimating risks when besides the index case other relatives are affected, which will influence the risk of recurrence.

Craniosynostosis

Premature fusion of cranial sutures (craniosynostosis) leads to craniostenosis; these two terms have been used interchangeably for a malformation occurring in ± 0.4 in 1000 newborns. The subject has been reviewed extensively by Cohen (1986) and his classification table is included in Chapter 9 of this book.

The anatomist and the surgeon tend to classify craniosynostosis as simple (one suture prematurely fused) or compound closure of more sutures. This is less informative to the geneticist, who is rather concerned with the overall pattern of anomalies. Primary craniostenosis is to be differentiated from secondary craniostenosis, the latter resulting from haematological (thalassemia, sickle cell disease) or metabolic (hypothyroidism, mucopolysaccharidoses) disorders and malformations (microcephaly, holoprosencephaly, etc.)

In isolated craniosynostosis, the patient has no other abnormalities as directly sequential to the craniosynostosis. In syndromic craniosynostosis, there are other defects of morphogenesis, as (poly)syndactyly, etc.

Simple synostosis, mostly (56%) of the sagittal sutures (occurring more in males) and in 18–30% of the coronal sutures (with slight predilection for females), is mostly sporadic, with 2–8%, respectively, of familial cases (Hunter & Rudd 1976, 1977). Autosomal dominant inheritance (with variation for type/number of sutures involved) is more frequent as autosomal recessive inheritance. This makes interpretation difficult in single cases, especially without data on the parents and relatives. Study of family photographs, including those of parents at very young age, may be very informative. If a parent and child are affected, the risk for subsequent children approaches 50% (Cohen 1986); if the parents (and family) are normal the risk is low. Normal parents with two affected children have a risk of recurrence of 25%. The risk to children of an affected patient (having normal parents) is presumed to be low. However, no extensive data are available and with improved neurosurgical results the fitness of patients will increase, with vertical transmission becoming more frequent in the future.

Sagittal stenosis may have a multifactorial origin in some cases, with a recurrence risk of ±1 in 50 to 1 in 70 (Hunter & Rudd 1976); this figure only applies when other genetic mechanisms have been excluded and the family history is negative.

ASSOCIATED ANOMALIES AND SYNDROMES IN CRANIOSYNOSTOSIS

There are 14 chromosomal, 31 monogenic, 3 environmentally induced, 10 'unknown genesis' and 6 miscellaneous syndromes among the 64 craniosynostosis syndromes, as listed in Cohen's table (Chapter 9). Associated anomalies in these syndromes are limb anomalies in 84% (syndactyly or polydactyly in 30%, limb deficiency in 23% and other limb defects in 32%), ear anomalies (38%) and cardiovascular malformations in 23% (Cohen 1986). The overall pattern of these malformations is an important consideration in arriving at a diagnosis.

Besides the well-delineated syndromes, associated anomalies are frequent. The coronal synostoses are more frequently associated with other defects than sagittal synostosis. A flow chart developed by Cohen (Chapter 9) may be a useful addition to the perusal of his diagnostic table.

The cloverleaf skull may be the most extreme end of the spectrum of craniosynostosis and may be associated with different syndromes (Cohen 1986).

Hypertelorism

Widely spaced eyes (hypertelorism) (Fig. 8.3) are to be differentiated from telecanthus (lateral displacement of the inner canthi, which may give a false impression of hypertelorism like in the Waardenburg syndrome (Fig. 8.4)). Sometimes a low nasal bridge may be another source of a false impression of hypertelorism. Measurement of inner and outer canthal distances will usually solve the problem (Smith 1982).

Hypertelorism may be associated with monogenic, multifactorial and chromosomal syndromes, and come to the attention of the plastic surgeon. The differential diagnosis is rather as wide as in craniostenosis-associated syndromes, and includes (among others) Aarskog's syndrome, acrodysostosis, the Coffin–Lowry syndrome, the cleft lip and palate sequence, the DiGeorge sequence, the fetal aminopterin syndrome, the fetal hydantoin syndrome, frontonasal dysplasia, Larsen's syndrome, multiple lentigines (leopard) syndrome, Noonan's syndrome, Opitz syndrome, oto-palatodigital syndrome, some of the acro-cephalosyndactylies (Apert, Pfeiffer, Saethre–Chotzen) Pena-Shokeir I syndrome, and some chromosomal syndromes.

Usually the pattern of malformation will suggest a certain type of diagnosis. Management and prognosis will be greatly influenced by the original condition and its variability, also as relevant to mental development (Smith 1982).

REFERENCES

Afzelius B A 1985 The immotile cilia syndrome: a microtubule-associated defect. CRC Critical Reviews in Biochemistry 19: 63–87

Baker C J, Rudolph A J 1971 Congenital ring constrictions and intrauterine amputations. American Journal of Diseases of Children 121: 393

Barlow S M, Sullivan F M 1982 Reproductive hazards of industrial chemicals. An evaluation of human and animal data. Academic Press, London

Bodian M, Carter C O 1963 A family study of Hirschsprung's disease. Annals of Human Genetics 25: 261–277

Bonaiti C, Briard M L, Feingold J et al 1982 An epidemiological and genetic study of facial clefting in France. I Epidemiology and frequency in relatives. Journal of Medical Genetics 19: 8–15

Bonaiti-Pellie C, Smith C 1974 Risk tables for genetic counseling in some common congenital malformations. Journal of Medical Genetics 11: 374–377

Boo-Chai K 1970 The oblique facial cleft: a report of 2 cases and a review of 41 cases. British Journal of Plastic Surgery 23: 352

Brent R L 1979 Effects of ionizing radiation on growth and development. Contributions to Epidemiology and Biostatistics 1: 147–183

Cohen M M Jr. 1978 Syndromes with cleft lip and cleft palate. Cleft palate Journal 15: 306–328

Cohen M M Jr. 1981 The patient with multiple anomalies. Raven Press, New York

Cohen M M Jr 1986 Craniosynostosis: diagnosis, evaluation and management. Raven Press, New York

David D J, Poswillo D, Simpson D 1982 The craniostenoses. Causes, natural history and management. Springer, Berlin

DeMyer W, Baird I 1969 Mortality and skeletal malformation from amniocentesis and oligohydramnios in rats. Cleft palate, club foot, microstomia and adactyly. Teratology 2: 33

Dey D L 1973 Oblique facial clefts. Plastic and Reconstructive Surgery 52: 258

Franklin J B, Brent R L 1964 The effect of uterine vascular clamping on the development of rat embryos three to fourteen days old. Journal of Morphology 115: 273

Fraser F C, Nora J J 1986 Genetics of man, 2nd edn. Lea & Fabiger, Philadelphia. pp 173–185

Friedman J M 1984 Does Agent Orange cause birth defects? Teratology 29: 193–221

Goodman R M, Gorlin R J 1977 Atlas of the face in genetic disorders. Mosby, St Louis

Graham J G, Miller M E, Stephan M J, Smith D W 1980 Limb reduction anomalies and early in utero limb compression. Journal of Pediatrics 96: 1052

Gunther G S 1963 Nasomaxillary clefts. Plastic and Reconstructive Surgery 32: 637

Harper P 1981 Practical genetic counseling. Churchill, Edinburgh

Harper P S 1979 Myotonic dystrophy. Saunders, Philadelphia. pp 170–206

Heinonen O P, Slone D, Shapiro S 1977 Birth defects and drugs in pregnancy. Publishing Science Group, Littleton

Holmberg P C, Hernberg S, Kurppa K et al 1982 Oral clefts and organic solvent exposure during pregnancy. International Archives of Occupational and Environmental Health 50: 371–376

Hunter A G W, Rudd N L 1976 Craniosynostosis. I Sagittal synostosis; its genetics and associated clinical findings in 214 patients who lacked involvement of the coronal suture(s). Teratology 14: 185–194

Hunter A G W, Rudd N L 1977 Craniosynostosis. II Coronal synostosis: its familial characteristics and associated clinical findings in 109 patients lacking bilateral polydactyly or syndactyly. Teratology 15: 301–310

Jost A 1961 Sur le role de la vasopressine et de la corticostimuline (ATCH) dans la production experimentale de lesions des extremities foetales (hemorragies, necroses, amputations congenitales). Comptes Rendus des Seances de la Société Biologie 4: 23

Kendrick F J, Field L E 1967 Congenital anomalies induced in normal and adrenalectomized rats by ammiocentesis. Anatomical Record 159: 353

Kennedy L A, Persaud T V N 1977 Pathogenesis of developmental defects included in the rat by amniotic sac puncture. Acta Anatomica 97: 23

Kino Y 1975 Clinical and experimental studies of the congenital constriction band syndrome, with an emphasis on its etiology, Journal of Bone and Joint Surgery 57a: 636

Lammer E J, Chen D T, Hoar R M et al 1985 Retinoic acid embryopathy. New England Journal of Medicine 313: 837–841

Levy H L, Waisbren S E 1983 Effects of untreated maternal phenylketonuria and hyperhenylalaninemia on the fetus. New England Journal of Medicine 309: 1269–1274

Lindhout D, Meinardi H 1984 Spina bifida and in-utero exposure to valproate. Lancet ii: 396

Martinet M 1958 Hemorragies embryonnaires par deficience en acide linoleique. Annales de Médecine Interne 53: 286

McKusick V A 1972 Heritable disorders of connective tissue. Mosby, St Louis. pp 1–30

McKusick V A 1988 Mendelian inheritance in man, 8th edn. Johns Hopkins, Baltimore

Mayou B J, Fenton O M 1981 Oblique facial clefts caused by amniotic bands. Plastic and Reconstructive Surgery 68: 675

Miller M E, Graham J M, Higginbottom M C, Smith D W 1981 Compression related defects from early amnion rupture: evidence for mechanical teratogenesis. Journal of Pediatrics 98: 292

Mossman K L, Hill L T 1982 Radiation risks in pregnancy. Obstetrics and Gynecology 60: 237–242

Otake M, Schull W J 1984 In utero exposure to A-bomb radiation and mental retardation; a reassessment. British Journal of Radiology 57: 409–414

Poswillo D 1966 Observations of fetal posture and causal mechanism of congenital deformity of palate, mandible and limbs. Journal of Dental Research 45: 584

Poswillo D E 1973 The pathogenesis of the first and second branchial arch syndrome. Oral Surgery 35: 302

Poswillo D E 1975 The pathogenesis of Treacher Collins syndrome (mandibulofacial dysostosis). British Journal of Oral Surgery 13: 1

Poswillo D E 1979 Etiology and pathogenesis of first and second branchial arch defects: the contribution of animal studies. Symposium on diagnosis and treatment of craniofacial anomalies, vol. 20.

Robert E, Guibaud P 1982 Maternal valproic acid and congenital neural tube defects. Lancet ii: 937

Roberts N J Jr, Michaelson S M 1985 Epidemiological studies of human exposure to radiofrequency radiation. International Archives of Occupational and Environmental Health 56: 169–178

Rollnick B R, Kaye C I 1986 Mendelian inheritance of isolated non-syndromic cleft palate. American Journal of Medical Genetics 24: 465–473

Rosett H L, Weiner L 1984 Alcohol and the fetus. A clinical perspective. Oxford University Press, New York

Saxen L, Holmberg P C, Nurminen M, Kuosma E 1982 Sauna and congenital defects. Teratology 25: 309–313

Schardein J L 1985 Chemically induced birth defects. Dekker, New York

Schinzel A 1984 Catalogue of unbalanced chromosome aberrations in man. de Gruyter, Berlin

Shepard T H, Fantel A G, Mirkes 1986 Megadoses of vitamin A. Teratology 34: 366

Shiota K 1982 Neural tube defects and maternal hyperthermia in early pregnancy: epidemiology of a human embryo population. American Journal of Medical Genetics 12: 281–288

Shprintzen R J, Siegel-Sadewitz V L, Amata J et al 1985 Anomalies associated with cleft lip, cleft palate or both. American Journal of Medical Genetics 20: 585–595

Singh S, Mathur M M, Singh G 1973 Congenital anomalies in rat fetuses induced by amniocentesis. Indian Journal of Medical Research 62: 394

Smith D W 1981 Recognizable patterns of human deformation. Saunders, Philadelphia

Smith D W 1982 Recognizable patterns of human malformation, 3rd edn. Saunders, Philadelphia

Spence M A, Westlake J, Lange K, Gold D P 1976 Estimation of polygenic recurrence risk for cleft lip and palate. Human Heredity 26: 327–336

Stewart R E, Prescott G H (eds) 1976 Oral facial genetics. Mosby, St Louis

Tenchini M L, Crimaudo C, Pacchetti G et al 1983 A comparative cytogenetic study on cases of induced abortions in TCDD exposed and non-exposed women. Environmental Mutagenesis 5: 73–85

Torpin R 1968 Fetal malformations caused by amnion rupture during gestation. Thomas, Springfield, Ill

Trasler D G, Walker B E, Fraser F C 1956 Congenital malformations produced by amniotic-sac puncture. Science 124: 439

Van der Meulen J C H 1985 Oblique facial clefts: pathology, etiology and reconstruction. American Journal of Plastic and Reconstructive Surgery 2: 212

Velasco Garcia D M 1980 Tratamiento de las hendiduras faciales tipo III, IV y V. III congreso ibero latino-Americano de Cirurgia plastica y constructiva y V congreso national, Valencia, June

Webster W S, Johnston M C, Lammer J L, Sulik K S 1986 Isotretinoin embryopathy and the cranial neural crest: an in vivo and in vitro study. Journal of Craniofacial Genetics and Developmental Biology 6: 211–222

Williams A R 1983 Ultrasound: biological effects and potential hazards. Academic Press, London

Wilson L F, Musgrave R H, Garret W, Conklin J E 1972 Reconstruction of oblique facial clefts. Cleft Palate Journal 9: 109

Classification

9. Classification of craniofacial malformations

J. Van der Meulen, R. Mazzola, M. Stricker, B. Raphael

'A new classification is needed from time to time as scientific evolution proceeds. The classification is usually based on new theories, but it remains always provisional' (J. W. von Goethe (1749–1832), *Schriften zur Naturwissenschaft*)

INTRODUCTION

Craniofacial malformations are relatively uncommon. The adopted terminology has always been far from satisfactory and consensus on the type of classification to be used has never been achieved.

Some authors have concentrated their efforts on the analysis of restricted areas of the face (Grünberg 1909, Zausch 1926, Stupka 1938, Scuderi 1954, Burian 1957, Kernahan 1957, Gunther 1963). Others have tried to classify all sorts of malformations on an anatomical basis (Greer Walker 1961, Duhamel 1966, Karfik 1966, Tessier 1976). Only a few workers took morphogenesis into consideration, even if the adopted system was mainly topographical (Sömmering 1791, Taullard 1961, De Myer 1967, Pfeiffer 1967, 1974, Sedano et al 1970, Mazzola 1976) (Fig. 9.1).

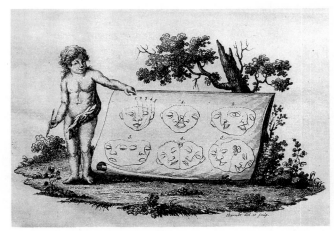

Fig. 9.1 Soemmering's classification.

The above considerations show the dualism between morphological (i.e. anatomico-clinical) and morphogenetic types of classification.

Identification

As a general rule no classification is possible without a correct identification of the elements to be classified. A classification must be consistent and leave as little room as possible for ambiguities. Careful analysis of similarities and differences between facial malformations constitutes a prerequisite and only then can order be created out of chaos.

Theoretically, one may identify craniofacial malformations according to pathogenesis, pathomorphology, topography and the time of developmental arrest.

PATHOGENESIS

As emphasized in the appropriate chapters of this book (biology, embryology, genetics, pathology), the complex mosaic of morphogenesis of the human face is the end result of a series of events, each one essential per se: genetic information, cell deposition, cell differentiation, cell proliferation, cell degeneration, and tissue remodelling all play a part.

Genetic information

Every cell has its own code, and when the genetic information is not correctly transmitted normal development does not take place.

Cell deposition

It has recently been demonstrated that the deposition of mesectodermal cells in the head–neck area occurs at a very early stage of development (Vermeij-Keers & Poelman 1980, Vermeij-Keers et al 1983, Smits-van Prooye 1986).

This theory implies that there is no need for the migration of neural crest cells (Ch. 3).

Cell differentiation

Normal development depends on the formation of different cell types (cytodifferentiation) or tissues (histo-differentiation). Once these cells or tissues are formed, they may interact with one another by induction to produce other varieties of tissue. This phenomenon is known as epithelio-mesenchymal interaction (e.g. bone formation and pneumatization).

Cell proliferation

The proliferation of cells and the formation of an extra-cellular matrix leads to an increase of tissue bulkiness or interstitial growth (e.g. formation of facial processes), while appositional growth refers to surface deposition (e.g. bone formation). The term 'differential growth' indicates that not all tissues develop at the same rate.

Cell degeneration

Death of some or groups of cells which have outlived their function (epithelial plate of Hochstetter) creates room for other cells and tissues to develop. Lack of cell degeneration seems to be one of the main causes of malformations such as a cleft of the lip (Ch. 3).

Tissue remodelling

Bone remodelling is determined by numerous factors, which may belong to two systems: a metabolic and a neuromuscular system. In a craniofacial malformation both groups may be involved. A bone, once formed, is composed of the minimum quantity of osseous tissue necessary to withstand the functional stress applied by neuromuscular activity. Changes in muscle–bone interaction are immediately followed by alterations in structure and shape of the bone (Wolf's law). Bassett & Becker (1962) have expressed this law in the following formulation: 'The form of a bone being given, bone elements place or displace themselves in the direction of functional pressures and increase or decrease their mass to reflect the amount of functional forces.'

Each one of the above mentioned systems may be disturbed, but we do not know to what extent such an interference is responsible for developmental arrest, nor do we have enough information about factors or agents which may cause such a disturbance. In fact, our understanding of chemical biology is still too rudimentary and, although phenocopies may be produced in animal models, the mech-

anism involved is not necessarily the same as in human beings. Extrapolation from one field of research to another is not justified: 'the phenomena must first be classified, each one on its own grounds before deductions, comparisons and generalizations can be attempted' (Holtfreter 1968).

At present the precise teratogenic potential of a factor is not known. A particular anomaly may develop due to different causative factors or agents (heterogeneity), while on the other hand a specific factor may produce a variety of malformations, depending on the time and the severity of the insult (pleiotropy).

A classification of anomalies based on their pathogenesis is therefore inadequate.

PATHOMORPHOLOGY

Malformations may also be identified by their appearance. When a malformation is examined and described, terms such as clefting, coloboma and microsomy are used, which cannot be defined with complete precision.

The use of improper terminology is, however, a source of confusion and may create the impression that these malformations have a different origin which, in fact, may not be true. De Myer (1975) considers a cleft to be 'a defect in apposition of structures along a junction'. This concept is easy to accept when it refers to a defect caused by failure of fusion of junctional structures. The concept becomes more difficult to accept when it refers to a median nasal or an oro-ocular cleft, which cannot be explained by classical embryological theories, and it can certainly not be applied to malformations like teleorbitism, Treacher Collins syndrome or hemifacial microsomia, not to mention nasal aplasia with or without proboscis, anophthalmia or microtia.

We have learned from embryology (Ch. 3) that a sharp distinction should be made between primary or true clefts, produced at an early stage of facial development (e.g. cleft lip, naso-ocular cleft), and secondary or pseudoclefts, which have their origin at a later stage of facial development (e.g. nasal clefts, oro-ocular clefts).

Secondary clefts only develop when the facial processes have fused. The fact that their appearance is different from malformations such as microsomia can easily be understood when one visualizes what may happen when growth is arrested in one skeletal area while it continues in the normal adjacent tissues. An hourglass deformity may be produced with the transition in the middle as the original site of the developmental arrest (Fig. 9.2) (Van der Meulen et al 1983). This part, behaving as a scar, will then prevent the surrounding tissues from expanding normally. As a result a series of V-shaped anomalies will develop, affecting the nose, the maxilla, the lips, the eyelids and the hairline. The character of these anomalies will vary with the area of skeletal involvement and the nature of the

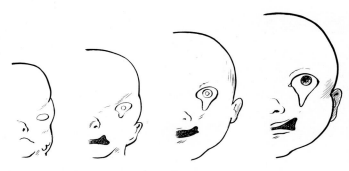

Fig. 9.2 The origin of secondary clefting.

adjacent tissues. The direction of these clefts, colobomas and peaks is predominantly in a craniocaudal direction.

The term dysmorphy applies to modifications in form, produced by a cleft, a coloboma or any other disruption. It only describes a clinical aspect and is insufficient when not related to a pathomorphogenic basis.

TOPOGRAPHY

Soemmering (1791) was, as far as we know, the first to conceive the idea of orientating defects or clefts along constant axes through the midline of the nose, the nostrils, the eyebrows and the maxilla, and to propose a system for identification (Fig. 9.1). Other authors based their classification of facial deformities on a clinical or anatomical judgement (Morian 1887, Davis 1935, Harkins et al 1962, Fogh-Andersen 1965, Karfik 1966). The majority of these systems are inadequate in several respects. Either conspicuous omissions are made, or they rely only on soft tissue landmarks.

An important contribution was made by Tessier (1976). With his great clinical experience based on the direct observation of numerous craniofacial malformations, Tessier argued that these anomalies are situated along definite axes. He emphasized for the first time the relationship between soft and bony tissue, stating that although the extent of their involvement may vary: 'a fissure of the soft tissue corresponds, as a general rule, with a cleft of the bony structures. The converse is also possible'. Tessier also suggested the term cleft as the common denominator in all craniofacial anomalies. He related these to the orbit, considering this structure to be common to the overlying cranium and to the underlying facial skeleton. In order to simplify the nomenclature he devised a very workable system in which the site of each malformation is assigned a number (0–14) depending on its relationship to the zero line (i.e. a vertical cleft in the midline of the face).

This system became widely accepted in a very short time, because the recording of the malformation was made easier and communications between observers were facilitated.

Although it is not our aim to object to the practical diagnostic validity of this classification, we feel that it is a descriptive, clinical system, not related to the morphogenesis of the anomaly. Understanding of the underlying pathology is in no way improved, while the origin of some of the clefts is not explained. As emphasized above, use of the word 'clefting' may even create confusion when a cleft does not exist.

Identification of anomalies by their localization is, however, important.

Unlike some congenital deformities of the hand, which defy classification, a craniofacial malformation remains recognizable, because it can be identified by comparing it to the facial characteristics of the embryo at a given stage of development (see Ch. 3).

CHRONOLOGY (Fig. 9.3)

Malformations may have their origin at different levels of development:

1. *During the stage of transformation* (see Ch. 3). A developmental arrest of the forebrain or its lateral extensions is associated with a deficiency of the interplacodal area and may even be incompatible with life. Distinction should therefore be made between malformations with or without cerebral involvement. The latter group will include the malformations which occur before fusion of facial processes has taken place, and therefore result in clefting (Fig. 9.4).
2. *During the stage of differentiation* (see Ch. 3). Abnormal or absent ossification is primarily characterized by osseous deficiency or dysostosis (Fig. 9.4). The resulting skeletal disharmony is frequently associated with muscular and cutaneous anomalies.
3. *During the stage of adaptation.* Premature ossification of sutures — synostosis — forms an obstacle to skeletal development in a direction perpendicular to the suture line (Virchow's law) (Fig. 9.4). This arrest is usually compensated for by hyperdevelopment in a direction parallel to the suture line. Muscles and skin are generally not directly involved.

These considerations allow us to identify malformations in relation to the underlying pathology with full appreciation of the fact that accurate delineation of these groups is not always possible and that some overlap may be observed.

By comparing one craniofacial malformation with another of the same category, an idea can finally be gained of the severity of the anomaly. It then becomes obvious that all of these malformations can be graded and related to the form at a certain stage of embryonic life. The earlier the developmental arrest the more severe the malformation.

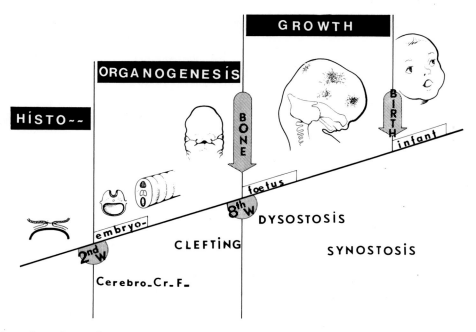

Fig. 9.3 The chronology of morphogenesis.

Classification philosophy

Modern knowledge of the normal development of the facial skeleton has increased our understanding of the underlying pathology. The application of clinical criteria used for identification has enabled us to classify all craniofacial anomalies in which the skeleton is predominantly involved. The basis of this classification (Van der Meulen et al 1983) was established by observation and categorization of a large number of patients with craniofacial malformations seen in the departments of plastic surgery of The University Hospitals of Grenoble (France), Nancy (France), Milan (Italy) and Rotterdam (the Netherlands), and by correlation of these anomalies with various stages of embryonic and fetal life.

It has been our aim to define a precise descriptive classification, both useful and truthful, while avoiding a cumbersome catalogue of the endless variations of clinical abnormalities. To achieve this a simplified nomenclature with a non-ambiguous terminology was used, the term 'Dysplasia' serving this purpose best.

Dysplasia or abnormal development of growth covers all pathogenic and clinical aspects of a malformation such as dysinduction, dysgenesis, dysmorphy and dystrophy, including qualitative or quantitative aspects.

The classification is founded on a pathomorphogenic basis, which includes a chronological and a topographical element. The chronological element is related to the various developmental stages at which a disturbance may occur and to the teratogenic mechanisms involved. The topographical element refers to the various anatomical sites and areas which may be affected.

The chronological element justifies differentiation into:
I. Cerebrocranial dysplasias
II. Cerebrofacial dysplasias
III. Craniofacial dysplasias

The term cerebro-cranial or cerebro-facial is used when the brain or its lateral optic extensions are implicated. The term cranio-facial applies when the brain and the eyes are not involved.

The chronological element allows further differentiation of this group into several categories, each related to specific developmental stages, such as the fusion of processes, the production of bones and the formation of sutures (Fig. 9.4).

Fusion of facial processes is prevented by the persistence of the epithelial plate (see Ch. 3). The resulting clefts are only seen in four locations:

1. latero-nasomaxillary
2. medio-nasomaxillary
3. intermaxillary
4. maxillo-mandibular.

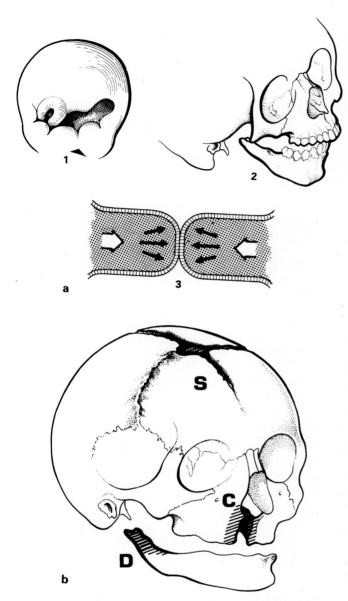

Fig. 9.4 (a) Types of skeletal deficiency related to the chronology of morphogenesis: (1) clefting; (2) dysostosis; (3) synostosis (b) Site of skeletal deficiency related to the chronology of morphogenesis. C = Clefting between facial processes; D = dysostosis of ossification centres; S = synostosis in desmocranium.

toses will affect a topography, analogous to that of the morphogenesis, implying that their distribution is ranged along a **craniofacial helix of dysostoses**. The concept of this helix and the idea to start its course on the lateral aspect of the craniofacial skeleton was developed (Van der Meulen et al 1983) when ranging of the whole spectrum of dysostosis in a logical order, beginning in the midline, proved to be impossible.

The following consideration also played a role. The importance of the sphenoid with its lateral extensions as a key structure for normal craniofacial development could thus be emphasized. Morphogenesis of the craniofacial skeleton starts with the formation of the middle and anterior cranial fossae, a process which is associated with a reduction in the interorbital distance. This process is followed by the development of the nasomaxillary complex, expanding forward, downward and laterally, and it is completed by the lengthening of the mandibular ramus, which is produced by this expansion.

The architectural design of the craniofacial skeleton can therefore be compared with a helix, the symbol of life in some cultures, and here symbolized by the letter S (Fig. 9.5). The ossification centres in the upper section of the helix form the anterior wall of the brain, while those in the middle section delineate the nasal aperture, the orbital cavity and the auditory meatus. The skeletal primordia in the lower section provide a floor for the oral cavity.

The formation of sutures is disturbed by deficient activity of sutural periosteum. This periosteal dysplasia, occurring at a later stage, compromises the normal arrangement of the skeletal parts by premature **synostosis**.

Combinations of dysostosis and synostosis are frequently observed producing a fourth category of craniofacial dysplasias.

The cartilaginous matrices are equally exposed to the impact of the malformation, quite often resulting in dyschondrosis. Awaiting further study and delineation, these abnormalities are provisionally classified in a fifth category of craniofacial dysplasias.

The classification is extended with a histological element upset which took place at the level of the skull base tissues. An additional group of dysplasias can thus be distinguished.

Arising at an early stage (before 17 mm C–RL) they are associated with bony defects or secondary dysostosis. We therefore incorporated medio-naso maxillary and latero-naso maxillary clefting in the classification of dysostosis as premaxillomaxillary and nasomaxillary dysplasia.

The production of bone is a key element in craniofacial morphogenesis. Ossification may be altered by deficient development of ossification centres. The resulting dysos-

IV. Craniofacial dysplasias with other origin. Bone may be affected by diseases which are characterized by hyperplasia. This category must be distinguished from dysostosis which is by definition hypoplastic.

Skin, nerves, muscles, and vessels may also participate in varying degrees, sometimes even taking a prominent place in the clinical manifestation of a final category of malformations, which frequently involves the craniofacial skeleton.

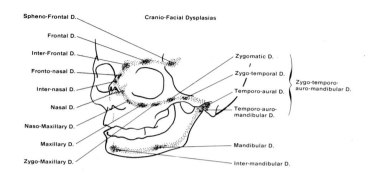

Fig. 9.5 Craniofacial helix with ossification centres.

CLASSIFICATION OF CRANIOFACIAL MALFORMATIONS

I CEREBROCRANIAL DYSPLASIAS
Anencephaly
Microcephaly
Others

II CEREBROFACIAL DYSPLASIAS
Rhinencephalic dysplasias
Oculo-orbital dysplasias

III CRANIOFACIAL DYSPLASIAS
(a) *With clefting*
Latero-nasomaxillary cleft
Medio-nasomaxillary
Intermaxillary clefting
Maxillo-mandibular cleft
(b) *With dysostosis* (Craniofacial helix)
Sphenoidal
Spheno-frontal
Frontal
Fronto-frontal
Fronto-nasoethmoidal
Internasal
Nasal
Premaxillo-maxillary and Intermaxillo-palatine
Naso-maxillary and maxillary
Maxillo-zygomatic
Zygomatic
Zygo-auromandibular
Temporo-aural
Temporo-auromandibular
Mandibular
Intermandibular
(c) *With synostosis*
Craniosynostosis
Parieto-occipital
Interparietal

Cranio-faciosynostosis
Interfrontal
Spheno-frontoparietal
Fronto-parietal
Fronto-interparietal
Faciosynostosis
Fronto-malar
Vomero-premaxillary (Binder)
Perimaxillary (post) (clefting)
Perimaxillary (ant.) (pseudo Crouzon)
Perimaxillary (total) (Crouzon)
(d) *With dysostosis and synostosis*
Crouzon
Acro-cephalosyndactlyly (Apert)
Triphyllocephaly (cloverleaf skull)
(e) *With dyschondrosis*
Achondroplasia

IV CRANIOFACIAL DYSPLASIAS WITH OTHER ORIGIN
(a) Osseous
Osteopetrosis
Cranio tubular dysplasia
Fibrous dysplasia
(b) Cutaneous
Ectodermal dysplasia
(c) Neurocutaneous
Neurofibromatosis
(d) Neuromuscular
Robin syndrome
Möbius syndrome
(e) Muscular
Glossoschizis
(f) Vascular
Haemangioma
Haemolymphangioma
Lymphangioma

CEREBROCRANIAL DYSPLASIAS (Fig. 9.6)

Simultaneous alteration of brain and cranium is strikingly manifested in the lethal condition named anencephaly. Cranial abnormalities reflecting deficient development of the brain are, however, also seen in: microcephaly, associated with harmonious reduction of the cranium; cranial asymmetry caused by cerebral cyst formation; and cranial defects due to abnormal ossification.

Anencephaly (Fig. 9.7).

According to Isidore Geoffroy St Hilaire (1832), anencephaly developed from absent closure of the neural tube (encephaloschizis).

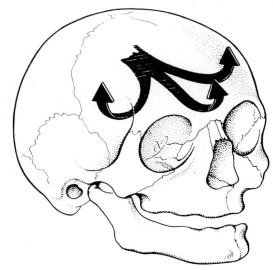

Fig. 9.6 Relationship between brain and cranium.

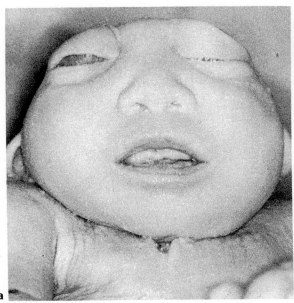

Fig. 9.7 Anencephaly: (a) frontal view; (b) lateral view.

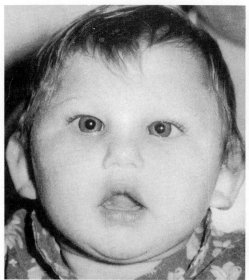
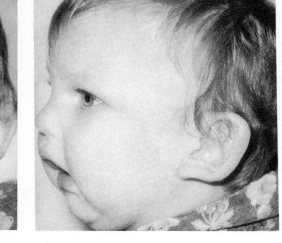

Fig. 9.8 Microcephaly: (a) frontal view; (b) lateral view.

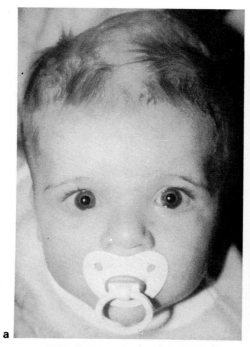

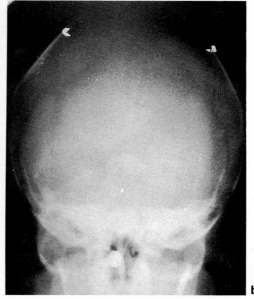

Fig. 9.9 Aplasia of the vault associated with herniation of the brain.

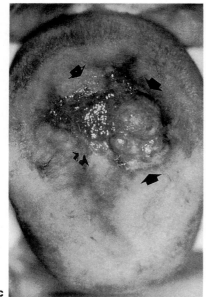

The vault of the skull is missing. The anterior brain structures are absent and replaced by a spongy vascular mass, named pseudencephaly or area cerebrovasculosa. The presence of normal eyes and optic nerves is, however, an indication that an exposed forebrain (exencephaly) existed originally, which degenerated as a result of inadequate protection.

Vogel & McClenahan (1952) stated that the destroyed parts of the brain are those normally supplied by the internal carotids, whereas the eyes and the brainstem are supplied by the ophthalmic and vertebral arteries, thus suggesting a vascular abnormality as a primary failure. This theory, however, has never been proven.

The incidence of anencephaly averages 1 per 1000 births in Europe, with enormous topographical variations which at present are unexplained.

Microcephaly (Fig. 9.8)

In this malformation the brain is reduced in size and enclosed in a small skull, while the cerebellum is of normal size. Over the age of 10 years, a head circumference under 46 cm is classified as microcephalic, but actually most authors require a cranial circumference greater than 3 standard deviations below the expected mean (always less than 43.2 cm maximum).

Microcephaly was known to Thomas Willus in the seventeenth century. It is always due to the reduced growth of the brain and not the smallness of the skull or the premature obliteration of the cranial sutures. In most of the cases the damage is prenatal.

Microcephaly may be primary (hereditary) or secondary to such factors as rubella or toxoplasmosis. Most infants have mental retardation and life expectancy is low.

Decades ago failure to distinguish between this condition and craniosynostosis induced surgeons to operate on infants with microcephaly, and Lannelongue (1890) described his craniotomy for this purpose.

Congenital defects of the skull (Fig. 9.9)

These defects are due to absence of bone, which is replaced by fibrous tissue. They are sometimes associated with protrusion of meninges and brain through the vault. Cranium bifidum occultum and cranioschizis are confusing terms used to describe these defects.

CEREBROFACIAL DYSPLASIAS (Fig. 9.10)

Rhinencephalic dysplasia

This condition is characterized by forebrain malformations and agenesis or hypodevelopment of the midline structures of the face (Fig. 9.8). The cerebral anomalies consist of the failure of the prosencephalon to divide: (1) transversely into telencephalon and diencephalon; (2) sagittally into cerebral hemispheres; and (3) horizontally into olfactory and optic bulbs. The facial defects include varying degrees of hypotelorism, absence or severe hypoplasia of the nose, the nasal cavity, nasal bones, lacrimal bones, ethmoid, vomer, septum, turbinates and premaxilla. Geoffroy St Hilaire (1832) was the first to divide these 'monstres cyclocephaliens' into two groups: those with a single orbit and those with two separate orbits. Kundrat (1882) coined the term 'arhinencephaly' for the second group, including less severe forms with absence of the rhinencephalon. He also reported the frequent association with trigonocephaly. An unbroken chain (Fig. 9.11) of faciocerebral malformations, from the severest form to the near-normal states, may be observed (Koelliker 1882, Schwalbe & Josephy 1909, Culp 1921, Yakovlev 1959, De Myer and Zeman 1963, De Myer 1975, Mazzola 1976, Cohen 1982, Fitz

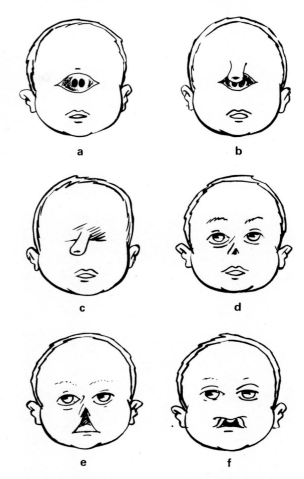

Fig. 9.11 Spectrum of cerebrofacial dysplasias: (a) cyclopia; (b) synophthalmus; (c) ethmocephaly; (d) cebocephaly; (e) without premaxilla; (f) with premaxilla.

1983). De Myer & Zeman (1963) have graded the facial defects according to their severity, in a series pathognomonic of the underlying brain anomaly ('the face predicts the brain').

MORPHOLOGY

Starting with cyclopia, representing the most severe example, the spectrum of faciocerebral anomalies, with hypotelorism, moves through ethmocephaly, cebocephaly, median cleft lip without a premaxilla, towards the normal state.

Cyclopia

Cyclopia (Fig. 9.12), described in Greek mythology (see Polyphemus in the *Odyssey*), represents one of the most striking examples of malformations ever reported in the literature (von Haller 1768, Soemmering 1791, Riviera

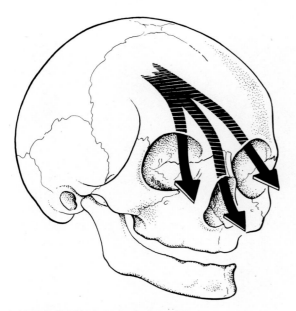

Fig. 9.10 Relationship between brain and face.

1793, Speer 1819, Raddatz 1829, Ahlfeld 1882) (see Fig. 1.12).

The forebrain here fails to divide into cerebral hemispheres (holoprosencephaly). The lateral ventricles are fused, and the falx, septum pellucidum and corpus callosum are absent or incomplete. Thalami, corpora striata and optic tracts are variously affected. The sphenoid is hypoplastic and there is only one optic canal. The olfactory bulbs and tracts are usually absent or rudimentary (arhinencephaly). Synophthalmus and synorbitism are observed.

The eyes, fused into a single or partially divided vesicle, are to be found in a single orbit, limited superiorly by a single frontal bone, laterally by the greater wings of the sphenoid and zygomatic bones, and inferiorly by the maxillary bones. The site of the fused olfactory placodes may be marked by a single proboscis located above the eye

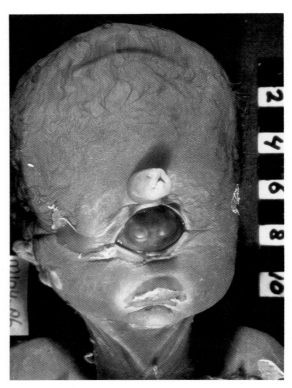

Fig. 9.13 Cyclopia associated with proboscis.

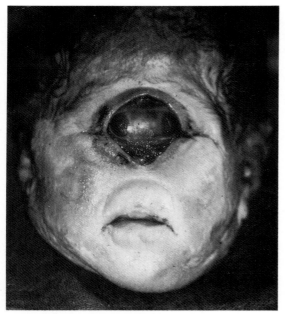

Fig. 9.12 Cyclopia.

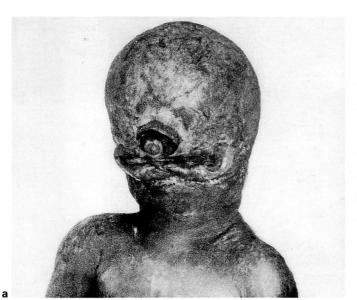

a

Fig. 9.14 Cyclopia associated with otocephaly.

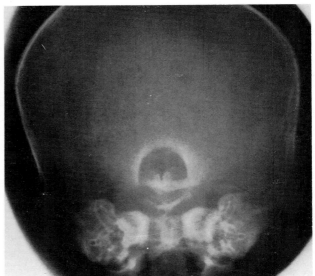

b

(Fig. 9.13). All the midline structures are absent. Cyclopia is occasionally associated with otocephaly (Fig. 9.14).

Ethmocephaly (ethmos = sieve)

Cerebral and facial malformations closely resemble those observed in cyclopia but the orbits are separated from each other. The optic nerves may bifurcate after a common

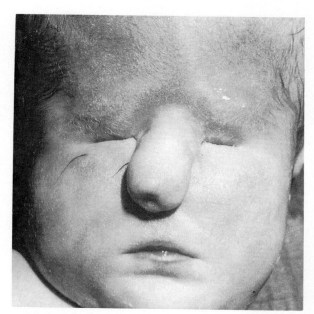

Fig. 9.15 Ethmocephaly.

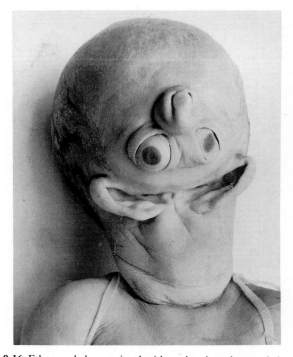

Fig. 9.16 Ethmocephaly associated with proboscis and otocephaly.

single origin. The nose is absent or substituted by a snout-like appendage (Fig. 9.15). The nasal cavity, nasal bones, ethmoid, vomer, septum, turbinates and premaxilla are all missing (Renner 1889). The condition is sometimes associated with otocephaly (Fig. 9.16).

Cebocephaly (cebos = monkey)

Cerebral anomalies consist of holoprosencephaly, absence of the falx, septum pelludicum, corpus callosum, olfactory bulbs and tracts (Fig. 9.17). The optic foramina, separated by a membrane, lie close together in a common bony canal.

Facial dysmorphism is characterized by severe hypotelorism and by hypodevelopment of the midline structures (nasal bones, ethmoid, vomer, septum, turbinates and premaxilla). The nose, rudimentary and flat, encompasses a unique nostril simplified into a blind pit.

Ocular, auricular, branchial, cardiac and urogenital malformations may be associated with all of the above deformities.

Premaxillary aplasia or hypoplasia

In the first type (Fig. 9.18) the cerebral anomalies involve semilobar holoprosencephaly, occasionally with a posterior interhemispheric fissure, and the absence of olfactory bulbs and tracts. The optic foramina, separated by a membrane, lie close together in a common bony canal. Hypotelorism is severe and wide palatal clefting is observed. The nose is flat and the columella as well as the philtrum are absent. The median cleft corresponds to the missing philtrum and is confluent with the single nasal opening. Hypertelorism is an abnormal finding (Fig. 9.19).

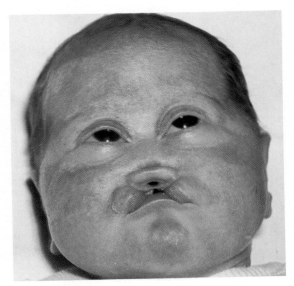

Fig. 9.17 Cebocephaly.

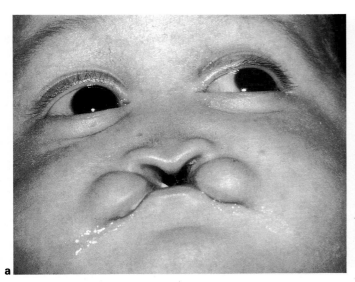 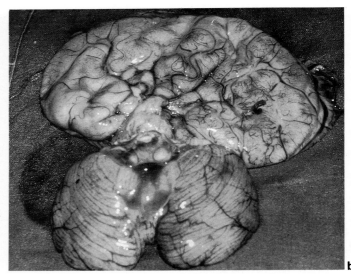

Fig. 9.18 Premaxillary aplasia associated with hypotelorism: (a) frontal view; (b) cerebral abnormalities consisting of cyst formation and holoprosencephaly.

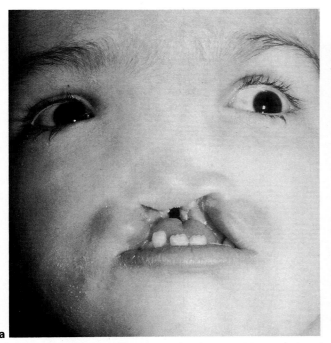 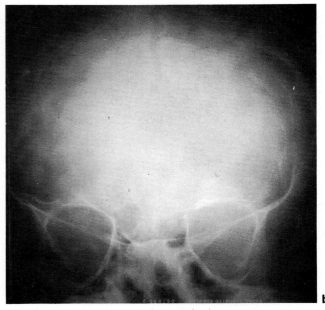

Fig. 9.19 Premaxillary aplasia associated with paradoxal hypertelorism due to encephalocele: (a) clinical view; (b) X-ray shows site of encephalocele.

In the second type (Fig. 9.20) cerebral anomalies vary in degree and include approximation of the lateral ventricles, absence of septum pellucidum, etc. (Fitz 1983). The cerebral lobes are well formed and brain development may be normal; hypotelorism is less severe, the nose is flat and palatal clefting is often present. Cardiovascular malformations are often associated.

This condition should not be confused with Binder's syndrome. Nasomaxillary dysostosis, first described by Binder (1962), is characterized by a slight degree of hypotelorism and a flat nose, short philtrum and columella, hypoplasia of the nasal spine and maxillary hypodevelopment. Although named by the author 'arhinencephaloid face', this dysmorphism belongs to the category of faciosynostoses (see Ch. 9, p. 244).

The above-mentioned classification is important from a prognostic point of view. Malformations such as cyclopia,

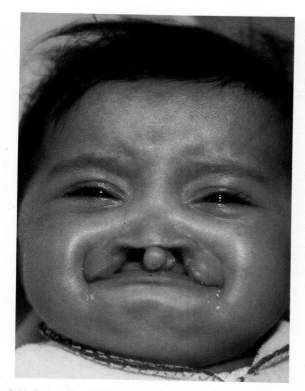

Fig. 9.20 Premaxillary hypoplasia associated with hypotelorism; distinction from bilateral cleft lip is required.

ethmocephaly and cebocephaly, with associated alobar holoprosencephaly, are not compatible with life, while patients showing facial dysmorphism with hypotelorism and absence of the premaxilla are usually severely mentally retarded and may die shortly after birth. Those with a hypoplastic premaxilla, having a normal or near-normal prosencephalon, usually live and benefit from surgical procedures which help them to integrate with society.

Oculo-orbital dysplasia

ANORBITISM AND MICROORBITISM

Complete absence of the orbit is exceedingly rare (Fig. 9.21). Orbital anomalies usually consist of changes in the dimension, the configuration and the position of the orbital skeleton. The orbital volume may be reduced by as much as 50% (Ellsworth 1967). The degree of microorbitism (Fig. 9.22) is proportional to the centrifugal force produced by the orbital contents.

Lateralization of the medial wall and caudalization of the roof and the floor of the orbit may be observed. In addition, there may be thickening of the lateral wall and flattening of the superoexternal angle. The optical nerve may be absent. The periocular muscles are usually present but differentiation and insertion may be defective. The conjuntival sac is small. The eyelids are reduced in size

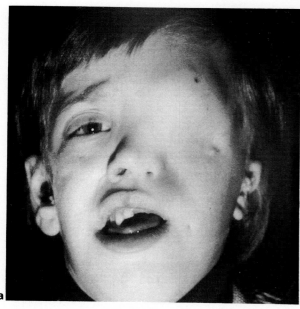

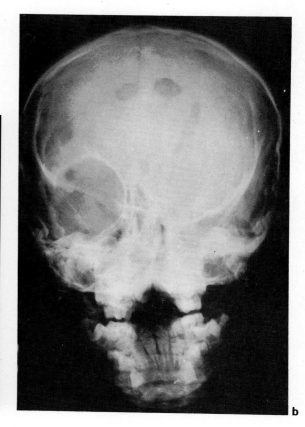

Fig. 9.21 Anorbitism forming part of major orbitonasal microsomia.

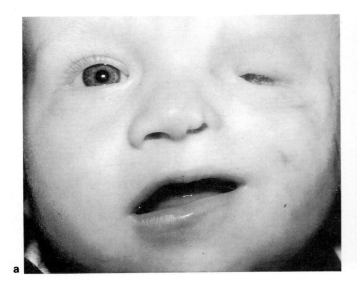

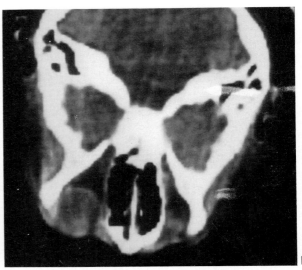

Fig. 9.22 Microorbitism forming part of minor orbitonasal microsomia.

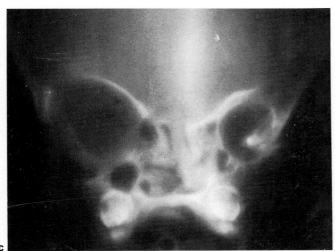

(microblepharon) while ptosis, hirsutism of the upper eyelid and hypertrichosis of the eyebrow may also be observed.

ANOPHTHALMIA AND MICROPHTHALMIA (Fig. 9.23)

This condition was recorded as early as 1654 by Bartholinus in his *Historiarum Anatomicarum*. A considerable number of unilateral as well as bilateral cases have been described since then and these reports show clearly that the anomaly may be associated with a great variety of other abnormalities — some of a cerebral nature, some craniofacial — while others may be located in different parts of the body.

For practical purposes the distinction between anophthalmia and microphthalmia should be made on a clinical basis. The term anophthalmia encompasses all those cases in which traces of ocular development are either absent or so small that differentiation between anophthalmia and extreme microphthalmia can only be established by histological examination. The term microphthalmia is reserved for those conditions in which the presence of some ocular development may be established by clinical means. The range, from complete anophthalmia to a minor degree of microphthalmia, is considerable and depending on the severity of the arrest a range of periocular malformations may also be observed.

These malformations may affect the orbit itself, the optic nerve, the periocular muscles, the eyelids and the eyebrow (see section on periocular dysplasias).

Differentiation

Anophthalmus and microphthalmus may be found in combination with many of the other dysplasias to be described in this classification, and sometimes also as part of one of the following syndromes:

Oculo-aurovertebral dysplasia (Goldenhar 1952)
Oculovertebral dysplasia (Weyers & Thier 1958)
Oculo-auromandibular dysplasia (Francois & Haustrate 1954)
Oculo-dentodigital dysplasia (Lohman 1920)
Mandibulo-oculofacial dysplasia (Hallerman & Streiff 1948, 1950)
Mandibulo-oculocranial dysplasia (Ulrich & Frenery-Dohna 1953)
Cervico-oculoacoustic dysplasia (Wildervanck 1960)
Cervico-oculofacial dysplasia with deafness (Franceschetti & Klein 1954)

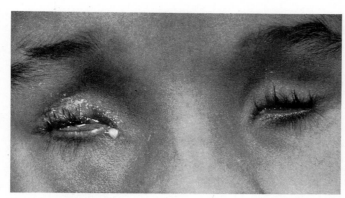

Fig. 9.23 Anophthalmia.

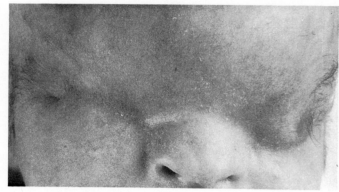

Fig. 9.24 Cryptophthalmia.

CRYPTOPHTHALMIA (Fig. 9.24)

Zehender et al (1872) have been credited with the first report on this rare malformation, which may occur unilaterally or bilaterally and is inherited in an autosomal recessive pattern.

The condition is usually characterized by complete fusion of the upper and lower eyelids and absence of the eyelashes. The eyebrows may be partially defective or absent. In addition the hairline is frequently abnormal. The cutaneous continuity between forehead and cheek is in fact a striking feature. Palpebral structures are deficient but the orbicularis and levator palpebrae muscles may be present.

The position of the eyeball is indicated by a swelling and eye movements can sometimes be seen. Reflex wrinkling of the palpebral remnants may be elicited by exposure to strong light.

On opening the skin over the eye, obliteration of the conjunctival sac is first observed. The eyeball may be disorganized or relatively well developed and covered anteriorly by transluscent tissue which is easily separated from the globe. Differentiation between cornea and sclera may be present but metaplasia of corneal epithelium into skin has also been observed.

The histopathology of this condition was reviewed by Francois (1965). Cryptophthalmia is frequently associated with other abnormalities involving the ear (auricular malformation and conduction loss), the nose (notching of the nostrils), the mouth (ankyloglossia), the limbs (syndactyly) and the genitalia.

Periocular dysplasia

The different structures of the anterior palpebral wall may show various abnormalities which are frequently seen, either as a solitary anomaly or in combination with one of the many skeletal dysplasias discussed in the ensuing sections, particularly those involving the orbit. Although not strictly belonging to the group of cerebrofacial dysplasias these malformations are closely related to the eye and are therefore described here. These anomalies involve the eyelids, the canthi, the sclera, the eyebrows and the nasolacrimal apparatus.

THE EYELIDS (Fig. 9.25)

Blepharoschizis

A coloboma can be defined as a defect in the lid affecting primarily the margin. All degrees may be found, varying from a simple notch in the eyelid rim to complete absence of the lid (ablepharon). The shape of the defect may be triangular or quadrilateral. The anomaly may be situated in the upper or the lower eyelid and may be either unilateral or bilateral.

Upper lid coloboma. The anomaly is usually situated in the inner half of the upper lid, lateral to the upper lacrimal punctum. The defect involves the whole thickness of the lid, the gap being about 1 cm in width, and is frequently associated with corneal exposure. Ulceration and corneal opacity are possible complications. When the coloboma is complete, eyelashes, tarsal plate and Meibomian glands stop abruptly at the rounded edges of the defect. The remainder of the lid has a normal appearance, although the medial side may show a swelling due to contraction of the underlying orbicularis muscle. The malformation is frequently associated with a defect in the upper orbital margin and irregularities of the eyebrow. Ocular malformations such as corneal opacity, epibulbar dermoid and iris coloboma may also be observed.

Lower lid coloboma. The defect is situated medially or laterally. Medially, a wide variety of forms may be seen, ranging from complete orbitofacial clefts with total corneal exposure to minor forms characterized by a notch. As a rule abnormalities of the lacrimal apparatus are also associated. Laterally, the defect is located at the junction of the lateral and middle third of the lid, giving the palpebral aperture its characteristic triangular shape. This condition

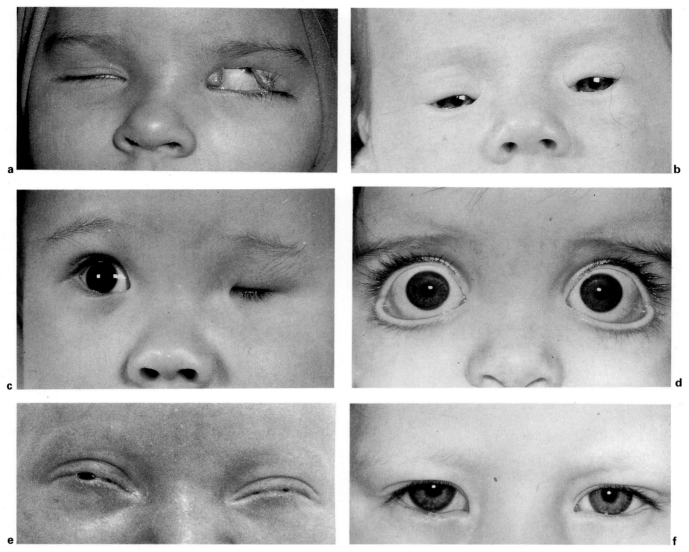

Fig. 9.25 Palpebral dysplasia: (a) blepharoschizis; (b) blepharophimosis; (c) microblepharon; (d) euryblepharon; (e) ankyloblepharon; (f) epiblepharon.

is typical of the Treacher Collins–Franceschetti–Klein syndrome. In these cases the coloboma is the expression of an underlying malar deficiency.

Eyelashes are usually present in the lateral third only and absent or abnormally formed over the remainder of the lid. The floating outer canthus is displaced downward (antimongoloid slant).

Mongoloid slant of the eyes is frequently combined with the A-pattern variety of concomitant squint, whereas anti-mongoloid slant of the eyes can be combined with the V-pattern variety of concomitant squint (Urrets Zavalia et al 1961).

Blepharophimosis

Among the features of a child, with blepharophimosis there is one which is particularly striking, viz. the total lack of 'relief' in the orbital region. This appearance seems to be caused by a flattening of the nasal root and the retrusion of the orbital roof. Further inspection of the eyelids, the palpebral fissure and the canthi reveals, however, a number of other anomalies which together with the skeletal abnormalities are responsible for the characteristic appearance of these patients.

Eyelids. The upper eyelid is shortened in all directions, simulating a microblepharon. The skin is thick and lacks its usual pliability. Hirsutism is frequently observed. Ptosis is always present. The tarsus is atrophic and the levator palpebrae muscle is either hypoplastic or missing. The absence of a fold is sometimes associated with an epiblepharon. The lower eyelid is equally lacking in skin and its temporal half may reveal some degree of ectropion. The orbicularis muscle is hypoplastic and not well differentiated, constricting the palpebral fissure, which is shortened and small. The canthi may be rounded. The medial canthi show lateral dystopia and telecanthus and the canaliculi appear lengthened. The insertion of the medial canthal tendon seems to be displaced in an anterior direction and telecanthus is frequently associated with epicanthus. The caruncle may thus be hidden from view. The lateral canthus shows medial dystopia.

Microblepharon

This is a rare malformation, characterized by shortening of the lids in all directions. The condition is generally associated with microphthalmia and microorbitism to some degree. It is also seen in blepharophimosis.

Euryblepharon

This anomaly is characterized by enlargement of the palpebral aperture, which is due to a deficiency of palpebral skin in a vertical direction.

Ankyloblepharon

This condition is characterized by partial fusion of the lid margins, through fine bands of fragile tissue. Fusion is rarely total.

Epiblepharon

Absence of a palpebral groove is the main feature of this anomaly. It is caused by maldevelopment of the palpebrotarsal insertion of the m. levator.

THE CANTHI (Fig 9.26)

Epicanthus

Epicanthus is defined as the condition in which a bilateral and symmetrical skin fold (epicanthal fold) runs in a vertical direction at the naso-orbital angle, overlapping in the severest forms the medial palpebral ligament.

Often present at birth, epicanthus gradually disappears in most instances as a result of the outgrowth of the nasal pyramid.

Prevalent in Asiatics, it is frequently associated with a flat nose and telecanthus in Down's syndrome and with ptosis in blepharophimosis.

One cause of the epicanthal fold seems to be the abnormal distribution of the orbicularis muscle. Instead of inserting wholly into the ligament some fibres pass circularly in front of the tendon, thus forming, with the overlying skin, the epicanthus.

Telecanthus

Telecanthus can be defined as the condition in which the distance between the medial canthi is increased.

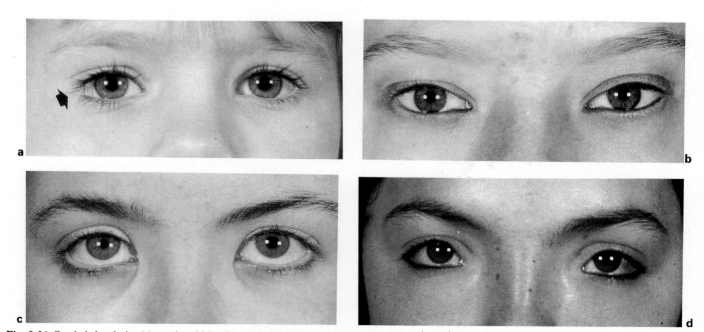

Fig. 9.26 Canthal dysplasia: (a) canthoschisis; (b) canthal dystopia (mongoloid obliquity); (c) epicanthus; (d) telecanthus.

Telecanthus is regarded as primary when the tendon of the orbicularis oculi m. is exceedingly long. The laterally displaced soft tissues of the canthal region overlap the conjunctiva, thus creating the illusion of hypertelorism, although the orbits are normally positioned. Primary telecanthus is a symptom characteristic of blepharophimosis and Waardenburg's syndrome.

Telecanthus is regarded as secondary when the entire ocular apparatus is laterally displaced or the canthi are mechanically separated.

Canthal dystopia

An abnormal position of the medial or lateral canthus is a frequent finding in craniofacial malformations.

Downward dislocation of the medial canthus is seen in abnormalities involving the nasomaxillary skeleton.

Downward dislocation of the lateral canthus is observed in malar hypoplasia (Treacher Collins' syndrome) and in a variety of syndromes with craniofacial dysostosis (antimongoloid slanting). In these conditions canthal dystopia may also be associated with ptosis.

Upward dislocation of the lateral canthus, or mongoloid slanting, is seen in sphenofrontal dysplasia or in plagiocephaly.

Canthoschizis

Clefting of the lateral canthus is a rare phenomenon. The condition can be observed as a separate entity or as a part of Goldenhar's syndrome, and is commonly associated with the presence of a scleral dermoid or lipoma.

THE SCLERA (Fig. 9.27)

The presence of a scleral dermolipoma on the lateral aspect of the eyeball is a condition sine qua non for Goldenhar's syndrome. The abnormality is, however, also seen as a separate entity or in combination with canthal clefting. Dermolipomas on the medial aspect are extremely rare.

THE EYEBROWS

Anomalies of the eyebrow are frequently observed. The malformation interrupts or distorts the normal pattern (configuration) and changes hair orientation. The position of the eyebrow marks the superior orbital margin and abnormalities of the skin may therefore be indicative of underlying skeletal deficiencies.

THE NASOLACRIMAL APPARATUS

Although some of the lacrimal fluid is removed by evaporation, most of the tears are carried away by the drainage system in the orbitonasal angle. Owing to its delicate anatomy this apparatus can only function well under normal conditions. The apparatus consists of:

1. a canaliculus, in the rim of each eyelid;
2. a sacculus, confined by the lacrimal groove on the one hand and the posterior and anterior insertion of the medial canthal tendon on the other;
3. an osseous canal that runs through the frontal process of the maxilla into the inferior nasal meatus.

Each of these parts may be affected, producing a whole range of anomalies. The malformations that may be observed are agenesis (partial or complete), stenosis or fistulae of the lacrimal canal, sac or canaliculi, and dystopia of the lacrimal puncta. Obstruction, frequently bilateral, is observed in 1–6% of all newborns. Fistulae are common — 1 per 2000 subjects according to Francois & Bacskulin (1969).

The relation between the site of the developmental arrest within the lacrimal apparatus and of that within the bony structures is obvious.

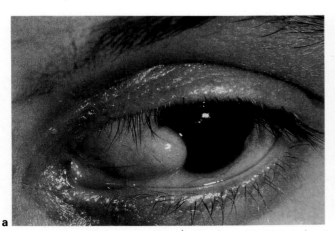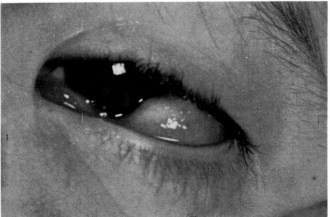

a   b

Fig. 9.27 Scleral dysplasia: (a) medial epibulbar dermoid; (b) lateral epibulbar dermoid.

Nasal aplasia is always associated with agenesis of the lacrimal canal, while the sac may be intact. The incidence with cleft lip and palate was found to be relatively high by Whitaker et al (1981).

Nasomaxillary and maxillary dysplasia are frequently characterized by agenesis and stenosis of the lacrimal apparatus, occasionally also by fistulae (Pichler 1911). Zygomatic dysplasia is often seen with dystopia of the lacrimal puncti or agenesis of the canaliculi. Examination of these patients requires an attempt to irrigate the lower canaliculus with a fluorescein-stained saline solution. If obstruction exists, as evidenced by the absence of fluorescein in the lower meatus of the nasal cavity, it can be visualized by X-ray photography after filling the lacrimal drainage system with lipiodol.

Recognition of anomalies is important, as obstruction frequently results in an infection of the conjunctiva and of the lacrimal sac. It is therefore a possible source of complications in craniofacial surgery.

CRANIOFACIAL DYSPLASIAS WITH CLEFTING
(Fig. 9.28)

True or primary clefts are caused by the persistence of epithelium between the borders of the facial processes, a phenomenon which is due to deficient epithelial cell degeneration. Their existence is therefore restricted to the following territories:

latero-nasomaxillary clefting — between the lateronasal and maxillary processes (naso-ocular clefts);
medio-nasomaxillary clefting — between the medionasal and maxillary processes (cleft lip);
intermaxillary clefting — between the palatine processes (cleft palate);
maxillo-mandibular clefting — between the maxillary and mandibular process (macrostomia).

The fact that similar terms are used to indicate not only the facial processes which develop at an early stage but also the bony units which develop at a later stage risks confusion for the reader. The maxillomandibular cleft, a true primary cleft, is not formed between the maxillary and mandibular bone but between the respective facial processes with the same names.

The nasomaxillary, both medio- and lateronasal, and the intermaxillary clefts, are always accompanied by osseous defects. These abnormalities will therefore be discussed in the section on dysostosis.

The maxillo-mandibular cleft rarely affects the bone and macrostomia is therefore discussed in the following section.

Maxillo-mandibular clefting

Clefting of the oral commissure, essentially a soft tissue defect affecting skin, muscle and mucosa, is usually called macrostomia. It may be unilateral or rarely bilateral. Its range of malformations varies from minor elongation of the oral angle to a wide cleft extending towards the tragal area (Fig. 9.29).

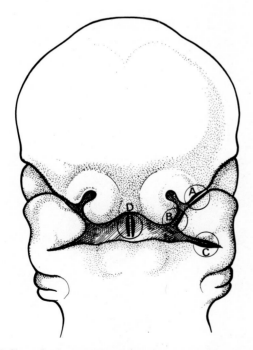

Fig. 9.28 Sites of primary (true) clefts: A latero-nasomaxillary; B medio-nasomaxillary; C maxillomandibular; D intermaxillary.

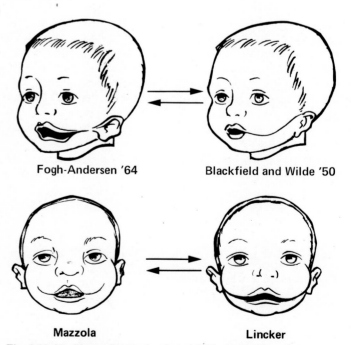

Fogh-Andersen '64   Blackfield and Wilde '50

Mazzola   Lincker

Fig. 9.29 Maxillomandibular dysplasia (clefting): selection of illustrations from the literature.

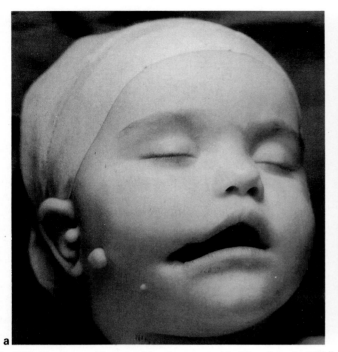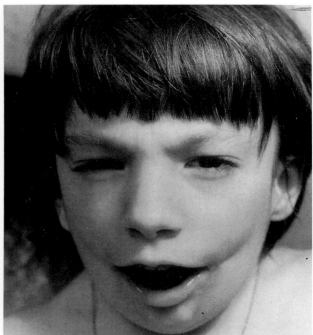

Fig. 9.30 Maxillomandibular clefting (macrostomia): (a) unilateral; (b) bilateral.

The parotid gland and duct which normally arise from the ectoderm of the stomodeal plate along a line which corresponds with the line of fusion of the maxillary and mandibular processes may be absent.

Macrostomia (Fig. 9.30) is rarely observed as an isolated malformation (Otto 1841, von Ammon 1842, Fergusson 1857, Grunberg 1909, Morgan 1882, Boo-Chai 1979). In the majority of cases it is associated with preauricular appendages or fistulae that may be found anywhere between the angle of the mouth and the tragus occasionally also with temporoaural and/or mandibular abnormalities. Facial paralysis is sometimes observed. The anomaly may also be seen in oculo-aurovertebral and cervico-otofacial dysplasia. The association with reductive limb anomalies has been reported by several authors (Grabb 1965, Black-field & Wilde 1950).

The incidence in large series of facial clefts analysed by several authors is as follows: Blackfield & Wilde (1950) 5 per 500; Fogh-Andersen (1965) 12 per 3988; Pitanguy & Franco (1967) 5 per 726; Popescu (1968) 14 per 1475.

CRANIOFACIAL DYSPLASIAS WITH DYSOSTOSIS

The craniofacial helix (Fig. 9.31)

In accordance with the thoughts expressed in the introduction to this chapter, the spectrum of anomalies belonging to this category have been ranged in a helix form, with its roots in the sphenoid, the key structure of the craniofacial skeleton. The pathway of the helix begins

with two branches: one lateral, originating at the junction of the greater wing of the sphenoid and frontal bone, and the other medial, emerging from the sphenoethmoidal junction. The two branches join each other at the root of the nose, where they separate briefly to provide space for the nasal aperture and then meet again in the maxilla, curving laterally. The course of the helix continues through the malar bone, the zygomatic arch and the temporal bone, where a medially directed turn is made. It

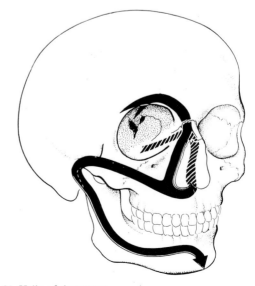

Fig. 9.31 Helix of dysostoses.

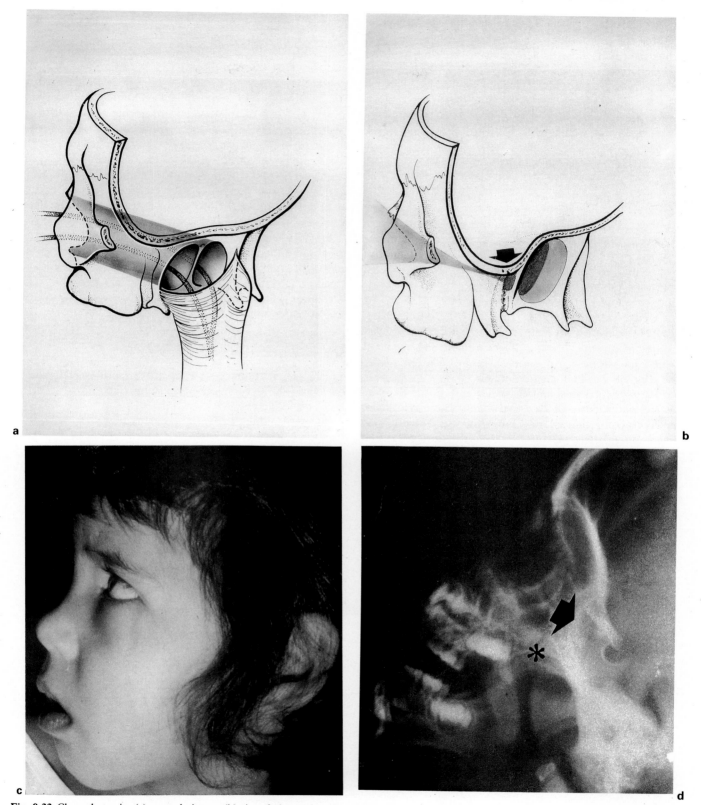

Fig. 9.32 Choanal atresia: (a) normal airway; (b) site of obstruction; (c) clinical view — note open mouth; (d) X-ray shows sphenoidal dysplasia and site of obstruction.

then passes through the mandible to end in the midline at the symphysis.

The upper half of the S encircles the orbit and the lower half the mouth. Dysplasias in the upper part of the S are sometimes associated with periocular dysplasias. Dysplasias in the middle part of the S (nasal, latero-nasomaxillary, maxillary) have been observed in combination with microphthalmia as well as with cleft lip. Dysplasias in the lower part of the S are frequently betrayed by the presence of periauricular pits and fistulae.

Sphenoidal dysplasia

The sphenoid controls the face in three different planes: the ethmoid anteriorly, the pterygoid inferiorly, and the alar processes laterally. It proves to be a fixed element of reference for the craniofacial architecture, an old concept put forward by anthropologists.

The sphenoid raises itself during growth. Penetrating like a wedge into the central portion of the cranial base, it elevates the cribriform plate, opens the angle of Welcker and develops its wings during this movement. The manner in which its position and dimensions are affected relates to the time of the malformative insult.

An early disturbance holds it in a low position as an undifferentiated bony block, restraining the development of the pterygoid, the palatine bone and the vomer. This form of sphenoidal dysostosis in its pure state results in choanal atresia (Fig. 9.32).

In some centrofacial malformations, an undifferentiated

mass of bone may be observed which corresponds to the sphenoethmoidal complex. This concerns undoubtedly a sphenoidal dysostosis, affecting the contiguous structures and therefore originating at an even earlier stage.

Rarely an osseous defect too may be observed, permitting the passage of a sphenoidal meningoencephalocele, a sphenopharyngeal meningoencephalocele passing through the sphenoid bone into the epipharynx, a spheno-orbital meningoencephalocele passing through the supraorbital fissure into the orbit or a sphenomaxillary meningoencephalocele passing through the supra- and infraorbital fissure into the pterygopalatine fossa. A late disturbance affects the dimensions of the sphenoid, resulting in shortness, mainly of a sagittal nature, and in a folded position of the alar expansion.

These sphenoidal dysplasias, practically always associated with synostosis, are responsible for the group of craniofacial malformations misnamed or erroneously called 'Croupert', which are discussed in the section on dysostosis and synostosis.

Sphenofrontal dysplasia (Fig. 9.33)

This malformation, located in the superolateral angle of the orbit, is rarely observed as a separate entity.

MORPHOLOGY (Figs. 9.34, 9.35)

The skeletal anomalies are characterized by retrusion of the upper part of the lateral wall and roof of the orbit, or

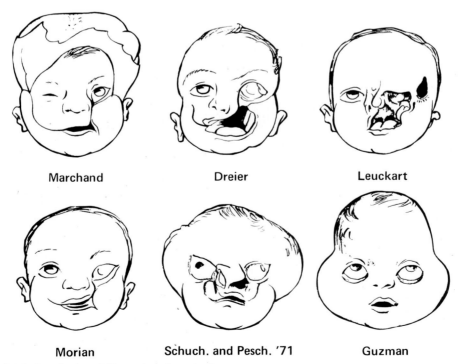

Marchand   Dreier   Leuckart

Morian   Schuch. and Pesch. '71   Guzman

Fig. 9.33 Sphenofrontal dysplasia: selection of illustrations from the literature.

sometimes by a defect behind the orbital rim. The soft tissue abnormalities may involve the lateral canthus, forming a canthoschizis, the upper eyelid, producing a coloboma (blepharoschizis), or an ablepharon, which introduces the risk of corneal clouding and ulceration. The eyebrow is distorted and the hairline may be irregular, forming a 'widow's peak'.

Sphenofrontal dysplasia is usually associated with nasomaxillary or maxillary dysplasia. In less severe cases the appearance of the malformation approaches that found in plagiocephaly. In severe bilateral cases a striking similarity may be observed to the bizarre trilobular configuration which is found in the cloverleaf skull.

Frontal dysplasia (Fig. 9.36)

MORPHOLOGY

Skeletal malformations in the frontal area are characterized by defects and irregularities in contour. From a clinical point of view two different types may be distinguished. The first relates to the presence of a bony defect, which involves the whole or part of the forehead and will correspond to a cerebromeningeal anomaly (meningoencephalocele) which is covered with a lipomatous mass. The second concerns an interruption of the superior orbital margin.

Soft tissue anomalies may affect the eyebrow, interrupting and distorting its pattern, the hairline, producing a widow's peak or cow's lick, and the skin, which may be deficient and covered with scattered spots or streaks of ectopic hair.

Colobomata of the upper eyelid are also common. The anomaly is frequently observed together with nasal, nasomaxillary or maxillary dysplasia and the pattern produced by this continuity is essentially a craniocaudal one. Variations, however, are possible, and the assignment of specific locations within the frontal bone does not seem to have a morphogenetic basis.

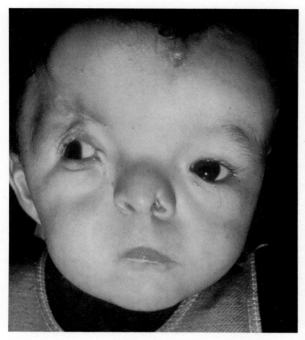

Fig. 9.34 Sphenofrontal dysplasia: note also nasomaxillary dysplasia.

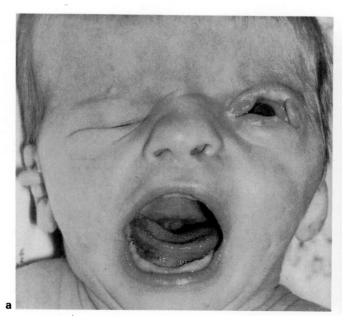

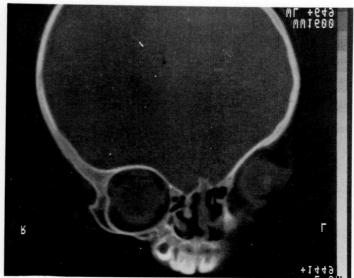

Fig. 9.35 Sphenofrontal dysplasia: (a) clinical view — note eyelid coloboma and hypertelorism; (b) CT scan.

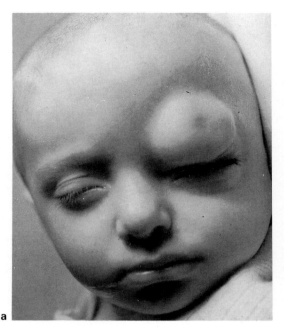 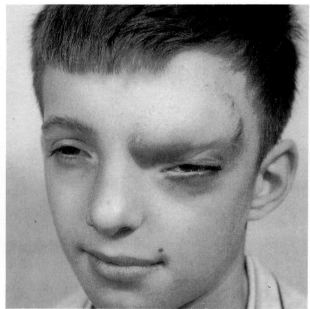

Fig. 9.36 Frontal dysplasia: (a) clinical view as a child — note defect in orbital roof and eyebrow distortion; (b) clinical view as an adult.

Fronto-frontal dysplasia (Fig. 9.37)

The definition fronto-frontal applies to the dysplasia in the middle of the forehead, so-called cranium bifidum occultum.

MORPHOLOGY

Skeletal abnormalities in the middle of the forehead may consist of bony defects or contour irregularities. A defect may result in protrusion of brain tissue and the meningoencephaloceles thus produced may be observed as a solitary malformation or, more frequently, in association with fronto-nasoethmoidal dysplasia. The soft tissue abnormalities may show skin atrophy in the midline (coup de sabre) and irregularities of the hairline (widow's peak).

Fronto-nasoethmoidal dysplasia

INTRODUCTION

The name frontonasal dysplasia has been given to a wide variety of malformations occurring in the frontonasal process. This term, however, is not specific enough. We believe it to be a misnomer, since it refers to all the structures between the eye and the maxillary process, and suggest that the word 'frontonasal' should be reserved for defects (including arrested growth) occurring at the junction of the frontal and nasal or ethmoidal bones.

The fact that the distance between the orbits may be abnormally large has been recognized since antiquity. The Homerian cattle with their wide foreheads were called *eury*

metopos. The term 'metopion' indicates the interorbital area.

Probably the first picture of a patient with a facies bovina was published by Giovanni Battista della Porta in 1586 in his *De Humana Physiognomonia* (Fig. 9.38). The art of metoposcopia was described by Gerolamo Cardano (1501–1576) in his book published posthumously in 1658 (Fig. 9.39). The term 'metopismus' was used to indicate the presence of a wide open metopic suture.

In 1904 J. Thomson was the first to draw attention to the resemblance between the craniofacial malformation of the 7-year-old Mary McDougal and that of a fetal skull.

MORPHOLOGY

David Greig (1924), physician and conservator of the Edinburgh Museum, examined Mary McDougal's skull after her death and coined the term hypertelorism, thinking it to be a specific syndrome. Later, in 1961, Greer Walker carefully distinguished between primary (or embryonic) and secondary hypertelorism.

Tessier (1967, 1972) stressed the differences between orbital hypertelorism, or teleorbitism, defined by him as a congenital condition in which the interorbital distance increases from the apex to the orbital rim, and hypertelorism caused by craniosynostosis. Converse et al (1970) differentiate between ocular hypertelorism, which is characterized by an increased divergence of the orbital axis from the midsagittal line, and pseudohypertelorism. The latter name refers to patients in whom the interpupillary distance and interorbital distance are normal, and an

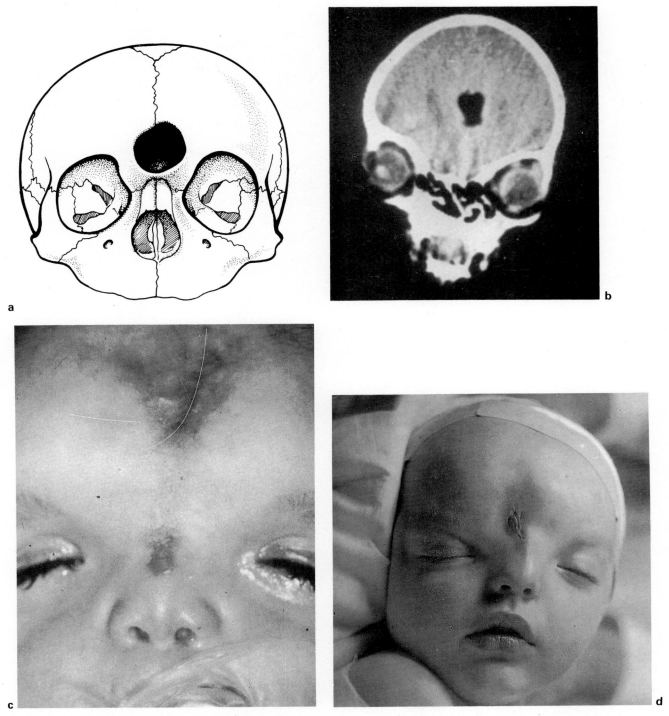

Fig. 9.37 Frontofrontal dysplasia: (a) defect between the frontal bones; (b) CT scan; (c) clinical view — note skin atrophy; (d) clinical view — note encephalocele.

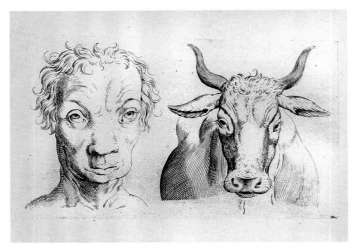

Fig. 9.38 Facies bovina (from G. B. della Porta 1586).

hypertelorism does not represent a syndrome but only one of the signs that may be observed in this area.

Dimension, configuration and position of the interorbital and orbital skeleton are intimately related and alterations in size, shape and site of one of these structures may therefore affect this relationship. An abnormally wide interorbital distance is, however, not automatically associated with divergence of the orbital axes and the lateral orbital walls.

We therefore suggest that distinction is made between orbital hypertelorism or teleorbitism, in which there is true lateralization of the orbits, and interorbital hypertelorism, in which no lateralization of the orbits is observed.

increase of the intercanthal distance is found. It tends, however, to obscure the fact that the distance between the orbits is indeed increased.

Classifying hypertelorism with its different aetiologies and varied appearances is apparently not as simple as one might believe. Accurate differentiation is, however, indicated if the type of malformation and its correction are to be matched. It should be based on the consideration that

CLASSIFICATION

The term hypertelorism per se is inexact and inadequate. The criteria by which assessment can be made are:

1. the distance measured between the dacrya (I.D.D.);
2. the distance measured between the ectocanthia at the site of insertion to the lateral orbital wall.

Interorbital hypertelorism is present when the I.D.D. is increased and the distance between the ectocanthia is normal. Orbital hypertelorism or teleorbitism exists when both distances are increased.

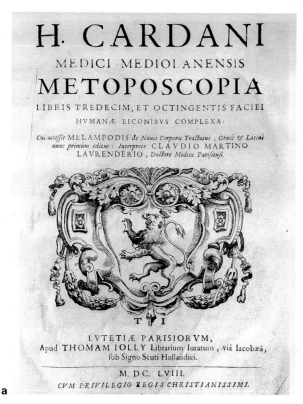

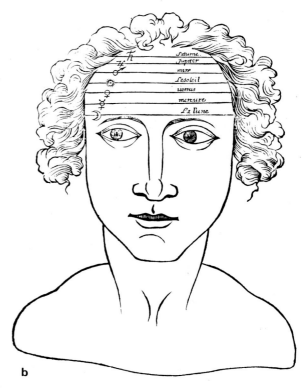

Fig. 9.39 (a) Title page of Cardano's book and (b) example of metoposcopia.

ASSESSMENT

The relation of the interorbital distance to the orbits themselves is in the divine proportion (Pacioli 1509, Rickets 1982) and our sense of cosmesis has therefore every right to be offended by abnormalities in this particular facial proportion. However, precise measurement of these anomalies has always been difficult.

Measurement of the interpupillary distance is unsatisfactory where strabismus is present and cooperation of the patient is poor.

Measurement of the intercanthal distance does not always reflect the position of the orbit and the globe in patients with telecanthus.

Günther (1933b) examined the normal distance between the dacrya and found an upper limit of 30 mm. This figure corresponds to a canthal index of 38 when the distance between the inner canthi is compared with that between the outer canthi and the result is expressed as a percentage:

$$\frac{\text{inner canthal distance}}{\text{outer canthal distance}} = \times\%$$

Euryopy is present when a value ranging from 30 to 34 mm is observed (Patry 1905). The term hypertelorism is used when an interorbital distance (I.O.D.) of more then 34 mm and a canthal index exceeding 42 mm are found.

Romanus (1953) advocated the use of an outer orbital (eyespan)–intercanthal (eyespace) index to measure the degree of hypertelorism. Dividing the external biorbital diameter measured between the most lateral points on the temporal margin of the orbital wall (O.O.D.) by the diameter joining the inner canthi (I.C.D.), he arrived at a normal value of 40.

$$\frac{\text{O.O.D.}}{\text{I.C.D.}} \times 1000 = 40$$

Tessier stressed the point that objective measurements of the interorbital distance should be taken between the lacrimal crests, the 'dacryons', recognizing that the value thus obtained may be 7–8 mm greater than that of more posterior measurements (Günther 1933b).

Along with Günther, Tessier (1972) distinguishes between three degrees of hypertelorism:

1st degree: 30–34 I.O.D.
2nd degree: 34–40 I.O.D.
3rd degree: > 40 I.O.D.

To accentuate the fact that the distance between these dacryons may not be the same as that measured in other parts of the interorbital space and to emphasize the difference with the values measured between the inner canthi, we propose the name 'interdacryal distance'. Thus I.D.D. is used in place of the interorbital distance or I.O.D. Average values for the distance between the dacryons, the canthi and the lateral orbital wall are presented in Fig. 9.40.

Marsh (1986) quantifies the position of the orbit by measuring the distance between the perpendicular plate of the ethmoid and the centroid of the globe, using axial and coronal analyses.

INTERORBITAL HYPERTELORISM

Interorbital hypertelorism may be observed in rare anomalies such as encephaloceles and pneumatoceles, or more

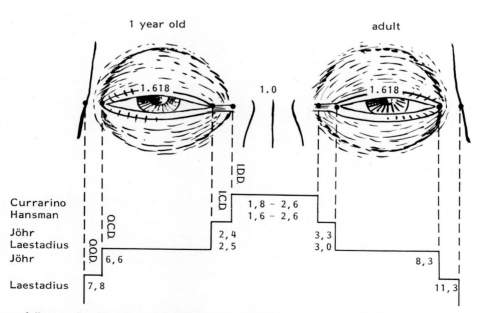

Fig. 9.40 Assessment of distances in orbital region by different authors: O.O.D. = outer orbital distance; O.C.D. = outer canthal distance; I.C.D. = inner canthal distance; I.D.D. = inner dacryal distance.

commonly in patients with craniosynostosis. These malformations affect the interorbital skeleton through alterations in the composition of its elements, the dimensions of its parts and the configuration of its walls; partial disorders characterized by anomalies along the surfaces of the medial orbital wall, posterior or anterior and superior or inferior to the insertion of the canthal tendon may thus be produced (Munro et al 1979).

Meningoencephaloceles

The term hernia cerebri was coined by Le Dran (1740) but it was Spring (1854) who was probably the first to publish a monograph on the subject.

The incidence of this anomaly shows wide variation. It is quite common in Thailand, about 1 in 6000 live births, (Charoonsmith and Suwanwela 1974), relatively common in some African countries such as Ethiopia and definitely rare in other parts of the world. A genetic base has never been established.

Patients with this malformation demonstrate swellings of varying size in the glabellar region. These swellings may be sessile or pedunculated. On palpation the mass may be solid and firm or soft and cystic. The contents of the cele mostly consists of glial tissue, often infiltrated with fibrous trabeculae (David et al 1984). The ventricular system is rarely involved. The skin over the mass may be thin and shiny or thick and wrinkled. Hyperpigmentation and hypertrichosis may be noted.

Telecanthus is usually pronounced. Downward dislocation of the insertion of the medial canthal tendon is frequently observed, producing a mongoloid slant, but the lateral orbital walls are in a normal position. Elongation of the nose is a cardinal feature of this condition.

The anomaly may be associated with abnormalities involving the brain, anterior angulation of the optic nerves and pituitary stalk and partial or complete occlusion of the foramen of Monro, which may result in hydrocephalus, ventricular dilatation, agenesis of the corpus callosum, cortical atrophy, mental retardation or generalized convulsions. Visual acuity may be decreased. Strabismus and lacrimal obstructions, resulting in epiphora and/or dacryocystitis, have been observed.

A classification of encephaloceles may be based on the location of the defect in the cranial base, on the site of the external orifice in the facial skeleton or on a combination of both. Von Meyer (1890) has classified encephaloceles on the basis that the cranial end of the defect is always at the junction of the frontal and ethmoidal bones (the foramen caecum) and he distinguishes between different types of frontoethmoidal dysplasia (nasofrontal, nasoethmoidal, naso-orbital).

We feel that further distinction between frontonasal and frontoethmoidal dysplasia is justified and propose the following classification: frontonasal, frontoethmoidal (medial and lateral), and ethmoidal.

Frontonasal or supranasal meningoencephaloceles (Fig. 9.41)

The encephalocele leaves the cranial cavity through the fonticulus frontalis between the developing frontal and nasal bones (Figs. 9.42, 9.43). The cribriform plate is usually tilted downwards, forming an angle of 45–50° with

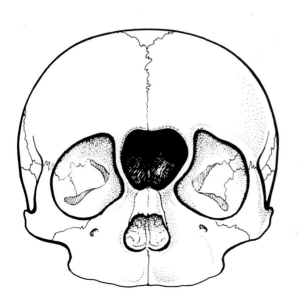
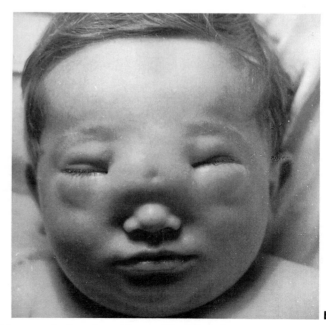

Fig. 9.41 Frontonasal dysplasia: (a) site of abnormality; defect is situated between the frontal nasal bones: (b) clinical view.

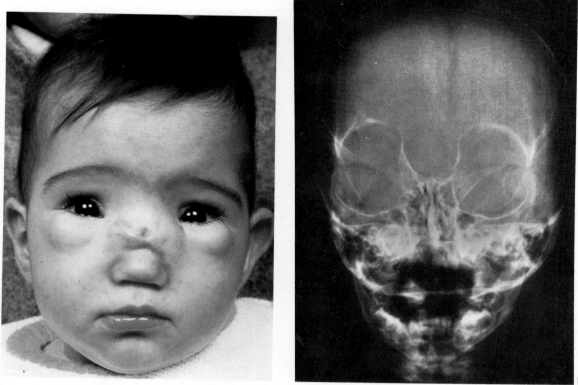

Fig. 9.42 Frontonasal meningoencephalocele: (a) clinical view; (b) X-ray — note abnormality in midline.

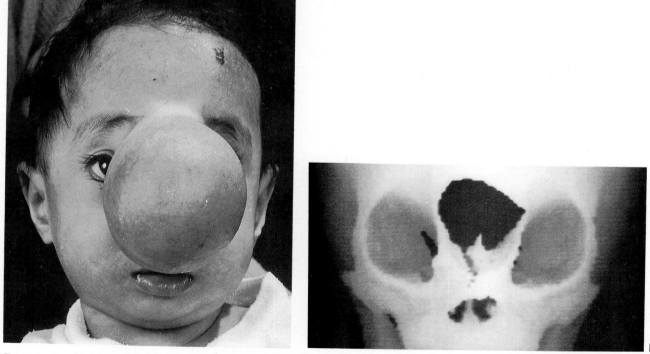

Fig. 9.43 Frontonasal meningoencephalocele: (a) clinical view; (b) 3-D reconstruction; note lowering of the cribriform plate (courtesy David David).

the orbital–meatal plane (David et al 1984). The nasal bones are attached to the inferior margin of the defect.

Medial frontoethmoidal or nasal meningoencephaloceles (Fig. 9.44).

The defect in the anterior cranial fossa is situated posterior to the frontonasal suture and anterior to the ethmoid. The mass protrudes between the nasal bones and the nasal cartilage, pushing the septum backwards and downwards. The pyriform aperture is displaced inferiorly. The lateral wall of the tunnel is formed by the intact medial wall of the orbit (Fig. 9.45).

Lateral frontoethmoidal or orbital meningoencephaloceles (Fig. 9.46)

The herniation in the cranial base is in the same position as that of the medial variation but the mass protrudes through holes in the medial wall of the orbit, in the frontal process of the maxilla or in the lacrimal bones, forming a paranasal swelling (Figs. 9.47, 9.48).

Ethmoidal or retronasal meningoencephaloceles (Fig. 9.49)

In this category the defect is situated in the ethmoidal bone. The cerebral mass remains intranasally and may even extend to the palate.

Craniosynostosis

This malformation is characterized by bulging of the superoposterior part of the medial orbital wall (Fig. 9.50) and by apparent deepening of the posterior part of the lateral wall. The distance between the dacrya is not necessarily increased and lateralization of the lateral walls of the orbit is frequently absent. Differentiation between

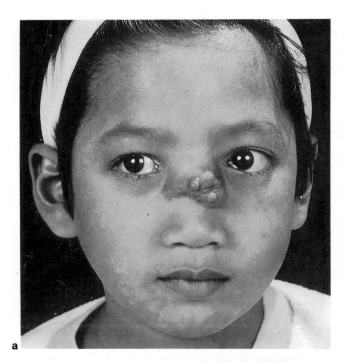

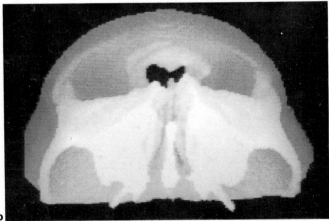

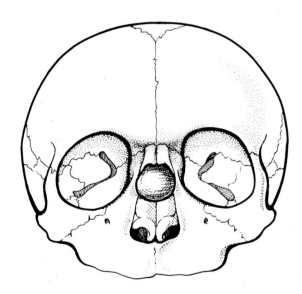

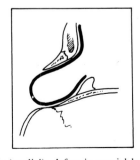

Fig. 9.44 Frontoethmoidal dysplasia (medial); defect in cranial base is situated between the frontal and ethmoidal bones. The meningo-encephalocele surfaces between the nasal bones and cartilages.

Fig. 9.45 Frontoethmoidal meningoencephalocele (medial): (a) clinical view; (b) 3-D reconstruction — note defect between the nasal bones and the cartilages (courtesy David David).

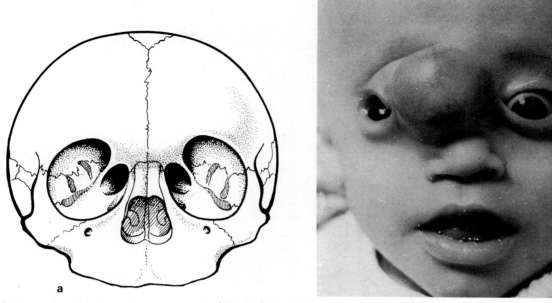

Fig. 9.46 Frontoethmoidal dysplasia (lateral): (a) site of abnormality: defect in cranial base is situated between the frontal and ethmoidal bones. The meningoencephalocele surfaces in the medial wall of the orbit or the medial canthal region; (b) clinical view of unilateral abnormality.

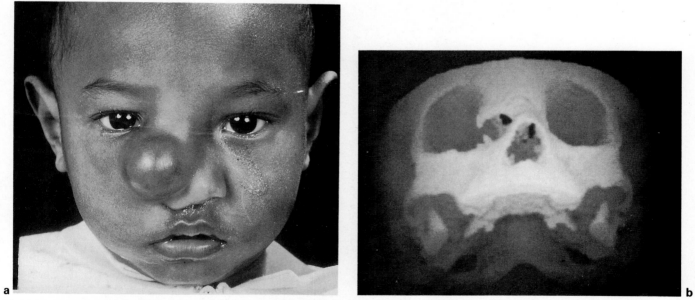

Fig. 9.47 Frontoethmoidal meningoencephalocele (lateral): (a) clinical view; (b) 3-D CT reconstruction shows defect in the anterior cranial fossa and the orbital abnormality (courtesy David David).

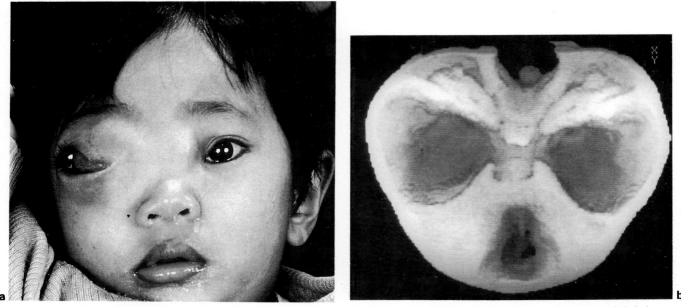

Fig. 9.48 Frontoethmoidal meningoencephalocele (lateral): (a) clinical view: interorbital hypertelorism is associated with severe exophthalmia; (b) 3-D reconstruction — note the small defect anterior to the cribriform plate (courtesy David David).

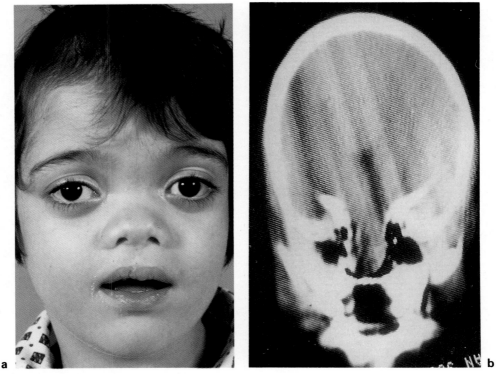

Fig. 9.49 Ethmoidal meningoencephalocele: (a) clinical view; (b) CT scan.

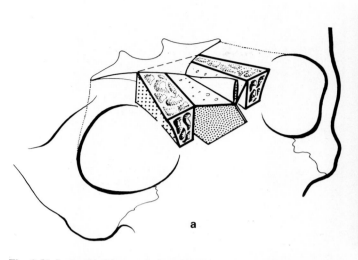

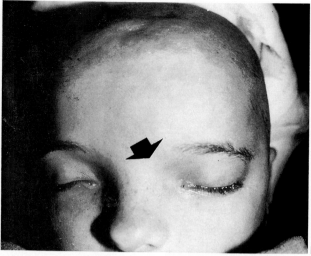

Fig. 9.50 Interorbital hypertelorism due to bulging of the superoposterior part of the medial orbital wall in patients with craniosynostosis: (a) site of abnormality indicated by arrows; (b) clinical view.

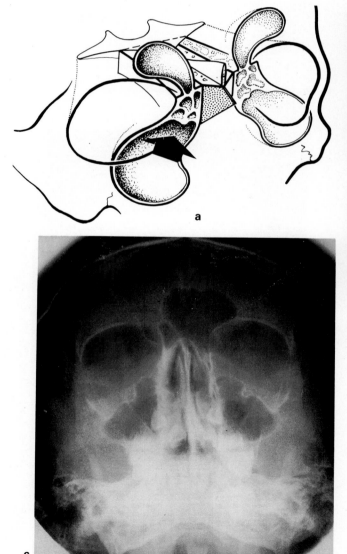

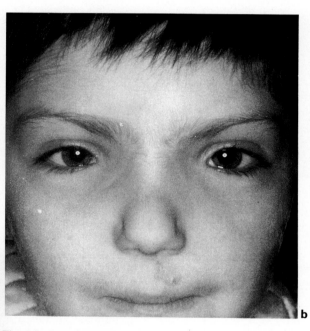

Fig. 9.51 Interorbital hypertelorism due to abnormal pneumatization of maxillary sinus: (a) site of abnormality indicated by arrow; (b) clinical view; (c) X-ray shows expansion of frontal sinus.

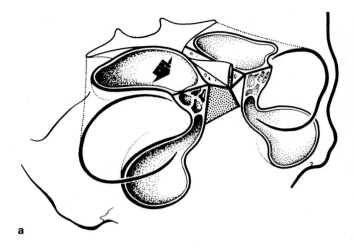

a

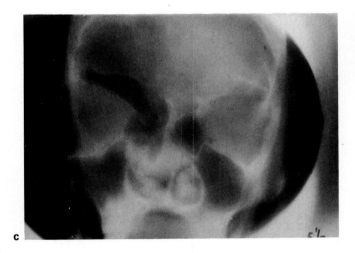

c

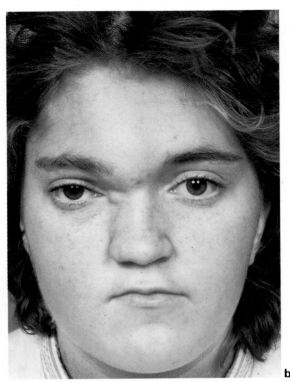

b

Fig. 9.52 Interorbital hypertelorism due to abnormal pneumatization of frontal sinus: (a) site of abnormality indicated by arrow; (b) clinical views; (c) X-ray shows expansion of frontal sinus.

orbital and interorbital variation is particularly important since it may influence the type of correction.

Pneumatoceles

A normal interdacryal distance is seen in combination with an increased interorbital distance in the superior or inferior part of the interorbital region. The anomaly is due to a ballooning of the maxilloethmoidal sinus (Fig. 9.51) or frontal sinus (Fig. 9.52).

Differentiation

Widening of the interorbital distance may also be secondary to the presence of a skeletal disease: fibrous dysplasia (Fig. 9.53) and craniotubular dysplasia (Fig. 9.54) are notorious examples. Trauma should finally be excluded as a possible cause.

ORBITAL HYPERTELORISM

This malformation is characterized by anomalies of the

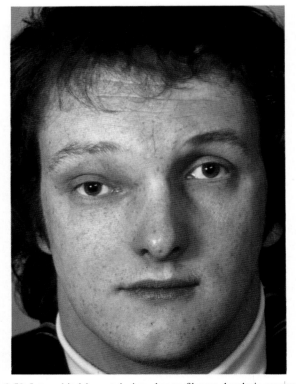

Fig. 9.53 Interorbital hypertelorism due to fibrous dysplasia protruding in superomedial part of the orbit.

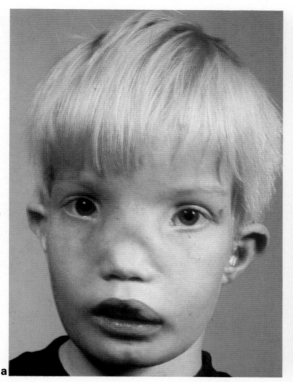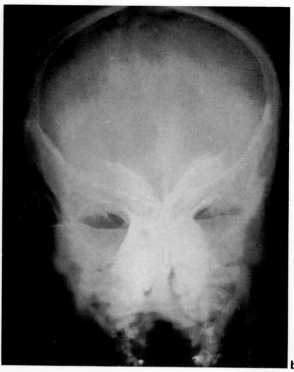

Fig. 9.54 Interorbital hypertelorism due to craniotubular dysplasia: (a) clinical view; (b) X-ray.

interorbital region and of the orbit itself. Teleorbitism may be symmetrical or asymmetrical.

Symmetrical teleorbitism (Fig. 9.55)

This anomaly is part of a great number of syndromes discussed in various textbooks (Salmon 1978, Smith 1982, Gorlin et al 1976). Many of these syndromes are associated with mental retardation. The majority of these patients are therefore never seen by the craniofacial surgeon.

Greig's syndrome or primary embryonic hypertelorism (Fig. 9.55) in combination with other skeletal abnormalities was the first to be described. The condition is rare. An incidence of about 1 in 100 000 births was reported by Gaard (1961). Its existence as a separate entity is, however, disputed by some authorities.

Cohen's syndrome or cranio-frontonasal dysplasia (Figs. 9.56, 9.57), in contrast, is much more common. Teleorbitism, internasal dysplasia and maxillary arching are the main characteristics of this condition, which is associated with premature coronal synostosis inherited as a dominant trait.

Asymmetrical teleorbitism (Fig. 9.58)

This abnormality is frequently observed. Its association with plagiocephaly was first observed by Fridoin (1885). Several varieties exist, depending on the position of the

two orbits in relation to each other and on the dimension of each of the orbits. Distinction may therefore be made between asymmetric teleorbitism with normal orbits, which is quite uncommon, or with an abnormal orbit — the majority.

The orbital anomalies involve alterations in the position of the orbit with valgization of its lateral wall and downward rotation of the orbitomeatal aperture. Alteration in dimension, e.g. microorbitism and configuration (craniosynostosis), may also be observed.

Teleorbitism may be the only abnormality in an otherwise normal face but frequently it is also associated with other anomalies. These may concern:

the brain (agenesis of the corpus callosum, V-shaped separation of the lateral Ventricles);
the forehead (widow's peak, meningoencephaloceles);
the eyebrow (dystopia, distortion);
the eyelids (colobomata, ptosis);
the eye (anophthalmia, microphthalmia, colobomata);
the eye muscles (strabismus);
the nose (internasal or nasal dysplasia).

The interorbital disorders usually consist of: widening of the crista galli, of the ethmoidal labyrinths, of the frontal processes of the maxilla and of the nasal bones; lowering of the cribriform plate ($N = 5$ mm below the level of the orbital roof); and thickening of the nasal septum. The

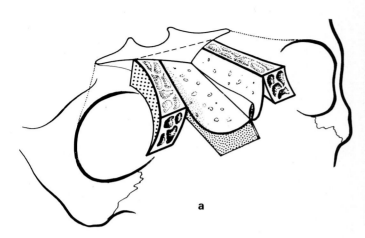

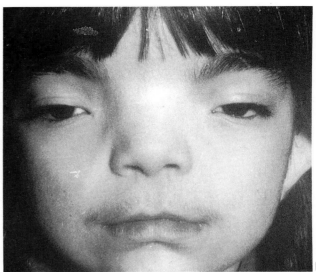

Fig. 9.55 Symmetrical teleorbitism in Greig's syndrome: (a) site of abnormality; (b) clinical view; (c) X-ray.

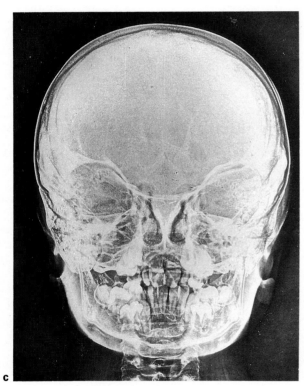

importance of each of these disorders is subject to changes in different patients and appears to be related to the pathogenesis.

PATHOGENESIS

Why lateralization is present in some patients and absent in others is probably due to the fact that growth and remodelling of the nasal capsule may be influenced by abnormal developmental conditions in and outside this structure. In normal development the interorbital distance

is reduced under the influence of the growing brain and eyes. This process is already completed in the 28-mm C–RL stage.

Orbital hypertelorism or teleorbitism has its origin in a period prior to the 28-mm C–RL stage (Vermeij-Keers et al 1984). Causes to be considered are, first, deficient remodelling or differentiation of the nasal capsule, which causes the future fronto-nasoethmoidal complex to freeze in its fetal form. As a result a morphokinetic arrest in the movement of the eyes towards the midline may be produced. This arrest may allow for further growth of the nasal capsule but not for further remodelling by narrowing and/or elongation of the structures involved. The interorbital distance and the angle between the lateral walls of the orbit ($N = 90°$) will remain abnormally wide, while the distance between the optic canals ($N = 20mm$) is not affected.

The second cause to be considered is deficient lateromedial movement of the orbit. Such a condition may be due to abnormalities in rate and direction of growth, affecting the brain, the eyes and the sphenoid. Greig found the greater wings of the sphenoid in Mary McDougal's skull to be small in relation to the enlarged lesser wings and considered this to be the 'fons et origo mali'.

Premature fusion of the sphenofrontal suture resulting in abnormalities determined by Virchow's law is another causative mechanism which must be considered. Abnormal development of the sphenoethmoidal synchondrosis may finally play a role.

Interorbital hypertelorism, by way of contrast, must have its origin in a period that follows medialization of the orbits and is evidently caused: by abnormal development of the fronto-nasoethmoidal complex, resulting in the

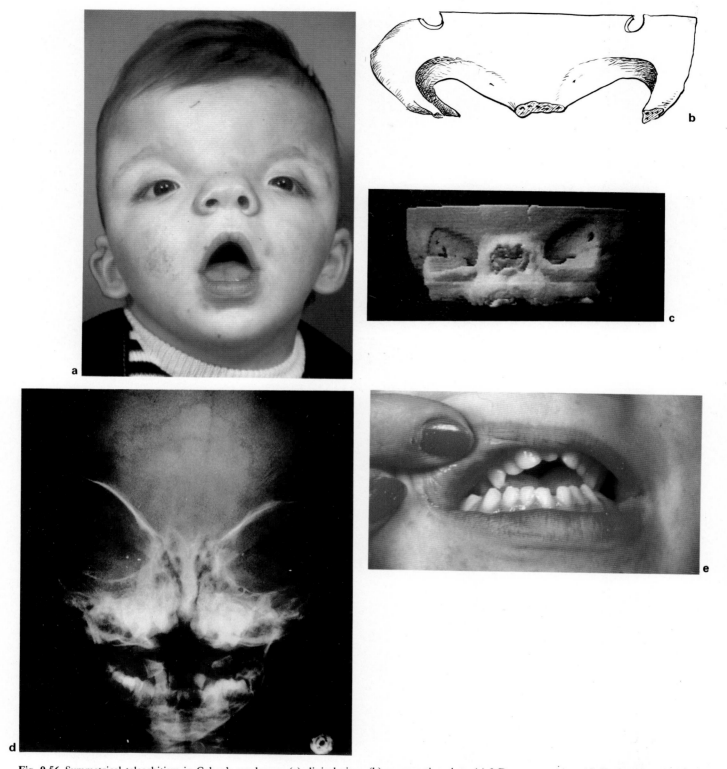

Fig. 9.56 Symmetrical teleorbitism in Cohen's syndrome: (a) clinical view; (b) peroperative view; (c) 3-D reconstruction; (d) X-ray; (e) oral view.

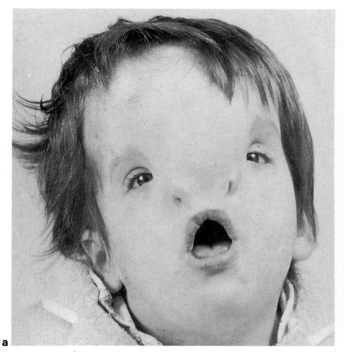

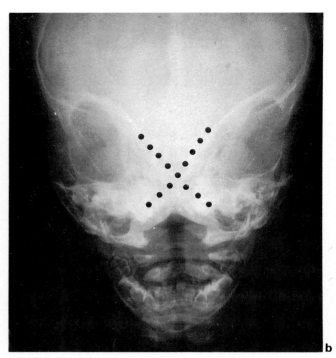

Fig. 9.57 Symmetrical teleorbitism; note similarity to Cohen's syndrome: (a) clinical view; (b) X-ray.

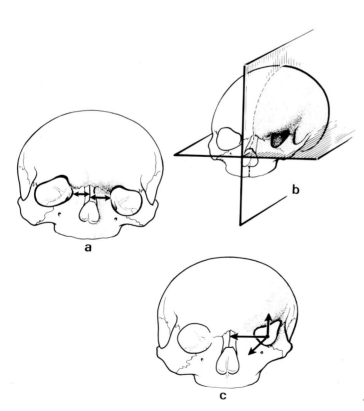

Fig. 9.58 Asymmetrical teleorbitism: (a) inferior and lateral displacement of orbit; (b) superior, posterior and lateral displacement of orbit.

protrusion of brain tissue in patients with encephaloceles; by abnormal expansion of the frontal and maxilloethmoidal sinus in pneumatoceles; or by abnormal medialization of the orbital roof in craniosynostosis.

Internasal dysplasia

Internasal dysplasia is also known by the following names: fronto-nasal dysraphia or dysplasia, median cleft face syndrome, doggenase, bifid nose, no. 0 cleft.

The early reports by Schenk (1609) and Bartholinus (1654) raise doubts about the nature of their observations. Borellus (1670) describes a certain Mauritian with two noses but it is not clear whether he refers to a case of nasal bifidity or to real duplication, since illustrations are absent. One of the oldest examples of this anomaly, reported by Gualthérie van Doeveren in 1765 (Fig. 9.59) can still be seen in the museum of the Department of Anatomy and Embryology of Leiden University. Although relatively rare, the condition has been described by many authors. Krikun (1972) of the Moscow Institute of Cosmetology, and Mazzola (1976) of Milan University were able to report on large series. Fogh-Andersen observed four cases in a group of 3988 facial clefts. Genetic transmittance as an autosomal dominant trait has been reported by Esser (1939), Boo-Chai (1965) and Mazzola (1976).

MORPHOLOGY

A whole spectrum of malformations (Fig. 9.60) may be

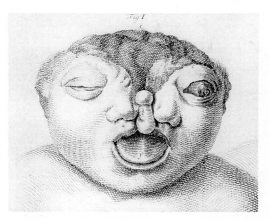

Fig. 9.59 Internasal dysplasia: specimen of severe malformation in the museum of the Department of Anatomy and Embryology at Leiden University (from G. van Doeveren 1765).

observed and the severity of the reported examples can be graded in a logical sequence. At one end is the patient with bifidity of the nasal tip or dorsum, sometimes associated with a median cleft lip or median notch of the Cupid's bow and with duplication of the labial frenulum. An excellent review of the observations made by many authors can be found in Millard's book (1977) on cleft lip and rare deformities (Figs. 9.60–9.62). Grooves and folds along the dorsum nasi are also occasionally observed.

At the other end of this spectrum we may find the monster with widely separated nasal halves and extreme orbital hypertelorism, including all the other anomalies caused by fronto-nasoethmoidal dysplasia, and occasionally even a trans-sphenoidal encephalocele with pituitary herniation (Fig. 9.63).

In contradiction to what is often stated in the literature, the premaxilla is not absent, although it may be retarded in development and bifid, like the remaining parts of the nose. The maxilla may show a keel-shaped deformity, with the incisors rotated upward in each half of the alveolar process. Sometimes a medial cleft of the palate is also found and this may extend upwards to the cribriform plate as an inverted V (Kazanjian & Holmes 1959).

The distance between the palate and the cranial base may be extremely short and in the remaining internasal space little else may be found but a cartilaginous mass. In its anterior part the septum may show differentiation into a Y-shaped duplication.

Frontonasoethmoidal dysplasia is present in the majority of cases. Günther (1933) observed orbital hypertelorism in every one of a group of 26 cases with internasal dysplasia.

Abnormalities in closure of the anterior neuropore (day 26) and persistence of epithelium in the internasal area may result in fistulae and cyst formation. Teratomas resemble this condition and distinction is therefore indicated (Fig. 9.64).

Nasal dysplasia

Nasal malformations are extremely rare. Reports are scattered throughout the literature, but many of these were collected by Mazzola in a recent review (1976).

Since embryologically the nose is made of two distinct

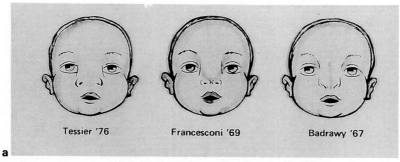

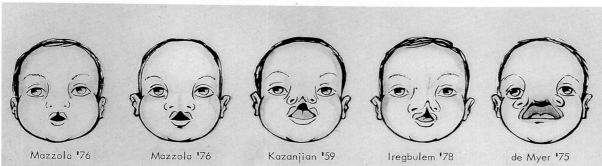

Fig. 9.60 Internasal dysplasia — selection of illustrations from the literature: (a) without medial cleft lip; (b) with medial cleft lip.

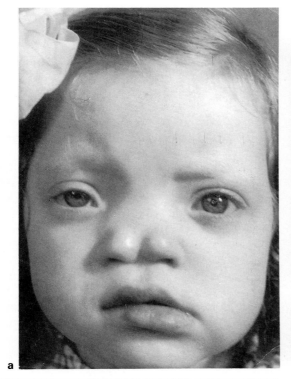

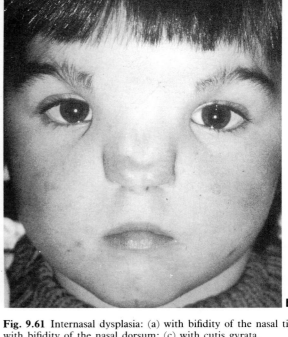

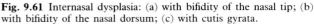

Fig. 9.61 Internasal dysplasia: (a) with bifidity of the nasal tip; (b) with bifidity of the nasal dorsum; (c) with cutis gyrata.

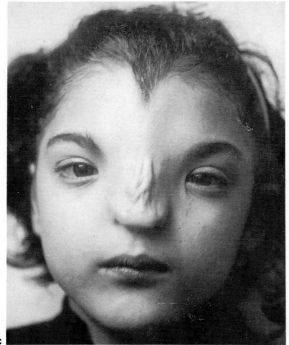

concept, four different types of nasal dysplasias can be distinguished: nasal aplasia, nasal aplasia with proboscis, nasoschizis, and nasal duplication.

NASAL APLASIA (Fig. 9.65)

'Naris sinistrae nullum vestigium adest, in sinistro latero nullum nasi cavum reperitur, cujus locum massa quaedam cartilaginae occupat'(Otto 1841).

This malformation is extremely rare and since Hensen's (1906) report only a small number of patients with this unilateral anomaly (Fig. 9.66) has been described. Davis (1935) observed four cases in a series of 948 facial clefts. Mazzola (1976) added five cases and reviewed the literature. Bilateral aplasia (arhinia) (Fig. 9.67) was probably first observed by Labat in 1833 but his description is not quite clear and an illustration is missing. We were able to trace 11 cases in the literature for which the term 'arhinia' should be used. Genetic transmittance has never been reported.

Morphology

Nasal aplasia is characterized by complete absence of one nasal half. The nasal cavity is missing and pneumatization of the maxillary ethmoidal and frontal sinuses has failed.

halves, and the majority of nasal malformations are restricted to one of these halves, it seems appropriate that the name 'nasal dysplasia' should only be used to indicate a unilateral malformation, while the word 'rhinal' should be applied when both halves are involved. Based on this

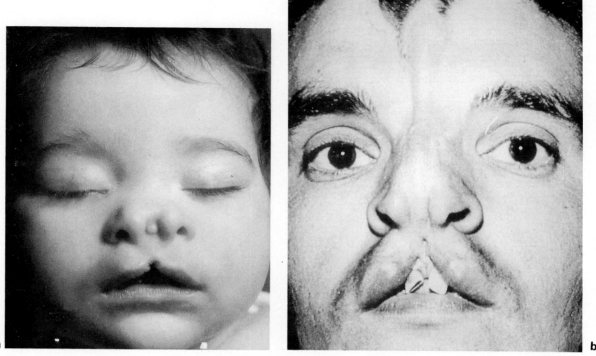

Fig. 9.62 Internasal dysplasia associated with medial cleft of the lip; (a) with bifidity of the nasal tip; (b) with bifidity of the nasal dorsum extending towards the forehead.

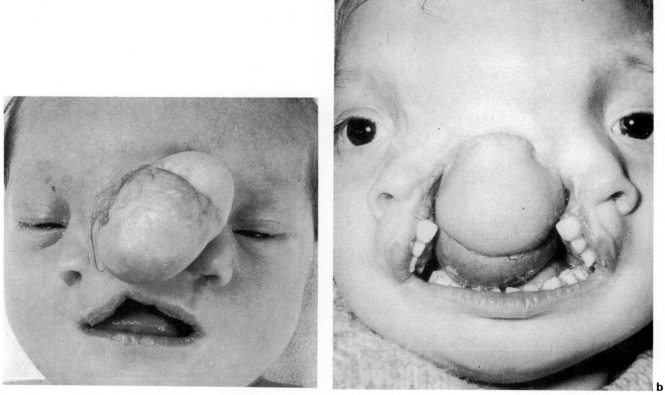

Fig. 9.63 Internasal dysplasia associated with encephalocele: (a) without cleft lip; (b) with cleft lip.

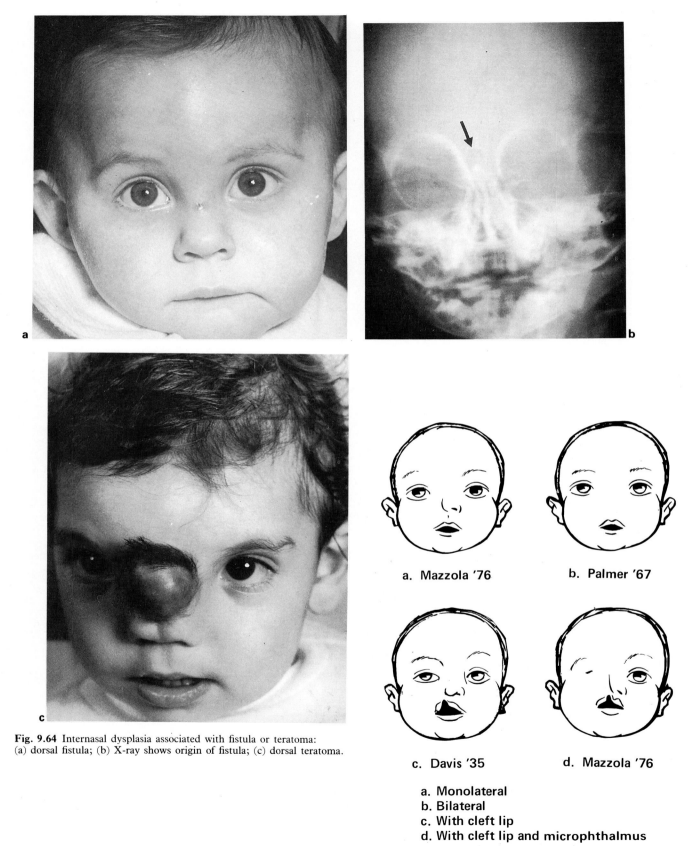

Fig. 9.64 Internasal dysplasia associated with fistula or teratoma:
(a) dorsal fistula; (b) X-ray shows origin of fistula; (c) dorsal teratoma.

a. Mazzola '76   b. Palmer '67

c. Davis '35   d. Mazzola '76

a. Monolateral
b. Bilateral
c. With cleft lip
d. With cleft lip and microphthalmus

Fig. 9.65 Nasal aplasia: selection of illustrations from the literature.

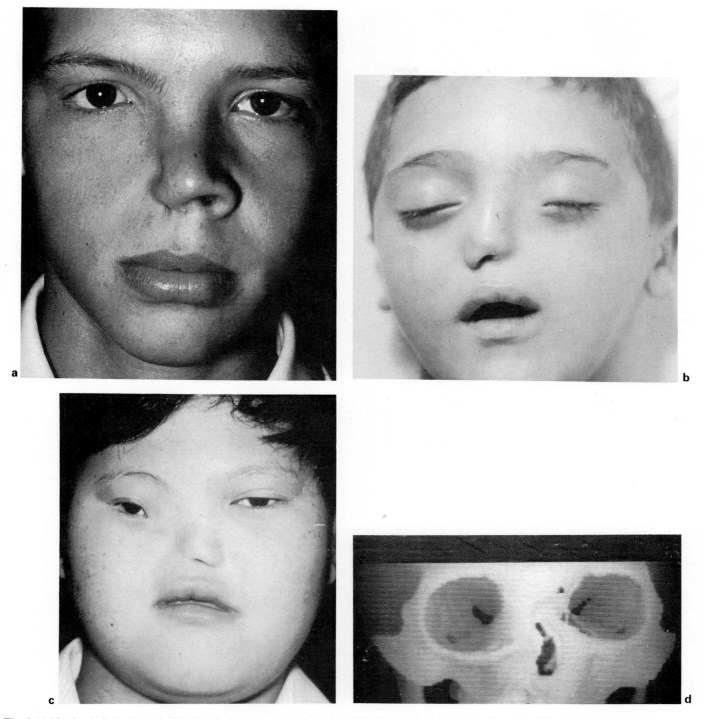

Fig. 9.66 Nasal aplasia (unilateral): (a) clinical view; note normal canthus; (b) clinical view; note telecanthus; (c) clinical view; note canthal dystopia; (d) 3-D reconstruction shows absence of nasal cavity on affected side (courtesy David David).

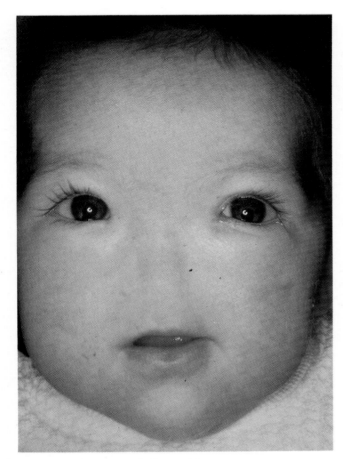

Fig. 9.67 Arhinia (courtesy G. Lemperle).

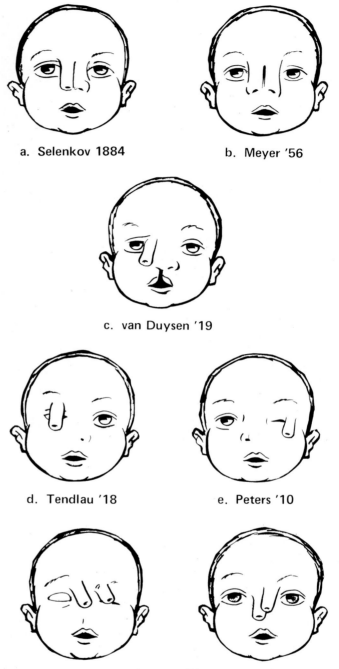

a. Selenkov 1884   b. Meyer '56

c. van Duysen '19

d. Tendlau '18   e. Peters '10

f. Rosen and Gitlin '59   g. Silverman and Cassini '65

a. Monolateral
b. Bilateral
c. With cleft lip
d. Dystopic proboscis (R)
e. Dystopic proboscis (L)
f. Bilateral with microphthalmus
g. Bilateral

Fig. 9.68 Nasal aplasia with proboscis: selection of illustrations from the literature.

Exploration reveals nothing but solid bone. There is no nasolacrimal duct and cyst formation or infection in the hypoplastic lacrimal system is frequently encountered (Fatin 1955). The affected half of the maxilla is hypoplastic and the palatal vault is high and acutely arched. The absence of one or more incisors and the resulting approximation of the canine teeth led Greer Walker (1961) to conclude that the premaxilla may also be absent in these patients. However, Bishop (1964) has described a case with arhinia and proboscis in which all the incisors were present, indicating that the premaxilla may be normal.

Non-erupted permanent incisors were also demonstrated by X-ray in a patient of Gifford et al (1972). X-ray examination in these cases demonstrates that the nasal bone, the cribriform plate and the olfactory bulbs are missing. Nasal aplasia is frequently associated with other malformations, such as cleft lip (Davis 1935), cleft palate (Schweckendiek & Hein 1973), microphthalmia (Berger & Martin 1969), coloboma of the lower eyelid (Berger & Martin) and coloboma of the iris (Gifford et al 1972). Thiefenthal (1910) reported a patient with orbital hypertelorism.

NASAL APLASIA WITH PROBOSCIS (Fig. 9.68)

Selenkow's (1884) case history of a patient with nasal aplasia and proboscis (Fig. 9.69) brings to mind the relatively recent period when plastic surgery was in its infancy and the general treatment of a patient was altogether different. Since his report little has been added to our knowledge of this condition.

Nasal aplasia with proboscis (Fig. 9.70) is rare and arhinia with proboscis even more so (Fig. 9.71) (Rosen & Gitlin 1959), (Silverman & Cassini 1971, Warkany

1971). Giraud et al (1976) reported an incidence of less than one per 100 000 newborns. Mazzola (1976) reviewed the literature.

Morphology

Except for the proboscis the characteristics of this malformation are essentially the same as those present in nasal aplasia. A lacrimal fistula was observed by Mahindra 1973. The origin of the proboscis is commonly found at the

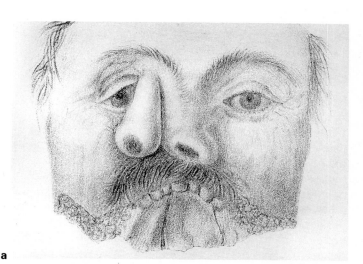

a

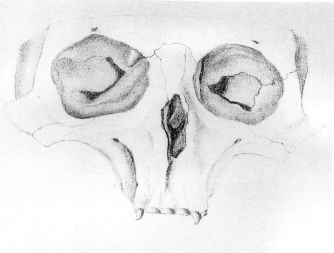

b

Fig. 9.69 Nasal aplasia with proboscis. Case recorded by Selenkow in 1884: (a) drawing of face; (b) drawing of skull.

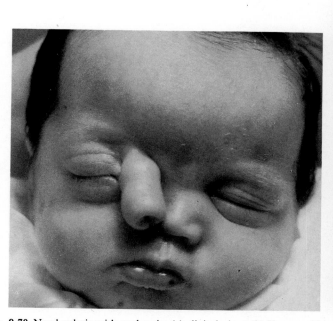

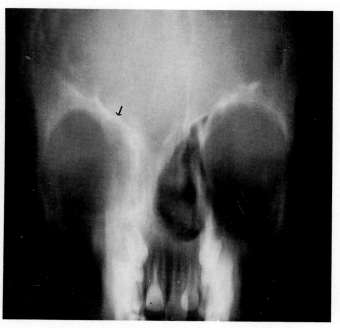

Fig. 9.70 Nasal aplasia with proboscis: (a) clinical view; (b) X-ray at 10 years of age shows absence of nasal cavity of the affected side and origin of the proboscis.

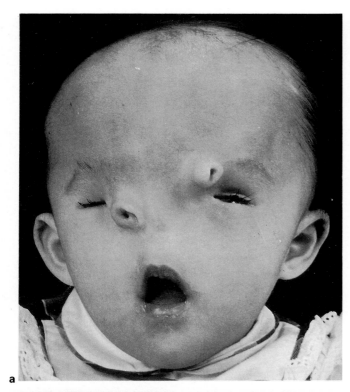

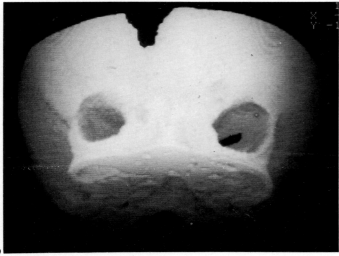

Fig. 9.71 Arhinia with probosces: (a) clinical view; (b) 3-D reconstruction shows total absence of nasal cavity and origin of the probosces (courtesy David David).

upper inner canthal region, and rarely at the upper outer margin of the orbit (Kundrat 1887, Peters 1910, Tendlau 1918).

Examination of the proboscis may reveal that the same tissues which are to be found in a normal nose are also present: hairs, sebaceous glands, sweat glands, striated muscle fibres, nerve fibres and cartilage can all be observed. There is, however, one major difference. The proboscis does not contain a cavity but rather a narrow

tract lined by mucosa and ending blindly at the dura mater or at the cranial base, where the cribriform plate and olfactory tract are missing. Tears have been known to come from this tract but their origin is not clear. They may have been produced by lacrimal gland tissue surrounding the tract (Zacherl 1920), or alternatively they may have come through a communication with the lacrimal apparatus (Smith 1950). A patent proboscis has been observed only once (Alves d'Assumpcão 1975).

Like nasal aplasia the same condition with proboscis may be associated with other deformities, such as colobomata of the iris and choroid (Seefelder 1910), of the retina (Tendlau 1918), upper eyelid (Peters 1910) and of the lower eyelid (Landow 1890). A cleft lip (van Duyse 1919) and microphthalmia or anophthalmia (Peters 1910) have also been reported occasionally.

Curiosities (Fig. 9.72)

Nature really becomes capricious when it produces an almost normal (Meyer 1956) or normal nose (Seefelder 1910) in combination with a proboscis. There are two theoretical explanations: one is a duplication of one nasal half, producing a normal nostril and a proboscis; the second is a combination of complete nasal duplication on one side of the face with nasal aplasia and proboscis on the other side. To make the developmental solution to this problem even more complex, nature also provides us with patients in which the same condition is observed as described above, in combination with a cleft lip (Kirchmayr 1906, McLaren 1955).

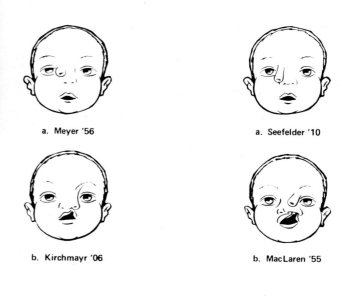

a. Meyer '56

a. Seefelder '10

b. Kirchmayr '06

b. MacLaren '55

a. Complete nose with proboscis
b. Complete nose with proboscis and cleft lip

Fig. 9.72 Accessory probosces: selection of illustrations from the literature.

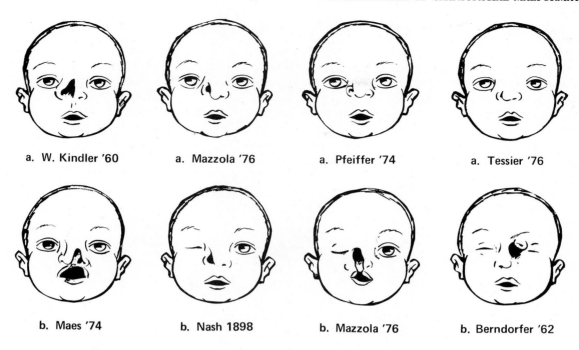

a. W. Kindler '60 a. Mazzola '76 a. Pfeiffer '74 a. Tessier '76

b. Maes '74 b. Nash 1898 b. Mazzola '76 b. Berndorfer '62

a. **Monolateral**
b. **With cleft lip and/or microphthalmus**

Fig. 9.73 Nasoschizis: selection of illustrations from the literature.

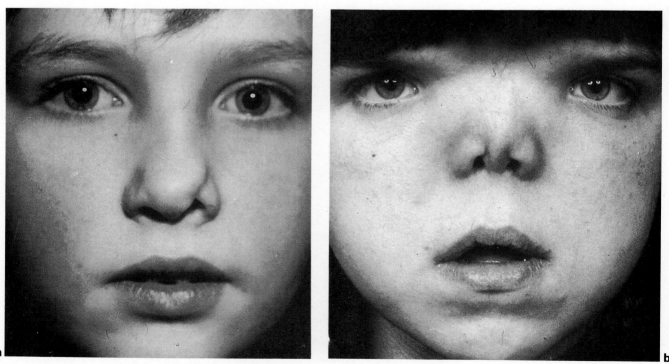

Fig. 9.74 Nasoschizis: (a) clinical view of unilateral abnormality; (b) clinical view of bilateral abnormality.

NASOSCHIZIS (Fig. 9.73)

Clefts of the nostril (no. 1 cleft in Tessier's classification) have long been referred to as lateral nasal clefts. Leuckart's case (1840) bears witness to the severity of the malformation, which may not be as rare as one might expect from the scarce literature on this subject. Frangenheim (1909) was able to collect no more than 13 cases. However, Mazzola (1976) added 14 cases of his own. Fogh-Andersen (1965) observed four cases in a group of 3988 facial clefts. A genetic basis has never been recorded.

Morphology

Nasoschizis is characterized by a cleft in one nostril, the septum and nasal cavity being normal. A cleft in the alveolar process between the first and second incisor and choanal atresia may, however, also be present. The severity of the malformation ranges from a simple notch in one or both alae (Fig. 9.74) to a more or less complete absence of nostrils and nasal bones. Complete absence of the nostril is inevitably associated with frontal, fronto-nasoethmoidal and internasal dysplasia. This means that

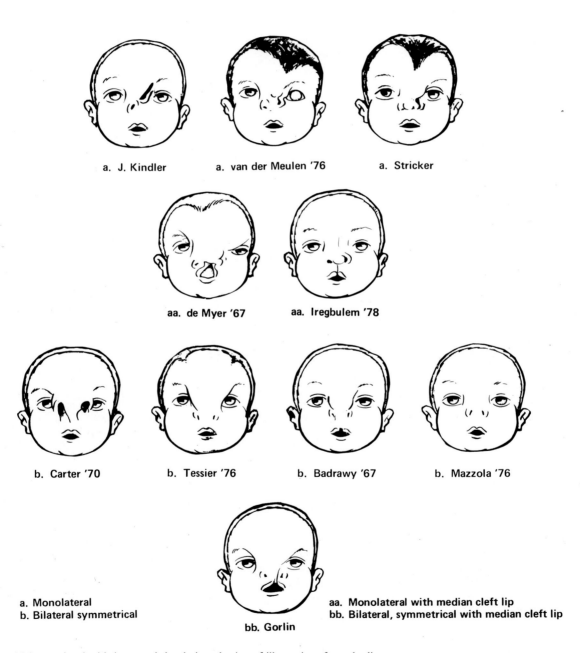

a. J. Kindler   a. van der Meulen '76   a. Stricker

aa. de Myer '67   aa. Iregbulem '78

b. Carter '70   b. Tessier '76   b. Badrawy '67   b. Mazzola '76

a. Monolateral
b. Bilateral symmetrical

bb. Gorlin

aa. Monolateral with median cleft lip
bb. Bilateral, symmetrical with median cleft lip

Fig. 9.75 Nasoschizis associated with internasal dysplasia: selection of illustrations from the literature.

CLASSIFICATION OF CRANIOFACIAL MALFORMATIONS 197

all the malformations described under these headings may be present.

In the same way, nasoschizis may also be found in combination with a cleft lip (Leuckart 1840), unilateral microphthalmia (Nash 1898) or bilateral ophthalmic dysplasia (Berndorfer 1962).

Bilateral cases of pure nasoschizis are extremely rare and are restricted to the presence of minor alar clefts, as were found in a patient described by Sedano et al (1970). This fact need not surprise us since severe bilateral nasal dysplasia will inevitably be associated with internasal dysplasia.

Combinations of nasoschizis and internasal dysplasia (Fig. 9.75) are rare. Unilateral cases (Fig. 9.76) have been described by Kindler (1889), Rosasco & Massa (1968) and Van der Meulen (1976). In some of these patients a keel-shaped deformity of the maxilla may also be observed, the apex of the keel being situated in a paramedian position. Unilateral as well as bilateral cases have been reported in combination with a median cleft lip (De Myer 1967, Millard & Williams 1968).

Accurate distinction between the various forms of nasoschizis is now possible by the 3-D reconstruction of CT scans (Figs. 9.77, 9.78).

NASAL DUPLICATION

Duplication of the nose occurs in different forms and different combinations.

Morphology

Comparison of the different examples in the literature (Fig. 9.79) clearly shows that grading is possible. The scale of variations can range from a supernumerary nostril in an otherwise normal nose to duplication of the upper face (diprosopia). The supernumerary nostril is usually the medial one. It may end blindly, be stenotic or open into a nasal cavity. In the milder cases there may be one continuous midline septum, while in the more severe cases duplication of the anterior part of the septum or full duplication (Bimar 1881; Fig. 9.80) may be observed (Mazzola 1976).

In facial duplication the following structures may be

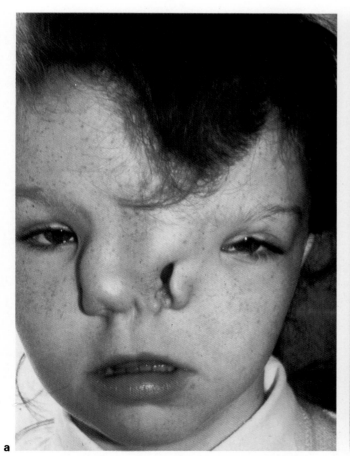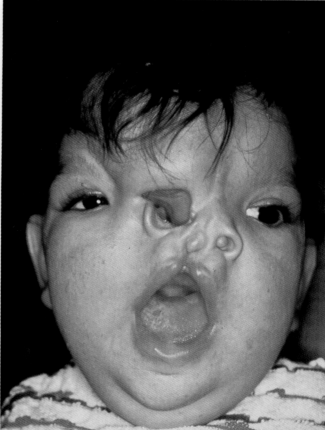

a   b

Fig. 9.76 Nasoschizis — note associated with internasal dysplasia: (a) clinical view — note widow's peak; (b) clinical view — note widow's peak and median cleft lip.

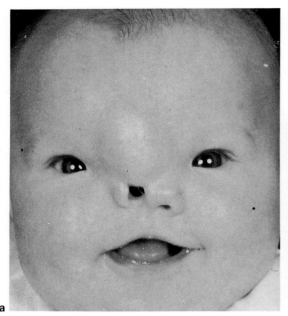
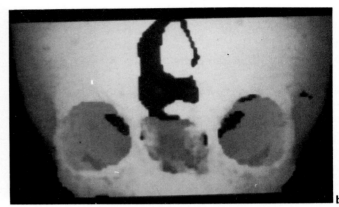

Fig. 9.77 Nasoschizis: (a) clinical view; (b) 3-D reconstruction — note defect extending into frontal bone (courtesy David David).

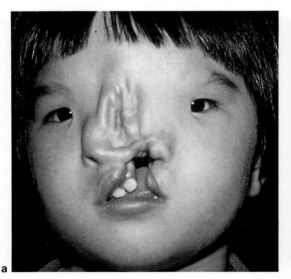
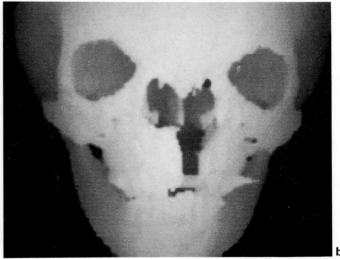

Fig. 9.78 Nasoschizis: (a) clinical view — note cleft lip and cutis gyrata; (b) 3-D reconstruction — note defect in maxilla (courtesy David David).

duplicated: the sphenoidal sinuses, the crista galli (Fig. 9.81), the cribriform plate, the nose and the premaxilla. As with internasal dysplasia, these structures are separated by a groove. In addition there may be rudimentary orbits with eyes and supplementary eyebrows (Obwegeser et al 1978).

The ethmoid may be composed of one central and two lateral masses. On the central mass a supplementary anterior cerebral lobe may be observed.

Unilateral as well as bilateral duplication has been reported by Blair (1931), who also recorded a case of unilateral duplication with internasal dysplasia. Combinations (Fig. 9.82) of nasal duplication and cleft lip, median or lateral, have recently been observed.

Holmes (1950) described a patient with nasal duplication and anophthalmus. When nasal duplication is found bilaterally, the dysplasia is known to produce hideous malformations.

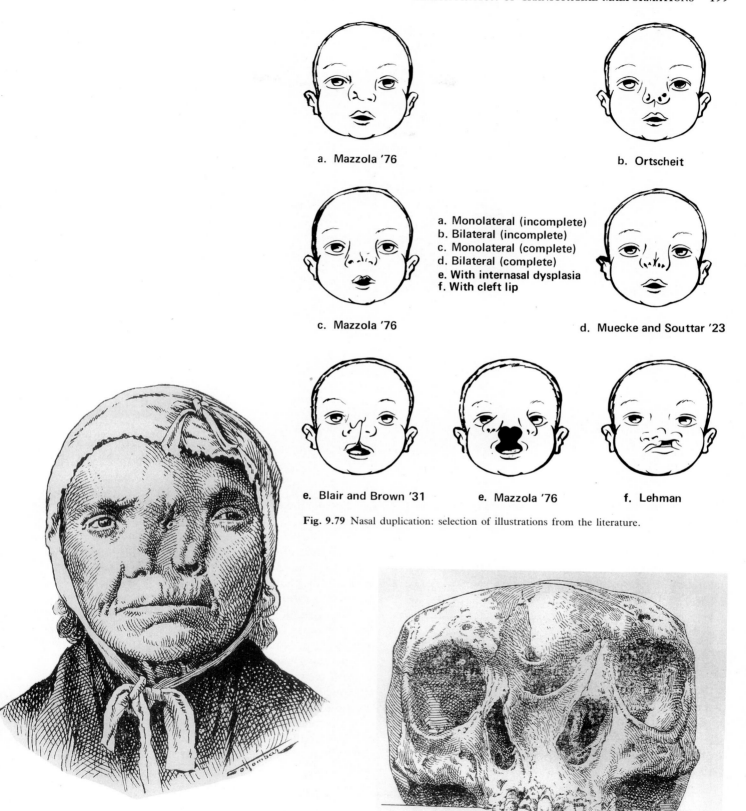

a. Mazzola '76

b. Ortscheit

a. Monolateral (incomplete)
b. Bilateral (incomplete)
c. Monolateral (complete)
d. Bilateral (complete)
e. With internasal dysplasia
f. With cleft lip

c. Mazzola '76

d. Muecke and Souttar '23

e. Blair and Brown '31

e. Mazzola '76

f. Lehman

Fig. 9.79 Nasal duplication: selection of illustrations from the literature.

Femme à deux nez.

a

b

Fig. 9.80 Nasal duplication. Case observed by D. Bimar and published in 1881 in the *Gazette Hebdomadaire* of Montpellier: (a) drawing of face; (b) drawing of skull.

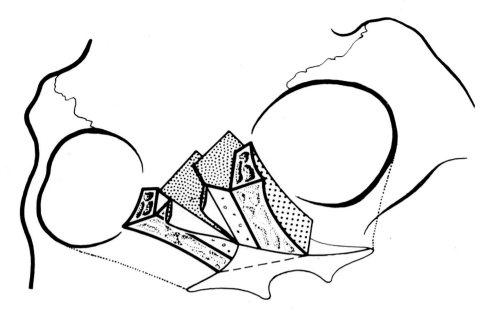

Fig. 9.81 Nasal duplication — note abnormality of crista galli.

Premaxillo-maxillary and intermaxillo-palatine dysplasia (cleft lip and palate) (Figs. 9.83 and 9.84)

The true clefts situated between the borders of the nasal and maxillary processes result in osseous defects, a genuine secondary dysostosis. The associated deformities are caused by the loss of balance which is due to the interruption of the muscular slings: anteriorly labionasal, posteriorly velopharyngeal.

The bony parts, separated by the cleft, are modified in their dimensions and their position. The dimensional alterations predominantly concern the horizontal plates of the maxilla and palatine bone (Fig. 9.85). The positional alterations primarily affect the vomeroseptal strut, which is deviated as a result of muscular imbalance, the position of the vomer sometimes becoming almost horizontal.

The alveolar borders are equally subject to the distracting effect of muscular interruption. The larger element is tilted superiorly; the smaller element is held backwards.

The impact of the cleft on the surrounding structures is not limited to the alveolar borders, but also involves the nasal pyramid. A medial deviation develops and the ipsilateral wall of the nasal roof takes a more horizontal position, creating a false impression of telecanthus.

The disruption of the buccal platform disturbs orality and linguomandibular posture. Indeed, the position of the tongue refers to the cleft disturbing lingual proprioception and inducing harmful habits.

Each cleft, small as it may be, generates a dysostosis, affecting the base of the pyriform aperture on the cleft side in premaxillo-maxillary dysplasia. In the same manner a cleft of the secondary palate affects the position and dimension of the maxillopalatine shelves, which shorten, become verticalized and retrude externally and superiorly from the sagittal axis.

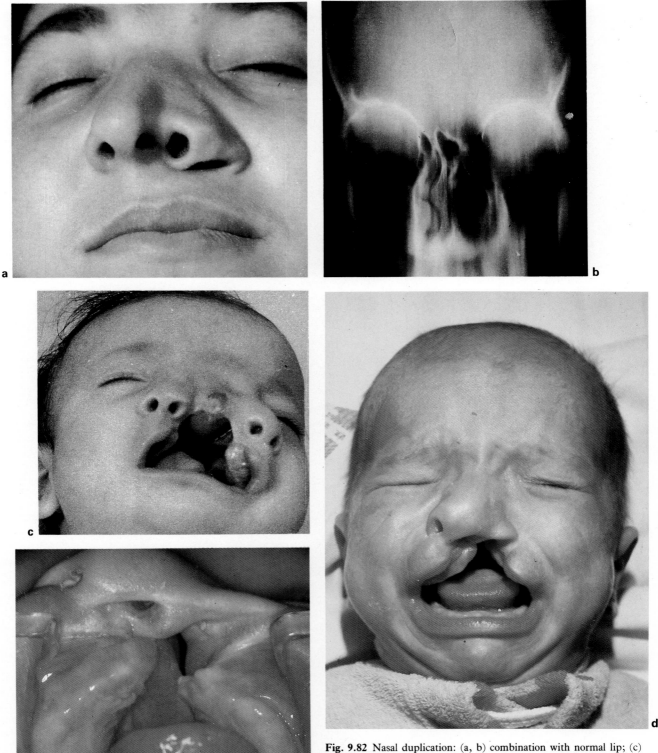

Fig. 9.82 Nasal duplication: (a, b) combination with normal lip; (c) combination with median cleft of the lip; (d, e) combination with unilateral cleft of the lip.

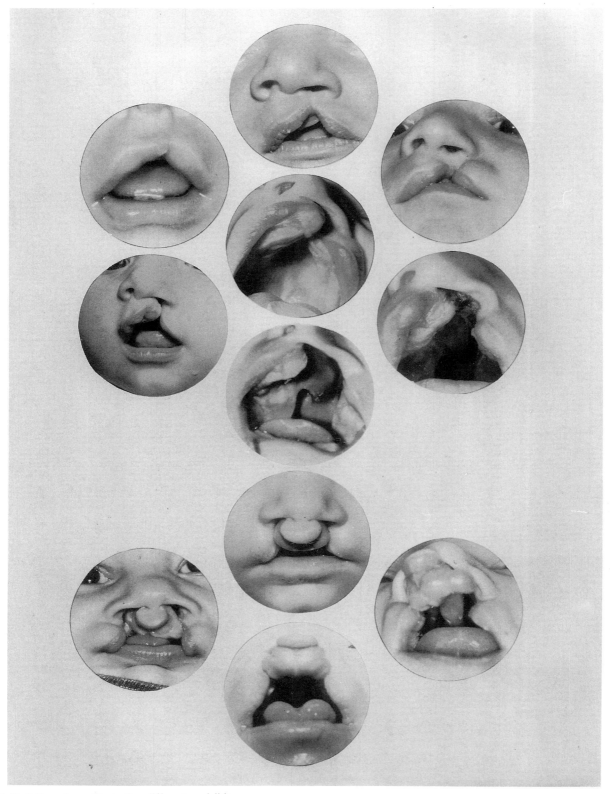

Fig. 9.83 Cleft lip: scheme illustrating different modalities.

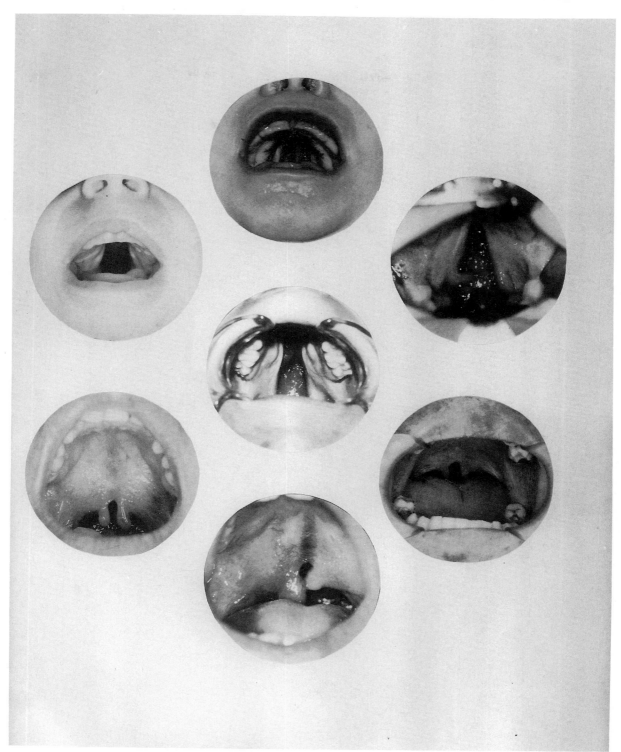

Fig. 9.84 Cleft palate: scheme illustrating different modalities.

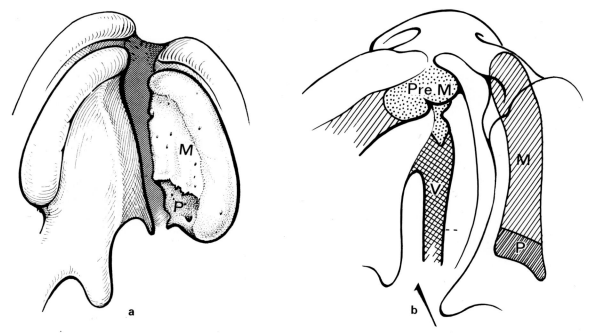

Fig. 9.85 Cleft palate: (a) angular distortion between the maxilla (M) and palatine bone (P); (b) bony area affected by the cleft.

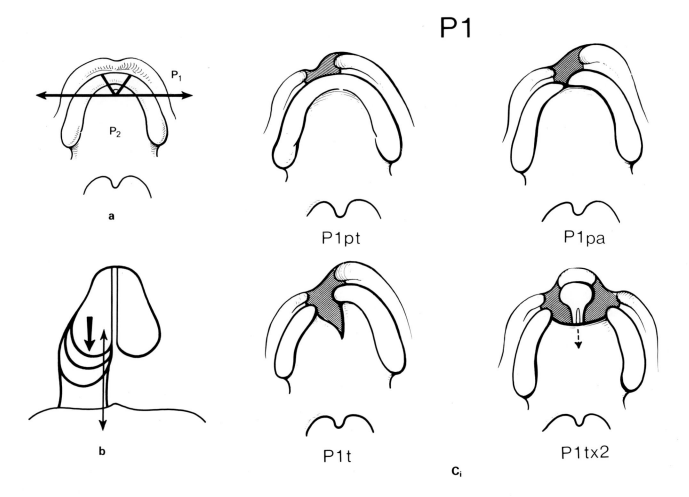

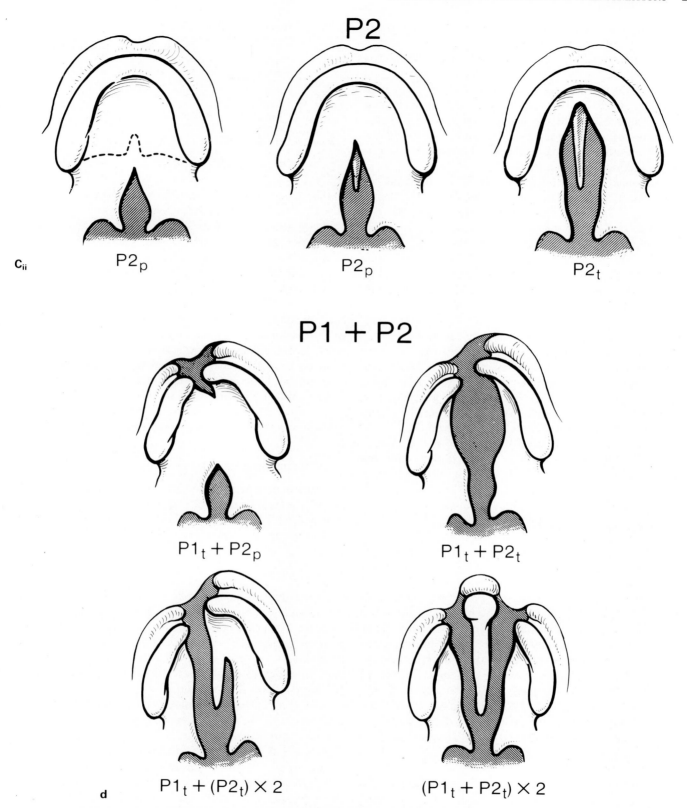

Fig. 9.86 Cleft palate. Classification of various types based on the distinction between a primary P_1 and secondary P_2 palate: (a) the two palatal areas; (b) the different degrees of bony involvement in cleft lips; (c) anomalies affecting the primary palate (P1)). P_1pL = partial lesion of primary palate affecting the lip, P_1pa = partial lesion of primary palate affecting the alveolus, P_1t = total lesion of primary palate, $P_1t \times 2$ = total lesion of primary palate (bilateral); (d) anomalies affecting the secondary palate (p2). P_2p = partial lesion of the secondary palate (two degrees), P_2t = total lesion of the secondary palate; (e) anomalies affecting primary and secondary palate ($P_1 + P_2$). $P_1 + P_2$ = common combinations of lesions affecting the primary and secondary palate.

The different degrees of severity form a wide range consisting of two categories. The key to a classification is embryological and based on the differentiation between a primary (P1) and a secondary (P2) palate.

In addition the morphological severity of the cleft, total or partial, is symbolized by capital and small letters, representing the lip and the alveolar process (Fig. 9.86). The anatomical disorder is associated with four functional disturbances affecting, respectively, alimentation, respiration, audition and phonation.

Alimentation is compromised initially by deficient suction. Masticatory problems only develop when dental eruption is complete. Occlusal disorders may become manifest during mixed dentition.

Respiration is disturbed by septal deviation, by the changes in the dimensions of the nasal fossa on the cleft side and by the alterations of the inspiratory valve. The inferior turbinate bears witness to the quality of respiration. Disturbed nasal respiration has repercussions on the drainage of the sinuses and on the aeration of the naso-pharynx, which plays a role in auditory function.

Audition. The patency of the Eustachian tube is quite frequently compromised in children with a cleft palate, but this disorder is not only determined by the cleft alone. Dysfunction of the tube interferes with the ventilation of the middle ear, causing a glue ear which eventually results in tympanic retraction with conductive hearing loss.

Phonation. The child and its parents are primarily preoccupied by the disturbance of phonation and this aspect therefore deserves discussion in a special chapter (Ch. 14).

Naso-maxillary and maxillary dysplasia

Although oblique facial clefts had been reported before, Laroche in 1823 was the first to differentiate between ordinary cleft lip or 'harelip' and clefts of the cheek. Further distinction was made by Pelvet in 1864, who separated oblique clefts involving the nose from the other cheek clefts. Drawing on Ahlfeld's work, Morian in 1887 collected 29 cases from the literature, contributing seven cases of his own. Morian recognized three different groups of oblique facial clefts. Since then excellent reviews have been written by Trendelenburg (1886), Grünberg (1909), Boo-chai (1970) and Millard (1977). The incidence of these rare conditions, all sporadic, is shown in Table 9.1.

Naso-maxillary and maxillary dysplasia have been classified according to:

1. the direction they take, which may be (oro)-naso-ocular (oculonasal), or oro-ocular (oculofacial); the latter type can be subdivided into oromedial, canthal and oro-lateral canthal, depending on the relationship of the defect to the infraorbital foramen;

Table 9.1 Incidence of oblique clefts

Ref.	Oblique clefts	Facial clefts	per thousand
Davis (1935)	5	944	5.4
Günther (1963)	4	900	4.4
Wilson (1972)			2.5
Rintala et al (1980)	11	3600	3.0
Fogh-Andersen (1965)	3	3988	0.75
Kubacek & Penkara (1974)	5	2880	1.7
Pitanguy & Franco (1967)	1	726	1.4

2. the period in which the development was disturbed, e.g. primary or secondary clefting;
3. the position of one dysplasia in relation to the other (Morian 1887: I, II, III; Tessier 1969, 1976: 3, 4, 5);
4. the areas in which the malformations have their origin: e.g. nasomaxillary and maxillary (medial and lateral) dysplasia.

Naso-maxillary and maxillary dysplasia may be associated with other craniofacial malformations, such as encephaloceles, hydrocephaly, widow's peak or cow's lick, hypertelorism, choanal atresia, anophthalmia and microphthalmia, colobomata of the iris or choroid and epibulbar dermoids. The combination with deformities such as constriction rings of the limbs, aplasia cutis congenita, clubfoot and ectopia vesicae has also been reported.

NASO-MAXILLARY DYSPLASIA (Fig. 9.87)

It is this malformation which is also known as the Morian I cleft, the Tessier no. 3 cleft or more commonly the naso-ocular cleft. The term nasomaxillary, which best describes the pathology, was coined by Günther (1963).

Morphology

Naso-maxillary dysplasias may be incomplete or complete. An incomplete or naso-ocular cleft (Figs. 9.87, 9.88) runs from the alar base which is drawn upward to the inferiorly dislocated medial canthus. There may be a fistula in the lacrimal canal. The lip is intact and the alar malformations resemble those found in patients with the Johanson–Blizzard syndrome.

The complete or oro-naso-ocular cleft (Figs. 9.87, 9.88) starts in the upper lip as an ordinary cleft and passes through the nasal aperture, skirting the foot of the distorted and superiorly dislocated ala nasi. The cleft then continues to the inner canthus, which is always drawn inferiorly. There is a retrusion of the maxilla, medial to the infraorbital foramen, and the frontal process may be deficient or absent. Morian (1887) was of the opinion that nasomaxillary dysplasia is characterized as a cleft located between the medial and lateral incisors. He based his view

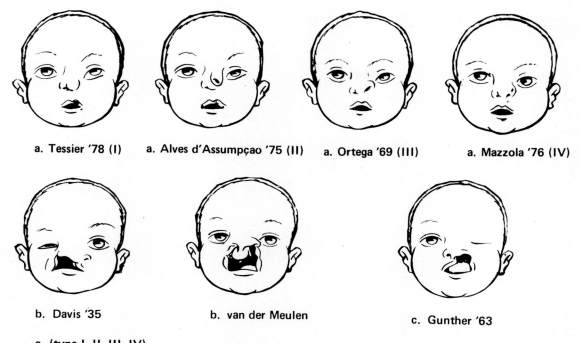

a. Tessier '78 (I)   a. Alves d'Assumpçao '75 (II)   a. Ortega '69 (III)   a. Mazzola '76 (IV)

b. Davis '35   b. van der Meulen   c. Gunther '63

a. (type I, II, III, IV)
b. Monolateral and bilateral with cleft lip
c. Monolateral with cleft lip and microphthalmus

Fig. 9.87 Nasomaxillary dysplasia: selection of illustrations from the literature.

on one personal observation, adding 18 case reports from the literature, in which there is little evidence to support this generalization. In contrast, Rintala et al 1980 observed that the alveolar cleft was always situated between the medial incisor and the canine tooth, while the lateral incisor was frequently missing. The complete cleft is frequently associated with a palatal cleft, but this defect is not obligatory. 3-D reconstruction of CT scans provides valuable information on the nature of the osseous defects (Figs. 9.89, 9.90).

Combinations with contralateral macrostomia were recorded by Pelvet (1864) and Kirmisson (1898). The nasolacrimal apparatus is absent in the majority of cases, but a patent duct may occasionally be found in less severe malformations.

MAXILLARY DYSPLASIA (medial)

Medial oro-ocular, Morian II or Tessier no. 4 cleft are some of the more commonly used terms for a malformation in that part of the craniofacial skeleton which is formed by the maxillary process. In the series reviewed by Morian, 12 cases belong to this type.

Morphology

The defect (Fig. 9.91) extends from an upper lip coloboma somewhere between philtrum and oral commissure to a lower eyelid coloboma. The intact but upward dislocated nares is avoided. The maxilla is always hypoplastic, resulting in severe retrusion of the rim of the pyriform aperture and the formation of a funnel-shaped concavity (infundibulum) in the medial and anterior part of the orbital floor.

A cleft may traverse the alveolus between the lateral incisor and canine tooth or, rarely, between two incisors as Morian reported. In Morian's cases, however, the incisor lateral to the cleft proved to be supernumerary. Not surprisingly, clefting of the palate, complete or partial, has also been reported by several authors.

Malformations of the nasolacrimal apparatus are found in the majority of patients but the duct may be patent in less severe cases. Unilateral as well as bilateral cases may occur. Choanal atresia has been observed by Davis (1935) and anopthalmia was reported by Miller et al (1973).

MAXILLARY DYSPLASIA (lateral)

This malformation is also known as the Morian III cleft and the lateral oro-ocular cleft. Morian includes the observations of Nicati (1822), Remacly (1864) and Fergusson (1857) (Fig. 9.92) in his review, but the illustration in Nicati's thesis leaves room for doubt as to the real nature of this case. Few examples of this dysplasia have been

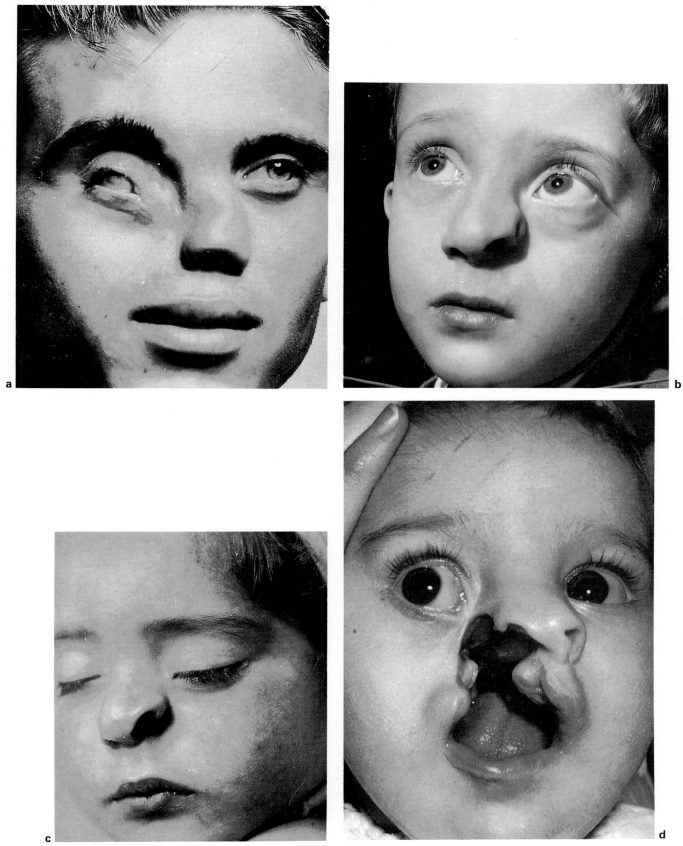

Fig. 9.88 Nasomaxillary dysplasia: (a) combination with nasal aplasia; (b) combination with nasal duplication; (c) without cleft lip; (d) with cleft lip.

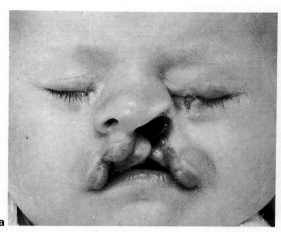
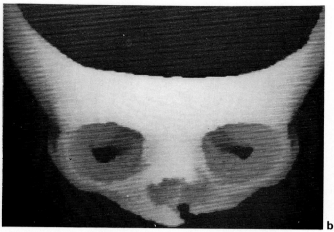

Fig. 9.89 Nasomaxillary dysplasia: (a) clinical view; (b) 3-D reconstruction shows osseous defect (courtesy David David).

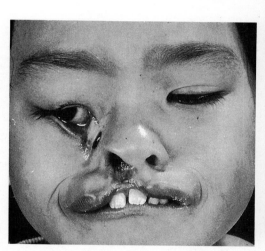
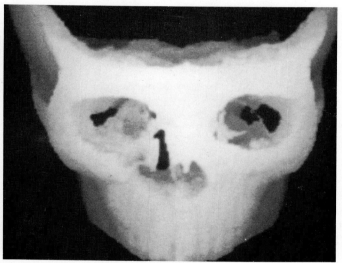

Fig. 9.90 Nasomaxillary dysplasia with cleft of the lip: (a) clinical view; (b) 3-D reconstruction — note combination with medial maxillary dysplasia (courtesy David David).

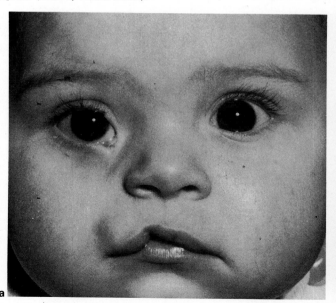
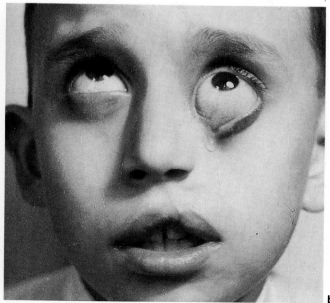

Fig. 9.91 Medial maxillary dysplasia (unilateral): (a) combination with medial canthal dystopia; (b) combination with medial canthal dystopia and lower eyelid coloboma.

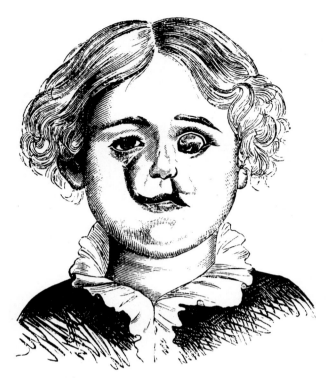

Fig. 9.92 Lateral maxillary dysplasia (unilateral). Case observed by Fergusson and published in *A practice of surgery* (1857). Note medial maxillary abnormality on opposite side.

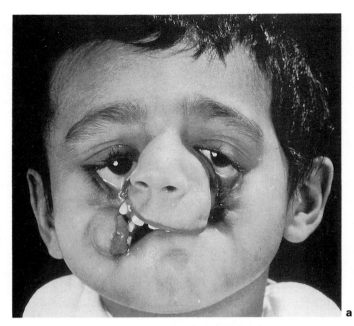

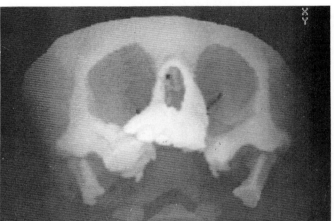

Fig. 9.93 Lateral maxillary dysplasia (bilateral): (a) clinical view; (b) 3-D reconstruction shows maxillary defects (courtesy David David).

reported, but the malformation may not be as rare as is usually thought, considering the resemblance to some of the Treacher Collins' patients, a fact previously noted by Tessier.

Morphology

The dysplasia starts on the lip, in or near the oral commissure, and arches upward to a coloboma in the lateral part of the lower eyelid (Fig. 9.93). Morian (1887) and Tessier (1976) observed that the bony defect on the orbital side was located at the zygomaxillary suture, while on the alveolar side it was situated between the canine tooth and the premolar. These findings suggest that the malformation is restricted to the maxilla, implying that we are dealing with a pure maxillary dysplasia. The similarity between the soft tissue malformation found in the lateral oro-ocular cleft and the Treacher Collins' syndrome is, however, so striking that there is reason to suspect that at least in some of these cases the zygoma is also involved. Duhamel (1966) in fact has stated that the maxillary dysplasia in patients with a lateral oro-ocular cleft is frequently associated with a malformation of the malar bone. Duke Elder (1958) even names these malformations zygomaxillary dysplasias or orotemporal clefts.

The diagnostic problems are probably best illustrated by one of Tessier's patients in which his clefts nos 5 and 6 run a parallel course from the lateral part of the lower eyelid to the corner of the mouth.

Maxillo-zygomatic dysplasia (Fig. 9.94)

Morphology

In the soft tissues this anomaly runs the same course as in lateral maxillary dysplasia, its position being somewhat more lateral.

Pitanguy's (1968) case with a bilateral cleft is probably unique. It is not clear from the description whether this is a case of maxillo-zygomatic dysplasia. Theoretically it might also be an example of lateral maxillary dysplasia.

Chavane (1890) reported a case (Fig. 9.95) with bilateral oro-ocular clefting in which the differences between lateral maxillary and zygomaxillary dysplasia are well described.

In the skeleton the defect is found between the maxilla and the zygoma, both of which may be hypoplastic. The defect extends into the infraorbital fissure and does not involve the alveolar process. It may be associated with a cleft in the soft palate (Chavane) or with choanal atresia.

Very few cases have been reported in the literature. In bilateral cases the clinical appearance resembles Treacher Collins' syndrome, requiring accurate differentiation.

Zygomatic dysplasia

Malar hypoplasia is the 'hall mark' of a malformation that was first described by Berry (1889) and later by Treacher Collins (1900). Today the malformation is commonly referred to as Treacher Collins' syndrome (Fig. 9.96).

Morphology

The facial appearance (Fig. 9.97) is characterized by the following features: flattening of the cheeks, antimongoloid angulation of the palpebral fissures, notching of the rim or even a coloboma of the lateral part of the lower eyelids, and absence or deficiency of eyelashes in the medial third of these eyelids and absence of the lacrimal canaliculus. When no other symptoms are found, it seems justified to speak of the 'incomplete form' that, with few exceptions, is found bilaterally. Malar hypoplasia may be associated with anomalies of the temporoaural complex (Fig. 9.98) and of the mandible, producing the complete form of the anomaly, which was first reported by Franceschetti & Zwahlen (1944). This cluster of malformations will be discussed under the name zygo-auromandibular dysplasia.

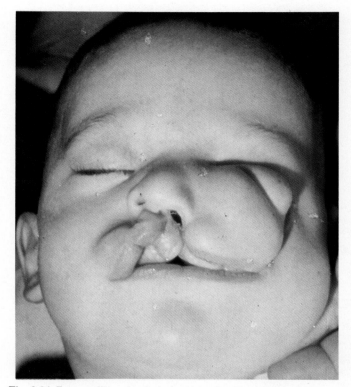

Fig. 9.94 Zygomaxillary dysplasia (courtesy Dr Chancholle).

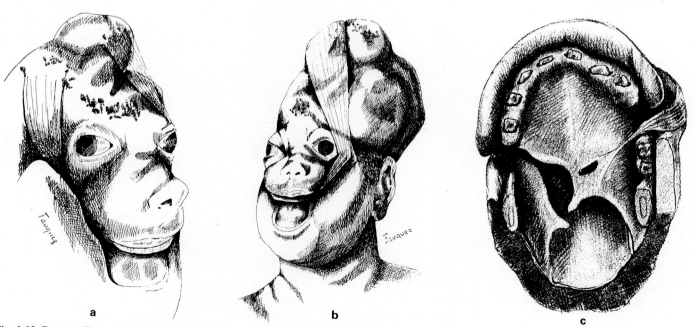

Fig. 9.95 Zygomaxillary dysplasia. Case recorded by Chavane in 1890: (a) zygomaxillary defect on the right side of the face; (b) maxillary defect on the left side of the face; (c) oral view illustrating differences between a and b.

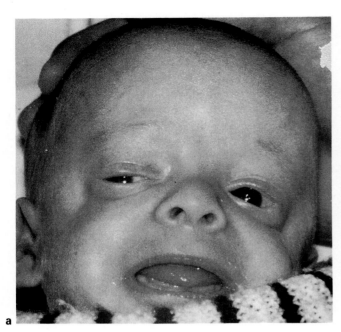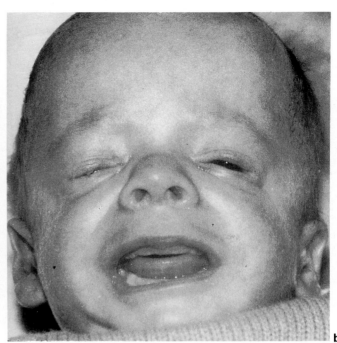

Fig. 9.96 Zygomatic dysplasia or Treacher Collins' syndrome in twins.

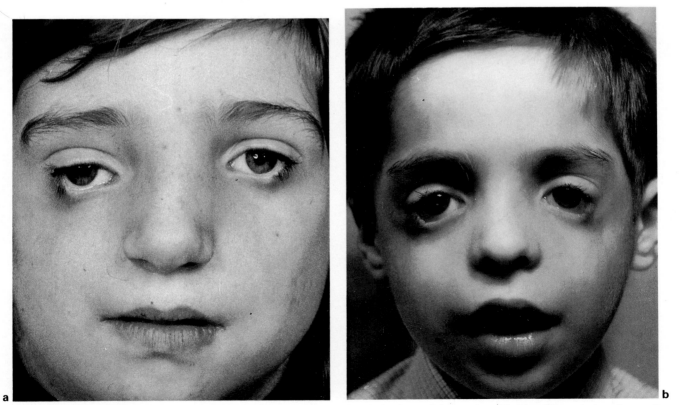

Fig. 9.97 Zygomatic dysplasias — note eyelid malformations: (a) absence of eyelashes in medial part of eyelid; (b) coloboma in lateral part of eyelid.

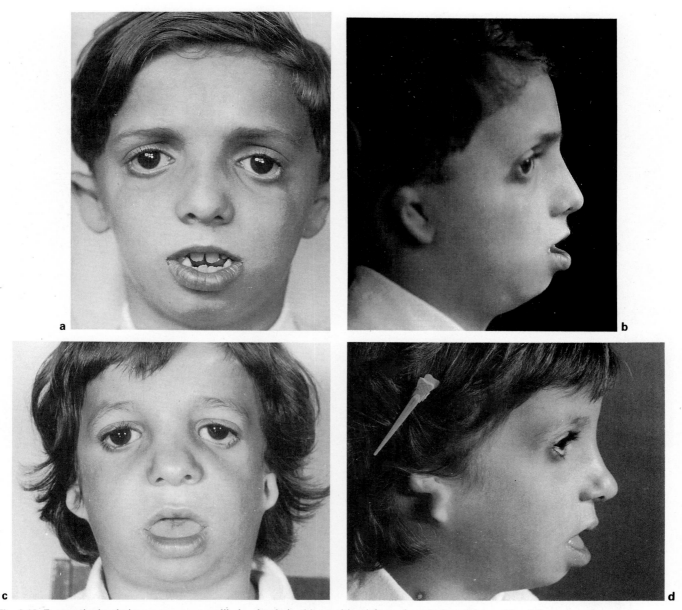

Fig. 9.98 Zygomatic dysplasia or zygo-auromandibular dysplasia: (a) transitional form, frontal view; (b) transitional form, lateral view; (c) complete form, frontal view; (d) complete form, lateral view.

The anomaly has also been observed in combination with limb deficiencies and is part of two syndromes: postaxial acrofacial dysostosis (Miller's syndrome), in which the digits as well as the ulnar and radial halves of the limb may be affected; and acrofacial dysostosis (Nager's syndrome), in which the limb deficiencies are restricted to the radial half.

Zygo-auromandibular dysplasia

Also known as mandibulofacial dysostosis, this bilateral anomaly represents a cluster of malformations produced by zygomatic temporoaural and mandibular dysplasia. In its complete form it was first described by Zwahlen (1944) in his thesis and immediately afterwards by Franceschetti & Zwahlen (1944). The condition is transmitted by a dominant gene with variable expression. Extensive reviews of the anomaly were published by McKenzie & Craig (1955) and by Rogers (1964) and Vatre (1971).

Morphology (Fig. 9.99)

The malar bone, the temporoaural complex and the lower jaw form the lower part of the craniofacial helix; the

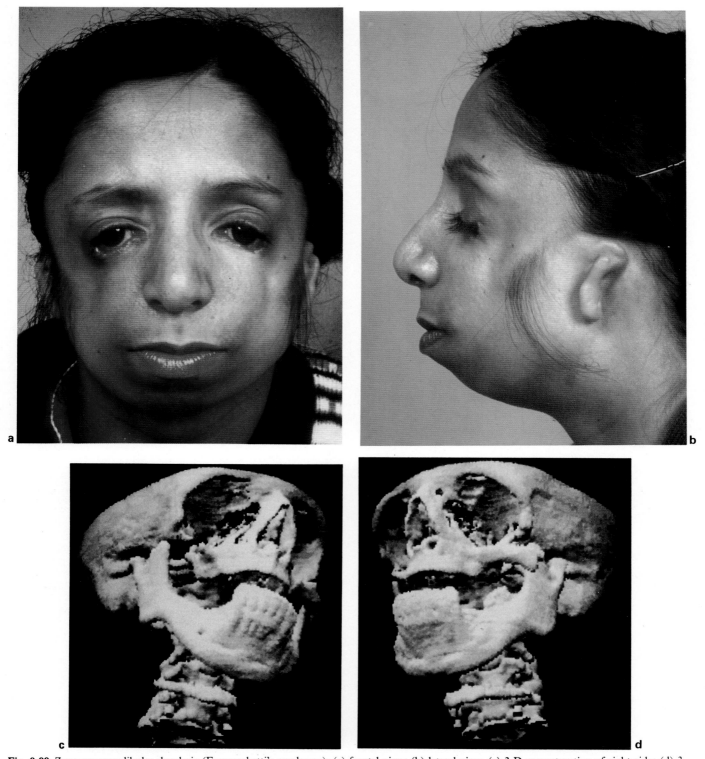

Fig. 9.99 Zygo-auromandibular dysplasia (Franceschetti's syndrome): (a) frontal view; (b) lateral view; (c) 3-D reconstruction of right side; (d) 3-D reconstruction of left side.

impact of malformations in these areas on the facial skeleton as a whole is therefore considerable.

The frontal appearance is marked by anomalies affecting the orbital region. Retrusion of the malar region, obliteration of the frontonasal angle and a receding chin give the patients a characteristic convex bird-like profile. Protrusion of the nose and the maxilla and the absence of a malar contour may produce an enophthalmic appearance (tunnel look).

The orbit. The orbital configuration is altered by the defect in the inferolateral angle and the caudal displacement of the superolateral angle. The orbits become egg-shaped, with their base superior and rotated medially and their apex inferior and rotated laterally. The orbital contents prolapse into the defect created by the deficiency in the malar bone.

Following careful dissection of the periorbit and respecting the infraorbital nerve which may pass directly from the cavity to the soft tissues, the superolateral surface of the maxilla, the greater wing of the sphenoid, the lateral pterygoid muscle and the coronoid process may become directly visible. A single temporomasseteric muscle is sometimes seen.

Inferolateral sloping of the orbits may be associated with: flattening of the cheeks; antimongoloid angulation of the palpebral fissures; shortening of these fissures due to laxity of the lateral canthi; and a coloboma of the lateral parts of the lower eyelid, sometimes continuing as a groove that may extend towards the angle of the mouth or more laterally. An impression of exophthalmia may be created when the eyelid coloboma is of a severe nature. Dystopic cilia along the edges of this groove, absence or deficiency of the eyelashes (madarosis) medial to the coloboma and atresia of the lacrimal canaliculus may also be present.

The maxilla. Forward projection of the maxilla caused by the skeletal discontinuity may be present. The frontonasal angle appears flattened. The posterior maxillary height is decreased and the anterior height is increased, resulting in a steep anteroinferior cant. An open bite related to shortening of the mandibular rami and premature posterior dental contact may be observed. Choanal atresia is not uncommon; cleft palate may also be noted.

The ear. An infinite variety of bilateral external ear malformations may be observed (Rogers 1964). Middle ear anomalies are usually more severe than in hemifacial microsomia (Caldarelli et al 1980) and the radiographic changes also differ. The attic is absent and the atticoantral space is reduced (Phelps et al 1981). Abnormalities of the inner ear are rare but have been reported (Sando et al 1968).

The mandible. Varying degrees of condylar hypoplasia may be observed. The coronoid process is usually normal. The mandibular angle is a characteristic feature and antegonial notching is considered to be syndrome-specific. Downward projection of the receding chin increases lower facial height and adds to the convexity of the facial profile. Downward and forward projection of the 'sideburns' is a salient feature of the condition.

The airway. Respiration of patients with this cluster of malformations is frequently compromised by the presence of choanal atresia and by lingual obstruction due to mandibular retrusion. As a result a sleep-apnoea syndrome may be observed, demanding treatment at an early stage. Zygo-auromandibular dysplasia is frequently associated with some of the malformations produced by maxillomandibular dysplasia, such as macrostomia, preauricular tags and sinuses. Periocular dysplasias such as microphthalmus and esophoria have also been reported.

Temporo-aural dysplasia

'Aural' signifies everything pertaining to the ear. With the word 'temporo-aural' we want to focus attention on the intimate developmental relationship in time and space between the temporal bone and the different aural structures. This relationship is expressed in a wide range of abnormalities in shape, size and site, affecting the external ear (Fig. 9.100) the auditory canal, the middle ear and the facial nerve.

Abnormalities involving the periaural tissues include fistulas, sinuses, cysts and tags. These anomalies may be found in the preauricular area along a line between the tragus and the angle of the mouth or below the ear in a direction passing from the auditory canal downward and forward below the parotid gland and the gonial angle of the mandible.

The average overall incidence of external ear anomalies was reported to be 1% in a study by Melnick & Myrianthopoulos (1979). The incidence of microtia is as low as 1.69% and that of preauricular sinus as high as 80.93%. The majority of these cases represent sporadic errors, but autosomal dominant and recessive inheritance may occur.

Morphology

The spectrum of external ear anomalies may be grouped as follows (Fig. 9.100):

1. Prominent ears.
2. Adherent ears. The retroauricular groove is absent in its superior part, resulting in 'cryptotia'.
3. Constricted ears (Tanzer 1978, Cosman 1978). This term includes cup ears and lop ears, which are anomalies caused by deficient development of the scapha and helix and are characterized by a vertical compression of the scapha and fossa triangularis.
4. Atretic ears (Meurmann 1957, Marx 1926). This group is generally referred to as 'microtia' or 'anotia' in its most severe form. Three grades of severity may by distinguished:

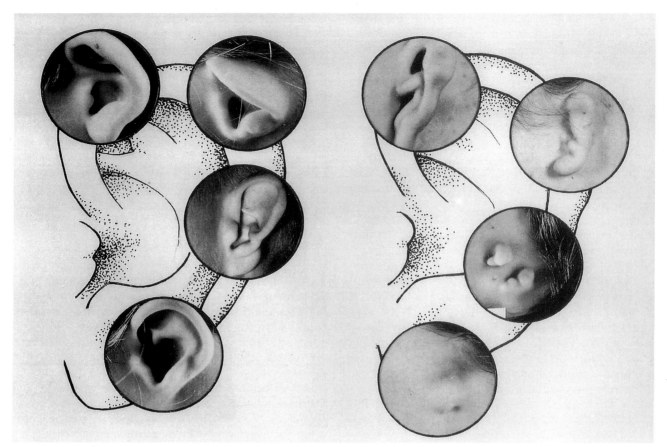

Fig. 9.100 Auricular dysplasias: spectrum of malformations: (a) constricted ears; (b) atretic ears.

Grade I: Hypoplasia of the auricle, including the concha, the anthelix, the scapha and the helix. Vertical compression of the scapha, and some stenosis of the auditory meatus may be observed. The auricular features are present and recognizable.

Grade II: Hypoplasia of the auricle is much more pronounced. The auditory canal is absent.

Grade III: Aplasia of the auricle. The lobule is malpositioned and abnormal.

Microtia is predominantly unilateral (86.5%, Bennun et al 1985), with a predilection for the right side and the male sex (Grabb 1965, Rolnick & Kaye 1983).

Facial paralysis was observed in conjunction with microtia in 12% of the cases studied by Bennun et al. Deviation of the velum towards the non-affected side was seen in 14% of these patients.

The cervicofacial branch is most commonly affected and the degree of involvement of the facial nerve and its bony canal correlates with the severity of microtia.

Differentiation

Abnormalities involving the temporoaural zone are frequently associated with malformations of adjacent structures. The mandible may be affected in 50% (Tanzer 1978) of patients with microtia, producing hemifacial microsomia or temporo-auromandibular dysplasia.

Bilateral involvement of the mandibules is observed in patients with the complete form of Treacher Collins' syndrome, resulting in zygo-auromandibular dysplasia.

The eye and the vertebrae may also be involved, although less frequently, and the following syndromes can be differentiated.

Aurovertebral dysplasia. This syndrome, consisting of external ear anomalies and vertebral malformations, was described by Weyers in 1966.

Oculo-aurovertebral dysplasia. In this syndrome the following malformations are found together: epibulbar dermolipomas, anomalies of the ear and vertebral dysplasia. The syndrome, now known as Goldenhar's syndrome, was first described by Van Duyse in 1882. He included a case report by Von Arlt made one year earlier. Oculo-aurovertebral dysplasia is frequently associated with malformations produced by zygomatic, mandibular or maxillomandibular dysplasias. The syndrome then resembles oculovertebral dysplasia. A combination of microphthalmia or anophthalmia and vertebral dysplasia was reported by Weyers & Thier (1958). This entity may also be associated with temporoaural (preauricular appendages) and maxillomandibular dysplasia (macrostomia).

Oculo-auromandibular dysplasia. The combination of microphthalmia or anophthalmia and malformations of the ear and mandible was recorded by Francois & Haustrate in 1954.

Cervico-oculoacoustic dysplasia. Originally described by Wildervanck (1960) this syndrome consists of another triad of typical malformations: abducens paralysis (with or without retractio bulbi), anomalies of the inner, the middle and occasionally the outer ear and Klippel-Feil's anomalad.

Cervico-oculofacial dysplasia with deafness. The similarity between the different syndromes described in the literature is even more obvious in a patient observed by Franceschetti & Klein (1954) with epibulbar dermolipomas, retractio bulbi, preauricular appendages, inner and middle ear deafness, mandibular dysplasia and Klippel-Feil's anomalad.

Branchio-otorenal dysplasia. Deafness, maxillomandibular dysplasia and renal anomalies are part of a syndrome reported by Melnick et al (1975) and Fraser et al (1978).

Comparison of all these syndromes provides evidence of a continuous spectrum of variations making delineation difficult or impossible. Epibulbar dermolipomas for instance have also been reported in the syndromes of Weyers and Thier and that of Wildervanck, while vertebral dysplasia may be minimal in Van Duyse's or Goldenhar's syndrome and in Wildervanck's syndrome. One spectrum of phenotypes appears to blend with the other.

Oto-palatodigital dysplasia. The combination of deafness, cleft palate and digital anomalies was recorded by Taybi (1962).

Temporo-auromandibular dysplasia

This combination of anomalies of the ear and the mandible is known by a variety of names, such as hemifacial microsomia (Gorlin & Pindborg 1964), otomandibular dysostosis (Obwegeser 1974), mandibular facial dysostosis (Roberts et al 1975), lateral facial dysplasia (Ross 1975), facial and craniofacial microsomia (Converse et al 1973, 1974).

According to Ballantyne (1894), the syndrome was already mentioned in the teratological tables written about seventh century BC by the Chaldeans of Mesopotamia (see Ch. 1). Centuries later, in 1654, Bartholinus reported on a child with the absence of an auditory orifice, and since then there have been many descriptions of patients that fall into this category. Thompson in 1845 was the first to emphasize the aetiological relationship between an arrest in the development of the first and second branchial arches with malformations of the face. The condition is usually restricted to one side of the face. Bilaterality, always asym-metrical and occurring with an incidence of 10–20%, has, however, been recorded by various authors (Meurman 1965, Grabb 1965, Dupertuis & Musgrave 1959, Converse (1973, 1974), Samuels et al (1974). Grabb (1965) reported an incidence of 1 per 5642 live births, Poswillo (1974) 1 per 3500 births. The majority of cases are sporadic.

Morphology

Facial asymmetry with deviation of the chin towards the affected side and ear anomalies are the 'hallmarks' of this entity (Fig. 9.101).

The temporoaural complex. All parts of this complex (Fig. 9.102) may be abnormal, making a wide spectrum of malformations possible. Auricular malformations are present in the majority of cases (75% in a study by Samuels et al 1983). Middle ear abnormalities are common. The tympanic cavity may be small and the ossicular chain disrupted or fused. Inner ear anomalies were not observed in 102 patients studied by Grabb (1965).

Pruzansky (1971) found no relation between the severity of the auricular malformations and the severity of hearing loss. Correlation between the degree of severity of temporoaural and mandibular malformations could, however, be established, although not necessarily in terms of gradation specificity (Caldarelli et al 1980). In their study, Caldarelli et al were also able to establish a correlation between the presence of auditory canal stenosis and the severity of microtia or the severity of mandibular malformations.

A similar relationship was observed between the presence of ossicular malformations and the severity of microtia or the severity of mandibular anomalies.

The zygomatic process of the temporal bone may be underdeveloped or absent, interrupting the zygomatic arch. Lack of pneumatization of mastoid air cells and different degrees of hypoplasia of the mastoid process are commonly observed. Any part of temporal bone other than the petrous bone which houses the inner ear may be involved (Grabb 1965).

The facial nerve. The condition may be aggravated by partial or complete facial palsy (Fig. 9.103), which was present in 26% in the study of Murray et al (1984).

The mandible. Both the horizontal and ascending ramus may be abnormal. The malformations are most severe in the condylar region (Fig. 9.104) and less severe near the middle sector, with flattening of the gonial angle and accentuation of the antegonial notch. Several classifications have been suggested.

Pruzansky (1969) distinguished between:

Grade I — slight reduction of the diameter of the hemi-mandible; normal anatomical features.

Grade II — important reduction of the diameter of the hemimandible. The condyle, the ascending ramus and the 'mandibular notch' are malformed.

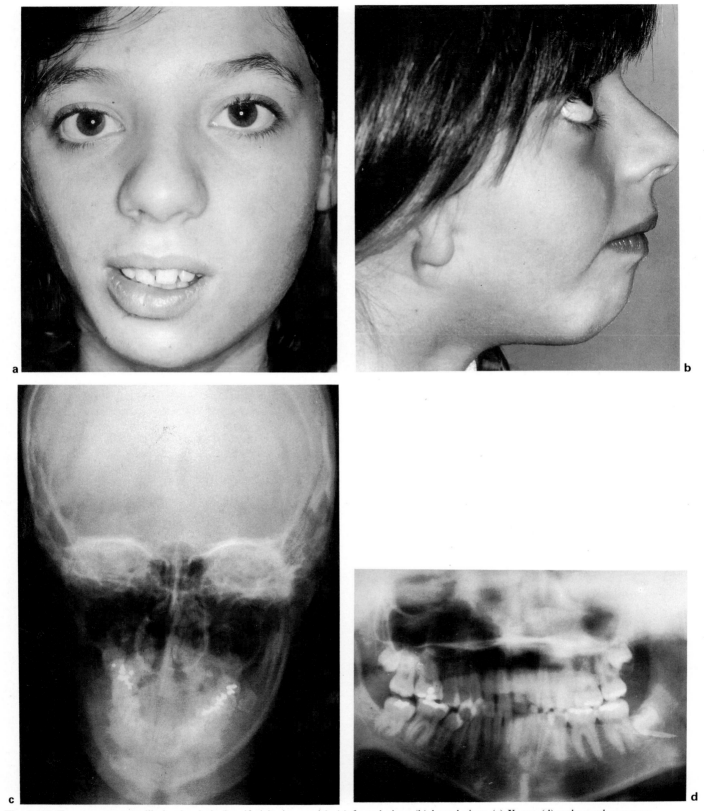

Fig. 9.101 Temporo-auromandibular dysplasia (hemifacial microsomia): (a) frontal view; (b) lateral view; (c) X-ray; (d) orthopanthomogram.

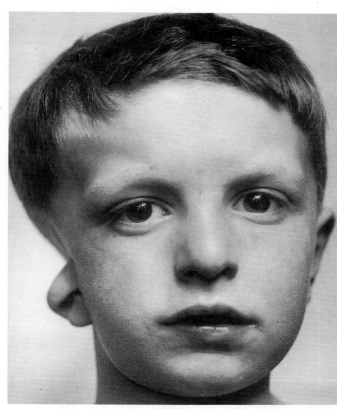

Fig. 9.102 Temporo-auromandibular dysplasia associated with malformation of the temporal region.

Grade III — the hemimandible is either absent or severely malformed and has lost all its anatomical characteristics.

Chierici (1983) focuses on the anomalies of the temporomandibular joint:

Grade I — absence of condylar cartilage and disc.
Grade II — absence of condylar head or condylar process.
Grade III — ankyloses of the temporomandibular joint.
Grade IV — absence of condylar process only.
Grade V — absence of condylar and coronoid process.

Maxilla and zygoma. Hypoplasia of the maxilla on the affected side is clearly demonstrated by obliquity of the occlusal plane. A depression and recession of the inferolateral angle of the orbit indicates involvement of the malar bone. Orbital dystopia may be observed. Lauritzen et al (1985) have considered all these aspects and suggest the following classification:

Grade I — the mandibular condyle is normal and the temporomandibular joint functional. Asymmetry is present and the degree of mandibular hypoplasia ranges from mild to severe.
Grade II — the mandibular condyle is missing, the glenoid fossa affected and the ascending ramus vestigial. The zygomatic arch is, however, present.

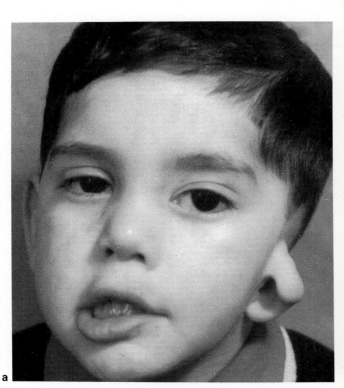

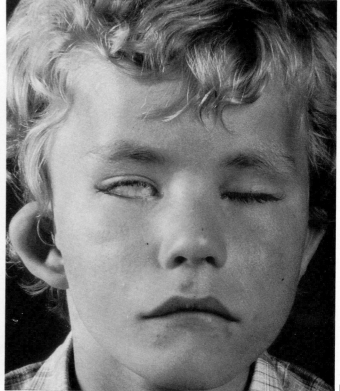

Fig. 9.103 Temporo-auromandibular dysplasia associated with neuromuscular alteration: (a) lower facial palsy; (b) upper facial palsy.

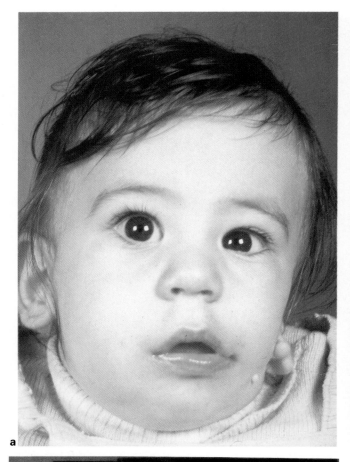

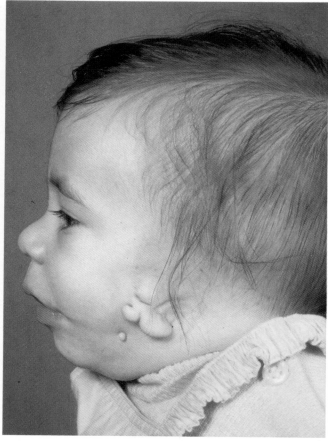

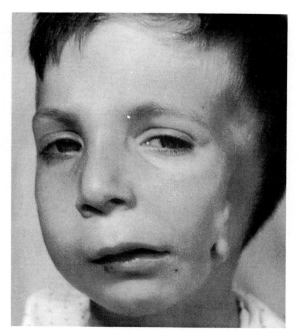

Fig. 9.104 Temporo-auromandibular dysplasia — note macrostomia and caudalization of auricular rudiments: (a) frontal view; (b) lateral view; (c) 3-D reconstruction shows skeletal abnormalities.

Fig. 9.105 Temporo-auromandibular dysplasia; hemifacial microsomia associated with macrostomia.

Grade III — the mandibular condyle, the glenoid fossa and ascending ramus are absent, and the zygomatic arch is hypoplastic or missing.

Grade IV — the inferior and lateral rims of the orbit are recessed in addition to the type III abnormalities.

Grade V — the orbit is hypoplastic and dystopic, in addition to the type IV defects.

It is apparent that a whole scale of variations may be possible, ranging from ear malformations of maximal severity, co-existing with jaw abnormalities that are scarcely apparent to minimal temporoaural malformations associated with characteristic maldevelopment of the mandibular ramus and condylar process (Converse et al 1973, 1974).

The soft tissues. The masticatory muscles, m. temporalis, masseter and pterygoid may be differentially hypoplastic. A fused mass may be observed on transverse CT scans, containing elements of each of these muscles. Hypoplasia of the lateral pterygoid is of particular importance since it allows the mandible, when opening, to deviate towards the affected side. Aplasia of the levator veli palatini, resulting

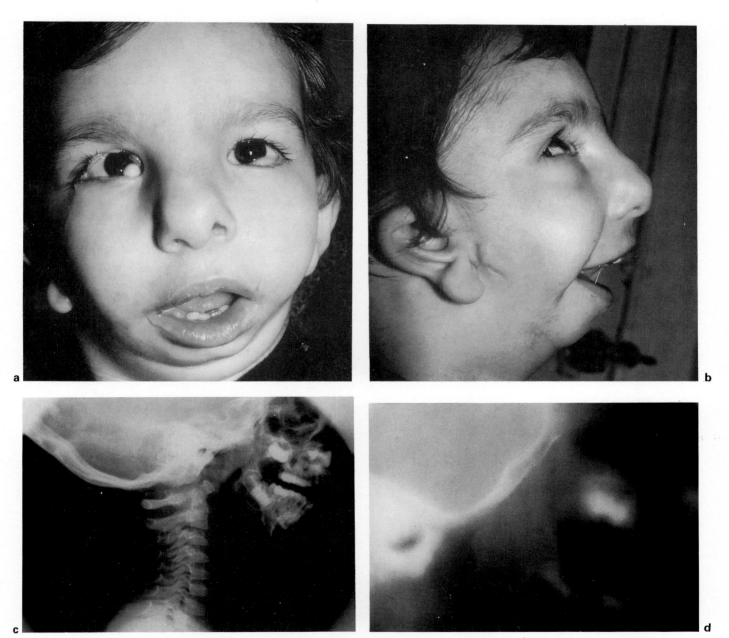

Fig. 9.106 Oculo-auriculovertebral dysplasia (Goldenhar's syndrome) associated with temperomandibular joint ankylosis and eyelid coloboma: (a) frontal view; (b) lateral view; (c) X-ray — note vertebral abnormality; (d) X-ray — note temperomandibular joint abnormality.

in abnormal elevation of the soft palate towards the unaffected side, was observed in 16% of the patients studied by Bennun et al (1985). Some degree of soft tissue deficiency is exhibited in all of these patients but the actual amount is difficult to assess and skeletal and soft tissue hypoplasia do not necessarily parallel each other. The condition may affect the skin, the subcutaneous tissues and superficial fascia. The parotid gland may be absent, producing a preauricular concavity. Macrostomia (Fig. 9.105), a short orotragal line and preauricular pits and tags of skin and cartilage were present in 16% of the cases studied by Grabb (1965).

Differentiation. Hemifacial microsomia may be associated with various other anomalies involving: (1) the orbital region (Tenconi & Hall 1983) — microphthalmia 6%, ptosis 6%, colobomas 12%, epibulbar dermoids 18%. Goldenhar's syndrome (Figs. 9.106, 9.107) serves as a perfect example; (2) the lip and palate 7% (Grabb 1965), 15% (Samuels et al 1983); (3) the vertebrae and ribs 11% (Grabb 1965); (4) the limbs 5% (Samuels et al 1983); (5) the cardiac system 10% (Samuels et al 1983). Cohen (1971) has therefore suggested that all patients with the syndrome should be evaluated for skeletal, cardiac and renal anomalies.

Mandibular dysplasia

Mandibular dysplasia involves the whole mandible. It is observed as a separate entity but its existence as such has never been recognized.

Morphology

The mandibular arch and body are reduced in all dimensions (Fig. 9.108). The alveolar process sometimes compensates for the malocclusion that may occur. The backward position of the chin is the main characteristic, causing confusion with Pierre Robin's syndrome.

This malformation may be associated with ocular dysplasia (microphthalmus, cataract) in the syndrome of Hallerman (1948) and Streiff (1950) named mandibulo-oculofacial dysplasia. Owing to the fact that this syndrome is often associated with a 'parrot-beaked' nose, one is reminded of a 'tête d'oiseau' or 'bird's face'. In this syndrome the anomalies of the mandible are restricted to the body, while the ascending ramus and temporomandibular joint are rarely involved (Van Balen 1961).

Combinations of ocular and cranial dysplasias are found in the syndrome of Ullrich & Fremery-Dohna (1953) (mandibulo-oculocraniofacial dysplasia).

Mandibular and reductive limb dysplasias, peromelia, hemimelia, hypodactylia, hypodactyly and brachydactyly are observed in Hanhart's syndrome (1950).

Hypoplasia of the mandible may occasionally be observed in patients with oculo-aurovertebral or oculo-vertebral dysplasia. In its most extreme and lethal form mandibular dysplasia is known as otocephalia (Fig. 9.109). This malformation, first described by Isidore Geoffroy St Hilaire in 1832, is characterized by the almost total absence of the lower jaw, resulting in medialization and convergence of the ears (Fig. 9.109) and microstomia (Josephy 1909).

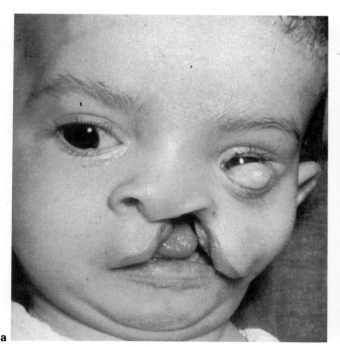
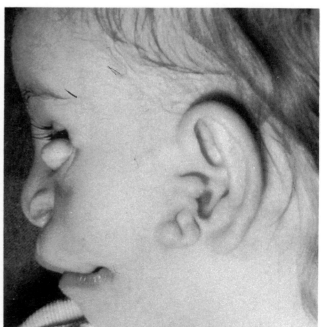

Fig. 9.107 Oculo-auriculovertebral dysplasia (Goldenhar's syndrome) associated with cleft lip: (a) frontal view; (b) lateral view.

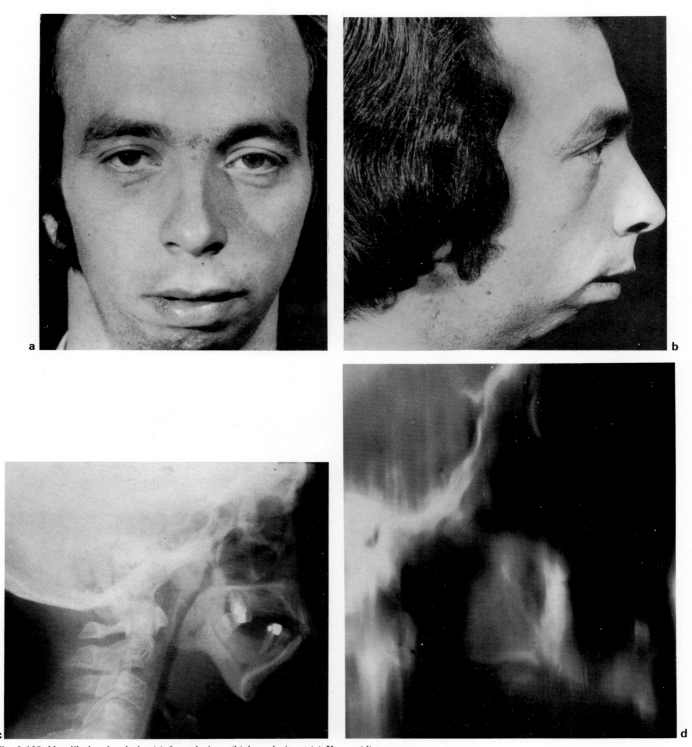

Fig. 9.108 Mandibular dysplasia: (a) frontal view; (b) lateral view; (c) X-ray; (d) tomogram.

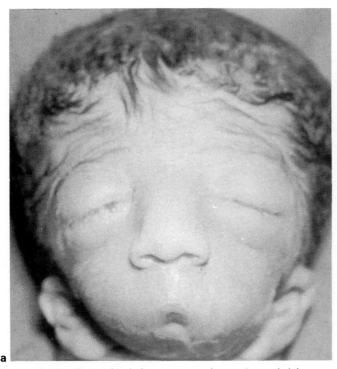
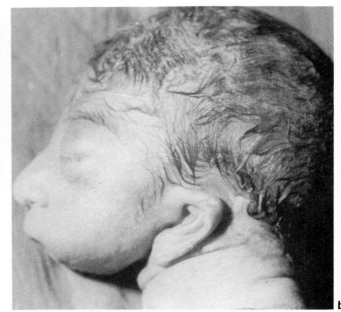

Fig. 9.109 Mandibular dysplasia: extreme variant or 'otocephaly'.

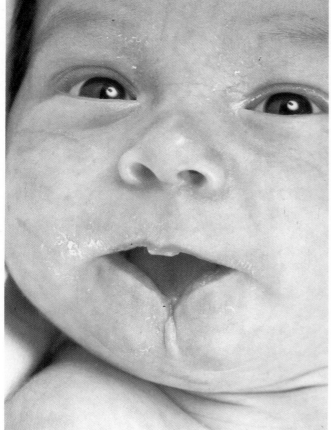
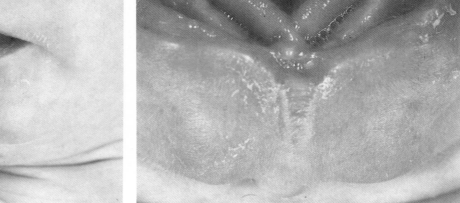

Fig. 9.110 Intermandibular dysplasia: (a) frontal view; (b) close-up.

Differentiation

Micrognathia should be distinguished from retrognathia, in which the mandible is held back by abnormal musculature (Pierre Robin's syndrome). This malformation probably has its origin in a neuromuscular deficiency and recovery is usually spontaneous within the first months of life (see p. 278).

Retrognathia and the Pierre Robin sequence are also observed in Stickler's syndrome (1965) (hereditary arthro-ophthalmopathy), which is characterized by ocular (myopia), temporoaural (deafness) and musculoskeletal (hypotonia) abnormalities.

The spectrum of malformations derived from the first mandibular arch may be extended with a series of oromandibular and oro-maxillomandibular dysplasias in which dysostosis, if present at all, is only of marginal importance.

Intermandibular dysplasia

This malformation (Fig. 9.110) completes the list of craniofacial dysplasias with dysostosis. A median cleft of the lower lip was first reported by Couronne in 1819 in a footnote. Since then it has been occasionally recorded in the literature (Parise 1862, Lannelongue 1879, Wolfler 1890).

The anomaly may vary from a small coloboma of the lower lip to a complete cleft of lip, mandible, and tongue, extending back to the glossoepiglottic ligament and downwards between the geniohypoglossus muscles to the sternal notch.

The helix of craniofacial dysostosis ends here. The so-called mentosternal dysraphies (Fig. 9.111) represent in our opinion the passage between the craniofacial sector and the other districts of the body. This malformation usually involves an osseous notch of the lower aspect of the symphysis, a cleft of hyoid bone and of the manubrium. A midline contracture of the neck is always present.

CRANIOFACIAL DYSPLASIAS WITH SYNOSTOSIS

Introduction

The clinical features of craniostenosis may be expressed in terms of dysmorphy and dysfunction.

Dysmorphy, a direct result of craniosynostosis, is chronologically the initial manifestation. It is obvious and the diagnosis is usually easy. The malformation varies, depending on the site and the number of sutures involved in the synostosis and on the alterations of growth, which are determined by Virchow's law. Craniostenosis is often associated with facial dysmorphy (craniofacial stenosis) and, less often, with malformations of the extremities. A number of clinical–anatomic forms, will be described in this chapter.

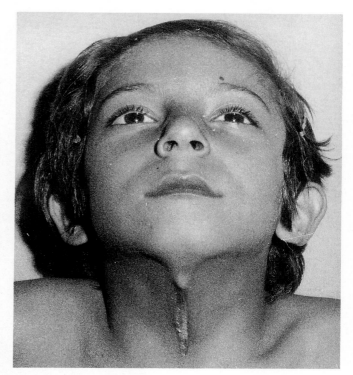

Fig. 9.111 Mentosternal dysplasia.

Dysfunction, a secondary manifestation of synostosis, may be evident from the outset but usually follows establishment of the dysmorphy. The clinical repercussions, common to all forms of craniostenosis, vary in expression and intensity depending on the anatomic type of dysmorphy. The function of important structures such as the brain, the eye and the airway may be disturbed.

There have been many attempts to create order out of the bewildering chaos of abnormally shaped skulls due to synostosis (Fig. 9.112). Our classification is inspired by that of Laitinen (1956) and also has a pathomorphogenical basis. Three groups of synostosis may be distinguished, dependent on the localization of the malformation in the craniofacial region: the craniosynostoses which almost exclusively concern the vault; the craniofacial synostoses which involve the upper third of the face, and part of the vault; and the faciosynostoses which are restricted to the face.

Craniosynostosis

PACHYCEPHALY (parieto-occipital)

Premature closure of the lambdoid sutures, or pachycephaly, is a rare entity. It is found isolated, associated with synostosis of the sagittal suture or as part of multiple synostoses. The first few cases of isolated bilateral lambdoid synostosis seem to have been described by Knudson & Flaherty (1960), who reported two cases without clinical

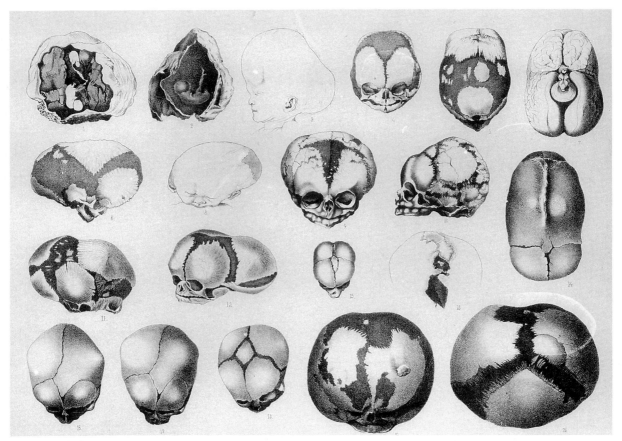

Fig. 9.112 Cranial syntostoses: first comprehensive table from Ahlfeld's *Atlas* (1880).

repercussions. The condition may, however, also be unilateral.

Morphology (Fig. 9.113)

When observed as an isolated feature, synostosis of the lambdoid suture is of little morphological consequence and is usually discovered fortuitously by X-ray studies. It causes hypoplasia and flattening of the occiput, with slight compensatory development of the ipsilateral anterior cranial region.

Radiographic features

Radiological examination confirms occipital hypoplasia with absence or stenosis of the lambdoid sutures. Lateral views show a depression localized to the parieto-occipital junction.

Craniometry

In isolated lambdoid synostosis there is little abnormality of skull size and axes. However, the longitudinal diameter is usually less than normal.

Associated synostoses

Lambdoid synostosis may be associated with sagittal synostosis. In these cases the occiput is small but rather projecting. The skull becomes pear-shaped, narrow posteriorly and prominent anteriorly.

Association with coronal synostosis is much less common. A case of unilateral lambdoid fusion associated with coronal synostosis was described by Weiss in 1969. Association with squamous synostosis has been reported by Matson (1969) and by Laitinen (1956). Lambdoid synostosis may finally be associated with multiple synostoses, particularly of the coronal and sagittal sutures: Laitinen reported three such cases.

The morphology is characterized by flattening of the occipital region and temporal fossa, with verticalization of the petrous bone in the Townes view.

Incidence

The incidence of pachycephaly is very low. In their studies, Bertelsen (1958) and Anderson & Geiger reported no cases of isolated lambdoid synostosis. Shillito & Matson (1968) reported 12 cases in a series of 525 craniostenoses:

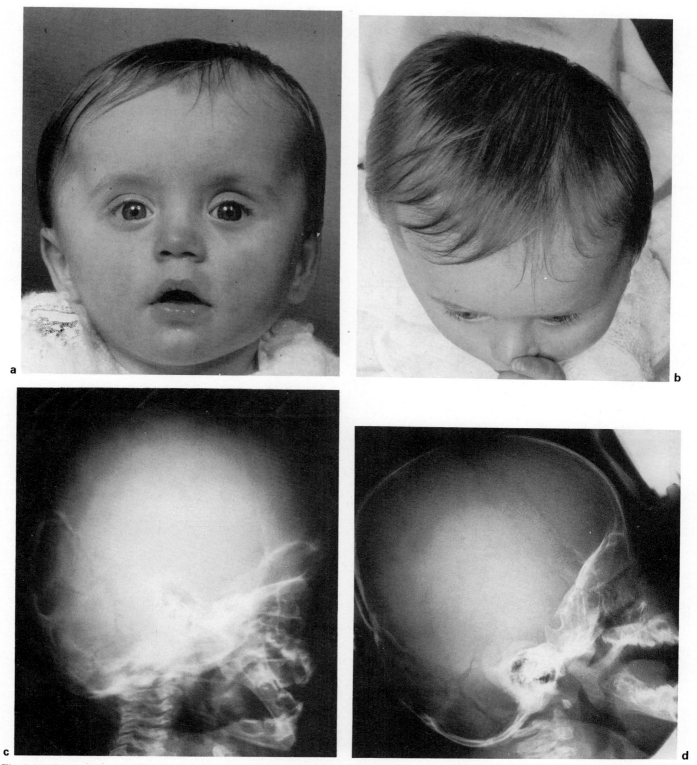

Fig. 9.113 Pachycephaly: (a) frontal view. A slight degree of plagiocephaly may be observed; (b) cranial view; (c) X-ray at 6 months of age; (d) X-ray at 12 months of age.

7 were unilateral and 5 bilateral. Lambdoid synostoses are most often associated with other synostoses, particularly of the sagittal suture: 2 cases in Laitinen's (1956) series, 3 cases in Anderson and Geiger's and 1 in the series of Montaut & Stricker (1977).

In the series of Montaut & Stricker no case of isolated lambdoid synostosis was observed. In contrast, there were: 6 cases of associated coronal and sagittal synostosis, 1 case of associated sagittal synostosis, and 1 case occurring in Apert's syndrome.

Finally, it should be noted that bilateral fusion of the lambdoid suture contributes to the picture of cloverleaf skull.

SCAPHOCEPHALY (interparietal)

Definition

The term scaphocephaly was coined in 1860 by von Bauer. It describes the elongated narrow shape of the skull, resembling the hull of a ship (Fig. 9.114). Virchow's law incriminates premature fusion of the interparietal sagittal sutures, which inhibits growth of the skull in breadth and is compensated by excessive longitudinal development.

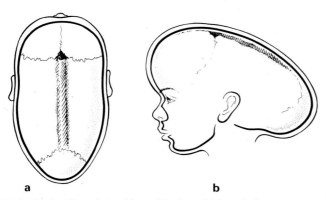

a   b

Fig. 9.114 Scaphocephaly: (a) cranial view; (b) lateral view.

Morphology (Fig. 9.115)

Viewed from in front, the skull is high and narrow, sometimes dominated by an interparietal median 'helmet crest' which gives it the appearance of an 'upturned keel'. This crest may be palpable along the length of the stenosed suture. Seen from the side, the skull is elongated from front to back with posterior occipital protrusion and excessive bulging of the frontal bones anteriorly.

Certain variations have been described: sphenocephaly (Fig. 9.116) (from the Greek *sphen* = wedge) is most common. It is characterized by prominence of the bregma and by frontal bossing. The forehead is wider than the very narrow occipital region. This deformity is attributed to patency of the anterior fontanelle and of the metopic suture.

In contrast, in leptocephaly (Fig. 9.117) (from the Greek *leptos* = thin) the skull is elongated while the forehead is narrow and does not protrude anteriorly. This appearance is related to relatively early closure of the anterior fontanelle and of the metopic suture.

Clinocephaly (Fig. 9.118) (from the Greek *clinos* = inclination) is an ambiguous term, indicating a variation with a depression of the cranial vault behind the bregma. The forehead is narrow and high.

Finally, the term bathmocephaly (from the Greek *batmos* = threshold) refers to parieto-occipital overdevelopment, with marked prominence of the occiput. In patients with scaphocephaly, there is little abnormality of the face in comparison with other forms of craniostenosis, and the changes are minor. The forehead is narrow and slightly bulging. There is no hypertelorism; exorbitism, although possible, is rare and not pronounced. There may be a vaulted palate.

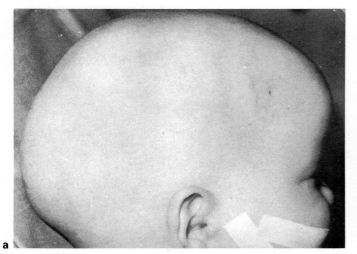

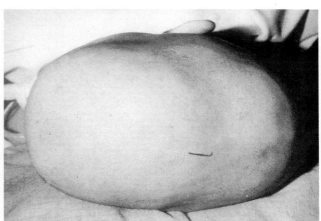

a   b

Fig. 9.115 Scaphocephaly: (a) lateral view; (b) cranial view.

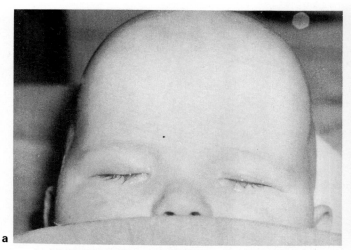

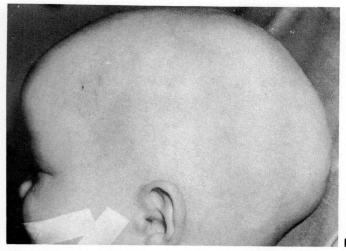

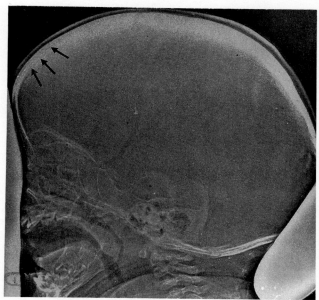

Fig. 9.116 Sphenocephaly: (a) frontal view; (b) lateral view; (c) X-ray; lateral view. Arrows indicate frontal bossing.

squamoparietal suture. The anterior fontanelle may be closed at the time of first examination but quite often remains open (in 56% of cases according to Shillito & Matson). Digital impressions are rare and not very marked, tending to be located in the posterior parietal region.

Craniometry

Cranial perimeter is usually slightly augmented with an average of 1.3. The cephalic index is low, the mean being 66.1 in the Adelaide series. The vertical index is increased in sphenocephaly.

Incidence

Figures given in the literature vary considerably. This type of craniostenosis is essentially morphological and rarely gives rise to complications. This accounts for the discrepancies noted in the literature. Where the authors refer to decompensated scaphocephaly, the incidence is low, ranging from 5.5% in the series of Bertelsen (1958) to 11.2% as reported by Choux (1977). There is a strong male preponderance in most series. The incidence given in the literature by various authors is: 57% by Anderson & Geiger (1965); 56% by Shillito & Matson (1968); 40% by Till (1975), 21% by Montaut & Stricker (1977); and 35% by David et al (1982). Hunter & Rudd (1977) noted a birth incidence of 1 in 4200 or 0.24 per thousand. David et al (1982) gave a somewhat lower figure: 0.12 per 1000 or 1 in 8500.

TRIGONOCEPHALY (INTERFRONTAL)

The term was coined by Welcker in 1862 to describe the

Associated malformations

Shillito & Matson (1968) found isolated minor malformations in 26% of cases. In 7.3% of cases there were multiple malformations. A relatively high incidence of 20.5% of associated malformations was also seen by Montaut & Stricker (1977). Examples of this are shown in (Figs. 9.119, 9.120).

Radiographic features

Lateral views of the skull reveal prominence of the occiput and of the frontal tuberosities. Seen from the front, the parietal bones are narrow and oblique, giving the vault the appearance of an arch in which the sagittal suture, synostosed and hyperosteotic, forms the keystone. The presence of temporal bulging may be explained by patency of the

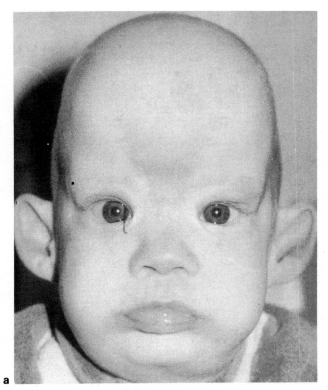

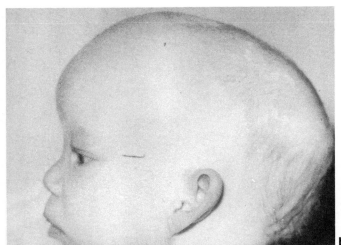

Fig. 9.117 Leptocephaly: (a) frontal view; (b) lateral view.

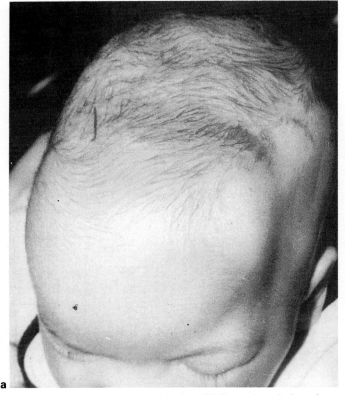

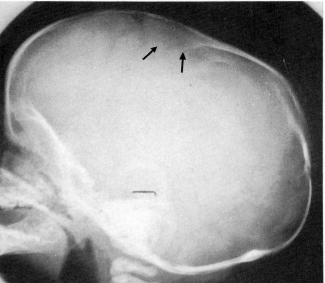

Fig. 9.118 Clinocephaly: (a) cranial view; (b) X-ray; lateral view. Arrows indicate bregmatic depression.

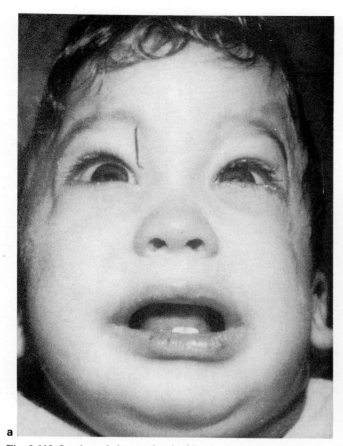

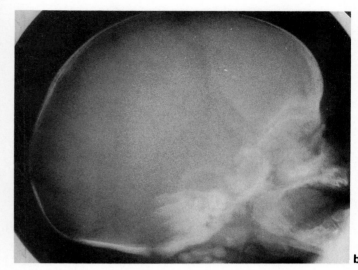

Fig. 9.119 Scaphocephaly associated with trigonocephaly: (a) frontal view; (b) X-ray.

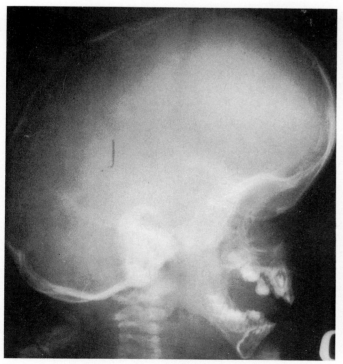

Fig. 9.120 Scaphocephaly associated with hydrocephalus.

cranial malformation which results from premature closure of the frontal suture. The frontal area becomes triangular (Fig. 9.121). This relatively rare type of craniostenosis does not lead to any appreciable reduction in cranial capacity. In fact, the metopic suture, physiologically functional until the age of 2 years and entirely closed at 8 years, plays only a minor part in the growth of the skull. The extent of skull malformation depends on how early the synostosis takes place; this usually occurs during intrauterine life.

Morphology (Fig. 9.122)

The cranial vault. The keel shape of the forehead is characteristic. This deformity is especially apparent in axial views and contrasts with the normal biparietal diameter. The mediofrontal angulation extends back as far as the anterior fontanelle in the form of a median ridge. This ridge, visible and palpable, corresponds to the fused frontal suture. The underdeveloped frontal eminences are directed forward and outward.

The face. The upper part of the face is greatly affected by the underdevelopment of the frontal eminences: the eyeballs are abnormally close as part of a varying degree

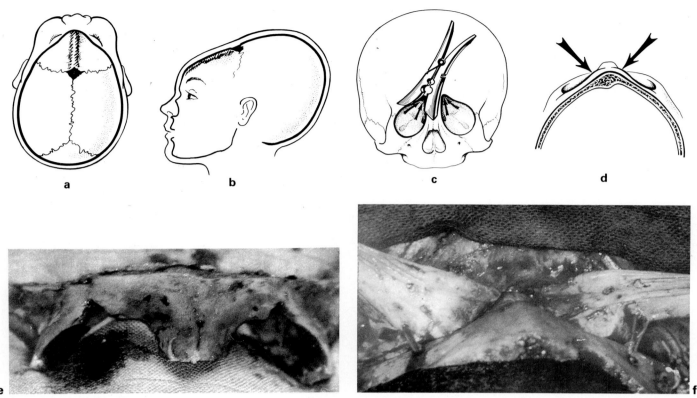

Fig. 9.121 Trigonocephaly: (a) cranial view; (b) lateral view; (c) orbital abnormality; (d) frontal abnormality; (e) anterior aspect of fronto-naso-orbital band; (f) superior aspect of fronto-naso-orbital band.

of hypotelorism; the eyebrows often appear raised in relation to the orbital arches, which seem to project because of the underlying frontal aplasia. The morphological diagnosis is easy except in some borderline cases, notably in the neonate where the fetal configuration with an angular forehead may persist. Some purely familial facial configurations, without craniostenosis, may also suggest trigonocephaly.

Associated malformations

The triad of trigonocephaly, arhinencephaly and hypotelorism was first reported by Kundrat (1882) and more recently by Currarino & Silverman (1960) and by Duggan (1970). The latter authors distinguish between two pathological entities: type 1 — simple trigonocephaly (primary craniosynostosis); and type 2 — trigonocephaly associated with cerebral malformations. This classification must be rejected in as much as it implies the possibility of a cerebral malformation inducing a secondary synostosis of the metopic suture, as asserted by Schueller (1929) and Riemenschneider (1957).

In almost all cases the craniostenosis is the primary event and the associated malformations are concomitant and fortuitous. There is, besides, no general agreement on their incidence. Park & Powers, (1920) as well as Shillito

& Matson (1968), consider that associated malformations are relatively rare in this type of craniostenosis (9%).

However, mental retardation remains fairly common, even in the absence of raised intracranial pressure: 6 cases out of 18 (Anderson et al 1962); 2 cases of mental impairment in 13 (Montaut & Stricker 1977); 1 case of slight mental retardation. These mental abnormalities may be secondary to compression of the frontal lobes by the anterior craniostenosis, which reduces their functional capacity (Anderson et al 1962). More often, there exist diffuse cerebral lesions which account for the relatively common mental retardation in this type of synostosis.

Epicanthus (Fig. 9.123), colobomata, strabismus, arched palate and polydactylism have also been recorded.

Radiographic features

The radiographic findings merely reflect the morphological abnormalities. The axial views recommended by Hirtz are of particular interest, as they bring out the triangular shape of the frontal region. The frontal suture is seen as a dense rectilinear ridge. However, a radiologically normal appearance of all or part of the suture does not exclude the diagnosis, as the suture may no longer be functional (Anderson et al 1962, Currarino & Silverman 1960).

In frontal views, the ethmoid is narrow; the orbits are

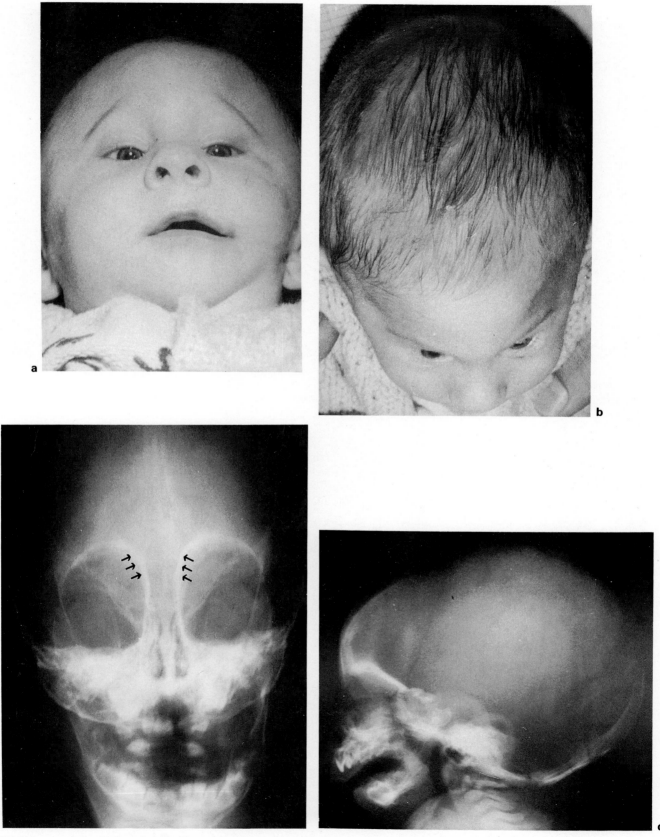

Fig. 9.122 Trigonocephaly: (a) frontal view; (b) cranial view; (c) X-ray. Frontal view shows hypotelorism and abnormal orbital configuration (arrows); (d) X-ray. Lateral view shows small frontal bone.

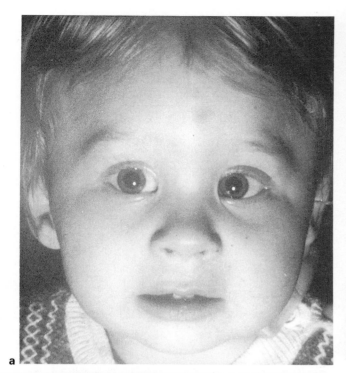

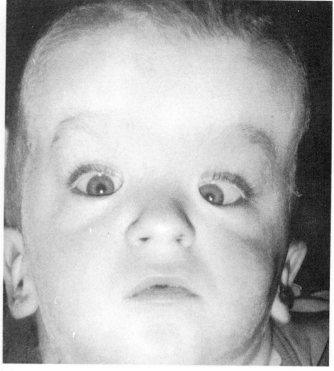

Fig. 9.123 Trigonocephaly: (a) minor degree of epicanthus; (b) major degree of epicanthus in patient with mental retardation; (c) agenesis of corpus callosum.

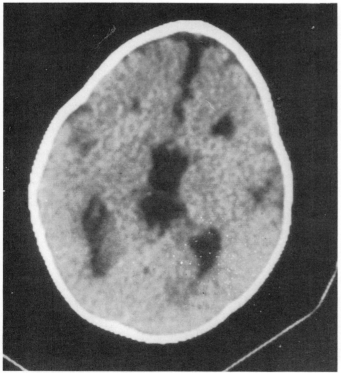

evident. They show a posterior concavity which contrasts with their normally rectilinear appearance. The frontal bone is low and very convex. The anterior fossa of the skull base is shortened; the crista galli is thickened or absent in cases of concomitant arhinencephaly.

CT scans sometimes show abnormalities in the rhinencephalic region, such as absence of the corpus callosum (Fig. 9.123) or cyst formation.

Cranio-faciosynostosis

PLAGIOCEPHALY (spheno-frontoparietal)

The term plagiocephaly (from the Greek *plagios* = slating), was coined by Virchow (1851) and refers to an asymmetric malformation secondary to fusion of one half of the coronal suture (Fig. 9.124). This synostosis is sometimes incomplete and occurs mainly in the inferior part, affecting the sphenotemporal suture (Seeger 1971).

Morphology

The vault. The malformation is characterized by frontal flattening on the affected side. Bulging of the ipsilateral temporal bone may be seen in addition. Palpation sometimes reveals a ridge corresponding to the obliterated

approximated, with their internal walls verticalized and rectilinear. Their shape is ovoid, sloping downwards and outwards, in contrast with the 'Mephisthophelean' deformity of brachycephaly.

In lateral views, the coronal sutures are abnormally

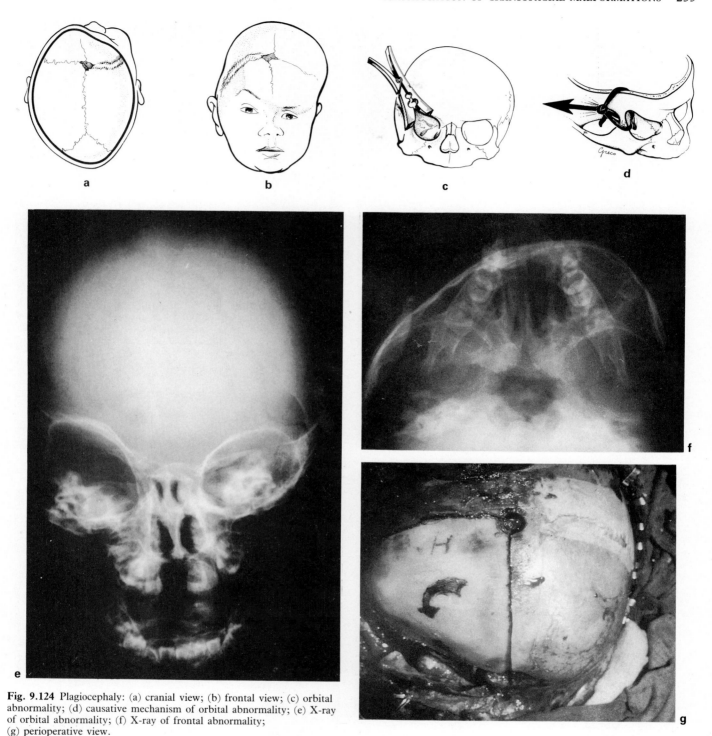

Fig. 9.124 Plagiocephaly: (a) cranial view; (b) frontal view; (c) orbital abnormality; (d) causative mechanism of orbital abnormality; (e) X-ray of orbital abnormality; (f) X-ray of frontal abnormality; (g) perioperative view.

suture. Quite often there is a compensatory expansion on the opposite side (Fig. 9.125) with frontal bossing and protrusion of the supraorbital ridge or bulging in the parietal region. Acrocephaly has also been observed (Fig. 9.126). The top of the skull is deviated. The anterior fontanelle is patent in 50% of cases.

The face. There is retrusion of the orbital arch on the affected side with steepening of the lesser wing of the sphenoid and ovalization of the orbital shape in a superolateral direction. The eyebrow and eyeball appear raised, and strabismus — usually convergent — may be observed (26% in Adelaide series). The nasal root is deviated

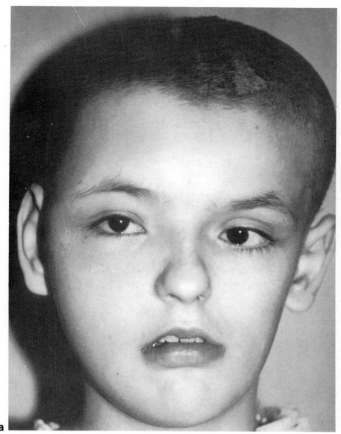 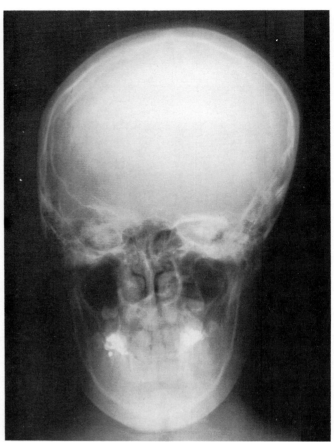

Fig. 9.125 Plagiocephaly associated with compensatory cranial expansion: (a) frontal view; (b) X-ray.

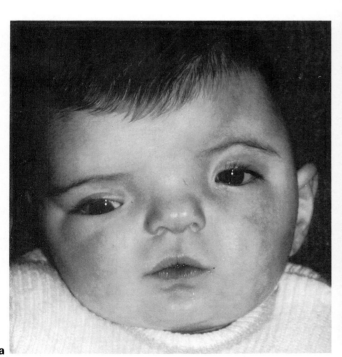 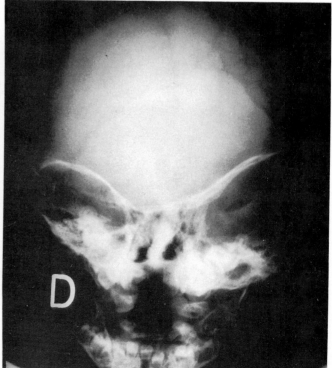

Fig. 9.126 Plagiocephaly associated with acrocephaly: (a) frontal view; (b) X-ray.

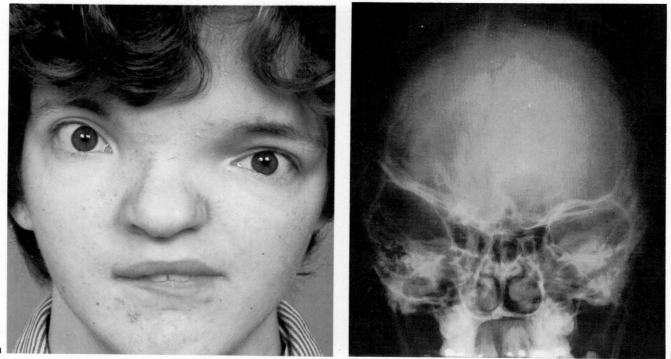

Fig. 9.127 Plagiocephaly associated with teleorbitism: (a) frontal view; (b) X-ray.

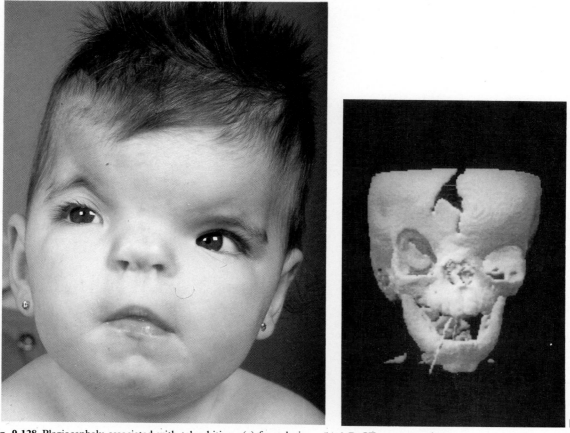

Fig. 9.128 Plagiocephaly associated with teleorbitism: (a) frontal view; (b) 3-D CT reconstruction.

towards the ipsilateral side owing to asymmetry of the nasal skeleton. Hypertelorism is not uncommon (Figs. 9.127, 9.128). The ear on the affected side is sited further forward and downward in comparison to the opposite ear. The hypoplasia sometimes extends to the middle third of the face and particularly to the malar bone. The maxillary bone may be affected (Rougerie et al 1972) with abnormalities of dental apposition. David et al (1982) distinguish between frontal plagiocephaly corresponding to unilateral coronal synostosis, occipital plagiocephaly caused by unilateral growth delay in the lambdoid zone and hemicranial plagiocephaly as an expression of unilateral growth disturbances involving the coronal, squamosal and lambdoid sutures.

Differentiation

Plagiocephaly must be distinguished from malformations secondary to birth injuries or to postural abnormalities, which are relatively common even in the absence of rickets. It must also be differentiated from cranial asymmetries: due to hypoplasia of one cerebral hemisphere, or to hyperplasia in abnormalities such as arachnoid cysts, Sturge–Weber syndrome, neonatal hydrocephalus and chronic subdural effusion in the neonate. The radiographic features and particularly the disappearance or sclerosis of a coronal hemisuture are thus of great importance in the diagnosis of this form of craniostenosis.

Associated malformations

These are rare, as is mental retardation.

Radiographic features

The radiographic findings have been well described by Faure et al (1967). Hirtz views are particularly helpful in demonstrating the asymmetric frontal eminences and the deviation of the nasal bones and/or the septum on the synostosed side. The lesser wing of the sphenoid is brought forward and its axis tends to become sagittal. The temporomandibular joint is pushed forward. The petrous bone is displaced anteriorly and acquires a transverse direction.

In the frontal view, the orbit on the side of synostosis in enlarged; its axis is oblique, upward and outward, and its roof is elevated. The flattened frontal eminence may show scattered cerebral imprints (Faure et al 1967), but this observation was not made in the Nancy series. The sagittal suture and the lambda are deviated towards the affected side. The lesser wing of the sphenoid is abnormally high and verticalized.

In the lateral views, the roof of the orbit is elevated on the diseased side, with shortening of the anterior fossa; the petrous bone is depressed, as is the temporomandibular

joint. The sphenotemporal suture, sometimes fused, is clearly shown in views of the optic grooves. Air encephalography was not performed in the Nancy series, but Foltz & Loeser (1975) noted deformation of the anterior horn of the affected side in two cases of plagiocephaly.

Craniometry

This circumference of the skull measures most commonly at the lower limit of normal. The longitudinal diameter is reduced. The biparietal diameter is slightly increased. The vertical diameter is also increased, but in a paramedian plane (Pugeaut 1968). The horizontal cranial index is at or slightly above the upper limit of normal.

Incidence

This type of malformation is rare — 7.7% in the Nancy series — but the prevalence varies in different series — 1.7% for Choux (1977) and 1.8% for Bertelsen — whereas Anderson & Geiger (1965) give a figure of 8.8%, Shillito & Matson (1968) of 12.7%, Rougerie et al (1972) and van der Werf (1966) each one of 14% and Till (1975) one of 16%.

BRACHYCEPHALY AND ACROBRACHYCEPHALY (frontoparietal)

Definition

The term brachycephaly refers to craniofacial dysmorphism secondary to premature bilateral coronal stenosis. According to Virchow's law, the skull is shortened in the sagittal plane and compensatory lateral development occurs in breadth or in height (Fig. 9.129).

Morphology

The vault. The skull is flattened from front to back. Where compensatory upward growth is allowed for by a patent sagittal suture, the upper part of the head is rounded and turricephalic. Delayed closure of the anterior fontanelle may cause the top of the skull to become pointed — acrocephaly. This deformity is the most common, hence the traditional term acrobrachycephaly (from the Greek *acros* = extremity) (Fig. 9.130). It may be characterized by prominence at the bregma with palpable hyperostosis and the appearance of a 'clown's hat' (Fig. 9.131). 'All combinations may occur, depending on the greater or lesser extent of compensatory upward growth and on the initial site of fusion at its upper end of the coronal suture (near the fontanelle) or at its opposite lower end' (Pujo 1960). The hairline is raised high up on the dome of the skull and the position of the ears appears lowered.

The face. Facial deformities are common. The forehead

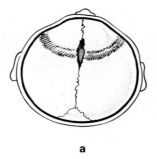
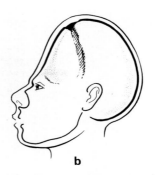

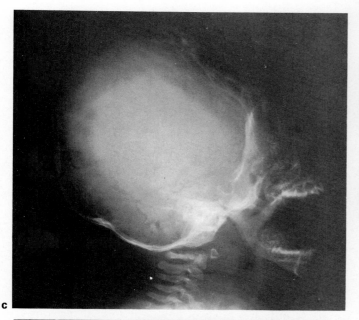

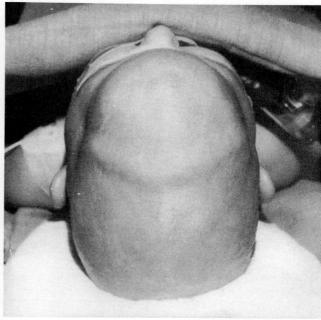

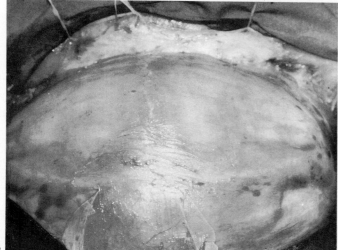

Fig. 9.129 Brachycephaly: (a) cranial view; (b) lateral view; (c) X-ray shows anteroposterior shortening of skull (brachycranium); (d) coronal ridge; (e) peroperative view of coronal suture.

may assume an antimongoloid obliquity. The lower face is usually normal.

Brain function

Signs of raised intracranial pressure are uncommon but mental retardation and blindness have been reported.

Associated malformations

These are quite common (Shillito & Matson 1968), particularly cleft palate and syndactyly.

Radiographic features

Lateral views disclose the absence of a coronal suture, which may leave a discreet trace or a line which is convex

is high, steep and flattened, sometimes even slightly concave. The orbital arches are hypoplastic and the eyeballs protuberant (prominent) in 50% of cases. Some degree of hypertelorism is common. The palpebral fissures

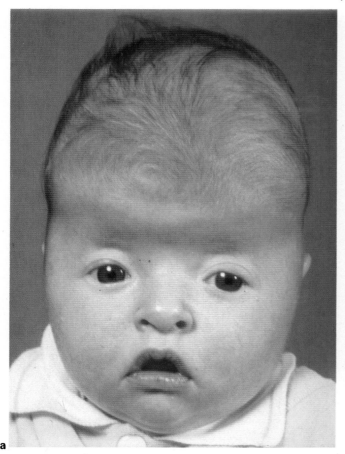 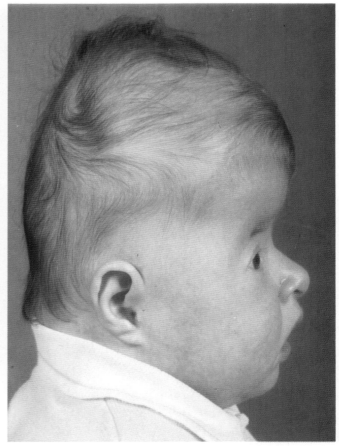

Fig. 9.130 Brachycephaly: (a) frontal view; (b) lateral view.

posteriorly. In some cases the upper bregmatic part of this suture may appear radiologically normal. The frontal eminences are poorly developed. The occipital bone is flat and the cerebriform impressions, which are not unusual, predominate in the frontal region and at the frontoparietal junction. The base is always deformed. The anterior fossa is short, more vertical than usual and concave upward and backward. The orbital cavities are shallow. The middle fossa is deep and appears to be pushed downward and forward.

Frontal views show the cranial vault to be wide and high, with the parietal eminences standing out. The lesser wings of the sphenoid are oblique upward, outward and forward, giving a 'Mephisthophelean' appearance.

Seeger & Gabrielsen (1971) stress the frequency of concomitant premature synostosis of the sphenofrontal suture, the basal prolongation of the coronal system of sutures.

Ossification of the sphenofrontal suture is frequently combined with that of the sphenoparietal and coronal sutures (Virchow 1851). Seeger & Gabrielsen found this association to be present in 12 out of 14 synostoses of the coronary sutures, 5 of them unilateral coronal synostoses. Seeger & Bertelsen point out that the coronal, sphenofrontal and sphenoparietal sutures and the sphenoethmoidal synchondrosis form a true sutural ring surrounding the skull from vault to base. The sphenofrontal suture can be seen in views of the optic groove.

Clinical and radiographic craniometry

The skull circumference is usually reduced but may be normal. In the Nancy series it was reduced in all cases, with a mean reduction of 3.9 cm. The width of the skull is approximately normal in this series. The sagittal diameter was routinely reduced by 3 to 1.5 cm as compared with normal figures, with a mean reduction of 2.2 cm. The horizontal cephalic index was increased, with a mean of 88.7 (89.3 in the Adelaide series). The height of the skull was greater than normal in 77% of cases and so was the vertical cranial index.

The deformations of the base caused basilar lordosis in all cases, with the nasal angle of Welcker increased to a mean value of 150° (range: 120–170°).

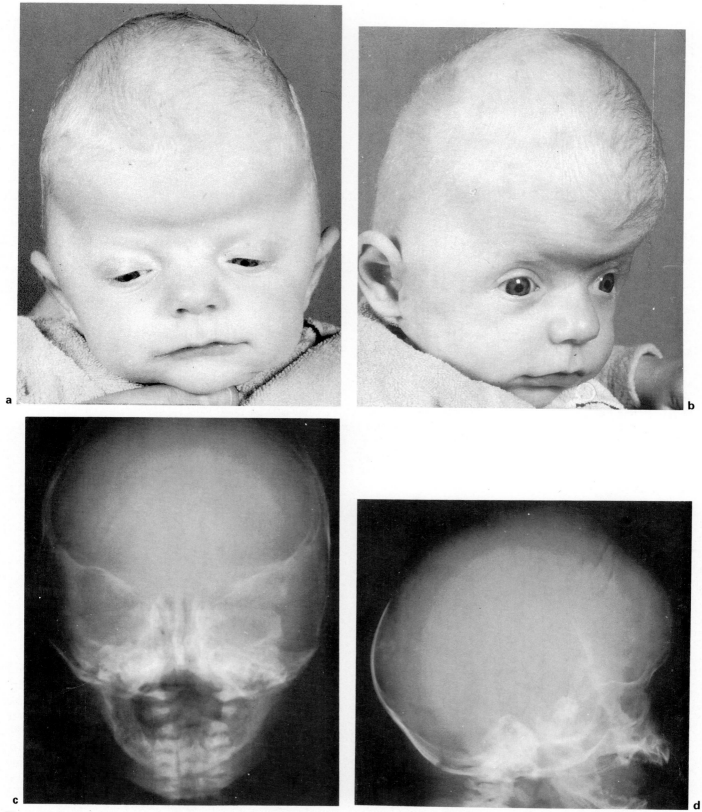

Fig. 9.131 Brachycephaly — note frontal bossing: (a) frontal view; (b) lateral view; (c) X-ray frontal view; (d) X-ray lateral view.

Incidence

The incidence of acrobrachycephaly reported by the French authors varies between 22% in the Nancy series and 33.8% observed by Monnet (1970). Similar percentages were recorded by other European writers: Müke (1972) 20.3%; Till (1979) 20.5%. American and Australian authors give much lower figures: Anderson and Geiger (1965) 8.8%; David et al (1982) 9.6%; Shillito & Matson (1968) 12.5%; Hunter & Rudd (1977) 15.4%. Bertelsen (1958) combined cases of oxycephaly and acrocephaly and reported an overall figure of 79%.

OXYCEPHALY (frontointerparietal)

Definition

Aristophanes (cited by Galen) used the term oxycephaly to describe heads with upward prolongation (from the Greek *oxus* = pointed). This term was long used as a synonym for craniostenosis in general and applied to all deformities of the skull.

According to Virchow (1851), oxycephaly means a pointed or sugarloaf head (Fig. 9.132), involving synostosis of the parietal bones with the occipital and temporal bones and compensatory development in the region of the anterior fontanelle. He included oxycephaly within the group of brachycephalies (cf. Virchow's classification).

Currently, the term oxycephaly is used to describe skull deformities related to multiple synostoses involving at least the coronal and sagittal sutures, with or without fusion of the lambdoid sutures and with compensatory upward development of the cranium.

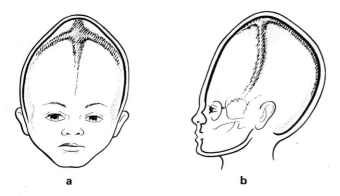

Fig. 9.132 Oxycephaly: (a) frontal view; (b) lateral view.

Morphology

The cranial vault. It is difficult to define the malformation of the skull since it varies more in relation to the order of sutural fusion than in relation to the number of sutures affected. Synostosis of the lambdoid sutures in the

context of oxycephaly alters the shape of the skull only slightly. However, three different types can be identified. The first type is oxycephaly, with a small ovoid skull and a convex top like a sugarloaf skull. The forehead is flat but receding (Fig. 9.133) rather than vertical, as in acrobrachycephaly. The second type is acrocephaly or turricephaly, approximating acrobrachycephaly. The obliteration of the coronal suture plays a predominant role as regards the general shape of the skull. The condition resembles that of simple coronal synostosis (Pugeaut 1968). Finally, global harmonious reduction of the various diameters may be seen. 'The diagnosis may then be missed or require distinction from "microcephaly"' (Rougerie et al 1972).

The face. Malformations are common and similar to those observed in acrobrachycephaly. The frontal eminences are not pronounced, the orbital arches are poorly developed and the forehead is vertical or receding; some degree of hypertelorism is not uncommon. Exopthalmia is frequent as a result of the reduced size of the orbits. 'The inward displacement of the lateral wall of the orbit is one of the main causes' (Djindjian 1952). There is antimongoloid slanting of the palpebral fissures. The ears are lowered, the nose wide, the palate often vaulted and the mouth small. Bertolotti (1910, 1914) has shown that the nasal bones are displaced downwards, as are the malar bones, so that the maxilla is curved anteriorly as in true superior prognathism.

Brain function

The malformation is compatible with normal intelligence but the risks of raised intracranial pressure, followed by mental retardation and blindness, are real and early surgery is therefore indicated.

Associated malformations

These are common (Shillito & Matson 1968) and include cleft palate and reductive limb anomalies, particularly of the digits (Tridon & Thiriet 1966).

Radiographic features

Anteroposterior and lateral views confirm the clinical impressions. The vault of the skull shows upward extension and a pointed appearance. The frontal sinuses are small or even absent. The sagittal and coronal sutures are fused, sometimes with synostosis of the lambdoid sutures. Some authors have stressed the thinness of the posterior part of the vault (Greig 1926), contrasting with frontal hyperostosis (Bertolotti 1910, 1914). The cerebriform depressions are very marked and often extend over the entire cranial vault.

The base of the skull is highly abnormal. The anterior fossa is shortened and verticalized. The middle fossa is

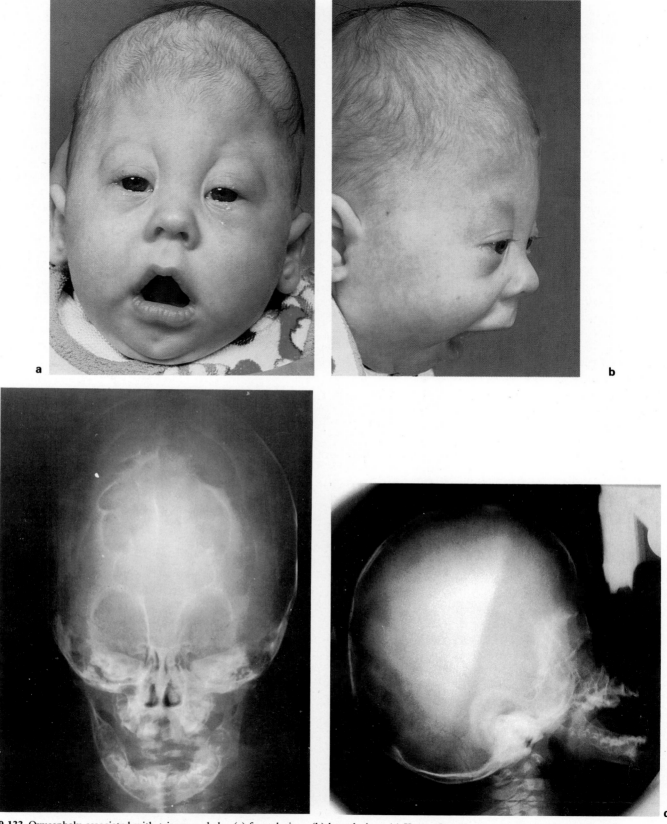

Fig. 9.133 Oxycephaly associated with trigonocephaly: (a) frontal view; (b) lateral view; (c) X-ray (frontal view) shows orbital abnormalities; (d) X-ray (lateral view) shows frontal retrusion.

depressed, with basilar lordosis, leading to a reduction in the height of the sphenoidal sinus, which is sometimes obliterated. The sella turcica appears depressed and angled backwards. The petrous bones are smaller in size. The posterior fossa is marked by the deep depression of the lateral sinuses. The orbits are reduced in their anteroposterior dimensions, whereas the vertical diameter is increased (Patry 1905, Smith 1974).

Craniometry

In most cases there is a marked reduction in the skull circumference (Bertelsen 1958), while the longitudinal and transverse diameters are reduced in 66% of cases (Ebel & Weidtman 1971).

In the Nancy series the mean difference from normal was −4 cm; the length was in all cases less than normal, with a mean of −2.1 cm. The width was slightly less than normal, with a mean of −0.68 cm. The horizontal cranial index was either normal or increased, with a mean of 84.

The cranial capacity was reduced. However, Hanotte (1898) and also Günther (1931) studying oxycephalic skulls, stated that they were of normal capacity. The basilar lordosis is comparable to that in brachycephaly, and sometimes greater. The angle of Welcker averages 148° The facial angle of Cloquet may be increased.

Incidence

The incidence of oxycephaly is relatively high in comparison with other malformations, ranging from 20% in the Nancy series (Montaut & Stricker) to an average of 12% in the combined Boston (Shillito & Matson) and Los Angeles (Anderson & Geiger) series.

Differences in systems of terminology and modes of selection are best expressed by the wide variation of incidence reported by Bertelsen (1958) — 79.9% — and David et al (1982) — 4.8%

Faciosynostosis

The examination of dry skulls may show the occurrence of isolated synostosis of the facial skeleton, affecting one or more sutures and responsible for localized deformities.

These faciostenoses had already been suspected in clinical cases. Indeed, Franceschetti in 1953 had drawn attention to the existence of inferior orbital retrusion and exorbitism, in the absence of occlusal and cranial abnormalities. The following typical forms may be observed in the face.

FRONTOMALAR SYNOSTOSIS (orbitostenosis)

Frontomalar retrusion affecting the lateral wall of the orbit results in backward sloping of the orbital contour. The

lateral canthus is loose and displaced downwards. The abnormality may therefore be confused with Treacher Collins' syndrome.

VOMERO-PREMAXILLARY SYNOSTOSIS (Binder's syndrome)

Maxillo-nasal dysostosis (Fig. 9.134) described by Binder (1962) produces a centrofacial nasomaxillary deformity which mainly affects the lower part of the nose and the premaxilla and is therefore fundamentally different from the malformation caused by hypochondroplasia.

In our opinion the malformation is due to an alteration of the inferior mesenchymal portion of the medial strut formed by the vomer pushing the premaxilla forward (Fig. 9.135). This vomero-premaxillary synostosis restricts sagittal projection and becomes evident by the presence of an anterior cross bite, by the retrusion of the pyriform aperture and the absence of the anterior nasal spine. The latter deformity is characterized by shortness of the columella and by separation of the philtral columns in their upper part.

The osseous deformities involve the chin, which is displaced downward and backward, and the cervical column, the centre of various anomalies.

THE PERIMAXILLARY SYNOSTOSES

Posterior perimaxillary synostosis

The perimaxillary sutural system is not always affected in its totality. Partial and posterior involvement is suspected in certain clefts in which the lateral maxillary element seems to be fused with the pterygoid, although proof of this is not available.

Anterior perimaxillary synostosis (pseudo Crouzon)

The description by Franceschetti in 1953 refers to the association of moderate exophthalmia with inferior orbital retrusion, a prominent forehead and marked digital impressions. Similar cases have been described by others but the majority of these seem to belong to the group of simple oxycephalies.

The definition of 'pseudo' Crouzon is based on the combination of moderate exorbitism and inferior orbital retrusion. Occlusion is normal.

Total perimaxillary synostosis (facial Crouzon)

Retromaxillism with exorbitism in the absence of cranial abnormalities or with discreet frontal flattening may be observed. These malformations are due to fusion of the posterior part of the perimaxillary sutural system. The case shown in the book by David et al (1982) provides an excellent example.

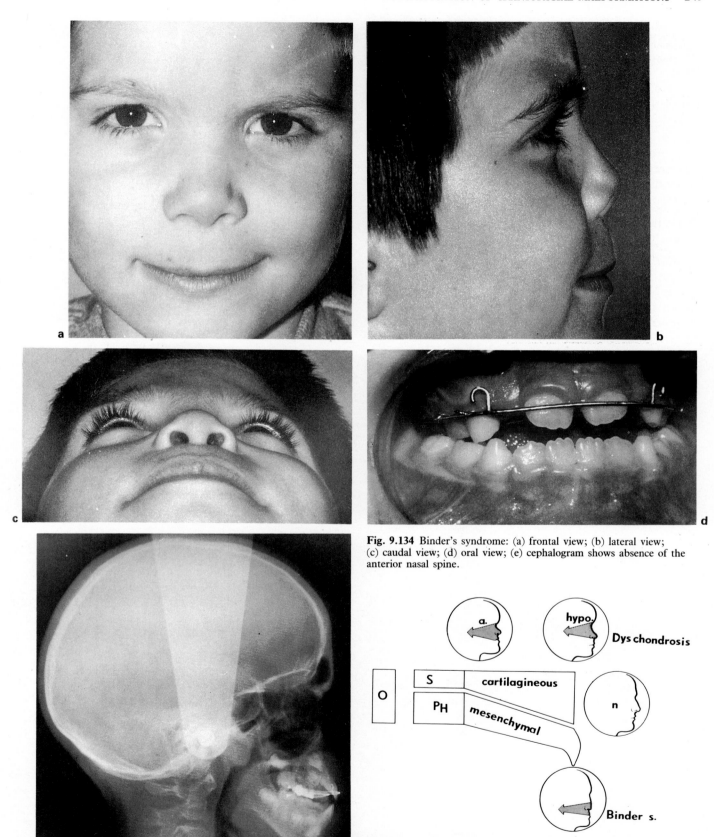

Fig. 9.134 Binder's syndrome: (a) frontal view; (b) lateral view; (c) caudal view; (d) oral view; (e) cephalogram shows absence of the anterior nasal spine.

Fig. 9.135 Causative mechanisms responsible for Binder's syndrome and nasal dyschondroses; an upper cartilaginous and a lower mesenchymal thrust can be distinguished. O = occipital; SPH = sphenoid.

This differentiation between the various types opens the discussion on Crouzon's syndrome in the section on dysostosis with synostosis.

CRANIOFACIAL DYSPLASIAS WITH DYSOSTOSIS AND SYNOSTOSIS

This group consists of the following three malformations: Crouzon; acrocephalosyndactyly (Apert); and triphyllocephaly (cloverleaf skull).

Reflections on 'Croupert'

The similarity between the abnormalities of the cranial base in the syndromes of Crouzon and Apert led Tessier to coin the term 'Croupert'. The temptation to simplify by grouping within this motley assembly of craniofacial dysostoses or cranio-faciostenoses is the more attractive as the therapeutic programme is analogous, at least in its goal: to disconnect the facial complex from the base of the skull so as to bring it forwards, together with the frontal bone, either in one piece or separately; and to free the stenosed cranium.

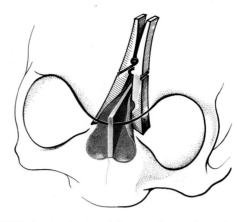

Fig. 9.137 Reduction in size of the nasopharynx is predominantly vertical in Crouzon's syndrome.

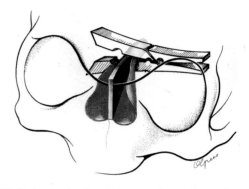

Fig. 9.138 Reduction in size of the nasopharynx is predominantly transversal in Apert's syndrome.

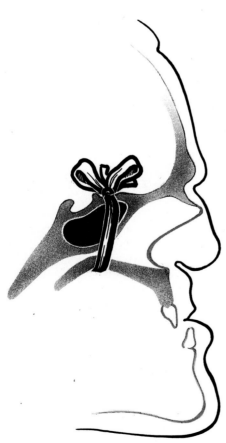

Fig. 9.136 Reduction in size of the nasopharynx.

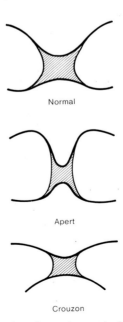

Normal

Apert

Crouzon

Fig. 9.139 Configuration of nasopharynx in Crouzon's and Apert's syndromes.

Retrusion of the facial massif and retromaxillism constitute the clinical features common to these malformations, but the term 'Croupert' does not do justice to the difference between the cranial and facial deformities of these syndromes, particularly where the nasopharynx is concerned (Figs. 9.136–9.139).

The cranium in Crouzon's syndrome is more harmonious and narrowing of the nasopharynx is only in an anteroposterior direction.

A dysostosis of the sphenoid seems to be the common denominator, aggravated by fusion of adjacent sutures extending towards the vault and the lateral sutures. For this reason we prefer to subdivide the syndrome of Crouzon, and separate it from the acrocephalosyndactylies.

The Crouzon syndromes

The term 'Crouzon' refers to a typical deformation but this anomaly may be due to various causes. Each of the resulting types corresponds to a specific topography of the lesion. Isolated or predominant facial forms are frequently observed. The developmental arrest affects the maxilla, the orbit and the vault.

The alterations mainly concern the sagittal dimensions of the face, and retrusion predominates. The orbital abnormalities in particular are worrisome because of the gravity of exorbitism.

We distinguish between five clinical forms:

the maxillary Crouzon (Fig. 9.140);
the 'pseudo' Crouzon with partial infraorbitary synostosis (Fig. 9.141);
the facial Crouzon, due to maxillary synostosis with mild cranial involvement. Two clinical forms can be distinguished: with exorbitism (Fig. 9.142a); without exorbitism (Fig. 9.142b).
the cranial Crouzon (Fig. 9.143) — a sphenoidal dysostosis with variable facial involvement. Sometimes even with almost normal occlusion as in the skull described by Kreiborg & Bjork (1982);
the craniofacial Crouzon (Fig. 9.144).

In contrast to Crouzon's syndrome, there is no facial Apert's syndrome. The malformations mainly affect the centrofacial area and are situated somewhat higher than in Crouzon's syndrome. Although concentrated along the midline, the facial abnormalities are distributed over three planes:

sagittally — centrofacial retrusion consists more of a tilt towards the sphenoid, which is pronounced in its upper part and mainly alters the root of the nose;
vertically — the maxilla assumes the form of an inverted V, resulting in infragnathy; the palate is narrow, simulating a cleft palate because of the usual fibromucosal peripheral hypertrophy;
transversely — plagiocephaly is common. The V-shaped basicranial deformation centred on the sphenoid is apposed at its apex by the reversed V of the maxillary and centrofacial areas.

Hypertelorism is frequently observed and is more evident because of the facial flattening.

The centrofacial abnormality involves mainly the nasopharynx and nasal fossa; the passages are narrow, the nasopharynx reduced and respiration is buccal, which aggravates the maxillary dysmorphism.

Interorbital hypertelorism can be seen in both syndromes. It is, however, somewhat disguised in Crouzon's syndrome by the extreme centrofacial retrusion and is more apparent in Apert's syndrome, with its large forehead and flared glabella.

CRANIOFACIAL CROUZON

Defined by Crouzon in 1912 in a mother and her daughter under the name of hereditary craniofacial dysostosis, this pathological entity is characterized by craniostenosis of the acrobrachycephalic or oxycephalic type, hypoplasia of the maxilla and exophthalmos (Fig. 9.145).

Morphology

The cranial vault. The morphology of the cranial vault varies. In his original paper, Crouzon described a deformity which features both scaphocephaly and trigonocephaly. However, the most characteristic type is represented by acrobrachycephaly (Bertelsen 1958) and oxycephaly (Chatelin 1914). Several sutures are always involved and a number of cases have been reported with asymmetric malformations. A very pronounced bregmatic boss ('clown's hat') may be observed. This prominence may extend as lateral ridges projecting over the fused coronal suture or as a median ridge descending towards the root of the nose (Pugeaut 1968, Maroteaux 1974). In other cases the skull is prolonged forwards by an anterior frontal prominence. The severity of the cranial malformations does not parallel that of the face.

The face. The malformations of the face lend the disease its characteristics. The face is flattened, sometimes concave. Two globular eyes give the patient a 'toadlike' appearance (Pugeaut 1968). This appearance is due essentially to hypoplasia of the maxilla, of the malar bone and of the orbital roof, resulting in a reduction in size of the orbital cavities. Exophthalmos, the cardinal sign described by Crouzon, is constant, often marked. Divergent strabismus or defective convergence is frequent. Hypertelorism may be present. Seen from in front the nasal root is flat, the dorsum and the nostrils are wide. In profile, the tip is

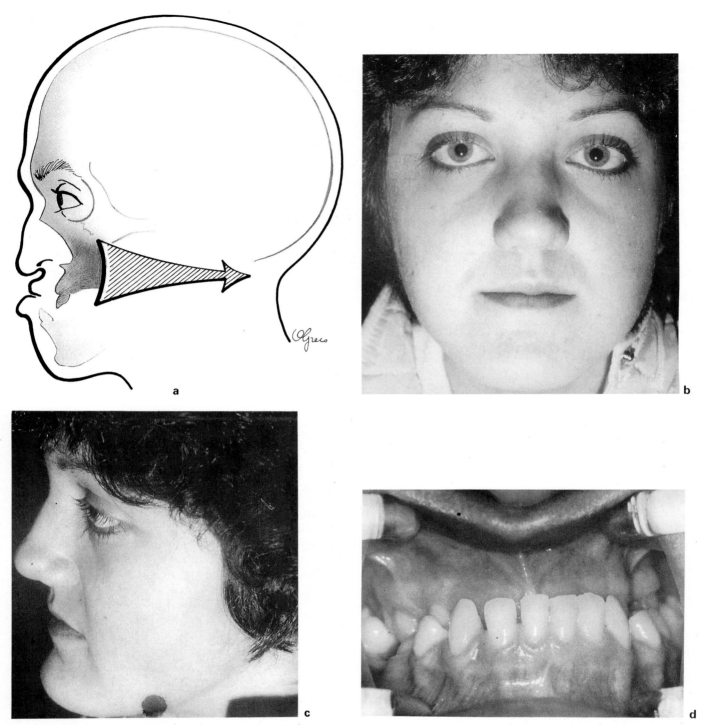

Fig. 9.140 Facial Crouzon (maxillary type or brachymaxilly): (a) diagrammatic representation; (b) frontal view; (c) lateral view — note minor exorbitism; (d) oral view — note severe retromaxillism.

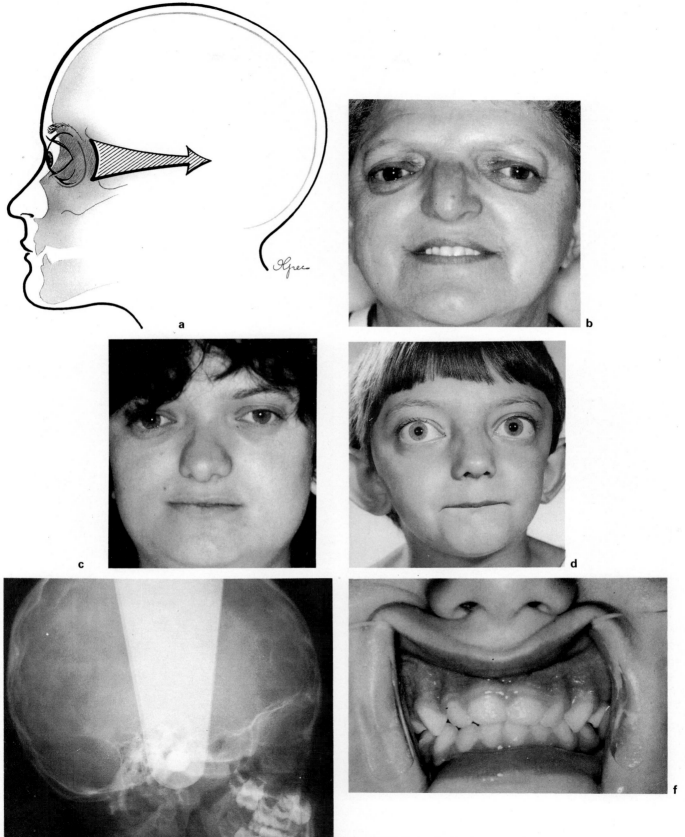

Fig. 9.141 Facial Crouzon (orbital type or 'pseudo' Crouzon): (a) diagrammatic representation; (b) grandmother with normal occlusion; (c) mother with normal occlusion; (d) son with normal occlusion; (e) oral view of son; (f) X-ray of son.

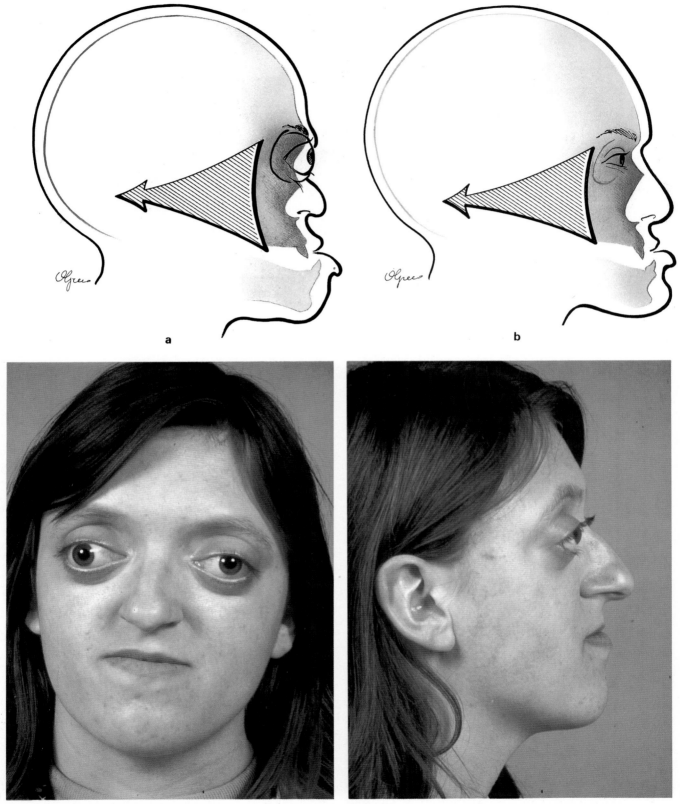

Fig. 9.142 Facial Crouzon: (a) with exorbitism (ai) frontal view; (aii) lateral view, (b) without exorbitism.

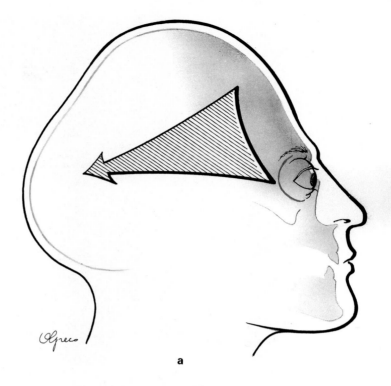

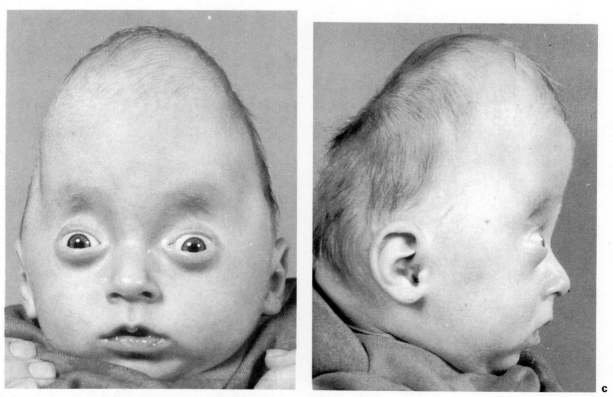

Fig. 9.143 Cranial Crouzon. Severe cranio-orbital malformation associated with normal occlusion: (a) diagrammatic representation; (b) frontal view; (c) lateral view. Note oxycephaly.

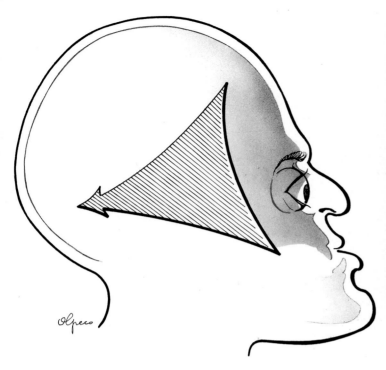

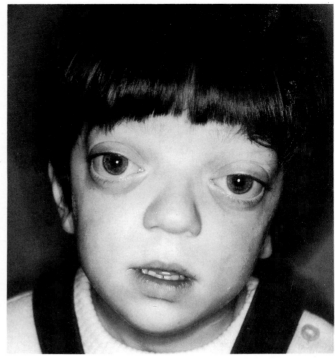

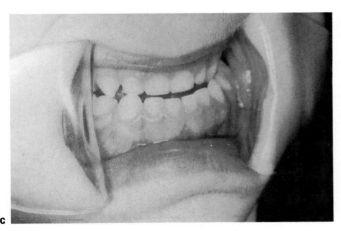

Fig. 9.144 Craniofacial Crouzon. Disproportion between minor degree of facial retrusion and severity of cranial involvement (augmentation of i.c.p.): (a) diagrammatic representation; (b) frontal view; (c) oral view.

protuberant and arched, like a 'parrot's beak', because of the recession of the maxillary bone. This faciostenosis gives the impression of prognathism despite a mandible which is normal or even reduced in size (de Gunten 1938). Not marked at birth, it tends to show up with growth. Malocclusion in varying degrees is the rule and dental malpositioning is common, sometimes with supernumerary or abnormal 'peg-top' teeth (Smith 1974). Caries is frequent. The palate is narrow and high and has an arched, pointed shape. Choanal atresia and stenosis of the auditory canal (Aubry 1935) may be observed.

Vision. Lack of skeletal protection may result in lagophthalmus, exposure keratitis or even dislocation of a globe.

Respiration. Constriction of the airways may result in chronic or intermittent respiratory problems, mouth breathing and snoring being the most common complaints.

Phonation. Speech may be affected by hyponasality and lack of resonance. Malocclusion will tend to distort phonation even more by disarticulation.

Hearing. Atresia of the auditory canal and obstruction of the Eustachian tube due to upper respiratory infections may both lead to hearing impairment.

Associated malformations

Additional abnormalities may affect: the spinal cord — syringomyelia (Moretti & Steffen 1959); the vertebrae — curvation, subluxation, fusion and reduction anomalies (Kreiborg 1981a,b, David et al 1982); and the limbs — cubital fusion or subluxation, digital anomalies (Tridon & Thiriet 1966).

Functional pathology

Brain function. A raised intracranial pressure may have several consequences. An increase in involutional impressions is often seen, papilloedema less frequently. The danger of visual failure from secondary optic atrophy is, however, real and narrowing of the optic canal as a possible causative mechanism should be excluded. Ventricular dilatation is

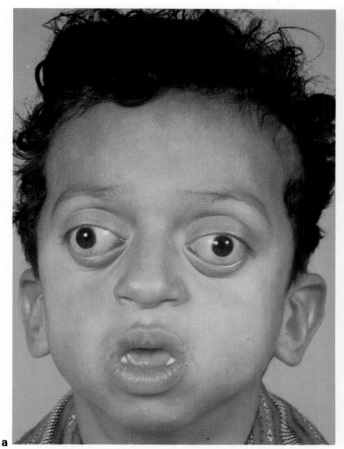

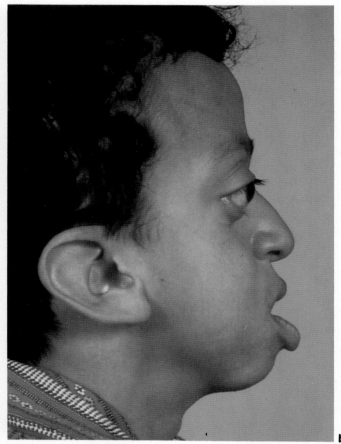

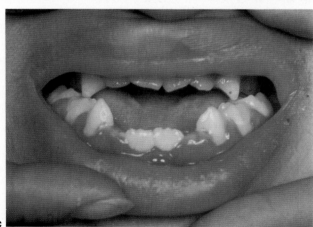

Fig. 9.145 Craniofacial Crouzon: (a) frontal view; (b) lateral view; (c) oral view.

an indication of hydrocephalus but its cause remains uncertain. It may represent a primary aqueduct stenosis or be secondary to compression of the basal cisterns of the cerebral aqueduct by a kyphotic deformity of the cranial base. Retardation is uncommon and its relationship to craniostenosis is difficult to prove, but there is some evidence that early surgery is beneficial in this respect. The incidence of epilepsy is equally low. The cases associated with syndactyly were classified by McKusik (1978) under the name of acrocephalosyndactyly of the Vogt type. The

combination with syndactyly has indeed been invoked by Cruveiller (1954) to support the identity of the two diseases (Maroteau 1974).

Radiographic features. The malformations of the vault vary in relation to the number of sutures affected, and are similar to those described in acrobrachycephaly or oxycephaly. A prominent bregma is the most constant finding; the frontal bone is either vertical or receding and thin. The coronal and often the sagittal sutures are obliterated; the cerebriform impressions are numerous and very marked, giving the cranium a 'hammered' appearance. The imprint of the lateral sinuses is clear. At the base of the skull the ethmoid bone forms a curve with an anteroinferior concavity. The lesser wings of the sphenoid are hypertrophied. The greater wings are reduced in width and length. The essential feature is the basilar kyphosis, exaggerated by diminution of the basilar angle of Welcker. This basilar kyphosis, which is not found in simple craniostenosis, gives the disease its true identity.

Craniometry. Measurements show that the skull is usually brachycephalic. The cranial circumference was less than normal in the Nancy series, the mean reduction being

−2 cm. The mean horizontal cranial index was close to that in brachycephaly: 79.3 for Bertelsen (1958). In the Nancy series the skull was brachycephalic, with a mean of 86.6. The reduced basal angle accounts for the basilar kyphosis, the mean being 109°. The facial angle may be increased by 8° to 10° (Berrada 1964).

Incidence of Crouzon. It is difficult to determine the incidence of Crouzon's diseases in the general context of the craniosynostoses. A number of authors include them in the acrobrachycephalies or oxycephalies (Shillito & Matson 1968, Anderson & Geiger 1965, Choux 1977), because of the cranial features. Others deny them any genuine anatomy, do not distinguish them from the Apert acrocephalosyndactylies, and give overall figures for these two conditions. The incidence ranges from 6.8% in the series of Bertelsen to 14.9% in the Adelaide series. The Nancy series included 21 cases of Crouzon's diseases in a total of 155 patients (13.5%).

Genetics

The heredofamilial nature of the condition was postulated in Crouzon's initial report of 1912. Many hereditary cases have been published since. Flippen (1950) studied the transmission of this dysmorphy over four generations and Dodge (1959) over three generations. Pinkerton and Pinkerton (1952) have reported a family in which the mother transmitted the abnormality to three of her five children. Rougerie (1974) reported two Crouzon families. In one of these, with seven children, there were two with Crouzon's disease, one with oxycephaly, one with complex craniostenosis and one with dysmorphism of the skull base. In the Nancy series there were 3 familial cases. Transmission appears to be of autosomal dominant nature with variable penetration. This mode of transmission has been demonstrated by Vulliamy and Normandale in a family with 14 members affected over four generations. The karyotype is invariably normal, both in our own cases as in those from the literature. However, sporadic cases remain the most numerous. In 1927, Roubinovitch and Crouzon reported two cases without either hereditary or familial features. Most of our own cases are of this type.

Apert's syndrome

This is a rare dysmorphy, for which Apert in 1906 suggested the term acrocephalosyndactyly to designate the association of a high skull flattened at the back and sometimes at the sides and excessively prominent in the superior frontal region (Fig. 9.146), with syndactyly of all four limbs (Fig. 9.147).

Apert described in his original paper the case of a 15-month-old girl observed in 1896, who presented with acrocephalosyndactyly associated with a bifid uvula and a cleft palate. He collected eight more cases from the literature, the first seemingly that of Troquart in 1886.

Since then, many studies have been devoted to this disorder, too tedious to list. Among the more important was the study by Park & Powers (1920) on acrocephaly and scaphocephaly with symmetrical malformations of the limbs, based on 30 cases from the literature. In 1960, Blank studied a series of 39 patients from the English language literature and listed 150 published cases.

Morphology

The craniofacial dysmorphy varies in severity and formes frustes are common. However, there is a distinct morphological type which distinguishes this syndrome from Crouzon's disease.

The cranial vault (Fig. 9.148). The malformation is mostly acrobrachycephalic in type. The occiput is flat and not clearly demarcated from the plane of the back of the neck. The vertex is at the level of the bregma or anterior to it, overhanging the forehead, which is steep, high and flat or slightly rounded. A vertical ridge in the middle of the forehead over the metopic suture and retrusion of the thick eyebrows reflect the skeletal abnormalities in the frontal region. Temporal bulging is due to the expansion of the middle cranial fossa, which results in obliteration of the temporal fossa and projection of the temporal muscle over the short zygoma. The auditory meatus is displaced inferiorly.

The face (Fig. 9.149). The appearance of the face is very specific. In contrast to Crouzon's disease, exophthalmus is usually less pronounced but severe exorbitism may be observed. The orbits are shallow. Downward slanting of the palpebral fissures with lateral canthal dystopia and moderate ptosis of the upper eyelids are usually present and may be explained by lateral and inferior rotation of the orbits. The medial orbital wall protrudes into the orbit and the lateral orbital wall is short. Hypertelorism may be marked and divergent strabismus is often associated. The bridge of the nose is flat and its root deeply furrowed. The tip is hooked as in Crouzon's syndrome. The mouth remains half open in the shape of an isosceles triangle. The upper lip is retracted, giving it a crossbow appearance. The cheeks are rounded while the dangling lower lip juts out. Maxillary retrusion is associated with a keel-shaped alveolar and dental crowding. Class III malocclusion with an open bite may be observed. The high ogival palate is divided by a midline furrow with a paramedian fold on each side. This furrow (Byzantine) may continue at the back as a cleft of the long soft palate (in 30% of cases according to Cohen 1971) of the uvula, a characteristic of the disease according to de Gunten (1938). Sebaceous gland diseases characterized by acne complete the picture.

The limbs. In Apert's original description all four limbs were affected. Syndactyly usually involves all the fingers and toes. The hands are reduced to a kind of 'spatula' with vertical grooves sketching the shape of the fingers. In other cases the fusion affects only the four fingers, leaving a free

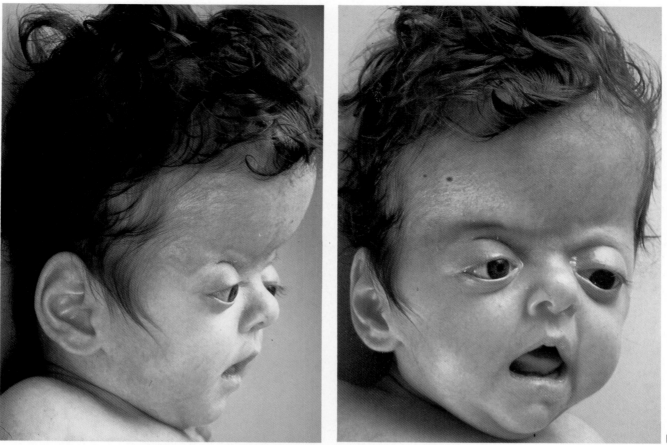

Fig. 9.146 Apert's syndrome: (a) frontal view — note frontal bossing; (b) lateral view.

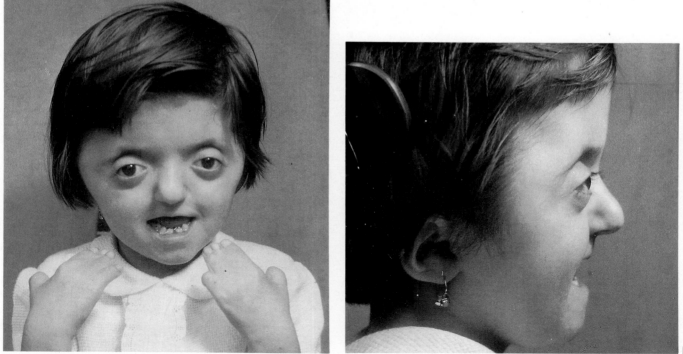

Fig. 9.147 Apert's syndrome: (a) frontal view — note malformations of hands; (b) lateral view.

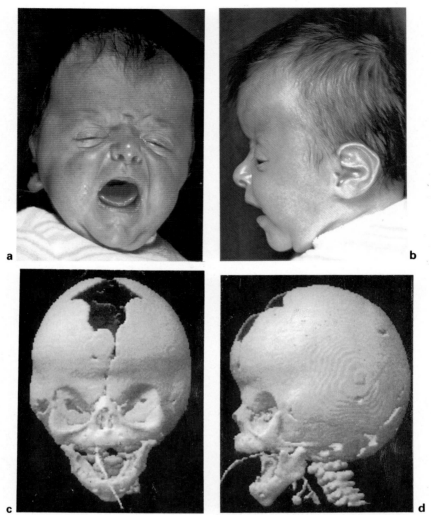

Fig. 9.148 Apert's syndrome: (a) frontal view; (b) lateral view; (c) 3-D reconstruction, frontal view; (d) 3-D reconstruction, lateral view.

thumb which is variably malformed. The fifth finger is sometimes spared (Park & Powers 1920). Like the fingers, the nails are ill-shapen. They are fused in a single mass but often there is a sketchy differentiation of the nails. Similar conditions are seen in the feet. In one of our cases there was symmetrical fusion of only the first two toes.

Functional pathology

Brain function. Mental retardation is commonly present, although there are exceptions. Many explanations may be offered but its real nature is still unclear. A raised intracranial pressure and hydrocephalus may contribute to this condition but they are certainly not solely responsible. A primary cerebral deficiency, communication and education problems due to hearing, speech and manual abnormalities and last but not least social ostracism are important factors to be considered.

Vision. Blindness may occur as a result of optic atrophy

or globar exposure. Binocular vision may be impaired owing to divergent strabismus.

Respiration. Speech may be affected in a similar way as in Crouzon's syndrome.

Hearing. Impairment of hearing may be due to ossicular fixation or to otitis media.

Associated malformations

In the face, cleft lip and palate have been described. Other, skeletal, malformations reported include: short humerus, radiohumeral synostosis, spinal malformations such as spina bifida (Wigert 1932) and synostosis of C1–C2 (Viallefont 1934), coxa valga, gena valgum and clubfoot (Tridon & Thiriet 1966). Visceral malformations have also been recorded: oesophageal atresia, pyloric stenosis, ectopic anus, congenital heart disease (Traissac 1962), polycystic kidneys (Hasse 1944).

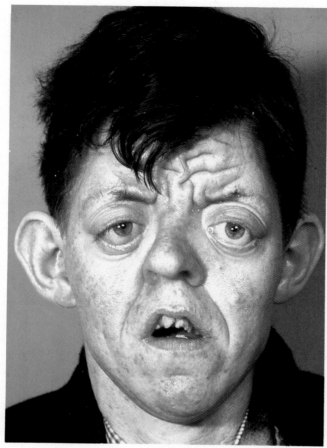

Fig. 9.149 Apert's syndrome — note trapezoidal configuration of upper lip and skin abnormalities.

Pathogenesis

The skull of patients with Apert's syndrome has now been examined on several occasions (Stewart et al 1977, Ousterhout & Melsen 1982). These studies demonstrate several abnormalities in the cranial base hitherto not recognized, although suspected, such as fusion of the spheno-occipital synchondrosis, of the sphenoid and vomer, and of the vomer and maxilla. These findings indicate a reduced growth potential of the cranial base to be at the origin of most of the skeletal abnormalities that may be observed.

Radiology

Lateral views show reduction of the anteroposterior diameter of the skull and excessive height to be prominent features. Digital markings are constant but less conspicuous than in Crouzon's disease. The posterior cranial fossa is deep and short. The posterior fontanelle and the lambdoid sutures are often absent. The anterior fossa is shortened. The clivus is short and vertical, the basal angle lordotic. The middle cranial fossa is short and deep, expanding anteriorly and inferiorly.

The fused coronal suture line is perceptible because of its increased density. Superiorly it exhibits a forward curvation, while inferiorly it extends to the steepened sphenoidal ridge and the sphenosquamous suture. The thickness of the vault is uneven and the frontal region may be very thin.

In frontal views, patency of the anterior fontanelle is a striking peculiarity. The sagittal and metopic sutures usually gape widely but additional synostosis of the sagittal and squamous sutures may be observed. The middle cranial fossa expands laterally and inferiorly. Also characteristic are the upward slanting of the lesser wings of the sphenoid and prolapse of the cribriform plate between the orbital roofs. The ethmoidal sinuses are hyperplastic and the interorbital distance somewhat increased.

In the hands, all the metacarpals are usually present but their arrangement and orientation are not always regular. The proximal phalanges of the four fingers are well indicated; the phalanges of the thumb are generally fused into a triangular or rectangular mass.

In the feet, the phalanges of the great toe are often fused; the disposition of the phalanges of the other toes is more or less fused, as in the hand.

Craniometry

This is very similar to the acrobrachycephalies. The skull circumference was reduced by a mean of 3 cm in the Nancy series. The anteroposterior diameter is greatly reduced and the transverse diameter increased, with a cephalic index above 90°. The angle of Welcker is also increased.

Incidence

Apert's syndrome is fortunately exceedingly rare. An incidence of 1 in 160 000 normal births was reported by Blank (1960). Tünte & Lenz (1967) counted 1 per 1 000 000 in their series.

Genetics

Transmission is by autosomal dominant mode but there are few known hereditary cases; three examples have been reported (Blank 1960, Hoover et al 1970, Weech 1927). Affected subjects rarely have children, in view of their dysmorphy and mental retardation.

Differentiation

The delineation of syndromes is a dynamic process. Some syndromes cease to exist as separate entities when more information is gained. Vogt's syndrome, Mohr's syndrome, Waardenburg's syndrome and Noack's syndrome are examples of entities whose validity is no longer recognized.

They are replaced by other syndromes hitherto unknown. At present 64 syndromes associated with synostosis are known. This list was compiled by Cohen (1986) and he has kindly given us permission to reproduce his master table (Table 9.2).

The majority of these syndromes are extremely rare or never referred for treatment because of mental retardation. Others and particularly those belonging to the group of acrocephalo-(poly)-syndactylies are more commonly seen and therefore deserve a short description.

Saethre–Chotzen (Fig. 9.150). This syndrome was first described by Saethre in 1931 and by Chotzen in 1932. It is characterized by facial asymmetry due to plagiocephaly and palpebral ptosis in combination with brachydactyly and partial syndactyly of the second interdigital space, sometimes extending to the third. Syndactyly, however, is not obligatory. A low-set hairline and teleorbitism are frequently observed. Radioulnar synostosis was reported by Bartsocas et al (1970), who described ten members of one family affected over three generations. Autosomal dominant inheritance appears to be evident.

Pfeiffer (Fig. 9.151). The combination of acrocephaly and digital anomalies was described by Rudolf Pfeiffer in 1964 in eight members of one family affected over three generations. The thumbs and first toes are broad and radially deviant, with a trapezoid configuration of the first phalanx. Brachydactyly and partial syndactyly affecting the second interdigital space, sometimes also the third, are observed. Hypertelorism and maxillary retrusion are common. The syndrome closely resembles Apert's syndrome, particularly when a trilobular configuration of the skull exists. Transmission is by autosomal dominant inheritance.

Carpenter (Fig. 9.152). The combination of acrocephaly and digital anomalies consisting of syndactyly of the third interdigital space and polysyndactyly of the feet was recorded by Carpenter in 1901. The syndrome was recognized as a distinct entity in 1966, when Tentamy reported one case and studied 12 cases previously described in the literature under the name of Laurence–Moon–Biedl syndrome. Multiple cranial synostoses and a facies resembling that in Apert's syndrome are the main features. Obesity and hypogonadism in the male, ocular malformations (microcornea or corneal opacity), ear abnormalities and mental retardation are commonly seen. The mode of transmission appears to be recessive. A somewhat similar type III has been described by Sakati et al (1971).

Jackson–Weiss (Fig. 9.153). The combination of craniosynostosis, maxillary retrusion and anomalies of the feet was recorded by Jackson et al in 1976. Medial deviation of the big toes and partial syndactyly of the first web space were the most constant features. Abnormalities of the thumb are characteristically absent. Transmission is by autosomal dominant inheritance.

Triphyllocephaly

The term triphyllocephaly was recently coined by David et al (1982) to describe the cloverleaf anomaly, which is characterized clinically and radiologically by hydrocephalus and a trilobular skull with synostosis of the lambdoidal and coronal sutures, permitting cerebral eventration through the open sagittal and squamosal sutures and a widely patent anterior fontanelle. Absence of craniosynostosis at birth or fusion of the sagittal metopic and squamosal sutures is, however, also observed.

Triphyllocephaly is observed as an isolated condition or as an expression of one of the syndromes described in this section; Crouzon, Apert, Pfeiffer, Carpenter, etc. Most commonly it is seen in thanatophoric dysplasia. Vrolik (1849) included an example of this anomaly (Fig. 9.154) in his book, but Holtermuller & Wiedemann (1960) were the first to provide a full description based on 13 cases, 12 of which had been described in the German literature under the title 'chondrodystrophic hydro-cephalus'. They introduced the term 'Kleeblattschädel' and defined the following anatomic and clinical characteristics of the malformation: a trilobed head with a low implant of the ears, hydrocephalus, facial malformations with hypertelorism, flattening of the bridge of the nose, an arched palate, micromelia and a poor prognosis.

Isolated cases had been described before this report. Most commonly, this malformation was included among the oxycephalies or among the 'Lückenschädel' or lacunar skulls. Sear (1937) classified them in his diagram in a specific group related to coronal and lambdoid synostosis and showed an illustrative radiograph in a baby aged 4 months. David et al (1947) reported a case in the context of multiple congenital malformations of a non-familial nature, impossible to classify. Berrada (1964) described in his thesis a case associated with Arnold-Chiari malformation. Other cases were recorded by Moscatelli et al (1968), Nawalkha & Mangal (1970), Schuch & Pesch (1971), Bonucci & Nardi (1972), etc.

Morphology

The cranial vault. Comings (1965) commented on the characteristic and 'almost extraterrestrial appearance' of the skull, which is trilobular, with a superior expansion and two low lateral expansions in the temporal regions (Fig. 9.155). The bulging superior 'lobe' is separated from the two inferior and lateral lobes by a constricted zone. The position of the superior expansion is more or less anterior, depending on whether the sagittal suture is still patent or only the anterior fontanelle and metopic suture remain open. The lateral expansions are related to nonclosure of the squamoparietal suture. The wide open anterior fontanelle is made tense by the concomitant hydrocephalus. There is extreme flattening of the occipital

Table 9.2 Master table of syndromes, as compiled by Cohen (1986)

Syndrome	Striking features other than craniosynotosis	Cranial suture especially involved	Syndrome	Striking features other than craniosynotosis	Cranial suture especially involved
Monogenically caused syndromes			Hunter's syndrome	Microcephaly, mental retardation, small oval face, almond-shaped eyes, droopy eyelids, small nose, small downturned mouth, minor acral skeletal anomalies, short stature; less commonly congenital heart defect, limited elbow extension	Coronal
Apert's syndrome	Proptosis, downslating palpebral fissures, strabismus, ocular hypertelorism, midface deficiency, highly arched palate, complete symmetric syndactyly of hands and feet minimally involving digitis 2–4	Coronal			
Crouzon's syndrome	Shallow orbits with proptosis, strabismus, midface deficiency	Coronal	Osteoglophonic dysplasia	Disproportionately short limbs, turribrachycephaly, severe craniofacial malformation, midface deficiency, multiple radiolucent metaphyseal defects, flattening and beaking of vertebral bodies, unerupted teeth	Multiple sutures
Pfeiffer's syndrome	Proptosis, strabismus, ocular hypertelorism, downslanting palpebral fissures, midface deficiency, broad thumbs and great toes, mild cutaneous syndactyly of fingers and toes (variable)	Coronal			
			San Francisco syndrome	Midface hypoplasia, ptosis of the eyelids, bulbous nose, small ears	Coronal
Saethre–Chotzen syndrome	Craniosynostosis, facial asymmetry, low-set frontal hairline, ptosis of the eyelids, deviated nasal septum, variable brachydactyly and cutaneous syndactyly, especially of the second and third fingers, normal thumbs and great toes, occasionally broad toes	Coronal	Tricho-dento-osseous syndrome	Kinky hair, enamel hypoplasia, taurodont molars, osteosclerosis	All sutures
			Vetruto's syndrome	Brachydactyly, absence of some middle or distal phalanges, aplastic or hypoplastic nails, symphalangis, synosotosis of some carpal and tarsal bones, hip dysplasia, pes planus	Coronal
Jackson–Weiss syndrome	Craniosynostosis with Pfeiffer-like, Saethre–Chotzen-like, or Crouzon-variant-like phenotype. Minimal manifestation consists of broad first metatarsals and fused tarsal bones. Pfeiffer-like great toes sometimes observed, but Pfeiffer-like thumbs not observed	Coronal			
			Autosomal recessive		
Berant's syndrome	Radioulnar synostosis	Sagittal	Carpenter's syndrome	Mental deficiency (but normal intelligence has been reported), preacial polysyndactyly of the feet, variable soft tissue syndactyly with brachymesophalangy of the hands, displacement of patellae, genua valga, congenital heart defects, short stature, obesity	All sutures
Frydman's trigonocephaly syndrome	Trigonocephaly, ridging of metopic suture, mild synophrys, ocular hypotelorism, normal intelligence, and low-frequency anomalies, such as preauricular tag, hemivertebra, and omphalocele	Metopic			
			Antley–Bixler syndrome	Brachycephaly, ocular proptosis, midface hypoplasia, dysplastic ears, radiohumeral synostosis, joint contractures, arachnodactyly, femoral bowing	Coronal
Greig's cephalopolysyndactyly	Scaphocephaly, frontal bossing, ocular hypertelorism, broad thumbs and halluces, pre- and postaxial polydactyly of hands and feet, variable syndactyly of fingers and toes	Variable sutures	Baller–Gerold syndrome	Radial aplasia, absent or hypoplastic carpal bones and preaxial digits	Coronal
			Baraitser's syndrome	Cleft lip and/or palate, choroidal coloboma, seizures, mental deficiency, short broad fingers and toes, mesomelia, dysplastic kidneys	Coronal

Table 9.2   Master table of syndromes, as compiled by Cohen (1986) (*cont'd*)

Syndrome	Striking features other than craniosyntosis	Cranial suture especially involved	Syndrome	Striking features other than craniosynotosis	Cranial suture especially involved
Christian's syndrome	Microcephaly, ocular hypertelorism, downslanting palpebral fissures, cleft palate, arthrogryposis	All sutures	Opitz trigonocephaly syndrome (C syndrome)	Ridged metopic area, narrow forehead, ocular hypotelorism, upslanting, palpebral fissures, epicanthic folds, strabismus, short broad nose, wide mouth, receding chin, wide alveloar ridge, attached frenum, short neck, widely spaced nipples, limb deformities, bridged palmar creases, redundant skin, deep sacral dimple, patent ductus arteriosus or other cardiac defect, cryptorchidism	Metopic
Cranioectodermal dysplasia	Dolichocephaly, frontal bossing, epicanthic folds, anteverted nares, everted lower lip, sparse slow-growing hair, microsontia, hypodontia, brachydactyly, soft tissue syndactyly of fingers and toes, clinodactyly, short narrow thorax, pectus excavatum, short limbs	Sagittal			
Elejalde's syndrome	Swollen face, epicanthic folds, ocular hypertelorism, hypoplastic nose, malformed ears, redundant neck tissue, gigantism at birth, short limbs, polydactyly, omphalocele, lung hypoplasia, cystic renal dysplasia, sponge kidney, redundant connective tissue in skin and many viscera, proliferation of perivascular nerve fibres	Coronal	Seckel's syndrome	Intrauterine growth deficiency, postnatal growth deficiency, microcephaly, mental retardation, prominent curved nose, receding chin, relatively large eyes, downslanting palpebral fissures, dysplastic ears, enamel hypoplasia, occasional cleft palate, fifth finger clinodactyly, retarded ossification	All sutures
			X-linked		
Gorlin–Chaudhry–Moss syndrome	Brachycephaly, midface deficiency, hypertrichosis, downslanting palpebral fissures, upper eyelid colobomas, patent ductus arteriosus, hypoplastic labia majora	Coronal	FG syndrome	Congenital hypotonia, severe mental Sagittal retardation, hyperactivity, short attention span, megalencephaly, dolichocephaly, ocular hypertelorism, downslanting palpebral fissures, epicanthic folds, strabismus, high, narrow palate, mild micrognathia, imperforate anus	Sagittal
Ives–Houston syndrome	Intrauterine growth retardations, perinatal death, marked microcephaly, fused elbows, short forearms usually containing only a single bone, hand anomalies with only two to four malformed digits	All sutures	Say–Meyer trigonocephaly syndrome	Trigonocephaly, ocular hypotelorism, short stature, developmental delay, other anomalies	Metopic
Lowry's syndrome	Prominent eyes, strabismus, highly arched or cleft palate, fibular aplasia, talipes equinovarus, simian creases	Coronal	**Monogenic; inheritance pattern unclear to date**		
			Armendares' syndrome	Microcephaly, retinitis pigmentosa, ptosis of the eyelids, malformed ears, mircorgnathia, highly arched palate, clinodactyly, simian creases, short stature	Coronal sagittal
Michel's syndrome	Corneal opacities, iris adhesions, primary telecanthus, ptosis of the eyelids, epicanthus inversus, limitation of upward gaze, short fifth fingers, skeletal anomalies, cleft lip and/or palate, deafness, mild mental retardation	Lambdoid	Cranio-frontonasal dysplasia	Brachycephaly, ocular hypertelorism, clefting of the nasal tip, skeletal anomalies, various abnormalities of the hands and feet	Coronal
			Thanatophoric dysplasia with cloverleaf skull	Large trilobular head, short-limbed dwarfism, short, thick, straight femora, narrow thoracic cage	Coronal, sagittal, lambdoid

Table 9.2 Master table of syndromes, as compiled by Cohen (1986) (*cont'd*)

Syndrome	Striking features other than craniosynotosis	Cranial suture especially involved	Syndrome	Striking features other than craniosynotosis	Cranial suture especially involved
Chromosomally caused syndromes			Deletion, short arm, chromosome 9	Mental deficiency, trigonocephaly, prominent forehead, upslanting palpebral fissures, flat nasal bridge, anteverted nostrils, long philtrum, micrognathia, highly arched palate, low-set ears, short broad neck, widely spaced nipples, hyperconvex fingernails, long fingers and/or toes, congenital heart defects	Metopic
Deletion, long arm, chromosome 1	Terminal deletion: growth deficiency, microcephaly, mental retardation, seizures, high-pitched cry, sparse, fine hair, flat nasal bridge, micrognathia, abnormal ears, short neck, abnormalities of hands and feet, hypospadias; interstitial deletion: microbrachycephaly; other abnormalities	Coronal			
Deletion, long arm, chromosome 3	Trigonocephaly, microcephaly, upslanting palpebral fissures, hypoplastic nose, broad nasal root, micrognathia, low-set posteriorly angulated ears, ventricular dilatation, absence of cerebellar vermis	Metopic	Deletion, long arm, chromosome 11	Growth deficiency, mental retardation, trigonocephaly, upslanting palpebral fissures, ptosis of the eyelids, carp-shaped mouth, thin lips, highly arched eyebrows, horizontal or downslanting palpebral fissures, pointed nasal tip, hypoplastic antihelices, low-set ears, hypoplasia of metacarpals and metatarsals	Metopic
Duplication, long arm, chromosome 3	De Lange-like phenotype with growth deficiency, microcephaly, mental retardation, seizures, hypertrichosis, synophrys, long eyelashes, broad nasal root, anteverted nostrils, long philtrum, highly arched or cleft palate, micrognathia, malformed ears, short or webbed neck, clinodactyly, congenital heart defects, genitourinary malformations and various skeletal anomalies	Coronal	Deletion, short arm, chromosome 12	Growth deficiency, mental retardation, microcephaly, narrow forehead, protruding occiput, highly arched eyebrows, horizontal or downslanting palpebral fissures, pointed nasal tip, hypoplastic antihelices, low-set ears, hypoplasia of metacarpals and metatarsals	Sagittal
Duplication, short arm, chromosome 5	Variable CNS anomalies, dolichocephaly, mental deficiency, respiratory difficulties, renal/urtal malformations, short great toes. Well-defined clinical picture has not emerged	Sagittal	Deletion, long arm, chromosome 13	Growth deficiency, mental retardation, microcephaly, frequent trigonocephaly, semilobar or lobar holoprosencephaly in some cases, prominent nasal bridge, ocular hypertelorism, ptosis of the eyelids, microphthalmia, iris coloboma, micrognathia, hypoplastic thumbs, talipes equinovarus, congenital heart defects, genital anomalies, imperforate anus	Metopic
Duplication, long arm, chromosome 6	Growth retardation, severe mental deficiency, acrocephaly, brachycephaly, carp-shaped mouth, micrognathia, short neck with unusual anterior webbing, joint contractures, clubfoot, male hypogenitalism, internal malformations uncommon	Coronal	Duplication, long arm, chromosome 13	Distal segment duplication: growth deficiency, mental retardation, hypotonia, seizures, microcephaly, prominent metopic ridge, trigonocephaly, long, upcurving eyelashes, microphthalmia in some instances, stubby nose, long philtrum, highly arched palate, hexadactyly, umbilical hernia, capillary haemangioma; proximal segment duplication: more severe growth deficiency, microcephaly, small mouth, micrognathia, clinodactyly, increase in nuclear projections in granulocytes	Metopic
Deletion, short arm, chromosome 7	Growth deficiency, psychomotor retardation, ocular proptosis, blepharoptosis, downslanting palpebral fissures, short nose, posteriorly angulated ears, transverse palmar creases and genital anomalies	Coronal, metopic			
Duplication, short arm, chromosome 7	Arachnodactyly, clubfoot, hip dislocation, choanal atresia. Phenotype not completely delineated at present	?			

Table 9.2 Master table of syndromes, as compiled by Cohen (1986) (*cont'd*)

Syndrome	Striking features other than craniosynotosis	Cranial suture especially involved	Syndrome	Striking features other than craniosynotosis	Cranial suture especially involved
Duplication, long arm, chromosome 15	Proximal segment duplication: mental deficiency, seizures, downslanting palpebral fissures, strabismus, low-set or posteriorly angulated ears, highly arched palate; duplication from unbalanced 12/15 translocation: cloverleaf skull, other anomalies	Multiple	Idaho syndrome	Scaphocephaly, strabismus, mental deficiency, congenital heart defect, umbilical hernia, complete anterior dislocations of tibia and fibula, talipes equinovarus, comptodactyly of fingers 2–5, deviation of fingers to ulnar side, proximally placed thumbs	Sagittal
Triploidy	Dysplastic calvaria, large posterior fontanelle, ocular hypertelorism, various eye defects from colobomas to micropthalmia, low nasal bridge, micrognathia, low-set malformed ears, syndactyly of the second and third fingers, congenital heart defects, genital anomalies, real anomalies; with dipoid/triploid mosaicism: body asymmetry	Metopic or coronal	Lopez–Hernandez syndrome	Pons–vermis fusion, cerebellar ataxia, trigeminal anaesthesia, parietal alopecia, midface deficiency, low-set posteriorly angulated ears, mental deficiency, short stature	Coronal
Environmentally induced syndromes			Lowry–MacLean syndrome	Microcephaly, seizures, prominent beaked nose, downslanting palpebral fissures, proptosis, glaucoma, cleft palate, delayed dental development, atrial septal defect, eventration of the diaphragm, narrow hyperconvex fingernails	All sutures
Aminopterin syndrome	Hypoplasia of cranial and facial bones, low-set ears, cleft palate, micrognathia, hypodactyly of feet, mild syndactyly of hands	Lambdoid, coronal			
Fetal hydantoin syndrome	Growth deficiency, mental deficiency, microcephaly, short nose, broad depressed nasal bridge, epicanthic folds, mild hypertelorism, ptosis of the eyelids, strabismus, sutural ridging, hypoplasia of nails and distal phalanges, cardiac anomalies, umbilical hernia	Sagittal or coronal	Sakati's syndrome	Turribrachycephaly, disproportionately small face, anomalous ears, patches of alopecia with atrophic skin, short limbs, polysyndactyly of feet, polysyndactyly of hands, congenital heart defect	All sutures
Retinoic acid embryopathy	CNS malformations, especially hydrocephaly, dysplastic calvaria, microtia/anotia, ocular hypertelorism, flat and low nasal bridge, micrognathia, cleft palate, conotruncal heart defects and aortic arch abnormalities, thymic defects	?	Shprintzen–Goldberg syndrome	Dolichocephaly, proptosis, Apert-like palate, micrognathia, abnormal ears, contractures of fifth fingers, clinodactyly of toes, arachnodactyly, diastasis recti, inguinal hernias, mitral valve prolapse, mental deficiency	Sagittal lambdoid
Syndromes of unknown cause			Thanos's syndrome	Exostoses of the skull, epibulbar dermoids, premature exfoliation of deciduous teeth, linear verrucous naevi of neck, scaly patches on hands	Coronal
COH syndrome	Cloverleaf skull, polymicrogyria, absent olfactory tracts and bulbs, duplication of thumbs, micropenis, bifid scrotum	All sutures	Wisconsin syndrome	Mental deficiency, upslanting palpebral fissures, microtia, short fourth metatarsals	Coronal
Hall's syndrome	Turner-like phenotype	Coronal			
Herrmann's syndrome	Microbrachycephaly, mental deficiency, anomalous ears, cleft lip and/or palate, symmetric limb reduction defects with absent finger 4 and 5, short forearms, valgus positioning of hands, ankylosis at knees and varus positioning of feet	Coronal			

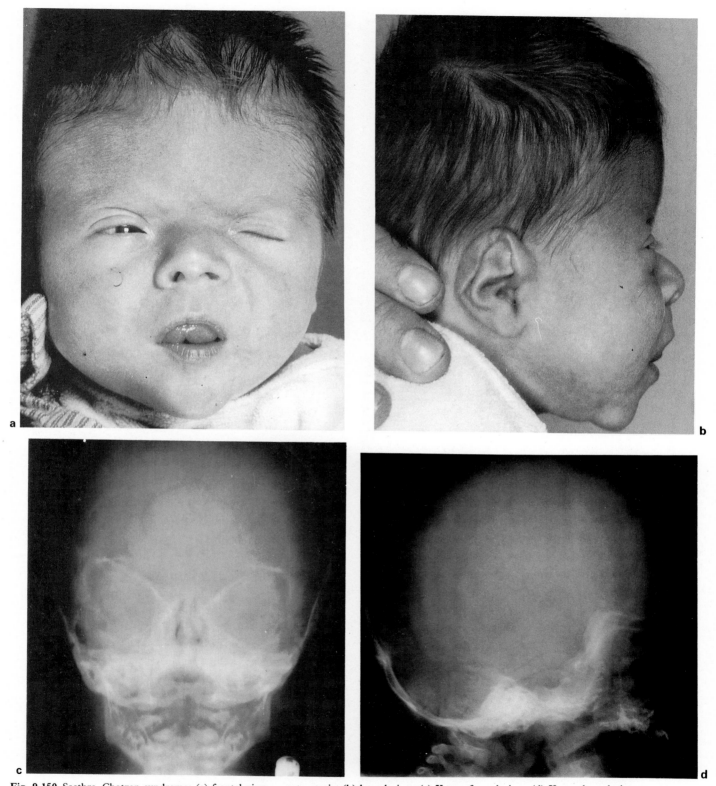

Fig. 9.150 Saethre–Chotzen syndrome: (a) frontal view — note ptosis; (b) lateral view; (c) X-ray, frontal view; (d) X-ray, lateral view.

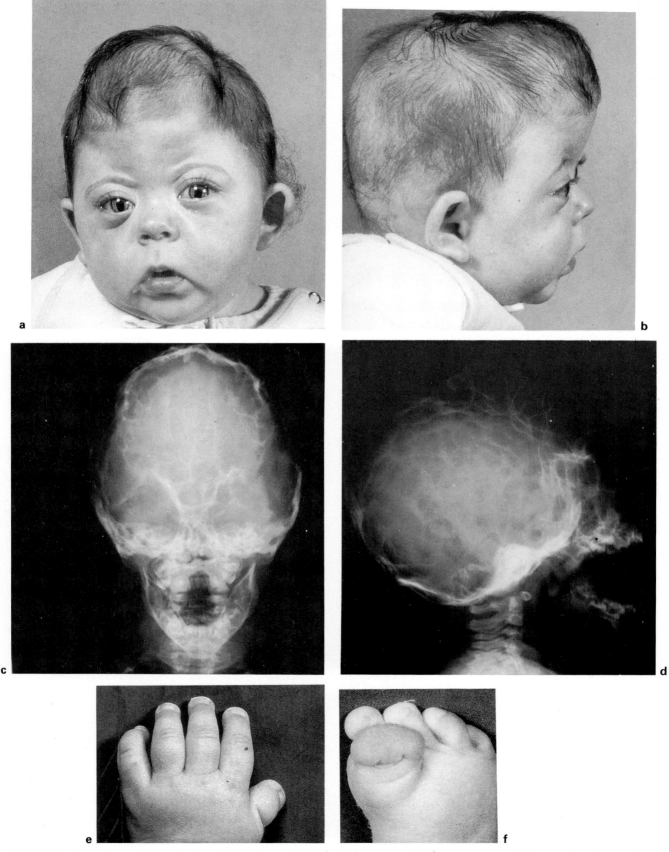

Fig. 9.151 Pfeiffer's syndrome: (a) frontal view; (b) lateral view; (c) X-ray, frontal view; (d) X-ray, lateral view; (e) characteristic abnormality of thumb; (f) characteristic abnormality of big toe.

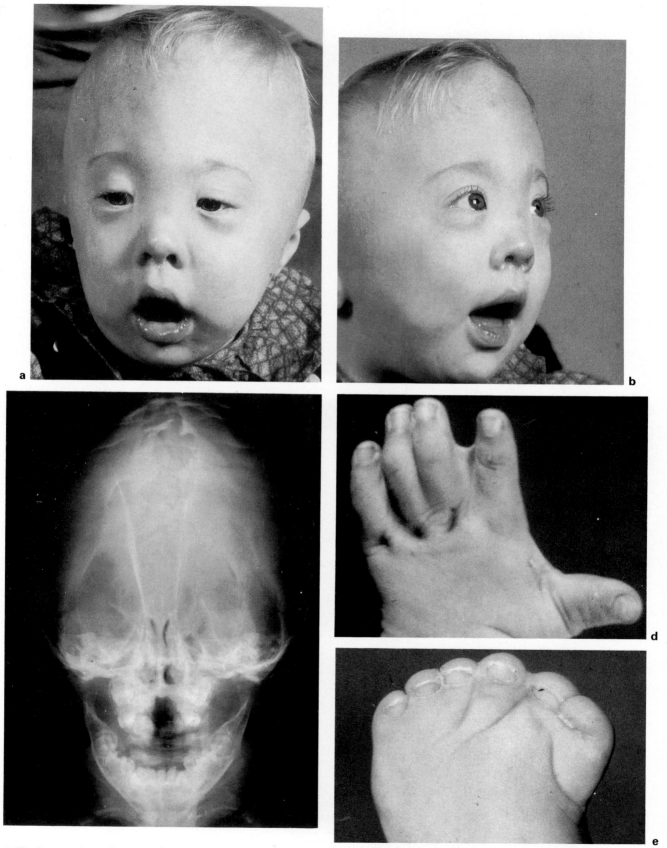

Fig. 9.152 Carpenter's syndrome: (a) frontal view; (b) lateral view; (c) X-ray, frontal view; (d) characteristic abnormalities of hands; (e) characteristic abnormalities of feet.

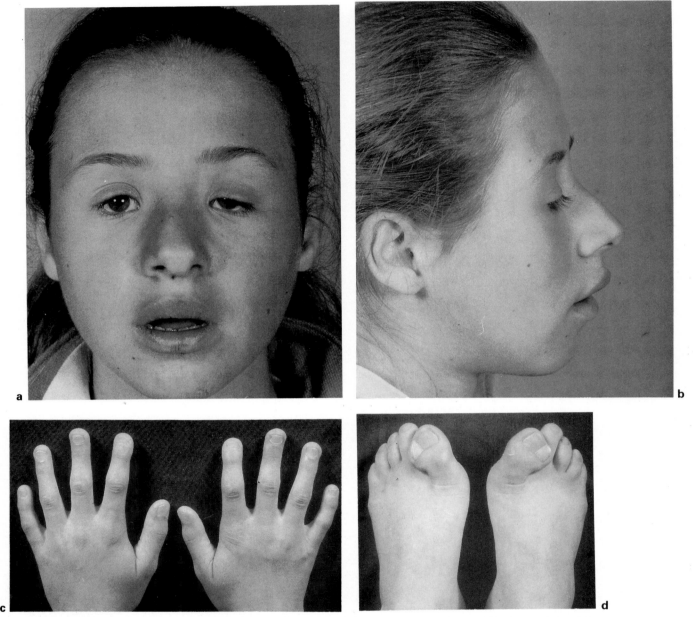

Fig. 9.153 Jackson–Weiss syndrome: (a) frontal view; (b) lateral view; (c) normal hands; (d) characteristic abnormalities of big toes.

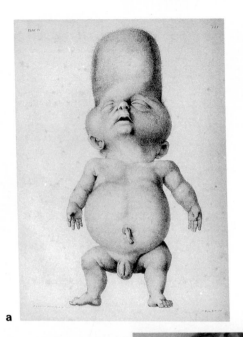

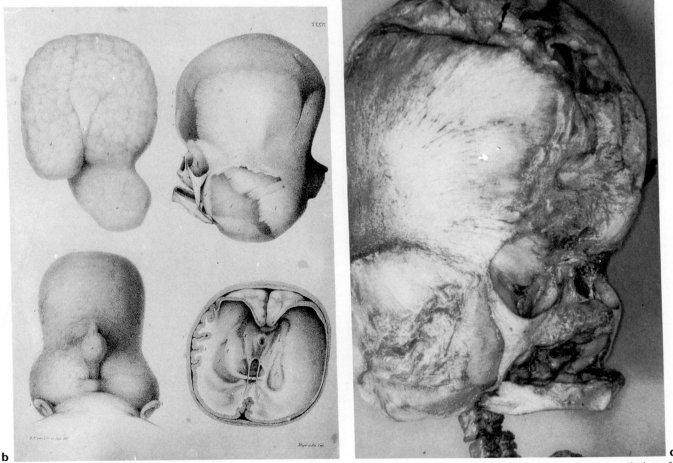

Fig. 9.154 Triphyllocephaly — illustrations from Vrolik's atlas (1849): (a) child with cloverleaf skull; (b) dissection of skull; (c) lateral view of skull now in Vrolik's collection (Leyden).

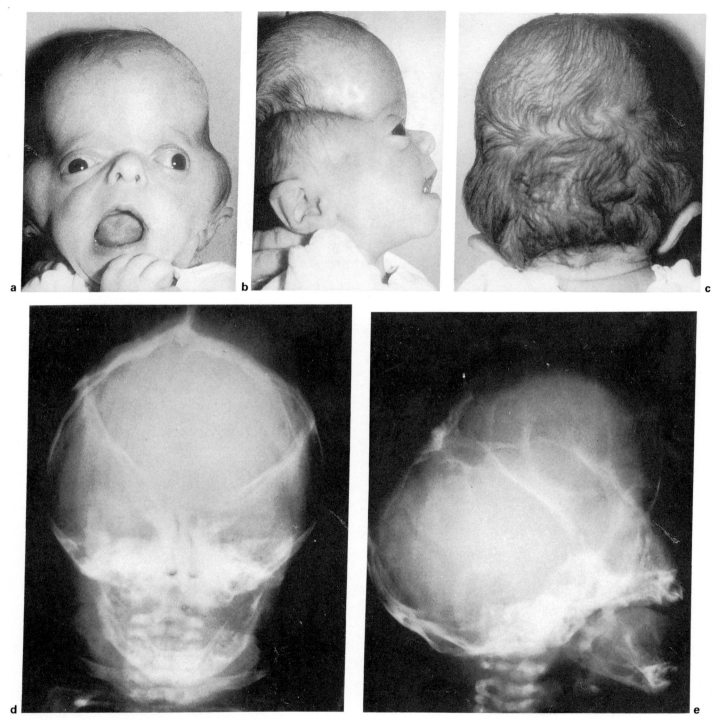

Fig. 9.155 Triphyllocephaly: (a) frontal view; (b) lateral view; (c) occipital view; (d) X-ray, frontal view show typical trilobular configuration; (e) X-ray, lateral view.

region and cutis verticis gyrata has been observed in this area (Warkany 1937). In some cases the veins of the scalp are dilated (Muller & Hoffman 1975).

The face. Retrusion of orbital roof, exorbitism, maxillary retrusion, severe downward displacement of ears and zygomatic arches, antimongoloid slanting, nasal flattening and an arched palate are the main characteristics of this abnormality, which may be observed in different degrees of severity (Fig. 9.156).

Associated malformations

In a case reported by Angle et al (1967), there were abnormalities of the vertebrae. In one of our cases, partial ankylosis of the elbows and vertebral fusion at C6–C7 was observed.

Radiographic features

In frontal views the cranial vault has a trilobed configuration with a lacunar pattern of the occipital and temporal plates. The anterior fontanelle is wide open and there is no evidence of bone over the outer portion of the lobes. The lesser wings of the sphenoid, very oblique and elevated, project at the junction of the superior and inferior lobes.

In lateral views the hourglass appearance tends to be especially pronounced when there is a stricture starting from the depressed occipital eminence and extending forward to the parietotemporal junction. The occiput is flat and the floor of the middle cranial fossa is severely lowered. The squamous parts of the temporal bones are everted and project beyond the aplastic occiput behind.

The lambdoidal and coronal sutures are usually closed. The cranial base shows lordosis with verticalization and shortening of the anterior fossa and aplasia of the orbital cavities.

The spheno-occipital synchondrosis is patent. The posterior cranial fossa is small and the face is hypoplastic.

Functional pathology

Children with this disorder have a marked degree of psychomotor retardation.

Hydrocephalus is always present and usually severe. When it is less marked the dilatation predominantly affects the temporal horns. This is a communicating hydrocephalus or, more rarely, a hydrocephalus related to aquaductal stenosis (one personal case and two cases of Feingold et al 1969). The pathogenesis of the hydrocephalus is controversial and not well defined. According to Angle et al (1967), there is extraventricular obstruction caused by the malformation at the base of the skull and particularly by the small size of the foramen magnum, which may be associated with invagination of the cerebellar tonsils. It will

be recalled that in Berrada's (1963) case there was an associated Arnold–Chiari malformation.

Muller & Hoffman (1975) mentioned the possibility of venous compression due to parieto-occipital aplasia and constriction involving the lateral sinus. In his case there was dilatation of the scalp veins. Resection of the parieto-occipital 'constriction band' appeared to have stabilized the hydrocephalus.

There is no primary cerebral lesion (Angle et al 1967, Holtermuller & Wiedemann 1960, Liebaldt 1964). Postmortem examination of one of our patients who died at the age of 11 days did not disclose any cerebral abnormality. The ventricles were moderately dilated, with the dilatation affecting mainly the temporal horns.

The brain was of normal weight (3320 g) but its shape was profoundly modified by the craniostenosis. There was considerable hypertrophy of the temporal lobes, which attained the sizes of the frontal and occipital lobes.

Pathogenesis

Some authors believe that there is abnormal ossification of the membranous bones, as shown by the lacunar aspect of the vault of the skull (Angle et al 1967). The hypothesis of abnormal enchondral ossification put forward by Burkhard is not in accordance with the fact that the basal synchondroses are normal. According to Partington et al (1971), however, chondrodysplasia may exist in some cases. This author classifies the cases in the literature and his own cases (27 in number) into three groups:

type I, with skeletal lesions, comprising 13 cases with cloverleaf skulls and chondrodysplasia or dwarfism incompatible with life, probably because of associated visceral lesions. Seven of these 13 cases were stillborn, 5 survived for a few days and 1 for 16 weeks. One of our cases was of this type;

type II, with minor skeletal lesions (e.g. ankylosis of the elbow) and a better prognosis. Of the 5 cases studied, 3 were alive at $4\frac{1}{2}$ months, 2 years and 14 years;

type III, with no skeletal lesions. Of 4 cases, 3 were alive at 6 months, 16 months and 8 years.

Thus, type II and type III cloverleaf skulls (a quarter of the total) have a better prognosis, with two-thirds surviving. The karyotype is normal in all cases. The prognosis is poor because of the mental abnormalities, which do not respond to treatment.

CRANIOFACIAL DYSPLASIAS WITH DYSCHONDROSIS

Achondroplasia

Achondrodysplasia, or deficient formation of enchondral bone was recognized as a separate entity by Parrot in 1878.

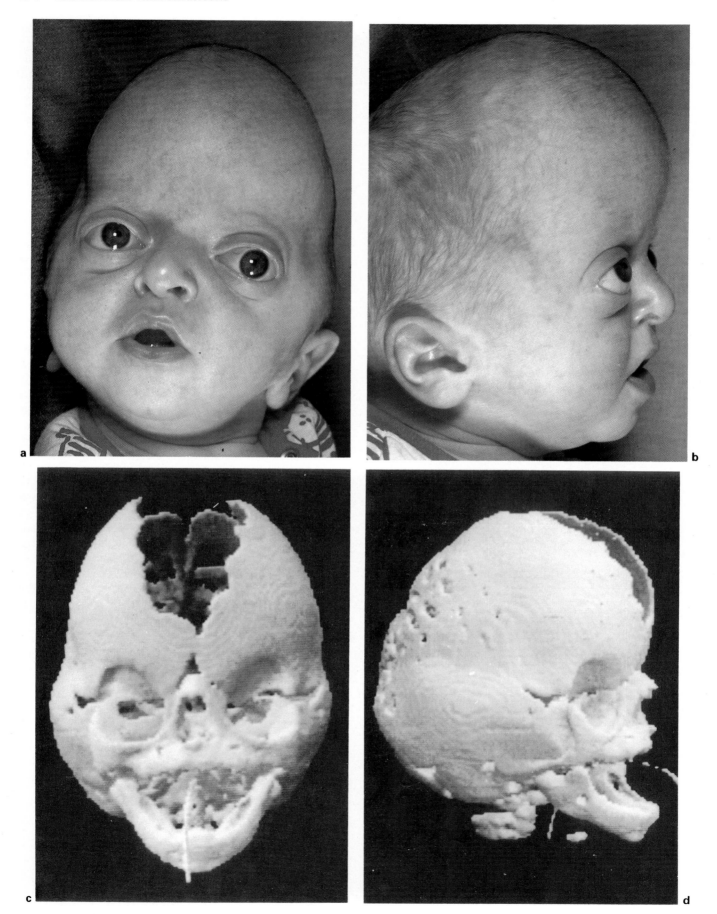

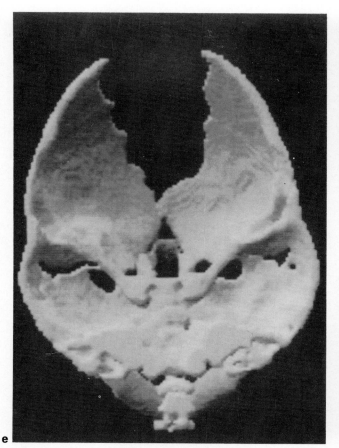

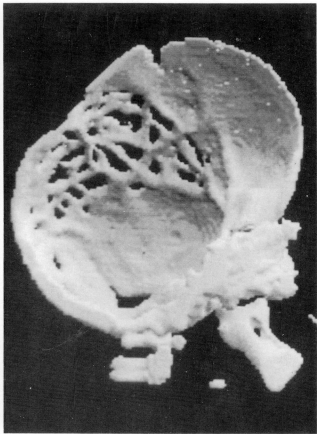

Fig. 9.156 Triphyllocephaly: (a) frontal view; (b) lateral view; (c) 3-D reconstruction, anterior view; (d) 3-D reconstruction, lateral view, (e) 3-D reconstruction, posterior view; (f) 3-D reconstruction, sagittal view.

A detailed description by Pierre Marie appeared in 1880. The disease occurs with an incidence of one in 10 000 live births (Mörch 1941) and is characterized by dwarfism, specific craniofacial dysmorphism, tripod hands and lumbar lordosis.

Familiality is observed in 20% of cases, and transmission is autosomal dominant. Homozygotic individuals are more severely affected. Rimoin et al (1970) have shown that the craniofacial malformations are caused by disturbed cartilaginous growth affecting the chondrocranium.

The skull is voluminous, the vault enlarged with a prominent occiput and a bulging forehead overhanging a small impacted nose. The middle third of the face is short. This is in contrast to the lower third, which is long and protruding. The upper lip is shortened and labial incompetence is associated with buccal respiration. Class III malocclusion is commonly seen.

Radiographic features

Lateral views show a small face suspended from the cranial balloon. The vault is thin and the frontal sinus is expanded. The cranial base is shortened, in particular the clivus, and the basal angle is more acute. Paradoxically, the anterior presellar branch of the basal compass is close to normal.

In a study of the anterior part of the cranial base by Cohen et al (1985) distinction is made between the frontal, the ethmoidal and sphenoidal segment, showing that the alterations predominantly affect the ethmoidal part and the cribriform plate and are partially compensated for by the sphenoid.

The maxilla is retruded and shortened in height. Relative promandibulism is observed.

Differentiation

The typical aspects of midfacial retrusion may be observed in some less severe anomalies. Hypochondroplasia frequently affects the nasomaxillary profile (Fig. 9.157) and must be differentiated from maxillary retrusion seen in Binder's syndrome and dyschondrosis due to trauma or infection (Fig. 9.158).

At present achondroplasia must be distinguished from

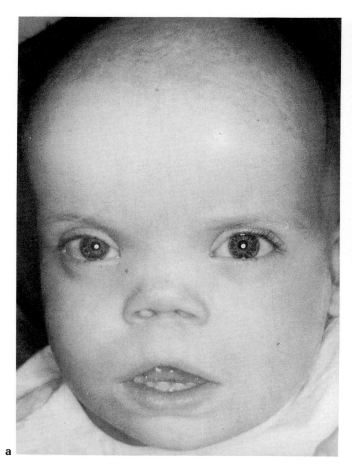

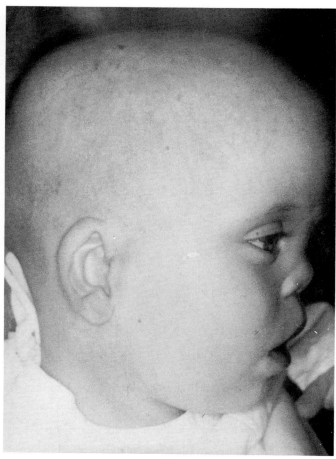

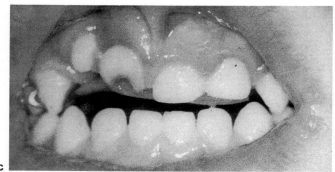

Fig. 9.157 Dyschondroplasia: (a) frontal view — note nasal retrusion; (b) lateral view; (c) oral view; (d) digital abnormalities of hands; (e) digital abnormalities of feet.

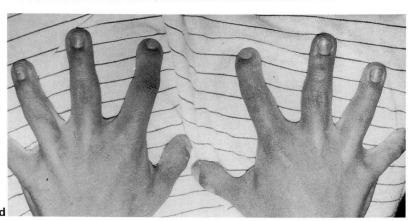

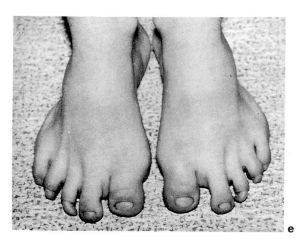

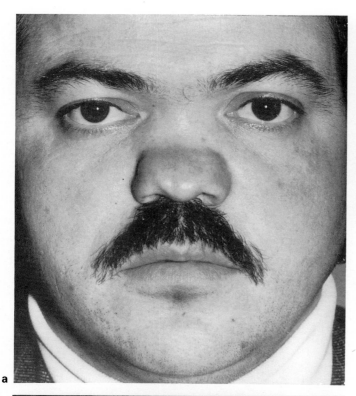

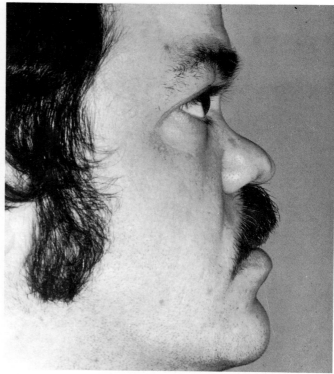

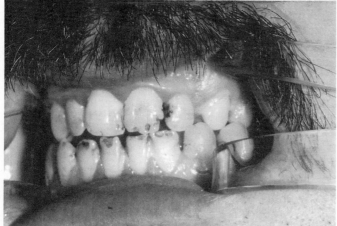

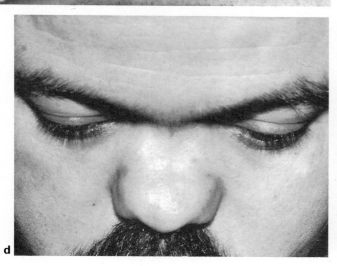

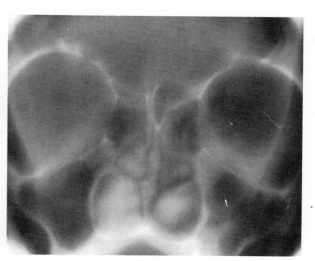

Fig. 9.158 Dyschondrosis — case illustrating diagnostic difficulties: (a) frontal view; (b) lateral view; (c) oral view; (d) superior view; (e) X-ray shows septal abnormality, which may be due to trauma or infection.

the following series of entities: diastrophic dysplasia, thanatophoric dysplasia, Jeune's syndrome, Ellis–van Creveld syndrome and achondrogenesis.

CRANIOFACIAL DYSPLASIAS WITH OTHER ORIGINS

OSSEOUS DYSPLASIAS

Osteopetrosis (Marble bones, Albers–Schönberg disease)

This rare disorder of the skeleton is characterized by thickening of bones, with a change in their normal structure. Recognized as a clinical entity by Albers-Schönberg in 1904, it has later been reported in many instances. The transmission is by autosomal dominant traits. Males and females are equally affected.

There is a striking contrast in body configuration: in fact, in its typical form, patients with osteopetrosis are small and underweight, with a macrocephaly. Frontal and parietal bossing is pronounced: exophthalmos is often present. The sclerotic and compact bone is responsible for narrowing of the cranial nerve foramina, resulting in blindness, strabismus, facial palsy and deafness.

Roentgenograms of osteopetrosis show increased density associated with absence of normal trabecular structure. This characteristic is particularly evident in long bones, where the medullary canal is either reduced or absent. A marked sclerosis of skull bones is a typical feature. Paranasal sinuses are poorly developed. The absence of bone marrow may be associated with severe anaemia.

Craniotubular dysplasia

This disease is represented by a group of genetic bone abnormalities which affect the craniofacial (Fig. 9.159) and tubular bones and is usually first observed in childhood. The craniofacial bones thicken, sometimes becoming rock-hard. Neural compression may result in loss of vision, nystagmus, deafness, peripheral facial nerve palsy, occlusion of the nasolacrimal duct, nasal obstruction and stenosis of the foramen magnum.

The tubular bones may show flaring of the metaphyseal areas, producing the so-called 'Erlen–Meyer flask' deformity and widening and sclerosis of the diaphyseal areas, giving rise to a 'policeman's stick' deformity.

Fibrous dysplasia

This disorder of bone formation answers to the description given by Jaffe (1964): 'fibrous tissue proliferation within the bone'. In the past this condition has frequently been confused with other osseous abnormalities, such as fibrocystic osteitis caused by hyperthyroidism, neurofibromatosis and osteitis fibrosa. The addition of the term 'craniofacial' by Ruppe in 1924 did not increase our knowl-

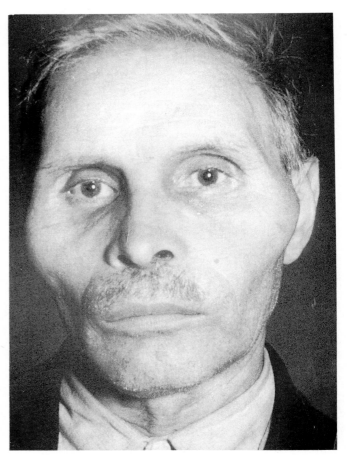

Fig. 9.159 Craniotubular dysplasia.

edge of this abnormality. At present fibrous dysplasia has been recognized as a separate entity, in accordance with the classification which is based on the evolution of the mesenchymal cell and the theory of the skeletoblast of Petrovic.

The disorder is not congenital and is usually first noticed in adolescence. Although it is therefore outside the scope of this book it deserves special mention because of the associated craniofacial deformities (Figs. 9.160, 9.161) (orbital, maxillary or mandibular), the neurological symptoms caused by compression and the craniofacial techniques used for correction.

Radiography may show cyst-like lesions or a more homogeneous 'ground glass' appearance with increased density and calcification.

In its typical form it is benign, although malignant transformation can exceptionally occur, either spontaneously or following imprudent radiotherapy.

CUTANEOUS DYSPLASIAS

Ectodermal dysplasia

These disorders affect a series of ectodermal derivatives, including the teeth, the sweat glands and the adnexa of the

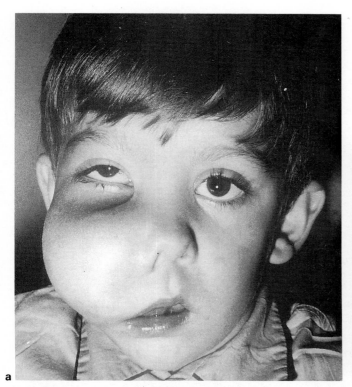

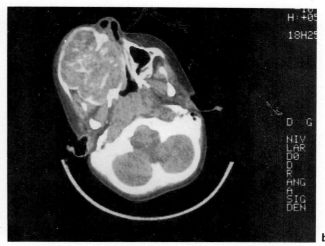

Fig. 9.160 Fibrous dysplasia: (a) frontal view; (b) CT scan shows skeletal abnormalities.

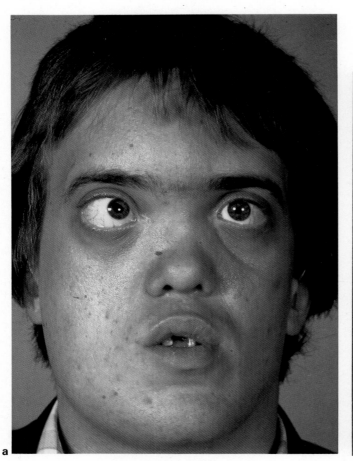

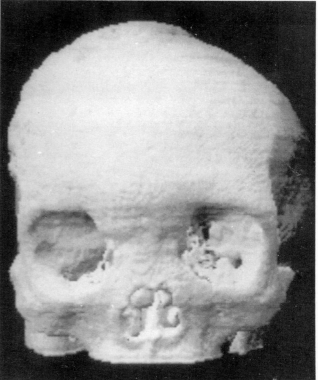

Fig. 9.161 Fibrous dysplasia: (a) frontal view; (b) 3-D reconstruction shows skeletal abnormalities.

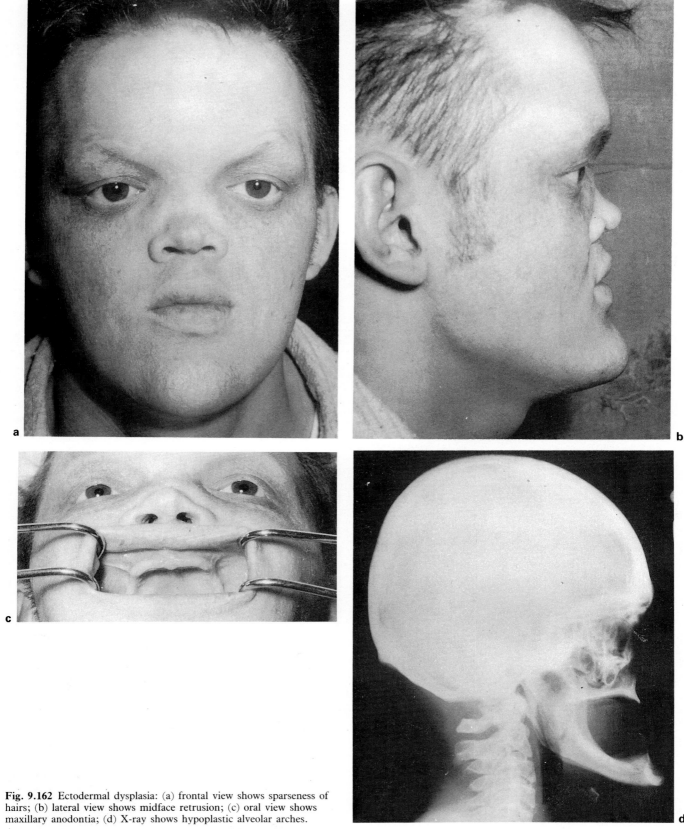

Fig. 9.162 Ectodermal dysplasia: (a) frontal view shows sparseness of hairs; (b) lateral view shows midface retrusion; (c) oral view shows maxillary anodontia; (d) X-ray shows hypoplastic alveolar arches.

skin (nails, hairs, sebaceous glands). Hypodontia, hypotrichosis and hypohidrosis are some of the characteristics. Ectodermal dysplasia (Fig. 9.162) is a typical sex-linked recessive trait. It occurs in males and is transmitted through females.

First described by Thurnan in 1848 the syndrome was later popularized by Touraine (1937). Facial deformities show the following features: the midface is retruded owing to deficient alveolar growth, which lends the face its aged appearance. Jaw and facial development are, however, essentially normal; the forehead is prominent and the nose flattened; the skin is thin and dry with multiple ridges; hairs are scarce and underdeveloped. The senile aspect is aggravated by a certain degree of dwarfism and mental retardation. Teeth disorders are implicated in many syndromes.

NEUROCUTANEOUS DYSPLASIA

Neurofibromatosis

Neurofibromatosis is characterized by neurofibromas or other neural tumours and by focal cutaneous hyperpigmentation (cafe-au-lait spots) caused by aggregation of melanoblasts in the basal layer of the epidermis. These elements, derived from the neural crest, are primarily affected. Mesenchymal elements, in particular the vessels and the skeleton, are secondarily involved. Collagen abnormalities may be observed. Craniofacial deformities occur in approximately 22% of cases. The lesion may be unilateral (Fig. 9.163) or bilateral (Fig. 9.164), diffuse or circumscript.

Skeletal malformations consist of macrocranium, interosseous cysts and perforating defects, expansion of the middle cranial fossa, hypoplasia of the lesser or greater wing of the sphenoid resulting in wide areas of communication between the cranial cavity and the orbit and downward displacement of the zygoma, the maxilla and the mandible on the affected side.

Soft tissue malformations correspond to the territorial pattern of a neurofibroma, which may affect the optic nerve, the trigeminal nerve, the facial nerve, etc. Buphthalmos, exophthalmos and musculocutaneous degeneration resulting in drift of the forehead, the palpebral complex, the nasolabial fold and the oral commissure are the main characteristics.

It is an autosomal dominant trait with full penetrance but variable expressivity. This differential expression is probably not intrinsic to the mutant gene but to local epigenic factors mediated by cellular interaction or to the time of the insult: the earlier, the more severe.

The frequency of neurofibromatosis has been documented as one case per 2500 to 3300 live births.

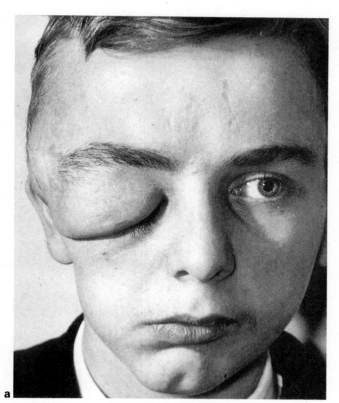

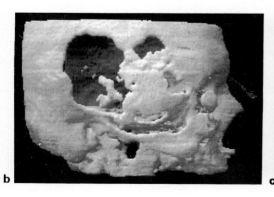

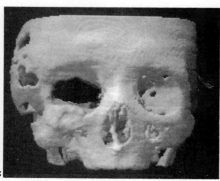

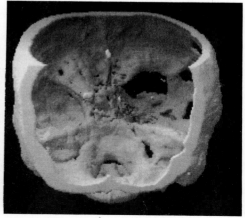

Fig. 9.163 Neurofibromatosis (unilateral): (a) Frontal view; (b) 3-D reconstruction shows defect in orbital roof.

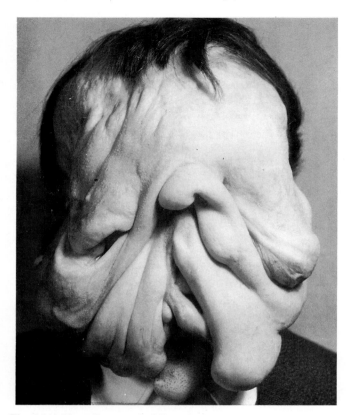

Fig. 9.164 Neurofibromatosis (bilateral).

NEUROMUSCULAR DYSPLASIA

Pierre Robin syndrome

The combination of micro-retromandibulism, glossoptosis, palatal clefting and respiratory troubles observed in the neonate is known as the syndrome of Pierre Robin (1929). It was, however, described previously by St Hilaire in 1832 and Lannelongue & Menard in 1891. To Tandler we owe a precise anatomical description in an autopsy report, published in 1899. Shukowski discussed the aetiology and characteristics of congenital inspiratory stridor in 1911.

Up until now the explanation and treatment of the syndrome have usually been based on mechanical concepts. The pathogenesis is a disturbance of muscular maturation of nervous origin and the syndrome of Robin (Fig. 9.165) therefore belongs to the category of muscular dysmaturations which affects the masticatory muscles, the tongue and the pharyngeal slings.

Swallowing is disturbed and the airway obstructed, resulting in the aspiration of secretion and food. The respiratory difficulties are further increased by the low and posterior position of the tongue.

A lateral radiographic soft tissue view shows the ptotic tongue to be positioned below the mandibular angle, pressing on the epiglottis.

The posterior position of the tongue quite frequently prevents the elevation of the palatal shelves, resulting in a secondary cleft of the palate with varying dimensions. Lingual protrusion is impossible. Clinical inspection shows three crests: mandibular, sublingual and lingual.

Retromandibulism is caused by deficient activity of the pterygoid muscle, which is unable to bring the mandible forward. Spontaneous improvement is common owing to progressive maturation of the affected muscles and after the sixth month the risk of asphyxia has virtually disappeared. It is therefore essential to help the child to pass through this difficult phase.

Mandibular growth is satisfactory in the majority of cases. Retromandibulism is spontaneously corrected and retrogenia disappears. Mandibular malformations are frequently associated with cardiac anomalies, which should be systematically looked for.

The clinical forms of Pierre Robin's syndrome are extremely variable and a frequent source of confusion in the less severe cases. Other mandibular malformations resemble the syndrome but the term Pierre Robin should not be applied when there is no abnormal tongue function. It may, however, be used in the absence of a palatal cleft.

Some authors wrongly distinguish between true and pseudo Robin. The answer to the question 'What is the Pierre Robin syndrome?' must be that the malformation is characterized by a functional disturbance of the tongue which may be associated with a palatal cleft. Neuromuscular deficiency is the causative factor, which is fortunately reversible. Micromandibulism, in contrast, does not represent a particular form of the Pierre Robin syndrome but true 'dysostosis' (see p. 222).

Muscular dysmaturation is also seen in arthrogryposis (Fig. 9.166), a closely related anomaly. This malformation is characterized by multiple joint contractures, muscular atrophy and osseous abnormalities. The causative mechanism, however, also affects the face.

Temporomandibular ankylosis is not uncommon, and suction and swallowing may be disturbed in the first month of life. Muscular rehabilitation with various forms of splinting is indicated to prevent permanent deformities. This goal, however, is not always possible since neuromuscular deficiency is more severe than that observed in Pierre Robin's syndrome.

Möbius syndrome

Congenital paralysis of the mimic muscles (Fig. 9.167) was described by Möbius in 1888. The abnormality results in a motionless face with a characteristic nasolabial grin. Strabismus due to involvement of the VIth cranial nerve may be observed in addition. Sometimes hypoglossia and microstomia too are seen.

Reductive limb anomalies are seen in 50% of the

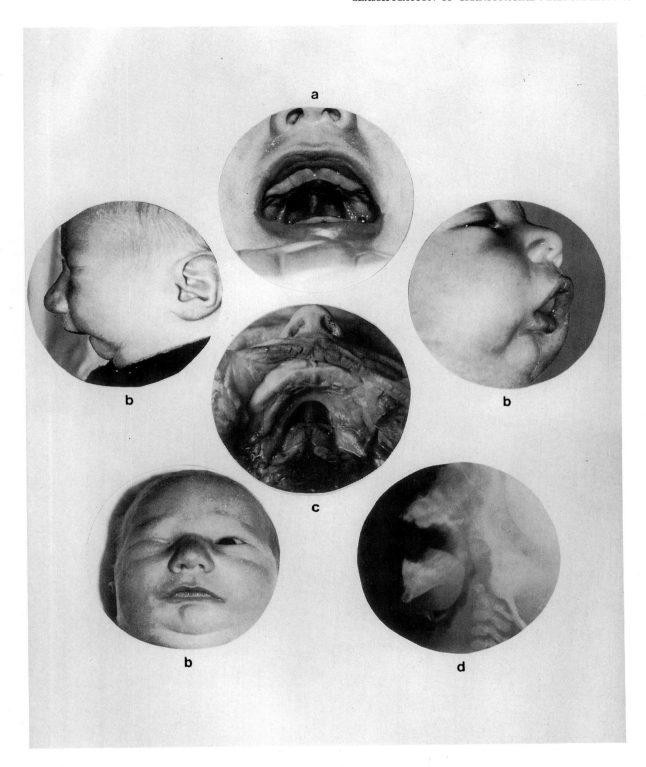

Fig. 9.165 Pierre Robin syndrome: (a) triple crest phenomenon; (b) retromandibulism; (c) glossoptosis and typical palatal defect; (d) X-ray shows low position of the tongue under the gonion.

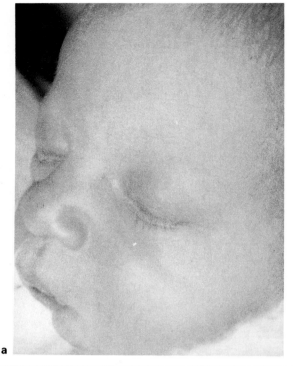

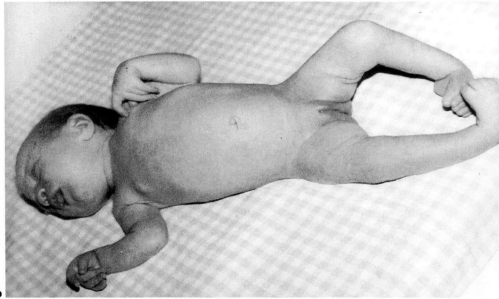

Fig. 9.166 Neuromuscular dysplasia associated with arthrogryposis.

patients. The malformation has its origin in the intracerebral nuclear part of the VIIth and VIth nerves. Facial paralysis is also observed in Charlie M's syndrome (Gorlin 1969), together with hypodontia and hypodactylia.

MUSCULAR DYSPLASIA

In patients with dysostosis, muscles are often modified, but a muscular malformation itself alters this structure in a more specific and quantitative way. The tongue is most commonly affected. It may be split (Fig. 9.168), ankylotic, reduced in size or even absent.

Glossoschizis

Clefting of the tongue in varying degrees of severity and different locations, tongue haematomas, hypertrophic frenula, medial cleft lip, cleft palate and limb anomalies

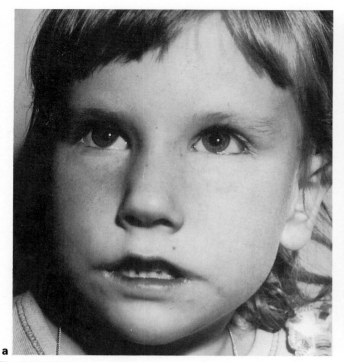
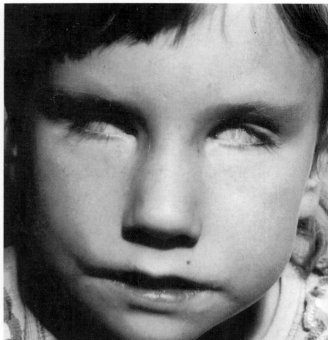

Fig. 9.167 Möbius' syndrome.

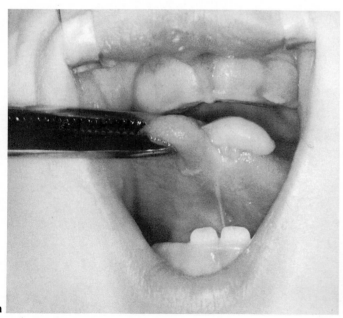
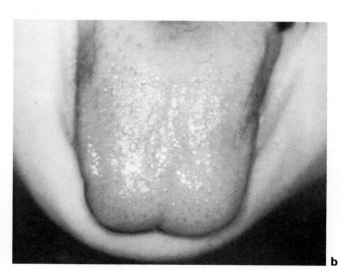

Fig. 9.168 Glossoschizis.

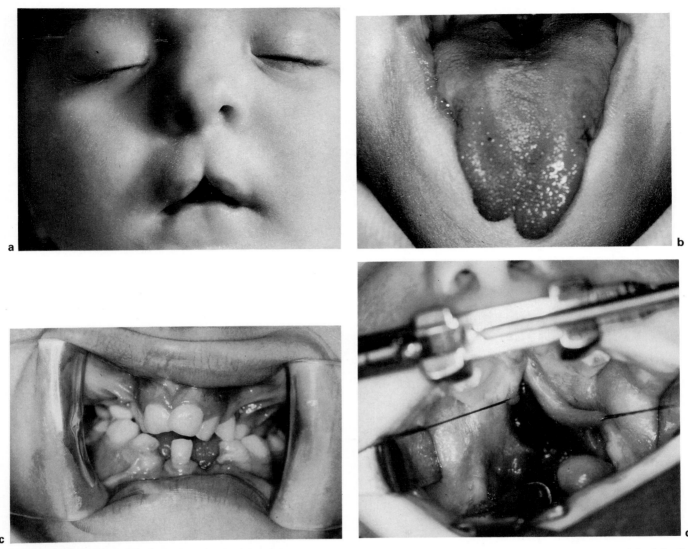

Fig. 9.169 Orofaciodigital syndrome (OFD): (a) median cleft of the lip; (b) glossoschizis; (c) dental abnormalities and frenula; (d) palatal cleft; (e) digital abnormalities.

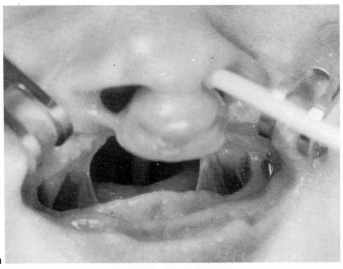

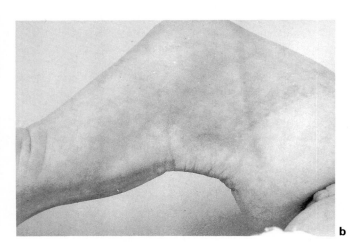

Fig. 9.170 Popliteal web syndrome: (a) ankyloglossia; (b) popliteal web.

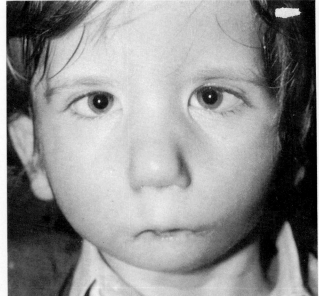

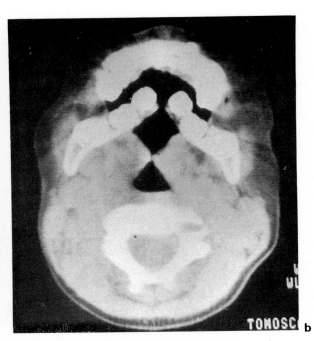

Fig. 9.171 Hanhart's syndrome — note acral and mandibular abnormalities: (a) frontal view; (b) CT scan shows mandibular abnormality; (c) acral abnormalities.

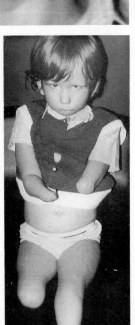

are the main features common to oro-faciodigital syndromes type I and II (OFD$_1$, OFD$_2$) (Fig. 9.169).

OFD$_1$, first described by Papillon-Leage & Psaume in 1954, has X-linked dominant inheritance; it is characterized by teeth anomalies (absence of the lower lateral incisors), anomalies of the oral region associated with unilateral polysyndactily and clinodactyly.

OFD$_2$, first recorded by Mohr in 1941, has autosomal recessive inheritance. Absence of the lower central incisors, bifid nasal tip, bilateral polysyndactyly and duplication of halluces distinguish type II from type I.

Ankyloglossia

This condition refers to a hypoplasia of the anterior third of the tongue (tuberculum impar). The tongue is then blocked within the floor of the mouth. Sometimes a fibrous intraoral band contracts the tongue to the palate (glosso-palatine ankylosis).

Ankyloglossia as a separate entity was first registered by Illera (1887). The presence of ankyloglossia, associated with limb anomalies, was recorded by Kettner in 1907. The combination of ankyloglossia with other craniofacial anomalies, such as fistulas, hypoglossia and cleft lip and palate, is well known. Trelat in 1869 described a case of ankyloglossia associated with popliteal webbing (Fig. 9.170).

Aglossia

De Jussieu (1718) is credited with the first report of a case of aglossia. The condition was recognized by Rosenthal in 1932, who gave the classical description of the association aglossia–adactylia. The mandible is altered and in some cases split along the midline, resembling the jaw of a snake. Hypoglossia must also be looked for in Hanhart's syndrome, which is characterized by the combination of micrognathia and limb anomalies (Fig. 9.171).

Mimic muscles

Absence of a single mimic muscle, in particular the depressor anguli oris, results in a deformity which becomes more apparent when the newborn is crying (asymmetric crying face) (Fig. 9.172). The anomaly is often associated with cardiovascular anomalies (in 50%); hence its name, cardiofacial syndrome (Cayler 1969).

A fibrous circumoral band is observed in the Freeman–Sheldon syndrome (Fig. 9.173), or whistling face deformity, also characterized by 'windmill vane' malformation of the hands.

VASCULAR DYSPLASIA

Vascular malformations are frequently seen in the cephalic extremity. They occur separately or in combination and

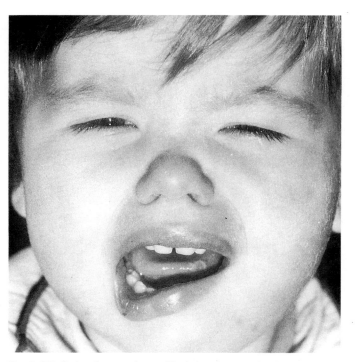

Fig. 9.172 Crying face syndrome (Cayler) — note oral palsy.

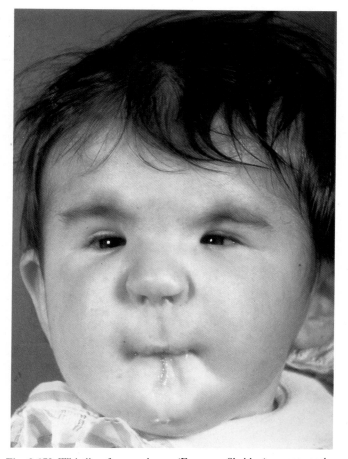

Fig. 9.173 Whistling face syndrome (Freeman–Sheldon) — note oral constriction.

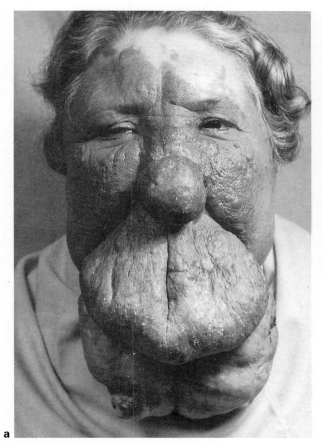
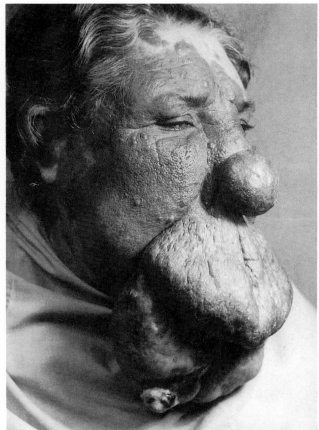

Fig. 9.174 Haemangioma.

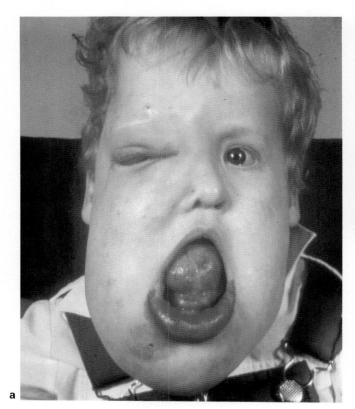
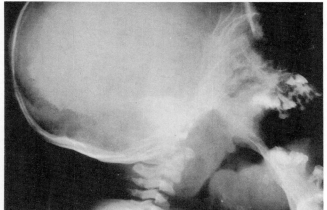

Fig. 9.175 Lymphangioma.

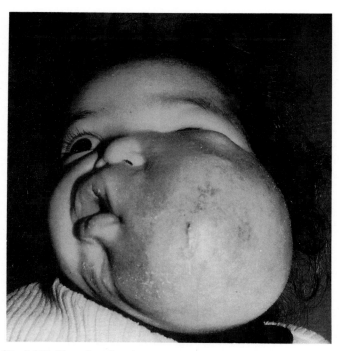

Fig. 9.176 Haemolymphangioma.

affect arteries, veins and lymphatics. The vascular system determines the trophic state and the growth of the irrigated territories. An increase in the flow will therefore result in hypertrophy of both the skeleton and the soft tissues. Craniofacial asymmetries of vascular origin are caused by:

Haemangiomas, with a rapid flow and extensive tissue involvement. These malformations may produce true tumours (Fig. 9.174).

Lymphangiomas, which are most common in the pelvi-buccal region (Fig. 9.175). In these cases the mandible is pushed forward by a dual mechanism: directly by the augmented flow, and indirectly by the thrust of the hypertrophic tongue (macroglossia).

Haemolymphangiomas, which are related to the nervous territories. Both the maxilla and the mandible may become hypertrophic (Fig. 9.176).

Arteriography is essential in these malformations, not only from a diagnostic but also from a surgical point of view, since it allows embolization, frequently indispensable, to be carried out before any surgical procedure is attempted. The correction of bony hypertrophy during the period of growth may finally prove to be quite problematical.

REFERENCES AND BIBLIOGRAPHY

Introduction

Ahlfeld P 1880–1882 Die Missbildungen des Menschen. Grunow, Leipzig

Barsky A J, Kahn S, Simon B E 1964 Principles and practice of plastic surgery, 2nd edn. McGraw-Hill, New York

Bassett C A L, Becker R O 1962 Generation of electrical potential by bone in response to mechanical stress. Science 137: 1063

Burian F 1957 Vzacne vrozene vady obliceje a lebky a jejich. Acta Universitatis Caroliniae, Praha

Davis W B 1935 Congenital deformities of the face. Types found in a series of one thousand cases. Surgery, Gynecology and Obstetrics 61: 201

De Myer W 1967 The median cleft face syndrome. Differential diagnosis of cranium bifidum occultum, hypertelorism and medial cleft nose, lip and palate. Neurology 17: 961

De Myer W 1975 Median facial malformations which predict brain malformations. Birth Defects 22: 155

Duhamel G 1966 Morphogénèse pathologique. Masson, Paris

Fogh-Andersen P 1965 Rare clefts of the face. Acta Chirurgica Scandinavica 129: 275

Gorlin R J, Pindborg J J 1964 Syndrome of the head and neck. McGraw-Hill, New York

Gorlin R J, Pindborg J J, Cohen M M Jr 1976 Syndromes of the Head and Neck, 2nd edn. McGraw-Hill, New York

Greer Walker D 1961 Malformations of the face. Livingstone, Edinburgh

Grünberg K 1909 Die Gesichtsspalten und die zu ihnen in genetischer Beziehung stehend anderweitigen Missbildungen des Gesichtes. In: Schwalbe E (ed) Die Morphologie der Missbildungen des Menschen und der Tiere, Teil III, Abt I. Fisher, Jena. p 113.

Gunther G 1963 Nasomaxillary cleft. Plastic and Reconstructive Surgery 32: 637

Harkins C S, Berlin A, Harding R, Longacre J J, Shodgrasse R 1962 A classification of cleft lip and cleft palate. Plastic and Reconstructive Surgery 29: 31

Holtfreter J 1968 Mesenchyme and epithelia in inductive morphogenetic processes. In: Fleischmajer R, Billingham R E (eds) Epithelial mesenchymal interactions. 18th Hahnemann Symposium Williams & Wilkins, Baltimore. p 1

Karfik V 1966 Proposed classification of rare congenital cleft malformations in the face. Acta Chirurgiae Plasticae 8: 163

Kernahan D A 1957 Types divers de malformations congénitales du nez. Annales de Chirurgie Plastique 2: 115

Mazzola R 1976 Congenital malformations in the frontonasal area: their pathogenesis and classification. Clinics in Plastic Surgery 3: 573

Millard D R 1977 Cleft craft, vol II. Bilateral and rare deformities. Little Brown, Boston p 781

Morian R 1887 Uber die schrage Gesichtsspalten. Archiv fur Klinische Chirurgie 35: 245

Pfeiffer G 1967 Die Entwicklungsstorungen des Gesichtsschadels als Klassifications problem. Deutsche Zahn- Mund- und Kieferheilkunde 48: 22

Pfeiffer G 1974 Systematik und Morphologie der Kraniofazialen Anomalien. Fortschritte der Kiefer und Gesichtschirurgie 18: 1

Scuderi R 1954 Malformazioni congenite del naso, della faringe e del cavo orale. In: Malformazioni congenite in O R L. Atti 43° Congresso Soc Ital Laring Otol e Rinol. Failli, Rome. p 1

Sedano H O, Cohen M M Jr, Jirasek J, Gorlin R J 1970 Frontonasal dysplasia. Journal of Pediatrics 76: 906

Smits-van Prooye A E 1986 Processes involved in normal and abnormal fusion of the neural walls in murine embryos. Thesis, Leidse Universiteit

Soemmering S T 1791 Abbildungen und Beschreibungen einiger Missgeburten. Universitatsbuchhandlung, Mainz

Stupka W 1938 Die Missbildungen und Anomalien der Nase und des Nasenrachnraumes. Springer, Vienna

Taullard J C 1961 El arco de cupido desde el punto de vista embriologico. La Semana Medica 118: 292, 314

Tessier P 1969 Fentes orbito-faciales verticales et obliques (colobomas), complètes et frustes. Annales de Chirurgie Plastique 14: 301

Tessier P 1976 Anatomical classification of facial, cranio-facial and latero-facial clefts. Journal of Maxillo-Facial Surgery 4: 69

Van der Meulen J C, Mazzola R, Vermeij-Keers C, Stricker M, Raphael B 1983 A morphogenetic classification of craniofacial malformations. Plastic and Reconstructive Surgery 71: 560

Vermeij-Keers C, Poelmann R E 1980 The neural crest: a study on cell degeneration and the improbability of cell migration in mouse embryos. Netherlands Journal of Zoology 30: 74

Vermeij-Keers C, Mazzola R, Van der Meulen J C, Stricker M 1983 Cerebrocranial, facial and craniofacial malformations: an embryological analysis. Cleft Palate Journal 20: 128

Virchow R 1857 Untersuchungen uber die Entwicklung der Schadelgruber in gesunden und krankhaften Zustand und uber den Einfuss derselben auf Schadelform, Gesichtsbildung und Gehirnbau. Reimer, Berlin

Warkany J 1971 Congenital malformations. Notes and comments. Year Book Medical Publishers, Chicago. p 594

Whitaker L A, Pashayan H, Reichman J 1981 A proposed new classification of craniofacial anomalies. Cleft Palate Journal 18: 161–176

Wolff J 1892 Das Gesetz der transformation der Knochen. Hirschwald, Berlin

Zausch F 1926 Die angeborenen Missbildungen und Formheler der Nase. In: Denker A, Kahler O (eds) Handbuch der Hals-Nasen-Ohrenheilkunde. Mit Einschluss der Grenzgebiete, vol 2 Springer, Berlin.p 354

Cerebrocranial dysplasias

Geoffroy St Hilaire I. 1832 Histoire générale et particulière des anomalies en l'organisation chez l'homme et les animaux . . . ou traité de tératologie. Baillière, Paris

Lannelongue O M 1890 De la craniectomie dans la microcephalie. Comptes Rendus des Seances de l'Academie des Sciences 110: 1382

Vogel F S, McClenahan J 1952 Anomalies of major cerebral arteries associated with congenital malformations and the brain. American Journal of Pathology 28: 701

Willus quoted by Stringaris M G 1929 Mikrencephalia. Ein beitrag 'zur Lehre und Kasuistik der Missbildungen. Zeitschrift fur Pathologic 37: 396

Cerebrofacial dysplasias

RHINENCEPHALIC DYSPLASIA

Bartholinus Th 1654 Historiarum Anatomicarum Rariorum. Hauboldt, Copenhagen. p 41

Binder K H 1962 Dysostosis maxillo-nasalis ein arhinen cephaler Missbildungscomplex. Deutsche Zahnarztliche Zeitschrift 17: 438

Cohen M M Jr 1982 An update on the holoprosencephalic disorders. Journal of Pediatrics 101: 865

Currarino G, Silvermann F N 1960 Orbital hypotelorism, arhinencephaly and trigonocephaly. Radiology 74: 206–217

De Myer W 1975 Median facial malformations and their implications for brain malformations. Birth defects: original article series, vol XI, no 7. 155–181, National Foundation

De Myer W, Zeman W 1963 A lobar holoprosencephaly (arhinencephaly) with median cleft lip and palate: clinical, electroencephalographic and nosologic considerations. Confinia Neurol 23: 1

De Myer W, Zeman W, Palmer C G 1963 Familiar alobar holoprosencephaly (arhinencephaly) with median cleft lip and palate. Neurology 13: 913

Duhamel B 1966 Morphogenese pathologique. Maisson, Paris

Fitz C R 1983 Holoprosencephaly and related entities. Neuroradiology 25: 225

Haller A 1768 Opuscula anatomici argumenti minorum, vol III. De monstris. Grasset, Lausanne

Koelliker Th1882 Uber das os intermaxillare des Menschen und die Anatomie der Hasenscharte und des Wolfrachens. Blochmann, Halle

Kundrat H 1882 Arhinencephalie als typische Art von Missbildung. Leuschner & Lubensky, Graz

Mazzola R F 1976 Congenital malformations in the frontonasal area:
their pathogenesis and classification. Clinics in Plastic Surgery 3: 573

Raddatz E J 1829 De cyclopia. Dissertatio inauguralis. Petschil, Berlin

Renner K 1889 Uber einen Fall von Cyclopie. Thesis. Halle

Riviera T 1793 Storia di un monocolo con alune reflessioni. Tomaso, Bologna

Schwalbe E, Josephy H 1909 Die cyclopie. In: Schwalbe E (ed) Die Morphologie der Missbildungen des Menschen und der Tiere, vol 3, Part I. Fischer, Jena. p 205

Soemmering S T 1791 Abbildungen und Beschreibungen einiger Missgeburten. Universitatsbuchhandlung, Mainz

Speer K 1819 De cyclopia. Halle

Vrolik W 1849 Tabulae ad illustrandam embryogenesis hominis et mammalium, tab 53–57. Londonck, Amsterdam

Yakovlev P I 1959 Pathoarchitectonic studies of cerebral malformations. III: Arrhinencephalies (hototelencephalies). Journal of Neurolathology and Experimental Neurology 18: 22

OCULO-ORBITAL DYSPLASIA

Ashley L M 1947 Bilateral anophthalmus in a brother and sister. Journal of Heredity 174

Avizonis P 1928 Uber Kryptopthalmus congenitus. Zeitschrift fur Augenheilkunde 64: 240

Azevedo E S, Biondi J, Ramalho L M 1973 Cryptophthalmus in two families from Bahia. Brazilian Journal of Medical Genetics 10: 389

Blessig E 1900 Fall einer seltenen Missbildung der Augen. Klinische Monatsblatter fur Augenheileunde 38: 652

Coover D H 1910 Two cases of cryptophthalmia. Ophthalmoscopy 8: 259

Dinno N D 1974 Edwards W C, Weiskopf B 1974 The cryptophthalmos-syndactyly syndrome Clinical Pediatrics 13: 219

Duke Elder S 1964 System of ophthalmology, vol III. Normal and abnormal development, parts 1 and 2. Kimpton, London

Ehlers N 1966 Cryptophthalmos with orbito-palpebral cyst and microphthalmos. Acta Ophthalmologica 44: 84

Ellsworth R M 1967 Orbital growth. In: Smith B, Converse J M (eds) Plastic and reconstructive surgery of the eye and adnexa. Mosby, St Louis

Franceschetti A, Klein D 1954 Dypmorphie cervico-oculofaciale avec surdite familiale. Journal de Genetique Humaine 3: 176

Francois J 1965 Syndrome malformatif avec cryptophthalmie. Ophthalmologica 150: 215

Francois J, Bacskulin J 1969 External congenital fistulae of the lacrimal sac. Ophthalmologica 159: 249

Francois J, Haustrate L 1954 Anomalies colobomateuses du globe oculaire et syndrome du premier arc. Annales d' Ocul: 187: 340

Goldberg H G 1912 Cryptophthalmos: congenital ankyloblepharon. Ophthalmic Record 21: 200

Goldenhar M 1952 Associations malformations de l'oeil et de l'oreille en particulier le syndrome dermoide epibulbaire — appendices auriculaires — fistula auris congenita et ses relations. Journal de Genetique Humaine 1: 243

Gupta S P, Saxena R C 1962 Cryptophthalmos. British Journal of Ophthalmology 46: 629

Gutman A 1909 Einseitiger Kryptophthalmus. Zentralblatt fur Praktische Augenheilkunde 33: 264

Hallerman W 1948 Vogelgesicht und Cataracta congenita. Klinische Monatsblatter fur Augenheilkunde 113: 315

Ide C H, Wollschlaeger P B 1969 Multiple congenital abnormalities associated with cryptophthalmia. Archives of Ophthalmology 81: 638

Key S N 1920 Report of a case of cryptopthalmia. American Journal of Ophthalmology 3: 684

Levine R S 1984 Powers T, Rosenberg H K et al 1984 The cryptophthalmos syndrome. American Roentgen Ray Society 143: 375

Lohmann W 1920 Beitrag zur Kenntnis des reinen Mikrophthalmus Archiv fur Augenheilkdunde 86: 136

Lurie I W, Cherstvoy E D 1984 Renal agenesis as a diagnostic feature of the cryptophthalmos–syndactyly syndrome. Clinical Genetics 25: 528

Magruder A G 1921 Cryptophthalmus. American Journal of Ophthalmology 4: 48

Meyer-Schwickerath G et al 1957 Mikrophthalmussyndrome. Klinische Monatsblatter fur Augenheilkunde 131: 18–30

Momma W G, Biermann B 1977 Cryptophthalmos: symptoms and treatment of a rare deformity, a case report. Journal of Maxillofacial Surgery 5: 208

Muthayya R E, Ramalingham T T 1949 Report of a case of bilateral cryptophthalmos. Proceedings of the All-India Ophthalmological Society 10: 81

Pflüger E 1872 Ein Fall von Colobom der Lider. Klinische Monatsblalfer fur Augenheilkunde 10: 250

Pichler A 1911 Traenennasengang und schraege Gesichtsspalte. Archiv fur Augenheilkunde 68: 172

Rochat G 1936 A contribution to the study of anophthalmia with description of a case. British Journal of Ophthalmology 28: 429

Schönenberg H 1973 Kryptophthalmus-Syndrom. Klinische Padiatrie 185: 165

Sinclair W 1918 A case of cryptophthalmos. Transactions of the Ophthalmological Societies of the UK 38: 142

Streiff E B 1950 Dysmorphie mandibulo-faciale (tete d'oiseau) et alterations oculaires. Ophthalmologica 120

Sugar H S 1968 The cryptophthalmos–syndactyly syndrome. American Journal of Ophthalmology 66: 879

Ulrich O, Fremerey-Dohna H 1953 Dyskephalie mit Cataracta congenita und Hypotrichose als typischer Merkmalskomplex. Ophthalmologica 125: 73

Urrets-Zavalia A, Solares-Zamora J, Olmos H R 1961 Anthropological studies on the nature of cyclovertical squint. British Journal of Ophthalmology 45: 578

Waring G O, Shields J A 1975 Partial unilateral cryptophthalmos with syndactyly, brachycephaly and anomalies. American Journal of Ophthalmology 79: 437

Weyers H, Thier C J 1958 Malformations mandibulo-faciales et delimitation d'un 'syndrome oculo-vertebral' Journal de Genetique Humaine 7: 143–173

Whitaker L A, Katowitz J A, Randall P 1974 The nasolacrimal apparatus in congenital facial anomalies. Journal of Maxillofacial Surgery 2: 59–63

Wildervanck L S 1960 Een cervico-oculo-acusticus syndrome. Nederlands Tijdschrift voor Geneeskunde 104: 52

Zehender W, Ackermann E, Manz K 1872 Eine Missbildung mit hautüberzogenen Augen order Kryptophthalmus. Klinische Monatsblatter Augenheilkunde 10: 225–234

Zinn S 1955 Cryptophthalmia. American Journal of Ophthalmology 40: 219

PERIOCULAR DYSPLASIA

Davidson 1875 Large coloboma of the upper eyelid. Medical Times and Gazette 50: 169

De Graefe 1858 Ein fall von Colobom beider Lider, der Nase und der Lippe. Archiv fur Ophthalmologie 4: 269

De Wecker L 1869 Beitrag zur congenitalen Spaltbildungen der Lider. Archiv fur Augenheilkunde und Ohrenheilkunde 1: 126

Gillette V 1873 Coloboma des yeux paupières supérieures. Union Médicale 60

Horner F 1864 Colobom des Augenlids. Zahlreiche Dermoidgeschwülste. Klinische Monatsblatter fur Augenheilkunde 1864: 190

Mayor 1808 Sur quelques maladies des yeux. Thesis, Montpellier. p 11

Seely 1871 A case of congenital fissure of the lids. Transactions of the American Ophthalmological Society 1871: 144

Talko J 1875 Zwei Fälle von congenitalen Coloboma palpebrarum. Klinische Monatsblatter fur Augenheilkunde 1875: 202

Tower P 1953 Coloboma of lower lid and choroid, with facial defects and deformity of hand and forearm. Archives of Ophthalmology 50: 333

Whitaker L A, Katowitz J A, Jacobs W E 1979 Ocular adnexal problems in craniofacial deformities. Journal of Maxillofacial Surgery 7: 55

Craniofacial dysplasias with clefting

INTERMAXILLARY AND MEDIO-NASO MAXILLARY CLEFTING (CLEFT LIP AND PALATE)

David J S, and Ritchie H P 1922 Classification of congenital clefts of the lip and palate. Journal of the American Medical Association 70: 1323

Fogh-Andersen P 1942 Inheritance of harelip and cleft palate. Busck, Copenhagen

Grabb W C, Rosenstein S W, Bzoch K R 1971 Cleft lip and palate. Surgical, dental and speech aspects. Little Brown, Boston

Harkins C S, Berlin A, Harding R, Longacre J J, Snodgrass R A 1962 A classification of cleft lip and cleft palate. Plastic and Reconstructive Surgery 29: 31

Kernahan D A 1973 On cleft lip and palate classification. Plastic and Reconstructive Surgery 51: 578

Kernahan D A, Stark R B 1958 A new classification for cleft lip and cleft palate. Plastic and Reconstructive Surgery 22: 435

Millard D R Jr 1976–1980 Cleft craft. The evolution of its surgery, vols 1–3. Little Brown, Boston

Ross R B, Johnston M C 1972 Cleft lip and palate. William & Wilkins, Baltimore. p 319

Stark R B 1954 The pathogenesis of harelip and cleft palate. Plastic and Reconstructive Surgery 13: 20

Veau V 1931 Division palatine. Masson, Paris. p 568

von Ammon F A 1842 De angeborenen chirurgischen Krankheiten des Menschen. Herbig, Berlin

MACROSTOMIA

Ahlfeld F 1875 Beitrage zur Lehre von der Zwillingen. Archiv fur Gynakologie 7: 210–286

Ballantyne J W 1895 Preauricular Appendages. Teratologia 2: 18–36

Benavent W J, Ramos-Oller A 1958 Micrognathia: report of twelve cases. Plastic and Reconstructional Surgery 22: 486–490

Blackfield H M, Wilde N J 1950 Lateral facial clefts. Plastic and Reconstructional Surgery 6: 62–78

Boo-Chai K 1969 The transverse facial cleft: its repair. British Journal of Plastic Surgery 22: 119–124

Clifford R H 1949 Unilateral macrostomia: case report. Annals of Surgery 130: 1098

Davies J 1949 Two cases of macrostomia described with some observations on the incidence of defective development of the mandibular arch in the sheep. British Dental Journal 86: 217–225

Davis W B 1935 Congenital deformities of the face. Types found in a series of one thousand cases. Surgery, Gynecology and Obstetrics 61: 201

Edington G H 1909 Macrostomia associated with clefts of soft palate. Glasgow Medical Journal 71: 338–341

Fergusson W 1857 A system of practical surgery, 4th edn. London. p 574

Fogh-Andersen P 1965 Rare clefts of the face. Acta Chirurgica Scandinavica 129: 275

Grabb W C 1965 The first and second branchial arch syndrome. Plastic and Reconstructive Surgery 36: 485

Grunberg K 1909 Die Gesichtsspalten und die zu ihnen in genetischer Beziehung stehend anderweitigen Missbildungen des Gesichtes. In: Schwalbe E (ed) Die Morphologie der Missbildungen des Menschen und der Tiere, Teil III, Abt I. Fischer, Jena. p 113

Kazanjian V H 1939 Congenital absence of the ramus of the mandible. Journal of Bone and Joint Surgery 21: 761

Keith A 1940 Concerning the origin and nature of certain malformations of the face, head and foot. British Journal of Surgery 28: 173–192

Mansfield O T, Herbert D C 1972 Unilat transverse facial cleft — a method of surgical suture. British Journal of Plastic Surgery 25: 29

May H 1962 Transverse facial clefts and their repair. Plastic and Reconstructive Surgery 29: 240–249

Meyer C 1835 De fissuris hominis mammaliumque congenitis. Accedit fissurace buccalis congenitae descriptio. Sittenfeld, Berlin

Morgan J 1882 Two cases of congenital macrostomia accompanied by malformation of the auricles and by the presence of auricular appendices. Medico-Chirurgical Transactions 65: 13

Otto A W 1841 Monstrorum sexcentorum descriptio anatomica. Hirt, Wratislaw

Pitanguy I, Franco T 1967 Nonoperated facial fissures in adults. Plastic and Reconstructive Surgery 39: 569

Popescu V 1968 Congenital transverse facial clefts. Stomatologia 15: 75

Powell W J, Jenkins H P 1968 Transverse facial clefts. Plastic and Reconstructive Surgery 42: 454–459

Ryshton M A, Walder F A 1936 Unilateral secondary facial clefts with excess tooth and bone formation. Proceedings of the Royal Society of Medicine 30: 79–82

Stark R B, Saunders D E 1962 The first branchial syndrome. The oralmandibular–auricular syndrome. Plastic and Reconstructive Surgery 29: 229

Craniofacial dysplasias with dysostosis

SPHENOIDAL DYSPLASIA

Baker M C 1953 Congenital atresia of posterior nares. Archives of Otolaryngology 58: 431

Blasberg B, Stool S, Oka S 1975 Choanal atresia. A cryptic congenital anomaly. Cleft Palate Journal 12: 409

Craig D H, Simpson N M 1959 Posterior choanal atresia with a report of ten cases. Journal of Laryngology and Otology 73: 603

Evans J N G, McLachlan R F 1971 Choanal atresia. Journal of Laryngology and Otology 85: 903

Flake C G, Ferguson C F 1964 Congenital choanal atresia in infants and children. Annals of Otology, Rhinology and Laryngology 73: 459

Freng A 1978 Congenital choanal atresia. Etiology, morphology and diagnosis in 82 cases. Scandinavian Journal of Plastic and Reconstructive Surgery 12: 261

Pracy R 1969 Posterior choanal atresia. In: Rickham P P, Johnston J H (eds) Neonatal surgery. Butterworths, London. p 145

Schwarz A A, Isaacs M J 1942 Congenital atresia of the posterior nares. Report of two cases. Archives of Otology 35: 603

Schwendt A 1889 Die angeborenen Verschlusse der hinteren Nasenoffnungen. Werner-Riehm, Basel

Singleton G T, Hardcastle B 1968 Congenital choanal atresia. Archives of Otolaryngology 87: 620

Stupka W 1938 Die Missbildungen und Anomalien der Nase und des Nasenrachenraumes. Springer, Vienna. p 154

Theogaraj S D, Hoehn J G, Hagan K F 1983 Practical management of congenital choanal atresia. Plastic and Reconstructive Surgery 72: 634

Wilson C P 1957 Treatment of choanal atresia. Journal of Laryngology and Otology 71: 616

SPHENO-FRONTO-NASOETHMOIDAL DYSPLASIA

Berliner M, Gartner, S 1940 Hypertelorism. Archives of Ophthalmology 24: 691

Blumenfeld R, Skolnik E M 1965 Intranasal encephaloceles. Archives of Otolaryngology 82: 527–531

Bojlen K, and Brems T 1938 Hypertelorism (Greig). Acta Pathologica Microbiologica Scandinavica 15: 217

Callister A 1943 Hypertelorism with facies bovinia. Rocky Mountain Medical Journal 40: 36

Cameron J 1931 Interorbital width. New cranial dimension. American Journal of Physical Anthropology 15: 509

Cardano H 1658 Metoposcopia. Jolly, Paris

Charoonsmith T, Suwanwela C 1974 Frontoethmoidal encephalomeningocele with special reference to plastic reconstruction. Clinics in Plastic Surgery 1: 27

Cockayne E A 1925 Hypertelorism. British Journal of Childhood Disorders 22: 265

Cohen M 1927 Orbital meningo-encephalocele associated with microphthalmia. Journal of the American Association 89: 746–749

Converse, J M, Ransohoff J, Mathews E S et al 1970 Ocular hypertelorism and pseudohypertelorism. Plastic and Reconstructive Surgery 45: 1

Costaras M, Pruzansky S 1982 Hypertelorism — pathogenetic mechanisms. Journal of Craniofacial Genetics and Developmental Biology 2: 19

Costaras M, Pruzansky S, Broadbent B H Jr 1982 Bony interorbital distance (BIOD), head size and level of the cribriform plate relative to orbital height: I. Normal standards for age and sex. Journal of Craniofacial Genetics and Developmental Biology 2: 5

Danoff D, Serbu J, French L A 1966 Encephalocele extending into the sphenoid sinus: report of a case. Journal of Neurosurgery 24: 684–686

David D J, Sheffield L, Simpson D, White J 1984 Fronto-ethmoidal meningo-encephaloceles: morphology and treatment. British Journal of Plastic Surgery 37: 271

Davis C Jr, Alexander E Jr 1959 Congenital nasofrontal encephalomeningoceles and teratomas. Journal of Neurosurgery 16: 365

della Porta G B 1586 De humana physiognomonia. Cacchio, Vico Equense

Fenger C 1895 Basal hernias of the brain. American Journal of Medical Science 109: 1–17

Finerman W B, Pick E I 1953 Intranasal encephalo-meningocele. Annals of Otology 62: 114–120

Fridolin J 1885 Studien ueber fruehzeitige Schaedel difformitaeten. Virschows Archiv Abteilung C 1885: 270

Friede R 1954 Über physiologische Euryopie und pathologischen Hypertelorismus Ocularis. Archives of Ophthalmology 155: 359

Gaard R 1961 Ocular hypertelorism of Greig: a congenital craniofacial deformity. American Journal of Orthodontics 47: 205

Gisselsson L 1947 Intranasal forms of encephalo-meningocele. Acta Oto-Laryngologica 35: 519–531

Gorlin R J, Pindborg J J, Cohen M M Jr 1964 Syndromes of the head and neck, second edition. McGraw-Hill, New York

Greer Walker D 1961 Malformations of the face. Livingstone, Edinburgh

Greig D M 1924 Hypertelorism: a hitherto undifferentiated congenital craniofacial deformity. Edinburgh Medical Journal 31: 560

Griffith B 1976 Frontonasal tumors: their diagnosis and treatment. Plastic and Reconstructive Surgery 57: 692

Gross H 1956 Der hypertelorismus. Ophthalmologica 131: 137

Günther H 1933a Hypertelorismus. Endokrinologie 13: 61–72

Günther H 1933b Konstitutionelle anomalien des augenabstandes und des interorbitalbreite. Virschows Archiv Abteilung A 290: 373

Hansman C F 1966 Growth of interorbital distance and skull thickness as observed in roentgenographic measurements. Radiology 86: 87

Ingraham F D, Matson D D 1943 Spina bifida and cranium bifidum IV. An unusual nasopharyngeal encephalocele. New England Journal of Medicine 228: 815

Johr P 1953 Tableaux de mensurations des distances oculaires et craniennes. Journal de Genetique Humaine 2: 247

Kahn E A, Crosby E C, Schneider R C et al 1969 Correlative neurosurgery, 2nd edn. Springfield. Thomas, pp 416–418

Kawamoto H K 1976 The kaleidoscopic world of rare craniofacial clefts. Order out of chaos (Tessier classification). Clinics in Plastic Surgery 3: 529

Laestadius N D, Aase J M, Smith D W 1969 Normal inner canthal and outer orbital dimensions. Journal of Pediatrics 74: 405

Le Dran H F 1740 Observations de Chirurgie. Osmont, Paris, p 1

Lewin M L 1976 Spheno-pharyngeal meningocele and cleft palate. Case repair with 12 years follow up. Cleft Palate Journal 13: 61

Mafee M F, Pruzansky S, Corrales M M et al 1986 CT in the evaluation of the orbit and the bony interorbital distance. American Journal of Neuroradiology 7: 265–269

Marsh J L, Vannier M W 1985 Comprehensive care for craniofacial deformities. Mosby, St Louis

Mood G F 1938 Congenital anterior herniations of brain. Annals of Otology 47: 391–401

Morin J, Hill J, Anderson J, Grainger R 1963 A study of growth in the interorbital region. American Journal of Ophthalmology 56: 895

Mortada A, El-Toraei I 1960 Orbital meningo-encephalocele and exophthalmos. British Journal of Ophthalmology 44: 309–314

Mustakalio M J 1946 On congenital sincipital encephalocele and its treatment, with special reference to the structure of the wall. Annales Chirurgie et Gynaecologiae (suppl. 2) 35: 1–56

Mustarde J 1963 Epicanthus and telecanthus. British Journal of Plastic Surgery 10: 346

Pacioli L 1509 Divina proportione. Paganini, Venice

Patry A 1960 Contribution à l'étude des lesions oculaires dans les malformations crâniennes specialement dans l'oxycephalie. Medical thesis, Paris

Peterson M O, Cohen M M, Sedano H O, Frericks C T 1971 Comments on fronto nasal dysplasia, ocular hypertelorism and dystopia canthorum. Birth Defects: original article series 7: 120

Pollock J A, Newton T H, Hoyt W F 1968 Transsphenoidal and transethmoidal encephaloceles: a review of clinical and roentgen features in 8 cases. Radiology 90: 442–453

Ricketts R M 1982 Divine proportion in facial esthetics. Clinics in Plastic Surgery 9: 401

Rickham P P 1969 Open myelomeningocele and encephalocele. In: Rickham P P, Johnston J H (eds) Neonatal surgery. Butterworths, London, p 481

Robinson R G 1957 Anterior encephalocele. British Journal of Surgery 45: 36–40

Romanus T 1953 Interocular–biorbital index. A gauge of hypertelorism. Acta Genetica 4: 117

Rosasco S A, Massa J L 1968 Fronto-nasal syndrome. British Journal of Plastic Surgery 21: 244

Salmon M A 1978 Developmental defects and syndromes. HM & M, Aylesbury, UK

Sedano H O, Cohen M M Jr, Jirasek J, Gorlin R J 1970 Frontonasal dysplasia, Journal of Pediatrics 76: 906

Smith D W 1982 Recognizable patterns of human malformation. Saunders, Philadelphia

Smith D W, Cohen M M 1973 Widow's peak scalp-hair anomaly and its relation to ocular hypertelorism. Lancet ii: 1127

Spring A 1854 Monographie de la hernie du cerveau et de quelques lésions voisines. De Mortier, Brussels

Strandberg B 1949 Cephalocele of posterior part of orbit: general survey, with report of a case. Archives of Ophthalmology 42: 254–265

Suwanwela C, Hongsaprabhas C 1966 Fronto-ethmoidal encephalomeningocele. Journal of Neurosurgery 25: 172–182

Suwanwela C, Suwanwela N 1972 A morphological classification of sincipital encephalomeningoceles. Journal of Neurosurgery 36: 201

Suwanwela C, Sukabote C, Suwanwela N 1971 Fronto-ethmoidal encephalomeningoceles. Surgery 69: 625

Tessier P 1972 Orbital hypertelorism. 1. Successive surgical attempts, material and methods, causes and mechanism. Scandinavian Journal of Plastic and Reconstructive Surgery 6: 135

Tessier P 1973 The definitive treatment of orbital hypertelorism by craniofacial or extra cranial osteotomies. Scandinavian Journal of Plastic and Reconstructive Surgery 7: 39

Tessier P 1976 Anatomical classification of facial craniofacial and lateral facial clefts. Symposium on Plastic Surgery in the Orbital Region, vol 20. Mosby, St Louis

Tessier P, Guiot G, Rougerie J, Delbet J P, Pastoriza J 1967 Osteotomies cranio naso orbito faciales — Hypertelorism. Annales de Chirurgie Plastique 12

Thomson J 1903–1904 Case reports. Transactions Medica Chirurgica of the Royal Society of Edinburgh 23: 208

Van der Meulen J C H, Vaandrager J M 1983 Surgery related to the correction of hypertelorism. Plastic and Reconstructive Surgery, 71: 6

Van Nouhuys J M, Bruyn G W 1964 Nasopharyngeal transsphenoidal encephalocele, craterlike hole in the optic disc and agenesis of the corpus callosum: pneumoencephalographic visualization in a case. Psychiatrie, Neurologie et Neurochirurgie 67: 243

Vermeij-Keers C, Poelmann R E, Smits-van Prooije, Van der Meulen J C 1984 Hypertelorism and the median cleft face syndrome. An embryological analysis. Ophthalmic Paediatrics and Genetics 4: 97

Von Meyer E 1890 Uber eine basale Hirnhernie in der Gegend der Lamina Cribrosa. Virchows Archiv Abteilung A 120: 309

Waardenburg P 1951 A new syndrome combining developmental anomalies of the eyelids, eyebrows and nose root with pigmentary defects of the iris and head hair and with congenital deafness. American Journal of Human Genetics 3: 196

Waardenburg P, Franceschetti A, Klein D 1961 Genetics and Ophthalmology. Thomas, Springfield

Whitaker L A, Katowitz J A, Jacobs W E 1979 Ocular adnexal problems in craniofacial deformities. Journal of Maxillofacial Surgery 7: 55

Wiese G M, Kempe L G, Hammon W M 1972 Trans-sphenoidal meningo hydroencephalocele: case report. Journal of Neurosurgery 37: 475

INTERNASAL DYSPLASIA

Badrawy R 1967 Midline congenital anomalies of the nose. Journal of Laryngology 81: 419

Baibak G, Bromberg B E 1966 Congenital midline defects of the midface. Cleft Palate Journal 3: 392–401

Bartholinus Th 1654 Historiarum anatomicarum rariorum. Hauboldt, Copenhagen. p 41

Bischoff C W 1898 Ein Fall von angeborener medianer Splatung der oberen Gesichtshälfte. Thesis, Bonn

Boo-Chai K 1965 The bifid nose, with a report of 3 cases in siblings. Plastic and Reconstructive Surgery 36: 626–628

Borellus P 1670 Historiarum et observationum medicophysicarum centuriae III. Francofurti et Lipsiae p 231

Bourgon, Derocque: 1908 Fissure médiane de la face. Revue d'Orthopedie Dento-Faciale 9: 219–224

Brejcha M, Fara M 1971 Osseous changes in middle clefts of the nose. Acta Chirugiae Plasticae 13: 141

Bumba J, Lucksch F 1927 Ein Fall von Doggennase. Virchows Archive Abteilung A 264: 554

Burian F 1960 Median clefts of the nose. Acta Chirurgiae Plasticae 2: 180

Bye H A S 1949 Mid-line congenital malformations of the nose. Journal of Laryngology and Otology 63: 596

Cohen M M, Sedano H O, Gorlin R J, Jrasek J E 1971 Fronto nasal dysplasia (median cleft face syndrome): comments on etiology and pathogenesis. Birth defects original series 7: 117

Dehesdin D, Andrieu-Guitrancourt J 1978 Les kystes dermoides congénitaux du nez par rapport aux gliomes et meningoceles. Pathogenie, incidences thérapeutiques. Annales de Chirurgie Plastique 23: 7

De Myer W 1967 The median cleft face syndrome. Neurology 17: 961

Dodge H Jr, Love J, Kernohan J 1959 Intranasal encephalomeningoceles associated with cranium bifidum. Archives of Surgery 79: 75

Esser E 1939 La fissure médiane du nez. Plastica Chirurgica 1: 40–51

Francesconi G, Fortunato G 1969 Median dysraphia of the face. Plastic and Reconstructive Surgery 43: 481–491

Galanti S 1961 Rara malformazione congenita del naso (due casi di naso bifido). Annals of Laryngology 60: 583

Günther H 1933 Hypertelorismus. Endokrinologie 13: 61

Gürsu K G 1967 Report on median cleft deformity. In: Fourth International Congress of Plastic Surgery, Rome. Excerpta Medica, Amsterdam.

Iregbulem L M 1978 Midline clefts of the upper lip. British Journal of Plastic Surgery 31: 63–65

Kazanjian V H, Holmes E M 1959 Treatment of median cleft lip associated with bifid nose and hypertelorism. Plastic and Reconstructive Surgery 24: 582–587

Kopp M M 1939 Two congenital nasal deformities: bifid nose and bulldog nose. Laryngoscope 49: 1128

Krikun L A 1972 Clinical features of median cleft of nose. Acta Chirurgiae Plasticae 14: 137

Kurlander G J, DeMyer W, Campbell J A 1967 Roentgenology of the median cleft face syndrome. Radiology 88: 473–478

Lehmann-Nitsche R 1901 Ein seltener Fall von angeborener medianer Spaltung der oberen Gesichtshälfte. Virchows Archiv Abteilung A 163: 126–134

McCaffrey T, McDonald T J, Gorenstein A 1979 Dermoid cysts of the nose: review of 21 cases. Otolaryngology and Head and Neck Surgery 87: 52

Mazzola R 1976 Congenital malformations in the frontonasal area: their pathogenesis and classification. Clinics in Plastic Surgery 3: 573

Mazzola R, Fittipaldi L 1970 Klassifikationsprobleme bei Nasenmissbildungen. Beurteilung über 200 Fälle. Verhandlungsbericht der IV. Tagung, Halle. p 26

Millard D R 1977 Cleft graft, vol. II. Bilateral and rare deformities. Little Brown, Boston. p 745

Millard D R Jr, Williams S 1968 Median clefts of the upper lip. Plastic and Reconstructive Surgery 42: 4

Muhlbauer W, Dittmar W 1976 Hereditary median dermoid cysts of the nose. British Journal of Plastic Surgery 29: 334

Pinto C J, Goleria K S 1971 The median cleft lip. In: Transactions of the 5th International Congress of Plastic Surgery. Butterworths, Australia. p 206

Sandifort E 1793 Museum anatomicum academiae Lugduno Batavae; vol I, sect VII. Monstra. Luchtmans, Leyden. p 300

Schenck J G 1609 Monstrorum Historia Memorabilis. Becker, Frankfurt. p 10

Scrimshaw G C 1967 Midline cleft lip and nose, 'true harelip': two interesting cases. In: Transactions of the 4th International Congress of Plastic and Reconstructive Surgery, Rome. Excerpta Medica, Amsterdam. p 472

Sercer A 1948 Das Syndrom der Dysplasie der Medianen Linie des Kopfes. Acta Oto-Laryngologica 36: 284

Soemmering S T 1791 Abbildung und Beschreibung einiger Misgeburten. Universitatsbuchandlung, Mainz. p 10

van Doeveren W 1765 Specimen observationum academicarum. Bolt & Luchtmans, Groningen. p 40

Vermeij-Keers C, Mazzola R F, Van der Meulen J C, Stricker M 1983 Cerebro-craniofacial and craniofacial malformations: an embryological analysis. Cleft Palate Journal 20: 128

Vermeij-Keers C, Poelmann R E, Smits van Prooje A E, Van der Meulen J C 1984 Hypertelorism and the median cleft face syndrome. An embryological analysis. Ophthalmic Pediatrics and Genetics 4: 97

Waever D F, Bellinger D H 1946 Bifid nose associated with midline cleft of upper lip. Acta Oto-Laryngologica 44: 480

Warkany J, Bofinger M K, Benton C 1973 Median facial cleft syndrome in half sisters. Dilemas in genetic counseling. Teratology 8: 273

Webster J P, Deming E G 1950 Surgical treatment of the bifid nose. Plastic and Reconstructive Surgery 6: 1

Wilkinson 1922 A case of bifid nose. Journal of Laryngology and Otology 37: 560

Witzel O 1882 Ueber die angeborene mediane Splatung der oberen Gesichtshalfte. Archiv fur Klinische Chirurgie 27: 893

Wolfler A 1890 Zur Casuistik der Medianen Gesichtsspalte. Archiv fur Klinische Chirurgie 40: 795

NASAL DYSPLASIA

Berndorfer A 1965 Besondere Kombinationsformen von Augen-, Nasen- und Mundmissbildungen mit Gehirndefekten. Archiv fur Kinderheilkunde 172: 160

Borellus P 1676 Historiarum et observationum medicophysicarum centruriae (IV). Francofurti et Lisiae Cent III. p 231

Denecke H J, Meyer R 1967 Plastic surgery of head and neck: corrective and reconstructive rhinoplasty. Springer, New York

Kernahan D A 1957 Types divers de malformations congénitales du nez. Annales de Chirurgie Plastique 2: 115

Mazzola R F 1976 Congenital malformations in the frontonasal area: their pathogenesis and classification. Clinics in Plastic Surgery 3: 573

Meyer R 1956 Ueber angeborene äussere Nasendeformitäten. Practica Oto-rhino-laryngologica 18: 399

Smith F 1950 Plastic reconstructive surgery: a manual of management. Saunders, Philadelphia

Stupka W 1938 Die Missbildungen und Anomalien der Nase und des Nasenrachenraumes. Springer, Vienna

Nasal aplasia

Berger M, Martin C 1969 L'arhinogénesis totale (absence congénitale d'une fosses nasales). A propos d'une observation exceptionelle. Revue de Laryngologie, Otologie, Rhinologie 90: 300

Blair V P 1931 Congenital atresia or obstruction of nasal air passages. Annals of Otology, Rhinology and Laryngology 94: 1021

Blair V P, Brown J B 1931 Nasal abnormalities, fancied and real. The reaction of the patient: their attempted correction. Surgical Gynecology and Obstetrics 53: 797

Fatin M 1955 A rare case of congenital malformation. Journal of the Egyptian Medical Association 38: 470

Gifford G H Jr, Swanson L, MaxCollumn D W 1972 Congenital absence of the nose and anterior nasopharynx. Report of two cases. Plastic and Reconstructive Surgery 50: 5

Greer Walker D 1961 Malformations of the face. Churchill Livingstone, Edinburgh

Labat L 1833 De la rhinoplastic dans le cas d'absence congenitale on accidentelle. Annales de Medecine Physiologiques 24: 619

Lütolf V 1976 Bilateral aplasia of the nose. Journal of Maxillofacial Surgery 4: 245

Otto A W 1841 Monstrorum sexcentorum dexcriptio anatomica. Vratislaviae. Fall 73, p 47, Taf IX Fig 3

Palmer C R, Thompson H G 1967 Congenital absence of the nose; a case report. Canadian Journal of Surgery 10: 83

Schweckendiek W, Hein J 1973 Seltene Nasenfehlbildungen: Eintseitige Aplasie in Kombination mit Gaumen Spalten. Fachartzt HNO D 3550 Marburg a.d. Lahn HNO 21 3: 73–76

Selenkoff A 1884 Ein Fall von Arhinencephalia unilateralis bei einem erwachsenen Manne. Virchows Archiv Abteilung A 95: 95

Thiefenthal G 1910 Totale Aplasie einer Nasenhälfte. Monatschrift fur Ohrenheilkunde 44: 1071

Wahby B 1903–1904 Congenital absence of nose and premaxilla. Journal of Anatomy 38: 49

Nasal aplasia with proboscis

Alves d'Assumpcö E 1975 Proboscis lateralis: a case report. Plastic and Reconstructive Surgery 55: 494

Aubrespy P, Giraud F, Derlon S, Oddo G, Bernard R 1968 Le proboscis: aspects majeurs, et formes degradées. Archives Française Pediatrie 25: 837

Biber J J 1949 Proboscis lateralis: a rare malformation of the nose, its genesis and treatment. Journal of Laryngology and Otology 63: 734

Binns J H 1969 Congenital tubular nostril (proboscis lateralis). British Journal of Plastic Surgery 22: 265

Bischoff 1898 Ein Fall von angeborener medianer Spaltung der Oberen Gesichtshaelfte. Inaugural dissertation

Bishop B W F 1964 Lateral nasal proboscis. British Journal of Plastic Surgery 17: 18

Boo-Chai K 1985 The proboscis lateralis. A 14-year follow up. Plastic and Reconstructive Surgery 75: 569

Bowe J J 1986 Lateral nasal proboscis. Case reports. Annals of Plastic Surgery 16: 250

Coetzee T S 1964 Proboscis lateralis, a rare facial anomaly. South African Journal of Laboratory and Clinical Medicine 10: 81

Chong J K, Crameer L M 1978 Proboscis lateralis: staged management with a four-year follow-up. Case report. Annals of Plastic Surgery 1: 225

Cotin G, Bodard M, Bouchenak B, Garabedian N 1982 Reconstruction de l'orifice et du vestibule narinaire dans le proboscis lateralis. Annales de Chirurgie Plastique 27: 144

Dasgupta G, Kacher S K, Bhan A K 1971 Proboscis. Journal of Laryngology and Otology 85: 401

Franklin P 1920 A case of lateral nasal proboscis. Proceedings of the Royal Society of Medicine 14: 48

Giraud F, Bureau H, Saracco J B, Mattei J F Magalon G, Fonta D 1976 Les formes dégrades de l'ectroprosopie. Journal de Génétique Humaine 24: 243–247

Grunberg 1913 Die Missbildungen des Kopfes 3, 1. Abt., S. 194. In: von Schwalbe E (ed) Die Morphologie der Missbildungen des Meschen und der Tiere. Fischer, Jena

Hartmann M 1938 Atiologie und Vererbungsproblem der angeborenen Missbildungen der Gesichts. Plastica Chirurgica 1: 52

Haymann 1903 Amniogene und erbliche Hasenscharte. Inaugural dissertation, Leipzig

Hein J 1972 Arhinia unilateralis als seltene Nasenfehlbildung. Dissertation, Marburg

Hensen 1906 Ein Beitrag zu den Gesichtsmissbildungen. Inaugural dissertation, Rostock

Hornicke 1907 Experimental erzeugte Missbildungen. Verhandlungen der Gesellschaft deutscher Naturforscher und Aerzte. 79 Versammlung zu Dresden, 15–21 September. 1907. Deutsche Medizinische Wochenschrift 1907: S. 1766

Kirchmayr L 1906 Ein Beitrag zu den Gesichtsmissbildung. Deutsche Zeitschrift fur Chirurgie 81: 71

Kirkpatrick T J 1970 Lateral nasal proboscis. Journal of Laryngology and Otology 84: 83

Kundrat K K 1887 Gesellschaft der Arzte in Wien. Sitzung vom 28 Januar 1887. Munchen, Medizinische Wochenschrift 1887: S. 90.

Landow M 1890 Uber einen seltenen Fall von Missbildung der Nase nebst einigen Bemerkungen über die seitlichen Nasenspalten. Deutsche Zeitschrift fur Chirurgie 30: 544

Mahindra S 1973 Lateral nasal proboscis. Journal of Laryngology and Otology 87: 177–180

McLaren L R 1955 A case of cleft lip and palate with polypoid nasal tubercle. British Journal of Plastic Surgery 8: 57

Meeker L H, Aebli R 1947 Cyclopean eye and lateral proboscis with normal one-half face. Archives of Ophthalmology 38: 159

Meyer M 1956 Ueber angeborene aeussere Nasendeformitaeten. Practica Oto-Rhino-Laryngologica 18: 399

Nessel E 1958 Proboscis lateralis als seltene. Nasenmissbildung HNO 7: 25

Ogura Y 1967 Half nose: a very rare congenital deformity. Journal of the Otorhinolaryngological Society of Japan 70: 2037

Ohura T 1974 Congenital deformities: proboscis lateralis. Clinics in Plastic Surgery 1: 116

Peters A 1910 Uber die bei Missbildungen des Gesichtes Vorkommende Rüsselbildung. Ber 36, Verh Ophth Ges, Heidelberg

Petit P, Lemoyne J, Guillaumat L, Barbadault J 1965 Malformations faciales congénitales avec proboscide unilatérale. Bulletin des Sociétés d'Ophthalmologie de France 65: 427

Rao P B 1963 Proboscis lateralis. Journal of Laryngology 77: 1028

Recamier J, Florentin M 1957 Un type exceptional de malformation congénital du nez. Annales de Chirurgie Plastique 2: 15

Rontal M, Duritz G 1977 Proboscis lateralis: a case report and embryologic analysis. Laryngoscope 87: 996

Rosen A, Gitlin G 1959 Bilateral nasal proboscis. Archives of Otolaryngology 70: 545

Seefelder R 1910 Kolobom des Augapfels und Rüsselbildung. Ber 36, Vers Ophth Ges, Heidelberg

Selenkow A 1884 Ein Fall von Arhinencephalia unilateralis bei einem erwachsenen Manne. Virchows Archiv Abteilung A 95: 95

Silverman F N, Cassini, 1971 vide Cohen M M et al: Holoprosencephaly and facial dysmorphia. Birth Defects: original series 7

Taruffi C 1890 Nuovo caso di Meso-rino-schisi nell'Uomo. Mem R Accad Sci Bologna Serie V, I: 227 1890.

Tendlau A 1918 Ein Fall von Proboscis Lateralis. Archiv fur Ophthalmologie 95: 135

Van Duyse G M 1919 Proboscide latérale et colobome oculaire atypique avec lenticone postérieur. Archives d'Ophthalmologie 36: 463

von Hippel: 1908 Die Missbildungen und angeborenen Fehler des Auges. In: Graefe-Saemisch (ed) Handbuch der gesamten Augenheilkunde 2, 1. Abt. Kapitel 9

Warkany J 1971 Congenital malformations. Yearbook Medical Publishers, Chicago

Zacherl H 1920 Ein Beigrag zu den Missbildungen des Gesichts. Archiv fur Klinisches Chirurgie 113: 374

Nasoschizis

Berndorfer A 1962 Ueber die seitliche Nasenspalte. Acta Oto-Laryngologica 55: 163

De Myer W 1967 The median cleft face syndrome. Differential diagnoses of cranium bifidum occultum, hypertelorism and medial cleft nose, lip and palate. Neurology 17: 961

Frangenheim P 1909 Zur Kenntnis der seitlichen Nasenspalten. Beitrage zur Klinischen Chirurgie 65: 54

Johanson A, Blizzard R 1971 A syndrome of congenital aplasia of the alae nasi, deafness, hypothyroidism, dwarfism, absent permanent teeth, and malabsorption. Journal of Pediatrics 79: 981

Kindler J 1889 Linksseitige Nasenspalte verbunden mit Defekt des Stirnbeins. Fisscher, Jena

Landow M 1890 Ueber Einen seltener Fall von Missbildung der Nase nebst einigen. Bemerkungen über die seitlichen Nasenspalten. Deutsche Zeitschrift fur Chirurgie 30: 544

Leuckart F S 1840 Untersuchungen über das Zwischenkieferbein des Menschen. Schweizerberart, Stuttgart

Mazzola R F 1976 Congenital malformations in the frontonasal area: Their pathogenesis and classification. Clinics in Plastic Surgery 3: 573

Nash W G 1898 Congenital absence of the right eye and fissure of the nose. Lancet i: 28

Rosasco S A, Massa J L 1968 Frontonasal syndrome. British Journal of Plastic Surgery 21: 244

Sedano H O, Cohen M M Jr, Jirasek J, Gorlin R J 1970 Frontonasal dysplasia. Journal of Pediatrics 76: 906

Stupka W 1950 The etiology of lateral nasal clefts. American Journal of Pathology 26: 1085

Van der Meulen J C 1976 The pursuit of symmetry in craniofacial surgery. British Journal of Plastic Surgery 29: 85–91

Van der Meulen J C, Moscona A R, Vaandrager J M, Hirshowitz B 1982 Pathology and treatment of nasoschizis. Annales de Plastic Surgery 8: 474–485

Nasal duplication

Bidault de Villier 1821 Observation de double nez. Journal Complémentaire 10: 183

Bimar 1881 Sur une difformité rare de la tête et de l'encéphale. Gazette Hebdomadaire de la Science Médicale 3: 171, 194, 291

Blair V P 1931 Congenital atresia or obstruction of nasal air passages. Annals of Otology, Rhinology and Laryngology 40: 1021

Erich J B 1962 Nasal duplication. Report of case of patient with two noses. Plastic and Reconstructive Surgery 29: 159

Goulian D, Conway H 1964 A rare case of facial duplication. Plastic and Reconstructive Surgery 33: 66–72

Holmes E M 1950 Congenital triple nares. Archives of Otolaryngology 52: 70

Lindsay B 1906 A nose with supernumerary nostrils, Transactions of the Pathological Society of London 57: 329

Mazzola R F 1976 Congenital malformations in the frontonasal area: their pathogenesis and classification. Clinics in Plastic Surgery 3: 573

Muecke F F, Souttar H S 1923–1924 Case of double nose. Proceedings of the Royal Society of Medicine 17: 8

Obwegeser H L, Weber G, Freihofer H P, Sailer H F 1978 Facial duplication — the unique case of Antonio. Journal of Maxillofacial Surgery 6: 179–198

Ortscheit M E 1923 Malformations du nez par cloisonnement de chaque narine. Bulletins et Mémoires de la Société Anatomique de Paris 93: 516

Regnault F 1901 La femme à deux nez et le polyzoisme tératologique. Bulletins et Memoires de la Société Anthropologique 2: 333

Tawse H B 1920 Supernumerary nostril and cavity. Proceedings of the Royal Society of Medicine 13: 1919–1920

Thompson St C 1919 Congenital deformity showing a nose with four nostrils. Journal of Laryngology 24: 207

NASOMAXILLARY AND MAXILLARY DYSPLASIA

Ahlfeld P 1880–1882 Die Missbildungen des Menschen. Grunow, Leipzig

Ask F, Van der Hoeve J 1921 Beiträge sur Kenntnis der Entwicklung der Tränenröhrchen unter normalen und abnormen Verhältnissen, letzteres an Fällen von offener schräger Gesichtsspalte. Graefe's Archive for Clinical and Experimental Ophthalmology 105: 1157

Bartels R J, O'Malley J E, Baker J L, Douglas W M 1971 Naso-ocular clefts. Plastic and Reconstructive Surgery 47: 351

Boo-Chai K 1970 The oblique facial clefts: a report of two cases and a review of 41 cases, British Journal of Plastic Surgery 23: 352

Braithwaite F, Watson J 1949 A report on three unusual cleft lips. British Journal of Plastic Surgery 2: 38

Chavanne G 1890 Malformation faciale (section par bride amniotique). Bulletin de la Société Anatomique de Paris 4: 137

Chiong A T, Guevara E S, Zantva R V 1981 Oblique facial clefts. Archives of Otolaryngology 107: 59

Cowell E M vide Greer Walker 1961

Dareste C 1891 Recherches sur la production artificielle des monstruosité. Reinwald, Paris

Davis W B 1935 Congenital deformities of the face. Types found in a series of one thousand cases. Surgery, Gynecology and Obstetrics 61: 201

Delpech J M 1828 Observations et réflexions sur l'operation de la rhinoplastique. In: Chirurgie clinique de Montpellier ou observations et réflecion tirées des travaux de chirurgie clinique de cette école. Gabon, Paris. p 221

Dey D L 1973 Oblique facial clefts. Plastic and Reconstructive Surgery 52: 258

Duhamel G 1966 Morphogenese pathologique. Masson, Paris

Duke Elder S 1958 System of ophthalmology. Kimpton, London

Ergin N O 1966 Naso-ocular cleft: a case report. Plastic and Reconstructive Surgery 38: 573

Fergusson W 1857 A system of practical surgery, 4th edn. London. p 574

Fogh-Andersen P 1965 Rare clefts of the face. Acta Chirurgica Scandinavica 129: 275

Francois J, Bacskulin J 1969 External congenital fistulae of the lacrimal sac. Ophtalmologica 159: 249

Garcia Velasco D M 1980 Tratamiento de las Hendiduras faciales Tipo III, IV, y V III congreso ibero Latino-Americano de Cirugia plastica y reconstructive y V congreso nacional, Valencia, June

Greer Walker D 1961 Malformations of the face. Livingstone, Edinburgh

Grünberg K 1909 Die Gesichtsspalten und die zu ihnen in genetischer Beziehung stehend anderweitigen Missbildungen des Gesichtes. In: Schwalbe E (ed) Die Morphologie der Missbildungen des Menschen und der Tiere. Teil III, Abt I. Fisher, Jena. p. 113

Guersant M P 1860 Gazette des Hôpitaux 28: 112

Gunter G 1963 Nasomaxillary clefts. Plastic and Reconstructive Surgery 32: 637

Harkins C S, Berlin A, Harding R L, Longacre J, Snodgrasse R M 1962 A classification of cleft lip and cleft palate. Plastic and Reconstructive Surgery 29: 31

Hovey L M vide Millard 1977

Hynes W vide Greer Walker 1961

Johanson A, Blizzard R 1971 A syndrome of congenital aplasia of the alae nasi, deafness, hypothyroidism, dwarfism, absent permanent teeth, and malabsorption. Journal of Pediatrics 79: 981

Karfik V 1966 Proposed classification of rare congenital cleft malformations in the face. Acta Chirurgiae Plasticae 8: 163

Karfik V 1969 Oblique facial cleft. In: Transactions of the Fourth Congress of the International Society of Plastic Surgery. Excerpta Medica, Amsterdam. p 105

Kawamoto H K, Wang M K H, Brandon Macomber W 1977 Rare craniofacial clefts. The Head and Neck. Reconstructive Plastic Surgery 1: 2116

Keith A 1909 Three demonstrations on congenital malformations of palate, face and neck. British Medical Journal 2: 310, 363, 438

Kilner P 1938 Unusual congenital malformations of the face. Revue de Chirurgie Structurale 8: 164

Kirmisson E 1898 Traité des maladies chirurgicales d'origine congénitale. Masson, Paris. p 101

Kraske P 1877 Zur casuistik der retardirten intrauterinen Verschmelzung von Gesichtsspalten. Archiv fur Klinisches Chirurgie 20: 396

Kubacek V, Penkava J 1974 Oblique clefts of the face. Chirurgiae Plasticae 16: 152

Kulmus J E 1732 Partus monstrosi historia. Thesis, Lipsia

Laroche G 1823 Essai d'anatomie pathologique sur les monstruosie ou vices de conformations primitifs de la face. Thesis, Paris

McEnery E T, Brenneman J 1937 Multiple facial anomalies. Journal of Pediatrics 11: 468

Mayou B J, Fenton O M 1981 Oblique facial clefts caused by amniotic bands. Plastic and Reconstructive Surgery 68: 675

Millard D R 1977 Cleft craft, vol II. Bilateral and rare deformities. Little Brown, Boston. p 781

Millard D R Jr, William S 1968 Median lip clefts of the upper lip. Plastic and Reconstructive Surgery 42: 4–14

Miller M E, Graham J M, Higginbottom M C, Smith D W 1981 Compression-related defects from early amnion rupture: evidence for mechanical teratogenesis. Journal of Pediatrics 98: 292

Miller S H, Wood A M, Abdul Haq M 1973 Bilateral oro-ocular cleft. Plastic and Reconstructive Surgery 51: 590

Morian R 1887 Über die schräge Gesichtsspalte. Archiv fur Klinisches Chirurgie 35: 245

Nicati C 1822 De labii leporini congeniti natura et origine. Utrecht and Amsterdam. p 63

Ortega J, Flor E 1969 Incomplete naso-ocular cleft. A case report. Plastic and Reconstructive Surgery 43: 630

Pelvet M 1864 Mémoire sur les fissures congénitales des joues. Gazette Médicale de Paris 19: 417

Pichler A 1911 Tränennasengang und schräge Gesichtsspalte. Archiv für Augenheilkunde 68: 172

Pitanguy I 1968 Facial clefts as seen in a large series of untreated adults and their later management. In: Longacre J J (ed) Craniofacial anomalies. Lippincott, Philadelphia. p 167

Pitanguy I, Franco T 1967 Nonoperated facial fissures in adults. Plastic and Reconstructive Surgery 39: 569

Ploner L 1957 Die schräge Gesichtsspalte. Fortschritte der Kiefer- und Gesichts-Chirurgie 3: 334

Politzer G 1937 Origin of facial cleft, harelip and cleft palate. Monatsschrift fur Ohrenheilkunde 71: 63

Poswillo D 1966 Observations of fetal posture and causal mechanisms of congenital deformity of palate, mandible and limbs. Journal of Dental Research (suppl) 458: 584–596

Potter J 1950 A case of bilateral cleft of the face. British Journal of Plastic Surgery 3: 209

Remacly 1864 De fissura genae congenita. Thesis, Bonn

Rintala A, Leisti J, Liesmaa M, Ranta R 1980 Oblique facial clefts. Scandinavian Journal of Plastic Surgery 14: 291–297

Rowlatt U 1979 Cleft lip and palate associated with amniotic band limb amputations in a 20 week human fetus. Cleft Palate Journal 16: 206

Sakurai E H, Mitchell D F, Holmes L A 1956 Bilateral oblique facial clefts and amniotic bands: a report of two cases. Cleft Palate Journal 3: 181

Schlenke J D, Ricketson G, Lynch J B 1979 Classification of oblique facial clefts with microphthalmia. Plastic and Reconstructive Surgery 63: 680

Schwenzer N 1974 Rare clefts of the face. Journal of Maxillofacial Surgery 2: 224

Stewart R, Mulick J, Kawamoto H K Jr, Thanos C 1976 A syndrome of multiple facial clefts, branchial arch anomalies and Streeters bands (abstract). Journal of Dental Research 55: 107

Takuya Onizuka M D et al 1978 Naso-ocular clefts. Three case reports. P.R.S. January 1978. vol. 118–122

Tessier P 1969 Fentes orbito-faciales verticales et obliques (colobomas), complètes et frustes. Annales de Chirurgie Plastique 14: 301

Tessier P 1976 Anatomical classification of facial, cranio-facial and latero-facial clefts. Journal of Maxillofacial Surgery 4: 69

Thomson H G, Sleightholm R 1985 Isolated naso-ocular cleft: a one-stage repair. Plastic and Reconstructive Surgery 76: 534

Tower P 1953 Coloboma of lower lid and choroid with facial defects and deformity of hand and forearm. Archives of Ophthalmology 50: 333

Trendelenburg F 1886 Verletzungen und chirurgische Krankenheiten des Gesichts. In: Von Bruns V (ed) Deutsche Chirurgie. Enke, Stuttgart. p 1

Van der Hoeve J 1930 Eye and amnion bands. Transactions of the Opthalmological Society of the UK 50: 237–243

Van der Hoeve J 1941 Aangeboren afwijkingen. Ned Tijds v Geneeskunde n. 4020 jaar

Van der Meulen J 1985 Oblique facial clefts: pathology, etiology and reconstruction. Plastic and Reconstructive Surgery 76: 212

Van Duyse M 1882 Bride dermoide oculo-palpebral et colobome partiel de la paupière. Annales d'oculistique 88: 101

Verlazquez J M 1975 Congenital facial malformations embryology. Classification. In: Transactions of the 6th International Congress of Plastic and Reconstructive Surgery Masson, Paris

Wilson L F, Musgrave R H, Garret W, Conklin J E 1972 Reconstruction of oblique facial clefts. Cleft Palate Journal 9: 109

Zachariades N et al 1985 The superior orbital fissure syndrome. Journal of Maxillofacial Surgery. 13: 125

ZYGO-TEMPORO-AUROMANDIBULAR DYSPLASIA

Axellson A, Brolin I, Engstrom H, Liden G 1963 Dysostosis mandibulo-facialis. Journal of Laryngology and Otology 87: 575

Behrents R G, McNamara J A Jr, Avery J K 1977 Prenatal mandibulofacial dysostosis (Treacher Collins syndrome). Cleft Palate Journal 14: 13

Berry G A 1889 Note on a congenital defect (? coloboma) of the lower lid. Ophthalmic Hospital Reports 12: 255

Briggs A H 1953 Mandibulo-facial dysostosis. British Journal of Ophthalmology 37: 171

Caldarelli D D, Hutchinson J C, Pruzansky S, Valvassori G 1980 A comparison of microtia and temporal bone anomalies in hemifacial microsomia and mandibulofacial dysostosis. Cleft Palate Journal 17: 103

Collins E T 1900 Case with symmetrical congenital notches in the outer part of each lower lid and defective development of the malar bones. Transactions of the Ophthalmological Society of the UK 20: 190

Cosman B 1978 The constricted ear. Clinics in Plastic Surgery 5

Dahl E, Bjoerk A 1981 Ossification defects and craniofacial morphology in incomplete forms of mandibulo-facial dysostosis. A description of two dry skulls. Cleft Palate Journal 18: 83–89

Farrar J E 1967 Mandibulofacial dysostosis. British Journal of Ophthalmology 51: 132

Franceschetti A, Klein D 1949 The mandibulo-facial dysostosis, a new hereditary syndrome, Acta Ophthalmologica 27: 144

Franceschetti A, Zwahlen P 1944 Un syndrome nouveau: la dysostose mandibulo-faciale. Bulletin der Schweizerischen Akadermie der Medizinischen Wissenschaften 1: 60

Franceschetti A, Brocher J E W, Klein D 1949 Dysostose mandibulofaciale unilatérale avec deformations multiples du séquelette (processus paramastoide, synostose des vertèbres, sacralisation, etc.) et torticolis clonique. Ophthalmologica 118: 796

Harrison S H 1951 Treacher Collins syndrome. British Journal of Plastic Surgery 3: 282

Harrison M S 1957 The Treacher Collins–Franceschetti syndrome. Journal of Laryngology and Otology 71: 597

Hövels O 1953a Zur systemmatik der Missbildungen des I. Visceralbogens unter besonderer Berucksichtigung der Dysostosis mandibulo-facialis. Zeitschrift fur Kinderheilkunde 73: 532

Hövels O 1953b Zur pathogenese der Missbildungen des I. Visceralbogens unter desonderer Berucksichtigung der Dysostosis mandibulo-facialis. Zeitschrift fur Kinderheilkunde 73: 568

Hurwitz P 1954 Mandibulo-facial dysostosis. Archives of Ophthalmology 51: 69

Johnston C, Taussig L M, Koormann C, Smith P, Bielland J 1981 Obstructive sleep apnea in Treacher-Collins syndrome. Anaesthesia 36: 196–198

Keerl G 1962 Zur formalen und causalen Genese der Dysostosis mandibulo-facialis. Ophthalmologica 143: 5

Klein D 1953 Genetic factors and classification of craniofacial anomalies derived form a perturbation of the first branchial arch. In: Craniofacial growth in man. A conference. Pergamon Press, Oxford

Klein D 1971 Genetic factors and classification of craniofacial anomalies derived from a perturbation of the first branchial arch. In: Craniofacial growth in man. A conference. Pergamon Press, Oxford. pp 193–204

Laplane R, Nenna A 1953 Un cas de dysostose mandibulo-faciale de Franceschetti. Archives Françaises de Pediatrice 10: 79

Leopold L H, Mahoney J F, Price M L 1945 Symmetric defects in the lower lids associated with abnormalities of the zygomatic processes of the temporal bones. Archives of Ophthalmology 34: 210

McKenzie J, Craig J 1955 Mandibulo-facial dysostosis (Treacher-Collins syndrome). Archives of Disease in Childhood 30: 391

Mann I 1943 Deficiency of the malar bones with defect of the lower lids (with notes of a similar case, treatment and suggestions by T. Pomfret Kilner). British Journal of Ophthalmology 27: 13

Marsh J L, Celin S E, Vannier M W, Gado M 1986 The skeletal anatomy of mandibulofacial dysostosis (Treacher Collins syndrome). Plastic and Reconstructive Surgery 78: 460–468

Miller M, Fineman R, Smith D W 1979 Postaxial acrofacial dysostosis syndrome. Journal of Pediatrics 95: 970

Nager F R, de Reynier J P 1948 Das Gehororgan bei den angeborenen Kopfmissbildungen. Practica Otorhinolaryngological (Suppl) 10: 1

O'Connor G B, Conwayt M E 1950 Treacher Collins syndrome (dysostosis mandibulo-facialis). Plastic and Reconstructive Surgery 5: 419

Phelps P D, Poswillo D, Lloyd G A S 1981 The ear deformities in mandibulofacial dysostosis (Treacher Collins syndrome). Clinical Otolaryngology 6: 15

Ploner L 1958 Dysostosis mandibulo facialis. Fortschritte der Kiefer- und Gesichts-Chirurgie 4: 133–139

Poswillo D 1966 Observations of fetal posture and causal mechanisms of congenital deformity of palate, mandible and limbs. Journal of Dental Research (Suppl) 458: 584–596

Poswillo D E 1973 The pathogenesis of the first and second branchial arch syndrome. Oral Surgery 35: 302

Poswillo D E 1974a Orofacial malformations. Proceedings of the Soceity of Medicine 67: 343

Poswillo D E 1974b Otomandibular deformity: pathogenesis as a guide to reconstruction. Journal of Maxillofacial Surgery 2: 64

Poswillo D 1975a Causal mechanisms of craniofacial deformity. British Medical Bulletin 31: 101

Poswillo D 1975b The pathogenesis of the Treacher Collins syndrome (mandibulofacial dysostosis). British Journal of Oral Surgery 13: 1

Roberts F G, Pruzansky S, Aduss H 1975 An x-radiocephalometric study of mandibulofacial dysostosis in man. Archives of Oral Biology 20: 265

Rogers B O 1964 Berry–Treacher Collins syndrome: a review of 200 cases (mandibulofacial dysostosis: Franceschetti–Zwahlen–Klein syndromes). British Journal of Plastic Surgery 17: 109

Rovin S, Dachi S F, Borewstein D B, Cotter W C 1964 Mandibular facial dysostosis a familial study of five generations. Journal of Pediatrics 65: 215–221

Sando I, Hemmingway W G, Morgan W R 1968 Histopathology of the temporal bones in mandibulofacial dysostosis (Treacher Collins syndrome). Transactions of the American Academy of Ophthalmology and Otolaryngology 72: 913

Synder C C 1956 Bilateral facial agenesis (Treacher Collins syndrome). American Journal of Surgery 92: 81

Straith C L, Lewis J R 1949 Associated congenital defects of the ears, eyelids and malar bones (Treacher Collins syndrome). Plastic and Reconstructive Surgery 4: 204

Tanzer R C 1971 Total reconstruction of the auricle. The evolution of a plan of treatment. Plastic and Reconstructive Surgery 47: 523

Tanzer R C 1975 The constricted (cup and lop) ear. Plastic and Reconstructive Surgery 55: 406–415

Tanzer R C 1977a Congenital deformities of the auricle. In: Converse J M (ed) Reconstructive plastic surgery, 2nd edition. Saunders, Philadelphia 1977.

Tanzer R C 1977b Congenital deformities. In: Converse J M (ed) Reconstructive plastic surgery, 2nd edition. Saunders, Philadelphia.

Tanzer R C 1978 Microtia — a long term follow-up of forty-four reconstructed auricles. Plastic and Reconstructive Surgery 61: 161

Treacher Collins E 1900 Case with symmetrical congenital notches in the outer part of each lower lid and defective development of the malar bones. Transactions of the Ophthalmological Society of the UK 20: 190

Vatre J L 1971 Etude génétique et classification clinique de 154 cases de dysostose mandibulo-faciale (syndrome de Franceschetti) avec description de leurs associations malformatives. Journal de Génétique Humaine 19: 17

Weyers H 1951 Zur Klinik und Pathologie der Dysostosis mandibulofacialis. Zeitschrift fur Kinderheilkunde 69: 207

Zwahlen P 1944 Un syndrome nouveau: la dysostose mandibulo-faciale. Thesis, Geneva

TEMPORO-AUROMANDIBULAR DYSPLASIA

Albers G D 1963 Branchial anomalies. Journal of the American Medical Association 183: 399

Alexander G, Benesi O 1921 Zur Kenntnis der Entwicklung und Anatomie de kongenitalen Atresie des menschlichen Ohres. Monatsschrift fur Ohrenheilkunde 55: 195

Altmann F 1949 Problem of so-called congenital atresia of the ear. Archives of Otolaryngology 50: 759

Altmann F 1950 Normal development of the ear and its mechanics. Archives of Otolaryngology 52: 725

Altmann F 1951 Malformations of the auricle and external auditory meatus. Archives of Otolaryngology 54: 115

Altmann F 1955 Congenital atresia of ear in man and animals. Annals of Otology, Rhinology and Laryngology 64: 824

Anson B J 1960 Early embryology of auditory ossicles and associated structures. Annals of Otology 69: 427

Arnot R S 1971 Defects of the first branchial cleft. South African Journal of Surgery 9: 93–98

Ballantyne J W 1894 The teratological records of Chaldea. Teratologia 1: 127

Ballantyne J W 1904 Manual of Antenatal pathology and hygiene (the embryo). Green, Edinburgh

Bartholinus T 1654 Historiarum anatomicarium et medicarum rariorem. Centuria VI. Historia 36. Copenhagen

Bast T H, Anson B J 1949 The temporal bone and the ear. Thomas, Springfield Ill

Bast T H, Anson B J, Richany S F 1956 The development of the second branchial arch (Reichert's cartilage, facial canal, and associated structures) in man. Quarterly Bulletin of the Northwestern University Medical School 30: 235

Batros G 1957 The facial nerve in surgery of congenital atresia of the ear. Annals of Otology, Rhinology and Laryngology 66: 173

Baum J L, Feingold M 1973 Ocular aspects of Goldenhar's syndrome. American Journal of Ophthalmology 75: 250

Belenky W M, Medina J E 1980 First branchial anomalies. Laryngoscopy 90: 28–39

Bennun R D, Mulliken J B, Kaban L B, Murray J E 1985 Microtia: a microform of hemifacial microsomia, Plastic and Reconstructive Surgery vol. 76: 864

Berkman M D, Feingold M 1968 Oculo-auriculo-vertebral dysplasia. Oral Surgery 25: 408

Bernard M 1824 Sur un vice d'organisation de l'oreille externe. Journal de Physiologie iv: 167

Bezold F, Joel F 1888 Ueber Atresia auris congenita. Zeitschrift fur Ohrenheilkunde 18: 278

Binny J F 1896 Remarks on some cases of deformity of the external ear. Annals of Surgery 24: 206–210

Birkett J 1857–1858 Congenital supernumerary and imperfectly developed auricles on the sides of the neck. Transactions of the Pathological Society of London ix: 448

Bonnafont 1843 Imperforation congenitale du conduit auditif. Annales de Chirurgie VIII: 160

Bourguet J, Mazéas R, Lehuerou Y 1966 De l'atteinte des deux premières fentes et des deux premiers arcs branchiaux. Annales Oto-Laryngologie 83: 317

Bowen D L, Collum M T, Rees D O 1971 Clinical aspects of oculo-auriculo-vertebral dysplasia. British Journal of Ophthalmology 55: 145

Brimie J F 1896 Remarks on some cases of deformity of the external ear. Annals of Surgery 14: 206

Byars I T, Anderson R 1951 Anomalies of the first branchial cleft. Surgery, Gynecology and Obstetrics 93: 755

Caldarelli D D, Hutchinson J C, Pruzansky S, Valvassori G 1980 A comparison of microtia and temporal bone anomalies in hemifacial microsomia and mandibulofacial dysostosis. Cleft Palate Journal 17: 103

Cantlie J 1891 Unilateral absence of ear, bilateral supernumerary auricles and developmental deformity of right side of face and features. British Medical Journal i: 1223

Canton E 1860 Arrest of development of lower jaw combined with malformation of external ear. Transactions of the Pathological Society of London 12: 237

Caronni E P 1971 Embryogenesis and classification of branchial auricular dysplasia. In: Transactions of the Fifth International Congress of Plastic and Reconstructive Surgery. Butterworth, Melbourne

Chierici G 1983 Radiologic assessment of facial asymmetry. In: Harvold E P (ed) Treatment of hemifacial microsomia. Liss, New York p 57

Chowne 1860 Congenital absence of the auricle and malformation of the external meatus. Lancet ii: 59

Christiaens L R, Walbaum J P, Farriaux J P, Fontain G 1966 A propos de deux cas de dysplasie oculo-auriculo-vertébrale, Pediatrie 21: 935

Coccaro P J, Becker M H, Converse J M 1975 Clinical and radiographic variations in hemifacial microsomia. Birth Defects 11: 314

Converse J M, Coccaro P J, Becker H, Wood-Smith D 1973 On hemifacial microsomia. The first and second branchial arch syndrome. Plastic and Reconstructive Surgery 51: 268

Converse J M, Wood-Smith D, McCarthy J G, Coccaro P J, Becker M H 1974 Bilateral facial microsomia. Plastic and Reconstructive Surgery 54: 413

Converse J M, McCarthy J G, Wood-Smith D, Coccaro P J 1977 Cranial facial microsomia. In: Converse J M (ed) Reconstructive plastic surgery, vol 4 Saunders, Philadelphia. p 2359

Cronin T D 1964 Deformities of the cervical region. In: Converse J M (ed) Plastic and Reconstructive Surgery. Saunders, Philadelphia p 1191

Davis E D 1912–1913 Postmortem specimen of unilateral deformity of the auricle, meatus and middle ear. Proceedings of the Royal Society of Medicine 6: 87

Dupertuis S M, Musgrave R H 1959 Experiences with the reconstruction of the congenitally deformed ear. Plastic and Reconstructive Surgery 23: 361

Eitner E 1920 Uber Unterpolsterung der Gesichtshant. Medizinische Klinik 16: 93

Eitner E 1936 Ein Fall von querer Gesichtsspalte mit Ohrmiszbildung. Monatsschrift fur Ohrenheilkunde 70: 714

Fagge C H 1903–1904 Specimen of maldevelopment of the external middle and internal ears in a stillborn infant. Journal of the Otological Society of the UK 5: 19

Figueroa A, Pruzansky S 1982 The external ear, mandible and other components of hemifacial microsomia. Journal of Maxillofacial Surgery 10: 200

Forster A 1865 Die Missbildungen des Menschen. Mauke, Jena

Francheschetti A, Klein D, Brocher J E 1959 Mandibulofacial dysostosis in the framework of the first branchial arch syndrome. Schweizerische Medizinische Wochenschrift 89: 478

Francois J 1961 Heredity in Ophthalmology. Mosby, St Louis

Francois J, Haustrate L 1954 Anomalies colobomateuses de globe oculaire et syndrome du premier arc. Annales Ocul 187: 340

Fraser A 1881 On the development of the ossicula auditus in the higher mammalia. Proceedings of the Royal Society 33: 446

Fraser F C, Ling D, Clogg D, Nogrady B 1978 Genetic aspects of the BOR syndrome — branchial fistulas, ear pits, hearing loss and renal anomalies. American Journal of Medical Genetics 2: 241

Fraser J S 1931 Maldevelopments of the auricle, external acoustic meatus and middle ear; microtia and congenital meatal atresia. Archives of Otolaryngology 13: 1

Frazer J E 1923 The nomenclature of diseased status by certain vestigial structures in the neck. British Journal of Surgery 11: 131

Gill N 1969 Congenital atresia of the ear: a review of surgical findings in 83 cases. Journal of Laryngology 83: 551

Goldenhar M 1952 Associations malformatives de l'oeil et de l'oreille en particulier le syndrome dermoide epibulbaire — appendices auriculaires-fistula auris congenita et ses relations. Journal de Génétique Humaine 1: 243

Gore D, Masson A 1959 Anomalies of first branchial cleft. Annals of Surgery 150: 309

Gorlin R J, Jeu K L, Jacobsen U, Goldschmidt E 1963 Oculoauriculovertebral dysplasia. Journal of Pediatrics 63: 991

Gould G M, Pyle W L 1937 Anomalies and curiosities of medicine. Sydenham, New York

Grabb W C 1965 The first and second branchial arch syndrome. Plastic and Reconstructive Surgery 36: 485

Grabb W C 1979 Some anomalies of the head and neck. In: Grabb W C, Smith D W (eds) Plastic Surgery, 3rd edn. Little Brown, Boston

Heaton G 1892 Remarks on congenital malformations of the auditory apparatus. Journal of Laryngology 6: 147

Hermann J, Optiz J M 1969 A dominantly inherited first arch syndrome. Birth Defects 5: 110

Hilson D 1957 Malformation of ears as sign of malformation of genito-urinary tract. British Medical Journal 2: 785

Hyndman O R, Light G 1929 The branchial apparatus. Archives of Surgery 19: 410

Ide C H, Miller G W, Wollschlaeger P B 1970 Familial facial dysplasia. Archives of Ophthalmology 84: 427

Jafek B W, Nager G T, Strife J, Gayer R W 1975 Cogenital aural atresia: an analysis of 311 cases. Transactions of the American Academy of Ophthalmology and Otolaryngology 80: 588

Kaban L B, Mulliken J B, Murray J E 1981 Three dimensional approach to analysis and treatment of hemifacial microsomia. Cleft Palate Journal 18: 90

Kaseff L G 1967 Investigation of congenital malformations of the year with tomography. Plastic and Reconstructive Surgery 39: 282

Kazanjian V H 1939 Congenital absence of the ramus of the mandible. Journal of Bone and Joint Surgery 21: 761

Kazanjian V H 1956–1957 Bilateral absence of the ramus of the mandible. British Journal of Plastic Surgery 9: 77

Klein D 1971 Genetic factors and classification of cranio-facial anomalies derived from a perturbation of the first branchial arch. In: Cranio-facial growth in man. A conference. Pergamon Press, Oxford. pp 193–204

Knapp H 1892 A case of supernumerary auricle with defective development of the side of the face. Archives of Otolaryngology 21: 438

Kravath R E et al 1980 Obstructive sleep apnea and death associated with surgical correction of velopharyngeal incompetence. Journal of Pediatrics 96: 645

Kruchinsky G V 1972 Classification of auricular anomalies and its significance for their surgical treatment. Acta Chirurgiae Plasticae 14: 225–233

Lannelongue M, Menard V 1891 Malformations de l'oreille externe et de l'oreille moyenne. In: Affections congénitales, vol 1. Asselin et Houzeau, Paris. p 515

Lauritzen C, Munro I R, Ross R B 1985 Classification and treatment of hemifacial microsomia. Scandinavian Journal of Plastic Surgery 19: 33

Lewin M 1950 Congenital malformations of the ear and mandible. Oral Surgery 3: 1115

Lockhardt R D 1929 Variations coincident with congenital absence of the zygoma. Journal of Anatomy 63: 233

Lodge W O 1957 Malformations of the auricle. Journal of Laryngology and Otology 71: 533

Lucae A 1864 Anatomisch-psysiologische Beitrage zur Ohrenheilkunde. Virchow's Archiv Abteilung A 29: 33

Lynch R C 1913 Congenital absence of both ears. Laryngoscope 23:1050

McKenzie J 1958 The first arch syndrome. Archives of Disease in Childhood 33: 477

Marx H 1926 Die Missbildungen des Ohres. In: Henke F, Lubarsch O (eds) Handbuch des Speziellen pathologische Anatomie und Histologie. Springer, Berlin. p 697

Meckel J F 1812 Handbuch der Pathologische Anatomie, vol 1 Leipzig. p 400

Melnick M, Bixler D, Silk K, Yune H, Nance W 1975 Autosomal dominant branchio-oto-renal dysplasia. Birth Defects (Original Article Series) 11: 121

Melnick M, Myrianthopoulos N C 1979 External ear malformations: epidemiology, genetics and natural history. Birth Defects 15: 1

Meurman Y 1957 Congenital microtia and meatal atresia. Archives of Otolaryngology 66: 443

Moos S, Steinbrugge H 1881 Anatomo-pathological conditions in a case of malformation of the right ear. Archives of Otology 10: 54

Morgan J H 1881 Two cases of congenital macrostomia accompanied by malformation of the auricles and by the presence of auricular appendages. Medical Times and Gazette 613: 1881

Morton J 1855 Case of congenital malformation. Glasgow Medical Journal 3: 167

Murray J E, Kaban L B, Mulliken J B 1984 Analysis and treatment of hemifacial microsomia. Plastic and Reconstructive Surgery 74: 186

Phelps P D, Lloyd G A S, Poswillo D E 1983 The ear deformities in craniofacial microsomia and oculo-auriculo-vertebral dysplasia. Journal of Laryngology and Otology 97: 995

Poswillo D E 1973 The pathogenesis of the first and second branchial arch syndrome. Oral Surgery 35: 302

Poswillo D E 1974a Orofacial malformations. Proceedings of the Society of Medicine 67: 343

Poswillo D E 1974b Otomandibular deformity: pathogenesis as a guide to reconstruction. Journal of Maxillofacial Surgery 2: 64

Potter E L 1937 An hereditary ear deformity transmitted through five generations. Journal of Heredity 28: 255

Pruzansky S 1969 Not all dwarfed mandibles are alike. Birth Defects 2: 120

Pruzansky S 1971a The challenge and opportunity in craniofacial anomalies. Cleft Palate Journal 8: 239

Pruzansky S 1971b Findings of hemifacial microsomia. Paper presented at the First International Symposium of Craniofacial Anomalies, New York

Randall P, Royster H P 1963 First branchial cleft anomalies. Plastic and Reconstructive Surgery 31: 497

Roberts F G, Pruzansky S, Aduss H 1975 An x-radiocephalometric study of mandibulo-facial dysostosis in man. Archives of Oral Biology 20: 265

Rocher H L, Fischer H 1929 L'agnénésie unilatérale et congènitale du corps du maxillaire inférieur. Vigots, Paris

Rogers B O 1968 Microtic, lop, cup and protruding ears: four directly related inheritable deformities. Plastic and Reconstructive Surgery 41: 208

Rollnick B R, Kaye C I 1983 Hemifacial microsomia and variants: pedigree data. American Journal of Medical Genetics 15: 233

Roosa S 1891 Treatise on the diseases of the ear. Wood, New York

Ross R B 1975 Lateral facial dysplasia (first and second branchial arch syndrome, hemifacial microsomia). Birth Defects 11: 51

Rowe N L 1972 Surgery of the temporomandibular joint. Proceedings of the Royal Society of Medicine 65: 383

Rune B, Selvik G, Sarnas K V, Jakobsson S 1981 Growth in hemifacial microsomia studied with the aid of Roentgen stereophotogrammetry and metallic implants. Cleft Palate Journal 18: 128

Samuels L, Lawson L I, Rowe L E 1983 Characteristics of patients with hemifacial microsomia at the craniofacial center. In Harvold E P (ed) Treatment of hemifacial microsomia. Liss, New York. pp 51–55

Sarnat B G, Engel M B 1951 A serial study of mandibular growth after removal of the condyle in the Macaca rhesus monkey. Plastic and Reconstructive Surgery 7: 364

Schwendt A 1891 Ueber congenitale missbildungen des Gehororgans in Verbindung mit branchiogenen Cysten und Fisteln. Archiv fur Ohrenheilkunde 32: 37

Setzer E S et al 1981 Etiologic heterogeneity in the oculoauriculovertebral syndrome. Journal of Pediatrics 98: 88

Sprintzen R J et al 1979 Pharyngeal hypoplasia in Treacher Collins syndrome. Archives of Otolaryngology 105: 127

Stark R B, Saunders D E 1962 The first branchial syndrome: the oro-mandibular-auricular syndrome. Plastic and Reconstructional Surgery 29: 229

Sugar H S 1967 An unusual example of the oculo-auriculo-vertebral dysplasia syndrome of Goldenhar. Journal of Pediatric Ophthalmology 4: 9

Summitt R 1969 Familial Goldenhar syndrome. Birth Defects 2: 106

Sutton J B 1887–1888 On some cases of congenital fissures of the mouth. Transactions of the Odontological Society of Great Britain 22: 97

Sykes P J 1972 Preauricular sinus: clinical features and the problems of recurrence. British Journal of Plastic Surgery 25: 175–179

Tenconi R, Hall B D 1983 Hemifacial microsomia: phenotypic classification, clinical implications and genetic aspects. In: Harvold E P (ed) Treatment of hemifacial microsomia.

Thompson A 1845 A description of congenital malformation of the auricle and external meatus of both sides in three persons. Proceedings of the Royal Society of Edinburgh 1: 443

Thomson A 1846–1847 Notice of several cases of malformations of the external ear, together with experiments on the state of hearing in such persons. Monthly Journal of Medical Science 7: 420

Tolleth H 1978 Artistic anatomy, dimensions, and proportions of the external ear. Clinics in Plastic Surgery 5: 337–345

Tomes C S 1872 Description of a lower jaw, the development of the left ramus which has been arrested. Transactions of the Odontological Society of Great Britain 4: 130

Toynbee J 1847 Description of a congenital malformation in the ears of a child. Monthly Journal of Medical Science 1: 738

Toynbee J 1851–1852 Congenital malformation of the external ear and meatus on each side. Transactions of the Pathological Society of London iii: 435

Toynbee J 1865 The diseases of the ear. Branchard & Lea, Philadelphia

Van Duyse D 1882 376 Macro Stomes. Congenitaux avec tumeurs preauriculaires et dermoide de l'oeil. Annales de la Société Médicale de Gand 60: 141

Vincent R W, Ryan R F, Longenecker C G 1961 Malformation of ear associated with urogenital anomalies. Plastic and Reconstructive Surgery 28: 214

Virchow R 1864 Ueber Missbildungen am Ohr und im Bereiche des ersten Kiemenbogens. Archives of Pathology and Anatomy 30: 221

Wenglowski R.: Ueber die Halsfisteln und Cisten. Arch. Klin. Chir. 100: 798, 1913

Weyers H.: Ueber die Koppelung einseitiger Anotie mit Wirbeldefekten (Auriculo-vertebrallis syndrom). Kinderarztliche Praxis, 34: 415, 1966.

Weyers, H.: Uber eine korrelierte Missbildung der Kiefer und Extremitätenakren. (Dysostosis acro-facialis). Fortschr. Röntgenstr. 77: 562, 1952.

Wenglowski R 1913 Ueber die Halsfisteln und Cisten. Archiv fur Klinische Chirurgie 100: 798

Weyers H 1952 Uber eine korrelierte Missbildung der Kiefer und Extremitätenakren. (Dysostosis acro-facialis). Fortschritte der Röntgenstrahlen 77: 562

Weyers H 1966 Ueber die Koppelung einseitiger Anotie mit Wirbeldefekten (Auriculo-vertebrallis syndrom). Kinderarztliche Praxis 34: 415

Weyers H, Thier C J 1958 Malformations mandibulo-facialis et délimitation d'un 'syndrome oculo-vertébral'. Journal de Génétique Humaine 7: 143–173

Wildervanck L S 1960 Een cervico-oculo-acusticus-syndrome. 24 december 1960. Nederlands Tijdschrift Geneeskunde 104: 52

Wilson T G 1959 A case of unilateral mandibulofacial dysostosis associated with agenesis of the homolateral lung. Journal of Laryngology and Otology 72: 238

Work W P, Proctor C A 1963 The otologist and first branchial cleft anomalies. Annals of Otology, Rhinology and Laryngology 72: 548

INTERMANDIBULAR DYSPLASIA

Couronne A 1819 Observation d'un bec-de-lièvre compliqué de fentes a la voûte palatine. Annales de la Société Médicale de Montpellier 6: 107

Davis A D 1950 Median cleft of the lower lip and mandible. Case report. Plastic and Reconstructive Surgery 6: 62

Eley R C, Farber S 1930 Hypoplasia of the mandible (micrognathy) as a cause of cyanotic attacks in the newly born infant: report of four cases. American Journal of Diseases of Children 39: 1167

Geoffroy Saint-Hilaire I 1832 Histoire generale et particulière des

anomalies en l'organisation chez l'homme et les animaux . . . ou traite de teratologie. Baillière, Paris

Hallermann W 1948 Vogelgesicht und Cataracta congenita. Klinische Monatsblatter fur Augenheilkunde 113: 315

Hanhart E 1949 Nachweis einer einfach-dominanten, unkomplizierten sowie unregel-massig-dominanten, mit Atresia auris, Palatoschisis und anderen Deformationen verbundenen Anlage zu Ohrmuschelverkermmerung (Mikrotie). Archiv der Julius Klaus-Stiftung fur Vererbungsforschung 24: 374

Hanhart E 1950 Uber die Kombination von Peromelie mit Mikrognathie, ein neues Syndrom beim Menschen, entsprechend der Akroteriasis congenita von Wriedt und Mohr beim Rinde. Archiv der Julius Klaus-Stiftung fur Vererbungsforschung 25: 531

Josephy H 1909 Octocephalie. In: Schwalbe E (ed) 'Die Morphologie der Missbildungen des Menschen und der Tiere, vol III/I. Fischer, Jena. p 247

Lannelongue M 1879 Sur un cas de bec de lièvre congénital médian et complet de la lèvre inférieure, compliqué d'une division de la machoire inférieure. Bulletin de la Société des Chirurgiens de Paris 5: 621

Monroe C W 1966 Midline cleft of the lower lip, mandible, tongue with flexion contracture of the neck. Case report and review of the literature. Plastic and Reconstructive Surgery 38: 312

Morton C B, Jordan H E 1935 Median cleft of lower lip and mandible, cleft sternum and absence of basihyoid. Archives of Surgery 30: 647

Parise 1862 Division de la lèvre inférieure et de la mandibule. Bulletin et Mémoires de la Société de Therapeutique 4: 269

Randall P, Hamilton R 1971 The Pierre Robin syndrome. In: Grabb W C, Rosenstein S W, Bzoch K R (eds) Cleft lip and Palate. Little Brown, Boston

Robin P 1923 Backward lowering of the root of the tongue causing respiratory disturbances. Bulletin of the Academy of Medicine 89: 37

Stickler G B, Belau P G, Farell F J et al 1965 Hereditary progressive arthroophthalmopathy. Mayo Clinic Proceedings 40: 433

Streiff E B 1950 Dysmorphie mandibulo-faciale (tête d'oiseau) et altérations oculaires. Ophthalmologica 120: 79

Ullrich O, Fremerey-Dohna H 1953 Dyskephalie mit Cataracta congenita und Hypotrichose als typischer Merkmalskomplex. Ophthalmologica 125: 73

Van Balen A Th M 1961 Dyscephaly with microphthalmos, cataract and hypoplasia of the mandible. Ophthalmologica 141: 53–63

Wolfler A 1890 Zur Casuistik der medianen Gesichtsspalte. Archiv fur Klinische Chirurgie 40: 795

Craniofacial dysplasias with synostosis

Acquaviva R, Tamic P M, Lebascle J Jr, Kerdoudi H, Berrada A 1966 Les craniostenoses en milieu marocain. A propos de 140 observations. Neurochirurgie 12: 561–566

Anderson B, Woodhall B 1953 Visual loss in primary skull deformities. Transactions of the American Academy of Ophthalmology and Otolaryngology 57: 497–516

Anderson F M, Geiger L 1965 Craniosynostosis: a survey of 204 cases. Journal of Neurosurgery 22: 229

Anderson H 1977 Craniosynostosis. In: Vinken P J, Bruyn G V (eds) Handbook of clinical neurology, vol 30. Elsévier, Amsterdam. pp 219–233

Anderson H, Gomes S P 1968 Craniosynostosis: review of the literature and indications for surgery. Acta Paediatrica Scandinavica 57: 47–54

Andre M 1972 Pronostic et resultats a long terme des opérations sur les craniostenoses prematurées. Lyon Medical 227: 1081–1093

Austin J H M, Gooding C A 1971 Roentgenographic measurement of skull size in children. Radiology 99: 641

Backman G 1908 Ueber die Scaphocephalie Bergmann, Wiesbaden

Berrada A 1964 Etude sur les craniostenoses en milieu marocain. A propos de 87 observations. Travail du centre de neurochirurgie de Casablanca. Thèse de Paris 16: 3

Bertelsen T I 1958 The premature synostosis of the cranial sutures. Acta Ophthalmologica (suppl) 51: 1–176

Bertolotti M 1910 Le syndrome radiologique de l'oxycephalie et des états similaires d'hypertension cérébrale. Contribution clinique, anatomique et antrophologique a la pathologie osseuse du crâne. Presse Medicale 18: 946–951

Bertolotti M 1914 Le syndrome oxycephalique ou syndrome de cranio-synostose pathologique. Presse Medicale 22: 332–334

Binder K H 1962 Dysostosis maxillo-nasalis, ein airhinencephaler Missbildungskomplex. Deutsche Zahnarztliche Zeitschrift 17: 438

Bolk L 1915 On the premature obliteration of sutures in the human skull. American Journal of Anatomy 17: 495–523

Bolk L 1919 Ueber pramature Obliteration der Nahte am Menschenschaedel. Zeitschrift fur Morphologie und Anthropologie 21: 1–22

Buchignani J S, Cook A J, Anderson L G 1972 Roentgenographic findings in familial osteodysplasia. American Journal of Roentgenology 116: 602–608

Carmel P W, Luken M G, Ascherl G F 1981 Craniosynostosis: computed tomographic evaluation of skull base and calvarial deformities and associated intracranial changes. Neurosurgery 9: 366–372

Choux M (quoted by Montaut & Stricker 1977)

Cohen M M Jr 1975 An etiologic and nosologic overview of craniosynostosis syndromes. Birth Defects 11: 137–189

Cohen M M Jr 1977 Genetic perspectives on craniosynostosis and syndromes with craniosynostosis. Journal of Neurosurgery 47: 886–898

Cohen M M Jr 1979 Craniosynostosis and syndromes with craniosynostosis. Incidence, genetics, penetrance, variability and new syndrome updating. Birth Defects 15: 13–63

Cohen M M Jr 1980 Perspectives on craniosynostosis. Western Journal of Medicine 132: 507–513

Cohen M M Jr 1982 The child with multiple birth defects. Raven Press, New York

Cronqvist S 1968 Roentgenologic evaluation of cranial size in children: a new index, Acta Radiologica: Diagnosis 7: 97

Currarino G, Silverman F N 1960 Orbital hypotelorism, arhinencephaly and trigonocephaly. Radiology 74: 206–217

David J D, Poswillo D, Simpson D 1982 The craniosynostoses: causes, natural history and management. Springler, New York

Delaire J, Gaillard A, Billet J, Landais H, Renaud Y 1963 Considérations sur les synostosis prématurées et leur conséquences au crâne et à la face. Revue de Stomatologie 64: 97–106

DeRossi G, Focacci C 1979 Early detection of craniosynostosis by [99m]Te-pyrophosphate bone scanning. Radiologica Diagnostica 20: 405–409

Djindjian R 1952 L'oxycephalie. Concours Medical 10: 863–870

Doerr W 1949 Ueber die geburtstraumatische Nahtsynostosis des kindlichen Schaedelsaches. Zeitschrift fur Kinderheilkunde 67: 96–122

Dominguez R, Oh K S, Bender T, Girdany B R 1981 Uncomplicated trigonocephaly. Radiology 140: 681–688

Duggan C A, Keener E B, Gay B B 1970 Secondary craniosynostosis. American Journal of Roentgenology 109: 277–293

Ebel K D, Weidtman V 1971 Die craniometrie pathologischer Schaedelformen. Radiologe 11: 291–295

Fairman D, Horrax G 1949 Classification of craniostenosis. Journal of Neurosurgery 6: 307–313

Faure C, Bonamy P, Rambert-Misset C 1967 Les craniostenoses par fusion prématurée unilatérale de la suture coronale. Annales de Radiologie 10: 32–42

Fishman M A, Hogan G R, Dodge P R 1971 The concurrence of hydrocephalus and craniosynostosis. Journal of Neurosurgery 34: 621–629

Foltz E L, Loeser J D 1975 Craniosynostosis. Journal of Neurosurgery 43: 48–57

Fridolin J 1885 Studien ueber fruehzeitige Schaedelformitaeten. Virchows Archiv Abteilung A 100: 266–273

Frydman M, Kauschansky A, Elian E 1984 Trigonocephaly: a new familial syndrome. American Journal of Medical Genetics 18: 55–59

Gates G F, Dore E K 1975 Detection of craniosynostosis by bone scanning. Radiology 115: 665–671

Gaudier B, Laine E, Fontaine G, Castier C, Farriaux J P 1967 Les craniosynostosis (étude de vingt observations). Archives Françaises de Pediatrie 24: 775–792

Gordon I R S 1966 Measurements of cranial capacity in children. British Journal of Radiology 39: 377

Gorlin R J 1982 Thoughts on some new old bone dysplasias. In: Papadatos C J, Bartsocas C S (eds) Skeletal dysplasias. Liss New York. pp 47–51

Graham J M, Smith D W 1980 Metopic craniostenosis as a consequence of fetal head constraint: two interesting experiments of nature. Pediatrics 65: 1000–1002

Graham J M, deSaxe M, Smith D W 1979 Sagittal cranial stenosis. Fetal head constraint as one possible cause. Journal of pediatrics 95: 747–750

Graham J M, Badura R J, Smith D W 1980 Coronal craniostenosis: fetal head constraint as one possible cause. Pediatrics 65: 995–999

Greig D M 1926 Oxycephaly. Edinburgh Medical Journal 33: 189–218, 280–302, 357–376

Günther H 1931 Der Turmschaedel als Konstitutionsanomalie und als klinisches Symptom. Ergebrisse der Inneren Medizin und Kinderheilkunde 40: 40–135

Haas L L 1952 Roentgenological skull measurements and their diagnostic applications. American Journal of Roentgenology 67: 197

Hanotte M 1898 Anatomie pathologique de l'oxycephalie. Thèse Médicale

Herzog T 1914 Beitrag zur Pathologie der Turmschaedels. Bruns Beitraege zur Klinischen Chirurgie 90: 464–489

Howel S C 1954 The craniostenosis. American Journal of Ophthalmology 37: 359–379

Hunter A G W, Rudd N L 1976 Craniosynostosis. I. Sagittal synostosis: its genetics and associated clinical findings in 214 patients who lacked involvement of the coronal suture(s). Teratology 14: 185–193

Hunter A G W, Rudd N L 1977 Craniosynostosis. II. Coronal synostosis: its familial characteristics and associated clinical findings in 109 patients lacking bilateral polysyndactyly or syndactyly. Teratology 15: 301–310

Ingraham F D, Matson D D 1954 Neurosurgery of infancy and childhood. Thomas, Springfield Ill

Ingraham F D, Alexander E Jr, Matson D D 1948a Clinical studies in craniosynostosis: analysis of 50 cases and description of a method of surgical treatment. Surgery 24: 518

Ingraham F D, Matson D D, Alexander E 1948b Experimental observations in the treatment of craniosynostosis. Surgery 23: 252–268

Kaufman B, David G J 1972 A method of intracranial volume calculation. Investigative Radiology 7: 533

King J 1942 Oxycephaly. Annals of Surgery 115: 488–506

Knudson H W & Flaherty R A 1960a (quoted by Montaut and Stricker 1977)

Knudson H W, Flaherty R A 1960b Craniosynostoses. American Journal of Roentgenology 84: 454–460

Kreiborg S, Bjoerk A 1981 Craniofacial asymmetry of a dry skull with plagiocephaly. European Journal of Orthodontics 3: 195–203

Kundrat K K 1882 Arhrinencephalie als typische Art von Nissbildung. Leuschner, Lubensky, Graz

Laitinen L 1956 Craniosynostosis: premature fusion of the coronal sutures. Annales Paediatriae Fenniae 2: 18

Matson D D 1969 Neurosurgery of infancy and childhood, 2nd edn. Thomas, Springfield, Ill

Mehner A 1921 Beitrage zu den Augenveranderungen bei der Schaedeldeformitat des sog. Turmschaedels mit besonderer Beruksichtigung des Roentgenbildes. Klinische Monatsblatter fur Augenheilkunde 61: 204

Michel J 1873 Beitrag zur Kenntnis der Entstehung der sogenannten Stauungspapille. Archiv fur vergleichende Ophthalmologie 14: 39–52

Monnet M P 1970 Craniosynostoses prématurées. Revue Lyonnaise de Medecine 19: 89–94

Montaut J, Stricker M 1977 Dysmorphies cranio-faciales: les synostoses prématurées (craniostenoses et facio-craniostenoses). Masson, Paris

Moss M L 1959 The pathogenesis of premature cranial synostosis in man. Acta Anatomica 37: 351

Müke R 1972 Neue Gesichtspunke zur Pathogenese und Therapie der Kraniosynostose. Acta Neurochirurgical 26: 191–250, 293–326

Nathan M H, Collins V P, Collins L C 1961 Premature unilateral

synostosis of the coronal suture. American Journal of
Roentgenology 86: 433–446

Park E A, Powers G F 1920 Acrocephaly and scaphocephaly with
symmetrically distributed malformations of the extremities.
American Journal of Diseases of Children 20: 235–315

Patry A 1905 Contribution a l'étude des lésions oculaires dans les
malformations crâniènnes. Spécialement dans l'oxycephalie. Thèse,
Faculté de Médecin, Paris

Pinkterton O D, Pinkterton F J 1952 Hereditary craniofacial dysplasia.
American Journal of Ophthalmology 35: 500–506

Pommerol F 1869 Recherche sur la synostose des os de crâne. Thèse
Médicale, Paris

Pruzansky S 1973 Clinical investigation of the experiments of nature.
ASHA 8: 62–94

Pruzansky S 1976 Radiocephalometric studies of the basicranium in
craniofacial malformations. In: Bosma J F (ed) Development of the
Basicranium. DHEW Publication no (NIH) 76–989, Bethesda.
pp 278–298

Pugeaut R 1968 Le problème neuro-chirurgical des craniostenoses.
Cahier de Médecin Lyonnais 44: 3343–3357

Pujo X P 1960 Contribution a l'étude des craniostenoses. Thèse
Médicale, Toulouse. p 25

Reiping A 1919 Zur Pathogenese des Turmschaedels. Deutsche
Zeitschrift fur Chirurgie 148: 1–51

Renier D, Sainte-Rose C, Marchac D, Hirsch J E 1982 Intracranial
pressure in craniostenosis. Journal of Neurosurgery 57: 370–377

Riemenschneider P A 1957 Trigonocephaly. Radiology 68: 863–865

Rougerie J, Derome P, Anquez L 1972 Craniostenoses et
dysmorphoses cranio-faciales. Principes d'une nouvelle méthode de
traitement et ses résultats. Neurochirurgie 18: 429–440

Schueller A 1929 Craniostenoses. Radiology 13: 377–382

Sear H R 1937 Some notes on craniostenosis. British Journal of
Radiology 10: 445–487

Seeger J F, Gabrielsen T O 1971 Premature closure of the
frontosphenoidal suture in synostosis of the coronal suture.
Radiology 101: 631–635

Shillito J Jr, Matson D D 1968 Craniosynostosis. A review of 519
surgical patients. Pediatrics 41: 829–853

Simmons D R, Peyton W T 1947 Premature closure of the cranial
sutures. Journal of Pediatrics 31: 528–546

Smith D W 1974 Types reconnaissables de malformations humaines.
Masson, Paris

Tait M V, Gilday D L, Ash J M, Boldt D J, Harwood-Nash D C E
1979 Craniosynostosis correlation of bone scans, radiographs and
surgical findings. Radiology 13: 615–621

Thoma R 1907 Synostosis suturae sagittalis cranii. Virchows Archiv
Abteilung A 188: 248–360

Till K 1975 Pediatric neurosurgery. Blackwell Scientific, London

Till K 1979 Craniosynostosis. In: Symon L (ed) Operative surgery:
neurosurgery, 3rd edn. Butterworth, Boston. pp 408–418

Tridon P, Thiriet M 1966 Malformations associées de la tête et des
extrémités. Masson, Paris

Van der Werf M A J M 1966 Les craniosynostoses. Thèse Médicale,
Amsterdam

Vargervik K, Miller A J 1982 Observations on the temporal muscle in
craniosynostosis. Birth Defects 18: 45–51

Virchow R 1851 Ueber den Cretinismus, namentlich in Franken, und
ueber pathologische Schaedelformen. Verhandlungen des
Physikalische-Medizinischen Gesellschaft zu Wurzburg 2: 230–270

von Bauer K E 1860 Die Macrocephalen im Boden der Krym und
Oesterreichs, verglichen mit der Bildungs – abweichung, welche
Blumenback Macrocephalus genannt hat. Memoires de l'Academie
Imperiale des Sciences de St Petersburg Sei. St Petersburg, VII
Serie, Band 2, No 6

Warkany J, Lemire R J, Cohen M M Jr 1981 Mental retardation and
congenital malformations of the central nervous system. Year book
Medical Publishers, Chicago

Weiss L 1969 (quoted by Montaut & Stricker) 1977

Welcker H 1862 Untersuchungen ueber Wachstum und Bau des
menslichen Schaedels, vol 1. Engelmann, Leipzig. pp 120–124

Willich E 1955 Ueber eine seltene Schaedelfehlbildung. Plagiocephalie
mit Dysostosis sphenoidalis. Archiv fur Kinderheilkunde
150: 279–289

Woon K C, Kokich V G, Clarren S K, Cohen M M Jr 1980
Craniosynostosis with associated cranial anomalies: a morphologic
and histologic study of affected like-sexed twins. Teratology
22: 23–35

Zuckerhandl E 1882 Fossae praenasales. Normale und pathologische.
Anatomischer Nasenhole 1: 48

Craniofacial dysplasias with dysostosis and synostosis

CROUZON'S SYNDROME

Anderson F M, Geiger L 1956 Craniosynostosis: a survey of 204 cases.
Journal of Neurosurgery 22: 229–240

Atkins F R B 1937 Hereditary craniofacial dysostosis or Crouzon's
disease. Medical Press and Circulair 195: 118–124

Aubry M 1935 Examen otologique de dix cas de dysostose. Revue
Neurologique 62: 302

Baldwin J L 1968 Dysostosis craniofacialis of Crouzon. A summary of
recent literature and case reports with involvement of the ear.
Laryngoscope 78: 1660–1676

Berrada A 1963–1964 Etude sur les craniostenoses en milieum
marocain. A propos de 87 observations. Thèse Médicale, Paris

Bertelsen T I 1958 The premature synostosis of the cranial sutures.
Acta Ophthalmologica (suppl) 51: 1–176

Bigot C 1922 L'acrocephalo-syndactylie. Thèse pour le doctorat en
médecine. Faculte de Médecine, Paris

Chatelin 1914 (quoted by Montaut & Stricker 1977)

Choux M 1978 Craniostenoses. Annexes de Pediatrie 25: 309–314

Crouzon O 1912 Dysostose craniofaciale héréditaire. Bulletin de la
Société de Médecine d'Hôpital 33: 545–555

Crouzon O 1915 Une nouvelle famille atteinte de dysostose crânio-
faciale héréditaire. Archives de Médecine de l'Enfant 18: 540

Crouzon O 1929 Une nouvelle famille atteinte de dysostose cranio-
faciale hereditaire. Annals of Medicine 25: 84

Crouzon O 1932 Sur la dysostose crânio-faciale héréditaire et sur les
rapports avec l'acro-cephalo-syndactylie. Bulletins et Mémoires de la
Société de Médecine d'Hôpital 48: 1568

Crouzon O 1936 Les dysostose prechordales. Bulletin de l'Académie de
Médecine 115: 696–700

Cruveiller J 1954 La maladie d'Apert–Crouzon. Thèse Médicale, Paris

David J D, Poswillo D, Simpson D 1982 The craniosynostoses: causes,
natural history and management. Springer, New York

de Gunten P 1938 Contribution a l'étude des malformations de la face
et des maxillaires dans la dysostose crâniofaciale. Annals of
Otolaryngology 57: 1056–1075

Devine P, Bhan I, Feingold M, Leonidas J C, Wolpert S M 1984
Completely cartilaginous trachea in a child with Crouzon syndrome.
American Journal of Diseases of Children 138: 40–43

Dodge H W Jr, Wood M W, Kennedey R L J 1959 Craniofacial
dysostosis: Crouzon's disease. Pediatrics 23: 98–106

Don N, Siggers D C 1971 Cor pulmonale in Crouzon's disease.
Archives of Disease in Childhood 46: 394–397

Flippen J H Jr 1950 Craniofacial dysostosis of Crouzon. Report of a
case in which the malformation occurred in four generations.
Pediatrics 5: 90

Franceschetti A 1953 Dysostose cranienne avec calotte cerebriforme
(pseudo-Crouzon). Confin Neurol 13: 161–166

Garcin M, Thurel R, Rudeaux P 1932 Sur un cas isole de dysostose
crâniofaciale (maladie de Crouzon) avec extradactylie. Bulletins de la
Société de Médecine de l'Hôpital 56: 1458–1466

Golabi M, Chierici G, Oosterhout D K, Vargervik K 1984
Radiographic abnormalities of Crouzon syndrome: a survey of 23
cases. Proceedings of Greenwood Genetic Centre 3: 102

Grenet H, Leveuf J, Issac G 1934 Etude anatomique de la maladie de
Crouzon. Bulletin de la Société Pediatrique 32: 343–350

Gunther G 1933 Dysostose crâniofaciale héréditaire. Endocrinologie
13: 255–260

Heuyer G 1951 A propos de la dysostose crânio-faciale (ou maladie de
Crouzon). Actualités Odonto-stomatologiques 16: 413

Jones K L, Cohen M M Jr 1973 The Crouzon syndrome. Journal of
Medical Genetics 10: 398–399

Juberg R C, Chambers S R 1973 An autosomal recessive form of craniofacial dysostosis (the Crouzon syndrome). Journal of Medical Genetics 10: 89–94

Kaler S G, Bixler D, Yu P 1982 Radiographic hand abnormalities in fifteen cases of Crouzon syndrome. Journal of Craniofacial Genetics and Developmental Biology 2: 205–213

Keats T E, Smith T H, Sweet D E 1975 Craniofacial dysostosis with fibrous metaphyseal defects. American Journal of Roentgenology 124: 271–275

Kreiborg S 1981a Crouzon syndrome. A clinical and roentgencephalometric study. Scandinavian Journal of Plastic and Reconstructive Surgery (suppl) 18: 1–198

Kreiborg S, Jensen B L 1977 Variable expressivity of Crouzon's syndrome within a family. Scandinavian Journal of Dental Research 85: 175–184

Kreiborg S, Bjoerk A 1982 Inscription of a dry skull with Crouzon's syndrome. Scandinavian Journal of Plastic and Reconstructive Surgery 245–253

Kreiborg S 1981b Craniofacial growth in plagiocephaly and Crouzon syndrome. Scandinavian Journal of Plastic and Reconstructive Surgery 15: 187–197

Lake M S, Kuppinger J C 1950 Craniofacial dysostosis (Crouzon's disease): report of three cases. Archives of Ophthalmology 44: 37–46

Leonard M A 1974 A sporadic case of apparent Crouzon's syndrome with extra craniofacial manifestations. Journal of Medical Genetics II: 206–215

Lutier F 1965 Le cadre elargi de la maladie de Crouzon. Presse Medicale 73: 1043–1046

McKusick V A 1978 Mendelian inheritance in man, 5th edn. Johns Hopkins University Press, Baltimore

Manns K J, Bopp K P 1965 Dysostosis craniofacialis Crouzon mit digitaler Anomalie. Medizinische Klinik 60: 1899–1910

Maximilian C, Dumiitriu L, Ionitiu D et al 1981 Syndrome de dysostose craniofaciale avec hyperplasie diaphysaire. Journal de Génétique Humaine 29: 129–139

Maroteau P 1974 Maladies osseuses de l'enfant. Flammarion Paris

Moretti G, Staeffen J 1959 Dysostose crânio-faciale de Crouzon et syringomyelie: association chez le frère et la soeur. Presse Medicale 67: 376–380

Peterson S J, Pruzansky S 1974 Palatal anomalies in the syndromes of Apert and Crouzon. Cleft Palate Journal 11: 394–403

Peterson-Falzone S J, Pruzansky S, Parris P J, Laffer J L 1981 Nasopharoryngeal dysmorphology in the syndromes of Apert and Crouzon. Cleft Palate Journal 18: 237–250

Pinkerton O D, Pinkerton F J 1952 Hereditary craniofacial dysplasia. American Journal of Ophthalmology 35: 500–506

Pugeaut R 1968 Le probleme neuro-chirurgical des crâniostenoses. Cahier Médicale Lyonnais 44: 3343–3357

Reddy B S N 1985 An unusual association of acathosis nigricans and Crouzon's disease. Journal of Dermatology 12: 85–90

Regnault F, Crouzon O 1927 Etude sur un cas de dysostose crânio-faciale héréditaire. Annales Medical de l'Enfant 43: 676–681

Roubinovitch & Crouzon O 1927 (quoted by Montaut & Stricker 1977).

Rougerie J, Derome P, Anquez L 1972 Crâniostenoses et dysmorphies crâniofaciales: principes d'une nouvelle technique de traitement et ses résultats. Neurochirurgie 18: 429

Schlapfer H 1939 Dyskephallie (Dysostosis craniofacialis-Maladie de Crouzon) bei zwei Schwestern. Klinische Monatsblatter fur Augenheilkunde 103: 469–477

Shiller J G 1959 Craniofacial dysostosis of Crouzon: a case report and pedigree with emphasis on heredity. Pediatrics 23: 107–112

Shillito J Jr, Matson D D 1968 Craniosynostosis. A review of 519 surgical patients. Pediatrics 41: 829–853

Smith D W 1974 Types reconnaissables de malformations humaines. Masson, Paris

Stanescu V, Maximillian C, Poenaru S et al 1963 Syndrome héréditaire dominant, reunissant une dysostose crânio-faciale de type particulier, une insuffiscance de croissance d'aspect chondrodystrophique et un épaississement massif de la corticale des os longes. Revue Française d'Endocrinologie Clinique 4: 219–231

Suslak E 1984 Crouzon's craniofacial dysostosis, periapical cemental dysplasia, and acanthosis nigricans: the pleitropic effect of a single gene? Society of Craniofacial Genetics, Denver, June 17

Tridon P, Thiriet M 1966 Malformations associées de la tête et des extrémités. Masson, Paris

Vogt A 1933 Dyskephalie (Dysostosis craniofacialis, Maladie de Crouzon 1912) und eine neuartige Kombination dieser Krankheit mit Syndaktylie der 4 Extremitaeten (Dyskephlodaktylie). Klinisches Monatsblatter fur Augenheilkunde 90: 441–460

Vuilliamy D G, Normandale P A 1966 Craniofacial dysostosis in a Dorset family. Archives of Disease in Childhood 41: 275–382

APERT'S SYNDROME

Apert E 1906 De l'acrocephalosyndactylie. Bulletin de la Société de Médecine 23: 1310–1330

Beaudoing A, Butin L P, Hadjian A J, Coulomb M 1967 Le syndrome d'Apert (acrocephalosyndactylie). Pediatrie 22: 723–724

Bigot C 1922 L'acrocephalo-syndactylie. Thèse pour le Doctorat en Médecine. Faculté de Médecine de Paris

Blank C E 1960 Apert's syndrome (a type of acrocephalo-syndactyly): observations on a British series of thirty-nine cases. Annals of Human Genetics 24: 151–164

Book J A, Hesselvink L 1953 Acrocephalosyndactyly. Acta Paediatrica. Scandinavica 42: 359–364

Buchanan R C 1968 Acrocephalosyndactyly, or Apert's syndrome. British Journal of Plastic Surgery 21: 406–418

Bull M, Escobar V, Bixler D, Antley R 1979 Phenotype definition and recurrence risk in the acrocephalosyndactyly syndromes. Birth Defects 15: 65–74

Caramia G, Venturelli D 1968 La sindrome di Apert. Clinical Pediatrics 50: 453–465

Cohen M M Jr 1972 Cardiovascular anomalies in Apert type acrocephalosyndactyly. Birth Defects 8: 132–133

Cohen M M Jr, Gorlin R J, Berkman M D, Feingold M 1971 Facial variability in Apert type acrocephalo-syndactyly. Birth Defects 7: 262

Cuttone J M, Brazis P T, Miller M T, Falk E R 1980 Absence of the superior rectus muscle in Apert's sydrome. Journal of Pediatric Ophthalmology 16: 349–354

de Gunten P 1938 Contribution à l'étude des malformations de la face et des maxillaires dans la dysostose crânio-faciale. Annals of Otolaryngology 57: 1056–1075

Dodson W E, Museles M, Kennedy J L Jr, Al-Aish M 1979 Acrocephalosyndactylia associated with chromosomal translocation. American Journal of Diseases of Children 133: 818–821

Dunn F H 1962 Apert's acrocephalosyndactylism. Radiology 78: 738–743

Elejalde B R, Giraldo C, Jiminez R 1977 Acrocephalopolydactylous dysplasia. Birth Defects 13: 53–67

Erickson J D, Cohen M M Jr 1974 A study of parental age effects on the occurrunce of fresh mutations for the Apert syndrome. Annals of Human Genetics 38: 89–96

Frerichs C T 1967 Apert's syndrome. Nebraska Medical Journal 52: 491–495

Genest P, Mortezai M A, Tremblay M 1966 Le syndrome d'Apert (acrocephalosyndactyly). Archives Françaises de Pediatrie 23: 887–897

Green S M 1982 pathological anatomy of the hands in Apert's syndrome. Journal of Hand Surgery 7: 450–453

Harris V, Beligere N, Pruzansky S 1977 Progressive generalized bony dysplasia in Apert syndrome. Birth Defects 14: 175

Hermann J, Opitz J M 1969 An unusual form of acrocephalosyndactyly. Birth Defects 5: 39–42

Hogan G R, Bauman M L 1971 Hydrocephalus in Apert's syndrome. Journal of Pediatrics 79: 782–787

Holmes E M (quoted by Montaut & Stricker 1977)

Hoover G H, Flatt A E, Weiss M W 1970 The hand and Apert's syndrome. Journal of Bone and Joint Surgery 52: 878–895

Kreiborg S, Prysdoe U, Dahl E, Fogh-Andersen P 1976 Clinical conference I. Calvarium and cranial base in Apert's syndrome: an autopsy report. Cleft Palate Journal 13: 296–303

Lacharetz M, Walbum C H, Tourgis R 1974 L'acrocephalo-synankie. A propos d'une observation avec synostoses multiples. Pediatrie 29: 169–177

Leonard C O, Daikoku N H, Winn K 1982 Prenatal fetoscopic diagnosis of the Apert syndrome. American Journal of Medical Genetics 11: 5–9

Mckusick V A 1978 Mendelian inheritance in Man, 5th edn. Johns Hopkins University Press Baltimore

Margolis S, Siegel I M, Choy A, Breinin G M 1978 Depigmentation of hair, skin, and eyes associated with the Apert syndrome. Birth Defects 14: 341–360

Maroteau P 1974 Maladies osseuses de l'enfant. Flammation, Paris

Mathur J S, Nema H V, Mehra K S, Dwivedi P N 1968 Apert's anomaly — a transition. Acta Ophthalmologica 46: 1041–1045

Ousterhout D K, Melsen B 1982 Cranial base deformity in Apert's syndrome. Plastic and Reconstructive Surgery 69: 254–263

Park E A, Powers G F 1920 Acrocephaly and scaphocephaly with symmetrically distributed malformations of the extremities. American Journal of Diseases of Children 20: 235–315

Peterson S J, Pruzansky S 1974 Palatal anomalies in the syndrome of Apert and Crouzon. Cleft Palate Journal 11: 394–403

Peterson-Falzone S J, Pruzansky S, Parris P J, Laffer J L 1981 Nasopharyngeal dysmorphology in the syndromes of Apert and Crouzon. Cleft Palate Journal 18: 237–250

Pillay V K 1964 Acrocephalosyndactyly in Singapore. A study of five Chinese males. Journal of Bone and Joint Surgery 46: 94–101

Roberts K B, Hall J G 1971 Apert's acrocephalosyndactyly in mother and daughter: cleft palate in the mother. Birth Defects 7: 262–263

Schauerte E W, St Aubin P M 1966 Progressive synostosis in Apert's syndrome (acrocephalosyndactyly) with a description of roentgenographic changes in the feet. American Journal of Roentgenology 97: 67–73

Scott C I 1972 The Apert syndrome with coarctation of the aorta. Birth Defects 8: 239–241

Solomon L M, Fretzin D, Pruzansky S 1970 Pilosebaceous abnormalities in Apert's syndrome. Archives of Dermatology 102: 381–385

Solomon L M, Cohen M M Jr, Pruzansky S 1971 Pilosebaceous abnormalities in Apert type acrocephalo-syndactyly. Birth Defects 7: 193–195

Solomon L M, Medenica M, Pruzansky S, Kreiborg S 1973 Apert syndrome and palatal mucopolysaccharides. Teratology 8: 287–292

Stewart R E, Dixon G, Cohen A 1977 The pathogenesis of premature craniosynostosis in acrocephalosyndactyly (Apert's syndrome): a reconsideration. Plastic and Reconstructive Surgery 59: 699–707

Traissac M 1962 (quoted by Montaut & Stricker 1977)

Tridon P, Thiriet M 1966 Malformations associées de la tête et des extrémités. Masson, Paris

Tünte W, Lenz W 1967 Zur Haeufigkeit und Mutationsrates des Aperts-Syndroms. Human Genetics 4: 104–111

Valentin B 1938 Die Korrelation (Koppelung) Missbildungen, erlautert am Beispiel der Acrocephalosyndactylie. Acta Orthopaedica Scandinavica 9: 235–316

Van den Bosch J, cited in Blank C E 1960 Apert's syndrome (a type of acrocephalosyndactyly): observations on a British series of thirty-nine cases. Annals of Human Genetics 24: 151–164

Verger P, Traissac M et al 1962 Acrocephalosyndactilie. Etude clinique et radiologique de deux cas chez des nouveaux nes. Archives Françaises de Pediatrie 18: 1076–1080

Waterson J R, DiPietro M A, Barr M 1985 Brief clinical report: Apert syndrome with frontonasal encephalocele. American Journal of Medical Genetics 21: 777–783

Weech A A 1927 Combined acrocephaly and syndactylism occurring in mother and daughter. Bulletin of Johns Hopkins Hospital 40: 73–76

Wigert 1932 Die Akrokephalosyndactylie weiters ueber die Allgemeine Skelett Veraenderungen. Acta Psychiatrika et Neurologika, fasc 1 et 2

Zippel H, Schuller K H 1969 Dominant vererbte Akrozephalosyndaktylie (ACS). Fortschritte der Roentgenstrahlen 110: 2340–2345

OTHER SYNDROMES

Allain D, Babin J P, Demarques J L et al 1976 Acrocephalosynankie, pseudomaphrodisme feminin et néphropathie hypertensive. Annales de Pediatrie 23: 277–284

Antley R, Bixler D 1975 Trapezoidocephaly, midfacial hypoplasia and cartilage abnormalities with multiple synostoses and skeletal factures. Birth Defects 11: 397–401

Antley R M, Bixler D 1983 Invited editorial comment: developments in the trapezoidocephaly–multiple synostosis syndrome. American Journal of Medical Genetics 14: 149–150

Antley R M, Hwang D S, Theopold W, Gorlin R J 1981 Further delineation of the C (trigonocephaly) syndrome. American Journal of Medical Genetics 9: 147–163

Anyane-Yeboa K, Gunning L, Bloom A D 1980 Baller–Gerold syndrome: craniosynostosis–radial aplasia syndrome. Clinical Genetics 17: 161–166

Armendares S, Antillon F, del Castillo V 1974 A newly recognized inherited syndrome of dwarfism, craniosynostosis, retinitis pigmentosa and multiple malformations. Journal of Pediatrics 85: 872–873

Armendares S, Antillon F, de Castillo V, Jimminez M 1975 A newly recognized inherited syndrome of dwarfism, craniosynostosis, retinitis pigmentosa and multiple congenital malformations. Birth Defects 11: 49–53

Asnes R S, Morehead C D 1969 Pfeiffer syndrome. Birth Defects 5: 198–203

Avoldelli G, Schinzel A 1982 Prenatal ultrasonic detection of humero-radial synostosis in a case of Antley–Bixler syndrome. Prenatal Diagnosis 2: 219–223

Baller F 1950 Radiusaplasie und Inzucht. Z Menschl Vererbungs Konstit Lehre 29: 782–790

Baraitser M, Rodeck C, Garner A 1982 A new craniosynostosis mental retardation syndrome diagnosed by fetoscopy. Clinical Genetics 22: 12–15

Baraitser M, Winter R M, Brett E M 1983 Greig cephalopolysyndactyly: report of 13 affected inviduals in three families. Clinical Genetics 24: 257–265

Bartsocas C S, Weber A L, Crawford J D 1970 Chotzen's syndrome. Journal of Pediatrics 77: 267–272

Beare J M, Dodge J A, Nevin N C 1969 Cutis gyratum, acanthosis nigricans, and other congenital anomalies: a new syndrome. British Journal of Dermatology 81: 241–247

Beighton P, Cremin B J, Kozlowski K 1980 Osteoglophonic dwarfism. Pediatric Radiology 10: 46–50

Benke P J 1984 The isotretinion teratogen syndrome. Journal of the American Medical Association 251: 3267–3269

Berant M, Berant N 1973 Radioulnar synostosis and craniosynostosis in one family. Journal of Pediatrics 83: 88–90

Bernheim A, Berger R, Vaugier G, Thieffry J C, Matck Y 1979 Patrial trisomy 6p. Human Genetics 48: 13–16

Bianchi D W 1984 FG syndrome in a premature male. American Journal of Medical Genetics 19: 383–386

Bianchi D W, Cirillo-Silengo M, Luzzatti L, Greenstein R M 1981 Interstitial delection of the short arm of chromosome 7 without craniosynostosis. Clinical Genetics 19: 456–461

Burn J, Martin N 1983 Two retarded male cousins with old facies, hypotonia and reserve constripation: Possible examples of the X-linked FG syndrome. Journal of Medical Genetics 20: 97–99

Carpenter G 1901 Two sisters showing malformations of the skull and other congenital abnormalities. Reports of the Society for the Study of Diseases in Children 1: 110–118

Carpenter G 1909 Case of acrocephaly with other congenital malformations. Proceedings of the Royal Society of Medicine II (part I) 45–53, 199–201

Carter C O, Till K, Fraser V, Coffey R 1982 A family study of craniostenosis, with probable recognition of a distinct syndrome. Journal of Medical Genetics 19: 280–285

Cassidy S B, Heller R M, Kilroy A W, McKelvey W, Engel E 1977 Trigonocephaly and the 11q-syndrome. Annals of Genetics 20: 67–69

Chotzen F 1932 Eine eigenartige familiare Entwicklungsstoerung. (Akrocephalosyndaktylie, Dysosis craniofacialis und Hypertelorismus). Monatsschrift Kinderheilkunde 55: 97–122

Christian J C, Andrews P A, Conneally P M, Muller J 1971 The adducted thumbs syndrome. An autosomal recessive disease with arthropryposis, dysmyelination, craniostenosis and cleft palate. Clinical Genetics 2: 95–103

Chudley A E, Houston C S 1982 The Greig cephalopolysyndactyly in a Canadian family. American Journal of Medical Genetics 13: 269–276

Clunie G J A, Mason J M 1962 Visceral diverticula and the Marfan syndrome. British Journal of Surgery 50: 51–52

Cohen M M Jr 1978 Syndromes with cleft lip and palate. Cleft Palate Journal 15: 306–328

Cohen M M Jr 1979a 'Syndromology's message for craniofacial biology'. Journal of Maxillofacial Surgery 7: 89–109

Cohen M M, Jr 1979b Craniofrontonasal dysplasia. Birth Defects 15: 85–89

Cohen M M Jr 1986 Craniosynostosis, diagnosis, evaluation and management. Raven Press, New York

Dallapiccola B, Zelante L, Cristalli P 1984 Diagnostic definition of the FG-syndrome. American Journal of Medical Genetics 19: 379–381

Daniel A, Ekblom L, Philips S, FitzGerald J M, Optiz J M 1985 NOR activity and centromere suppression related in a de novo fusion tdic (9 : 13) (p. 22 : p. 13) chromosome in a child with del (9p) syndrome. American Journal of Medical Genetics 22: 577–584

David J D, Poswillo D, Simpson D 1982 The craniostenoses. Springer, Berlin

Delozier C D, Antley R M, Williams R et al 1980 The syndrome of multisynostosic osteodysgenesis with long-bone fractures. American Journal of Medical Genetics 7: 391–403

dePablo C E, Sagredo J M G, Ferro M T, Ferrando P, Roman C S 1980 Interstitial deletion in the long arms of chromosome 1: 46 XY, del (1) (pter q 22 : q25 qter). Journal of Medical Genetics 17: 483–486

Der Kaloustain V 1972 Acrocephalopolysyndactyly type II (Carpenter's syndrome). American Journal of Diseases of Children 124: 716–718

DiLiberti J H, Farndon P A, Dennis N R, Curry C J R 1984 The fetal valproate syndrome. American Journal of Genetics 19: 473–481

Dingman R O 1956 A syndrome of craniofacial dysostosis. Report of two cases. Plastic and Reconstructive Surgery 18: 113

Duncan P A, Klein R M, Wilmot P L, Shapiro L R 1979 Greig cephalosyndactyly syndrome. American Journal of Diseases of Children 133: 818–821

Eastman J R, Escobar V, Bixler D 1978 Linkage analysis in dominant acrocephalosyndactyly. Journal of Medical Genetics 15: 292

Eaton A P, Sommer A, Kontras S B, Sayers M P 1974 Carpenter syndrome — acrocephalopolysyndactyly, type II. Birth Defects 10: 249–260

Elejalde B R, Giraldo C, Jimenez R, Gilbert E F Acrocephalopolydactylous dysplasia. Birth Defects 13: 53–67

Escobar V, Bixler D 1977a Are the acrocephalosyndactyly syndromes variable expressions of a single gene defect? Birth Defects 13: 139–154

Escobar V, Bixler D 1977b The acrocephalosyndactyly syndromes: a metacarpophalangeal pattern profile analysis. Clinical Genetics 11: 295–305

Escobar V, Bixler D 1977c Metacarpophalangeal pattern profile analysis as a tool to identify gene carriers in the acrocephalosyndactyly syndromes. Birth Defects 13: 299

Escobar V, Brandt I K, Bixler D 1977 Unusual association of Saethre–Chotzen syndrome and congenital adrenal hyperplasia. Clinical Genetics 11: 365–371

Evans C A, Christiansen R L 1976 Cephalic malformations in Saethre-Chotzen syndrome. Radiology 121: 399–403

Falk R E, Crandrall B F, Sparkes R S 1977 Profound growth failure and minor congenital anomalies in a child with a small chromosomal delection: 46 XX, del (1) (pter qter). Clinical Research 25: 176a

Fernhoff P M, Lammer E J 1984 Craniofacial features of isotretinoin embryopathy. Journal of Pediatrics 105: 595–597

Fitch N 1982 Albright's hereditary osteodystrophy: a review. American Journal of Medical Genetics 11: 11–29

Fitch N, Levy E P 1975 Adducted thumb syndromes. Clinical Genetics 8: 190–198

Flatz S D, Schinzel A, Doehring E, Kamran D, Eilers E 1984 Optiz trigonocephaly syndrome: report of two cases. European Journal of Pediatrics 144: 183–185

Fontaine G, Farriaux J P, Blanckaert D, Lefebre C 1977 Un nouveau syndrome polymalformatif complexe. Journal de Génétique Humaine 25: 109–119

Francke U, Gonzalez y Rivera E L, Delgado C G, Ramos M G 1977 Saethre–Chotzen syndrome (SCS) with additional abnormalities in a Mexican family. Birth Defects 13: 241

Fraser F C, Preus M 1984 Aminopterin syndrome sine aminopterin. David W. Smith Workshop on Malformations and Morphogenesis, Boca Raton, June 7–10

Frias J L, Felman A H, Rosenbloom A L, Finkelstein S N, Hoyt W E, Hall B D 1978 Normal intelligence in two children with Carpenter syndrome. American Journal of Medical Genetics 2: 191–199

Friedman J M, Hanson J W, Graham C B, Smith D W 1977 Saethre–Chotzen syndrome: a broad and variable pattern of skeletal malformations. Journal of Pediatrics 91: 929–933

Fryns J P, Goeck W, van der Bergher H 1977 The Greig polysyndactyly–craniofacial dysmorphism syndrome. European Journal of Pediatrics 126: 283–287

Fryns J P, Noyen G, van der Berghe H 1981 The Greig polysyndactyly-craniofacial dysmorphism syndrome: variable expression in a family. European Journal of Pediatrics 136: 217–220

Fuks A, Rosenmann A, Chosack A 1978 Pseudoanodontia, cranial deformity, blindness, alopecia and dwarfism: a new syndrome. Journal of Dentistry in Children 52: 155–157

Furlong J, Kurezynsky T W, Hennessy J R 1985 A new Marfanoid syndrome with craniosynostosis (unpublished manuscript)

Gagliardi A R T, Gonzalez C H, Pratesi R 1984 GAPO syndrome. Report of three affected brothers. American Journal of Medical Genetics 19: 217–223

Gallazzi F, Salti R, Marianelli L, La Causa C 1980 La syndrome di Saethre–Chotzen. Minerva Pediatrica 32: 325–328

Gellis S S, Feingoldt M 1968 In: Atlas of mental retardation syndromes. Publ 26, US Department of Health Education and Welfare, Washington, DC

Gerold M 1959 Frakturheilung bei einen seltenen Fall kongenitaler Anomalie der oberen Gliedmaessen. Zentralblatt fur Chirurgie 84: 831–834

Gnamy D, Farriaux J P 1971 Syndrome dominant associant polysyndactyly, pouces en spatule anomalies faciales et retard mental (une forme particulière de l'acrocephalo-polysyndactylie de type Noack). Journal de Génétique Humaine 19: 299–316

Goldberg M J, Pashayan H M 1976 Hallux syndactyly–ulnar polydactyly–abnormal ear lobes: a new syndrome. Birth Defects 12: 225–266

Gollop T R, Fontes L R 1985 The Greig cephalopolysyndactyly syndrome: report of a family and review of the literature. American Journal of Medical Genetics 22: 59–68

Goodman R M 1965 Family with polysyndactyly and other anomalies. Journal of Heredity 56: 37–38

Goodman R M, Stenberg M, Shem-Tov Y, Bat-Miriam Katznelson M, Hertz M, Rotem Y 1979 Acrocephalopolysyndactyly type IV: a new genetic syndrome in 3 sibs. Clinical Genetics 15: 209–214

Gorlin R J, Whitley C 1984 Growth retardation, alopecia, pseudo-anodontia and optic atrophy. The GAPO syndrome. Proceedings of the American Society of Human Genetics 35 Oct 31–Nov 3

Gorlin R J, Chaudhry A P, Moss M L 1960 Craniofacial dysostosis, patent ductus arteriosus, hypertrichosis, hypoplasia of labia majora, dental and eye anomalies. Journal of Pediatrics 56: 778–785

Gorlin R J, Cervenka J, Pruzansky S 1971 Facial clefting and its syndromes. Birth Defects 7: 3–49

Grawfurd M d'A, Kessel F, Libermann M, Mckeown J A, Mandalia P Y, Ridler M A C 1979 Partial monosomy 7 with interstitial delections in two infants with differing congenital abnormalities. Journal of Medical Genetics 16: 453–460

Greitzer L J, Jones K L, Schnall B S, Smith D W 1974 Craniosynostosis–radial aplasia syndrome. Journal of Pediatrics 84: 723–724

Hall J G 1974 Craniofacial dysostosis — either Stanescu dysostosis or a new entity. Birth Defects 10: 521–523

Hall J G, Reed S D, Sells C J, Hanson J W 1980 Autosomal recessive acrocephalosyndactyly revisited. American Journal of Medical Genetics 5: 423–424

Hanson J W, Smith D W 1975 The fetal hydantoin syndrome. Journal of Pediatrics 87: 285–290

Hanson J W, Myrianthopoulos N C, Harvey M S, Smith D W 1976 Risks to the offspring of women treated with hydantoin anticonvulsants, with emphasis on the fetal hydantoin syndrome. Journal of Pediatrics 89: 662–668

Hermann J, Pallister P D, Optiz J M 1969 Craniosynostosis syndromes. Rocky Mountain Medical Journal 66: 45–56

Hodach R J, Viseskul C, Gilbert E F 1975 Studies of malformation syndromes in man XXXVI: the Pfeiffer syndrome, association with Kleeblattschaedel and multiple visceral anomalies. Case report and review. Zeitschrift fur Kinderheilkunde 119: 87–103

Hoger P H, Bolthauser E, Hitzig W H 1985 Craniosynostosis in hyper-IgE syndrome. European Journal of Pediatrics 144: 414–417

Hootnick D, Holmes L B 1972 Familial polysyndactyly and craniofacial anomalies. Clinical Genetics 3: 128–134

Hornstein L, Soukup S 1981 A recognizable phenotype in a child with partial duplication 13q in a family with t(10q : 13q). Clinical Genetics 19: 81–86

Hunter A G W, McAlpine P J, Rudd N L, Fraser F C 1977 A 'new' syndrome of mental retardation with characteristic facies and brachyphalangy. Journal of Medical Genetics 14: 430–437

Jackson C E, Weiss L, Reynolds W A, Forman T F, Peterson J A 1976 Craniosynostosis, mid-facial hypoplasia, and foot abnormalities: an autosomal dominant phenotype in a large Amish kindred. Journal of Pediatrics 88: 963–968

Jaffer Z, Beighton P 1983 Syndrome identification, case report 98: arachnodactyly, joint laxity and spondylolisthesis. Journal of Clinical Dysmorphology 1: 14–18

Keller M A, Jones K L, Nyhan W L, Francke U, Dixon B 1976 A new syndrome of mental deficiency with craniofacial, limb and anal abnormalities. Journal of Pediatrics 88: 589–591

Kelly R I, Borns P F, Nichols D, Zackai E H 1983 Osteolophonic dwarfism in two generations. Journal of Medical Genetics 20: 436–440

Keutel J, Kindermann I, Mockel H 1970 Eine wahrscheinlich autosomal recessiv vererbte Skeletmissbildung mit Humeroradialsynostose. Humangenetik 9: 43–53

Khajavi A, Lachman R S, Rimoin D L et al 1976 Heterogeneity in the campomelic syndromes: long and short bone varieties. Birth Defects 12: 93–100

Kopyse Z, Stanska M, Ryzko J, Kulezyk B 1980 The Saethre–Chotzen syndrome with partial bifidy of the distal phalanges of the great toes. Human Genetics 56: 195–204

Kreiborg S, Pruzansky S, Pashayen H 1972 The Saethre–Chotzen syndrome. Teratology 6: 287–294

Kunze J, Park W, Hansen K H, Hanfeld F 1983 Adducted thumb syndrome: report of a new case and diagnostic approach. European Journal of Pediatrics 141: 122–126

Kurezynski T W 1983 Auralcephalosyndactyly: a new hereditary craniosynostosis syndrome. Proceedings of the American Society of Human Genetics 34, Oct 30–Nov 2

Kwee M L, Lindhout D 1983 Frontonasal dysplasia, coronal craniosynostosis, pre- and postaxial polydactyly and split nails: a new autosomal dominant mutant with reduced penetrance and variable expression. Clinical Genetics 24: 200–205

Lacheretz M, Walbum C H, Tourgis R 1974 L'acrocephalosynankie. A propos d'une observation avec synostoses multiples. Pediatrie 29: 169–177

Ladda R L, Stoltzfus E, Gordon S L, Graham W P 1978 Craniosynostosis associated with limb reduction malformations and cleft lip/palate: a distinct syndrome. Pediatrics 61: 12–15

Lenz W 1975 Zur Diagnose und Atiologie der Akrocephalosyndaktylie. Zeitschrift Kinderheilkunde 79: 546–558

Levin L S, Perrin J C S, Ose L, Dorst J P, Miller J D, McKusick V A 1977 A variable syndrome of craniosynostosis, short thin hair, dental abnormalities and short limbs: craniodermal dysplasia. Journal of Pediatrics 90: 55–61

Lewin M L 1953 Facial and hand deformity in acrocephalosyndactyly. Plastic and Reconstructive Surgery 12: 138

Lichtenstein J, Warson R, Jorgenson R, Dorst J P, McKusick V A 1972 The tricho-dento-osseous (TDO) syndrome. American Journal of Human Genetics 24: 569–582

Lippe B M, Sparkes R S, Fass B, Neidengard L 1981 Craniosynostosis and syndactyly: expanding the llq- chromosomal deletion phenotype. Journal of Medical Genetics 18: 480–483

Lopez-Hernandez A 1982 Craniosynostosis, ataxia, trigeminal anesthesia and parietal alopecia with pons–vermis fusion anomaly (atresia of the fourth ventricle). Report of two cases. Neuropediatrics 13: 99–102

Lowry R B 1972 Congenital absence of the fibula and craniosynostosis in sibs. Journal of Medical Genetics 9: 227–229

Lowry R B, McLean J R 1977 Syndrome of mental retardation, cleft palate, eventration of diaphragm, congenital heart defect, glaucoma, growth failure and craniosynostosis. Birth Defects 13: 203–228

McKeen E A, Mulvihill J J, Levine P H, Dean J H, Howley P M 1984 The concurrence of Saethre–Chotzen syndrome and malignancy in a family with in vitro immune dysfunction. Cancer 54: 2946–2951

KcKusick V A 1971 Mendelian inheritance in man, 3rd edn. Johns Hopkins University Press, Baltimore

McKusick V A 1978a Mendelian inheritance in man, 5th edn. Johns Hopkins University Press, Baltimore

McKusick V A 1978b Medical genetic studies of the Amish. Johns Hopkins University Press, Baltimore

McLoughlin T G, Krovetz L J, Schiebler G L 1966 Heart disease in the Laurence–Moon–Biedl–Bardet syndrome. A review and report of three brothers. Journal of Pediatrics 65: 388–399

McPherson E, Hall J G, Hickman R 1976 Chromosome 7 short arm delection and craniosynostosis. A 7p-syndrome. Human Genetics 35: 117–123

Majewski F, Goecke T 1982 Studies of microcephalic primordial dwarfism I: an approach to a delineation of the Seckel syndrome. American Journal of Medical Genetics 12: 7–21

Marschall R E, Smith D W 1970 Frontodigital syndrome: a dominantly inherited disorder with normal intelligence. Journal of Pediatrics 77: 129–133

Martsolf J T, Cracco J B, Carpenter G G, O'Hara A E 1971 Pfeiffer syndrome. American Journal of Diseases of Children 121: 257–262

Merlob P, Grunebaum M, Reisner S H 1981 A newborn infant with craniofacial dysmorphism and polysyndactyly (Greig's syndrome). Acta Pediatrica Scandinavica 70: 275–277

Minami R, Olek K, Wardenbach P 1975 Hypersarcosinemia with craniostenosis–syndactylism syndrome. Human Genetics 28: 167–171

Moffie D 1950 Une famille avec oxycephalie et acrocephalosyndactyly. Revue Neurologique 83: 306–312

Mohr O L 1939 Dominant acrocephalosyndactyly. Hereditas, 25: 193–203

Motegi T, Ochuchi M, Othaki C et al 1985 A craniosynostosis in a boy with a del(7)(9p15, 3p21,3): assignment by deletion mapping of the critical segment for craniosynostosis to the mid-portion of 7p21. Human Genetics 7: 160–162

Moynahan E J, Wolff O H 1967 A new neurocutaneous syndrome (skin, eye, brain) consisting of linear nevus, bilateral lipodermoids of the conjunctiva, cranial thickening, cerebral cortical atrophy and mental retardation. British Journal of Dermatology 79: 651–652

Murray J C, Johnson J A, Bird T D 1985 Dandy-Walker malformation: etiologic heterogeneity and empiric recurrence risks. Clinical Genetics 28: 272–283

Naveh Y, Friedman A 1976 Pfeiffer syndrome: report of a family and review of the literature. Journal of Medical Genetics 13: 277–280

Nelson M M, Thompson A J 1982 The acrocallosal syndrome. American Journal of Medical Genetics 12: 195–199

Noack M 1959 Ein Beitrag zum Krankheitsbild der Akrozephalosyndactyly (Apert). Archiv fur Kinderheilkunde 160: 168–170

Oberklaid F, Danks D M 1975 The Optiz trigonocephaly syndrome. American Journal of Diseases of Children 129: 1348–1349

Optiz J M, Kaveggia E G 1974 Studies of malformation syndromes of man XXXIII: the FG0-syndrome. An X-linked recessive syndrome of multiple congenital anomalies and mental retardation. Zeitschrift fur Kinderheilkunde 117: 1–18

Optiz J M, Patau K 1975 A partial trisomy 5p syndrome. Birth Defects 11: 191–200

Optiz J M, Johnsons R C, McCreadie S R, Smith D W 1969 The C

syndrome of multiple congenital anomalies. Birth Defects
5: 161–166

Optiz J M, Kaveggia E G, Adkins W N Jr et al 1982 Studies of
malformation syndromes of humans XXXIIIC: the FG-syndrome —
further studies on three affected inviduals from the GF-family.
American Journal of Medical Genetics 12: 147–154

Orbelli D J, Lurie I W, Goroshenko J L 1977 The syndrome
associated with the partial D-monosomy. Case report and review.
Human Genetics 13: 296–308

Orye E, Craen M 1975 Short arm deletion of chromosome 12. Report
of two new cases. Human Genetics 28: 335–342

Owen R H 1952 Acrocephalosyndactyly. A case with congenital cardiac
abnormalities. British Journal of Radiology 25: 103–106

Palacios E, Schimke R N 1969 Craniosynostosis–syndactylism.
American Journal of Roentgenology 106: 144–155

Pantke O A, Cohen M M Jr, Witkop C J et al 1975 The
Saethre–Chotzen syndrome. Birth Defects 11: 190–225

Pedersen C 1976 Partial trisomy 15 as a result of an unbalanced 12/15
transcolation in a patient with cloverleaf skull anomaly. Clinical
Genetics 9: 378–380

Pelias M, Superneau D W, Thurmon T F 1981 Brief clinical report: a
sixth report (eighth case) of cranio-synostosis radial aplasia
(Baller–Gerold) syndrome. American Journal of Medical Genetics
16: 133–139

Pfeiffer R A 1964 Dominant erbliche Akrozephalosyndactylie.
Zeitschrift Kinderheilkunde 90: 301–320

Pfeiffer R A 1969 Associated deformities of the head and hands. Birth
Defects 5: 18–34

Pfeiffer R A, Seemann K B, Tuente W, Gussone J, Klemm E 1977
Akrozephalopolysundactylie (Akrozephalo-syndaktylie, Typ II
McKusick) (Carpenter-Syndrome). Bericht ueber 4 Faelle und eine
Beobachtung des Typs von Marshall-Smith. Klinische Paediatrie
189: 120–130

Preus M, Alexander W J, Fraser F C 1975 The C-syndrome. Birth
Defects 11: 58–62

Preus M, Vetemans M, Kaplan P 1986 Diagnosis of chromosome 3
duplication q23-qter, delection p25-pter in a patient with C
(trigonocephaly) syndrome. American Journal of Medical Genetics
23: 935–943

Pruzansky S, Pashayan H, Kreiborg S, Miller M 1975
Roentgencephalometric studies of the premature craniofacial
synostoses: report of a family with the Saethre–Chotzen syndrome.
Birth Defects 11: 226–237

Pruzansky S, Costaras M, Rollnick B R 1982 Radiocephalometric
findings in a family with craniofrontonasal dysplasia. Birth Defects
18: 120–138

Reich E W, Cox R P, MacCarthy J C, Becker M H, Genieser N B,
Converse J M 1977 A new heritable syndrome with frontonasal
dysplasia and associated extracranial anomalies. In: Littlefield J W
(ed) Fifth International Conference on Birth Defects. Excerpta
Medica, Amsterdam. p 243

Reynolds J F, Haas R J, Edgerton M T, Kelly T E 1982
Craniofrontonasal dysplasia in a three-generation kindred. Journal of
Craniofacial Genetics and Development Biology 2: 233–238

Riccardi V M, Hassler E, Lubinsky M S 1977 The FG-syndrome:
further characterization. Report of a third family, and of a sporadic
case. American Journal of Medical Genetics 1: 47–58

Robert E, Bethenod M, Bourgeois J 1984 Le syndrome
d'Antley–Bixler. Journal de Génétique Humaine 32: 291–298

Robertson K P, Thurmon T F, Tracy M C 1975
Acrocephalosyndactyly and partial trisomy 6. Birth Defects
11: 267–271

Robinow M 1984 Comments on Pfeiffer syndrome and case report 113.
Journal of Clinical Dysmorphology 2: 7

Robinow M, Sorauf T J 1975 Acrocephalosyndactyly, type Noack, in a
large kindred. Birth Defects 11: 99–106

Robinson A 1962 Ataxia–telangiectasia presenting with craniostenosis.
Archives of Disease in Childhood 37: 652–655

Robinson L K, Powers N G, Dunklee P, Sherman S, Jones K L 1982
The Antley–Bixler syndrome. Journal of Pediatrics 101: 201–205

Robinson L K, James H E, Mubarak S J, Allen E J, Jones K L 1985
Carpenter syndrome: natural history and clinical spectrum.
American Journal of Medical Genetics 20: 461–469

Saath A A, Juliar J F, Harm J, Brough A J, Perrin E V, Chen H 1976
Triploidy syndrome. A report of two live-born (69, XXY) and one
still-born (69, XXX) infants. Clinical Genetics 9: 43–50

Saethre H 1931 Ein Beitrag zum Turmschaedelproblem (Pathogenese,
Erblichkeit und Symptomologie). Deutsche Zeitschrift fur
Nervenheilkunde 117: 533–555

Sakati N, Nyhan W L, Tisdale W K 1971 A new syndrome with
acrocephalopolysyndactyly, cardiac disease, and distinctive defects of
the ear, skin and lower limbs. Journal of Pediatrics 79: 104–109

Saldino R M, Steinbach H L, Epstein C J 1972 Familial
acrocephalosyndactyly (Pfeiffer syndrome). American Journal of
Roentgenology 116: 609–622

Sanchez J M, Negrotti T C 1981 Variable expression in Pfeiffer
syndrome. Journal of Medical Genetics 18: 73–75

Sargent C, Burn J, Baraitser M, Pembrey M E 1985 Trigonocephaly
and the Optiz C syndrome. Journal of Medical Genetics 22: 39–45

Sax C M, Flannery B D, Dineen M K, Brown J A 1984
Craniofrontonasal dysplasia: a seminal mutation with similarities to
the mouse T-locus. Proceedings of the American Society of Human
Genetics 35, Oct 31–Nov 3

Saxena S, Sharma J C, Garg O P 1981 Carpenter's syndrome: report of
a case. Indian Journal of Pediatrics 37: 627–628

Say B, Meyer J 1981 Familial trigonocephaly associated with short
stature and development delay. American Journal of Diseases of
Children 135: 711–712

Schinzel A 1982 Acrocallosal syndrome. American Journal of Medical
Genetics 12: 201–203

Schinzel A, Schmidt N 1980 Hallux duplication, postaxial polydactyly,
absence of the corpus callosum, severe mental retardation and
additional anomalies in two unrelated patients: a new syndrome?
American Journal of Medical Genetics 6: 241–249

Schinzel A, Hayashi K, Schmid W 1976 Further delineation of the
clinical picture of trisomy for the distal segment of chromosome 13.
Human Genetics 32: 1–12

Schinzel A, Savodelli G, Briner J, Figg P, Massini C 1983
Antley–Bixler syndrome in sisters: a term newborn and a prenatally
diagnosed fetus. American Journal of Medical Genetics 14: 139–147

Schinzel A, Woodly M, Burck U 1984 Acrocephalosyndactyly: how
many different syndromes? Proceedings Greenwood Genetic Centre
3: 102

Schmid W, d'Apuzzo V, Rossi E 1979 Trisomy 6q25-6qter in a
severely retarded 7-year-old boy with turricephaly, bowshaped
mouth, hypogenitalism and club feet. Human Genetics 46: 279–284

Schonenberg H, Scheidhauer E 1966 Ueber zwei ungewoehnliche
Dyscranio-Dysphalangien bei Geschwistern (Atypische
Akrozephalosyndaktylie) und fragliche Dysencephalia
splanchnocystica. Monatsschrift fur Kinderheilkunde
114: 322–327

Schutten H J, Schutten B, Mikkelsen M 1978 Partial trisomy of
chromosome 13: case report review of literature. Annals of Genetics
21: 95–99

Scott C R, Bryant J I, Graham C B 1971 A new craniodigital syndrome
with mental retardation. Journal of Pediatrics 78: 658–663

Sells C J, Hanson J W, Hall J G 1979 The Summit syndrome:
observation on a third case. American Journal of Medical Genetics
3: 27–33

Sensenbrenner J A, Dorst J P, Owens R P 1975 New syndrome of
skeletal, dental and hair anomalies. Birth Defects 11: 372–379

Shprintzen R J, Goldberg R B 1982 A recurrent pattern syndrome of
craniosynostosis associated with arachnodactyly and abdominal
hernias. Journal of Craniofacial Genetics and Development Biology
2: 65–74

Sklower S L, Willner J P, Cohen M M Jr, Feingold M, Desnick R J
1979 Craniosynostis–radial aplasia: Baller–Gerold syndrome.
American Journal of Diseases of Children 133: 1279–1280

Slover R, Sujansky E 1979 Frontonasal dysplasia with coronal
craniosynostosis in three sibs. Birth Defects 15: 78–83

Smith D W 1974 Syndromes II. In: Motulsky A G, Lenz W (eds)
Birth defects: Proceedings of the Fourth International Conference.
Amsterdam, Excerpta Medica. p 309

Spear S L, Mickle J P 1983 Simultaneous cutis aplasia congenita of the
scalp and cranial stenosis. Plastic and Reconstructive Surgery
71: 413–417

Summit R L 1969 Recessive acrocephalosyndactyly with normal intelligence. Birth Defects 5: 35–38

Sunderhaus E, Wolter J R 1968 Acrocephalosyndactylism. Journal of Pediatric Ophthalmology 5: 118–120

Temtamy S A 1966 Carpenter's syndrome: acrocephalopolysyndactyly: an autosomal recessive syndrome. Journal of Pediatrics 69: 11–120

Temtamy S A, Louttfy A H 1974 Polysyndactyly in an Egyptian family. Birth Defects 10: 207–215

Temtamy S, McKusick V A 1969 Synopsis of hand malformations with particular emphasis on genetic factors. Birth Defects 5: 125–184

Thanos C, Stewart R E, Zonana J 1977 Craniosynostosis, bony extoses, epibular dermoids, epidermal nevus and slow development. Syndrome Identification 5: 19–21

Thompson E, Pembrey M 1985 Seckel syndrome: an overdiagnosed syndrome. Journal of Medical Genetics 22: 192–201

Thompson E M, Baraitser M, Hayward R D 1984 Parietal foramina in Saethre–Chotzen syndrome. Journal of Medical Genetics 21: 369–377

Thompson E M, Baraitser M, Lindenbaum R H, Zaidi Z H, Kroll J S 1985 The FG-syndrome: 7 new cases. Clinical Genetics 27: 582–594

Tommerup N, Nielsen F 1983 A familial reciprocal translocation t(3 : 7) (p21,1 : p13) associated with the Greig polysyndactyly–craniofacial anomalies syndrome. American Journal of Medical Genetics 16: 313–321

Tridon P, Thiriet M 1966 Malformations associées de la Tête et des extrémités. Masson, Paris

Turleau C, Grouchy J 1981 Trisomy 6qter. Clinical Genetics 19: 202–266

Turner H 1931 Endocrine clinic: diabetes insipidus. Laurence–Moon–Biedl syndrome. Journal of Oklahoma State Medical Association 24: 148–155

Valentin B 1938 Die Korrelation (Koppelung) von Missbildungen, erlautert am Beispiel der Akrozephalo-syndaktylie. Acta Orthopaedica Scandinavica 9: 235–316

Vanek J, Losan F 1982 Pfeiffer's type of acrocephalosyndactyly in two families. Journal of Medical Genetics 19: 289–292

Ventruto V, Di Girolamo R, Festa B, Romano A, Sebastio G, Sebastio L 1976 Family study of inherited syndrome with multiple congenital deformities: symphalangism, carpal and tarsal fusion, brachydactyly, craniosynostosis, strabimus, hip osteochondritis. Journal of Medical Genetics 13: 394–398

Vogt A 1933 Dyskephalie (Dysostosis craniofacialis, Maladie de Crouzon 1912) und eine neuartige Kombination dieser Krankheit mit Syndaktylie der 4 Extremitaeten (dyskephalodaktylie). Klinische Monatssblatter fur Augenheilkunde 90: 441–460

Waardenburg P J 1934 Eine merkwuerdige Kombintion von angeborenen Missbildungen: Doppelseitiger Hydrophtalmus verbunden mit akrophalosyndactylie, Herzfehler, Pseudohermaphroditismus und anderen Abweichungen. Klinische Monatsblattes fur Augenheilkunde 92: 29–44

Walbaum R 1983 Antley–Bixler syndrome. Journal of Pediatrics 104: 799

Warkany J, Frauenberger G S, Mitchell A G 1937 The Laurence–Moon–Biedl syndrome. American Journal of Diseases of Children 53: 455–470

Wilson G N, Hieber V C, Schmickel R D 1978 The association of chromosome 3 duplication and the Cornelia de Lange syndrome. Journal of Pediatrics 93: 783–788

Wilson G N, Dasouki M, Barr M B Jr 1985 Further delineation of the dup(3q) syndrome. American Journal of Medical Genetics 22: 117–123

Woolf R M, Georgiade N G, Pickrell K L 1959 Acrocephalosyndatyly. Plastic and Reconstructive Surgery 24: 201

Woon K C, Kokich V G, Clarren S, Cohen M M Jr 1980 A new syndrome with craniosynostosis in a pair of twins: a morphologic and histologic study of the calvaria and cranial base. Teratology 22: 23–25

Young I, Harper P S 1982 An unusual form of familial acrocephalosyndactyly. Journal of Medical Genetics 19: 286–288

TRIPHYLLOCEPHALY

Angle C R, McIntire M S, Moore R C 1967 Cloverleaf skull:

Kleeblattschaedel-deformity syndrome. American Journal of Diseases of Children 114: 198–202

Berrada A 1963–1964 Etude sur les craniostenoses en milieu morocain. A propos de 87 observations. Thèse Médicale, Paris, no 182,

Bonucci E, Nardi F 1972 The cloverleaf skull syndrome: histological, histochemical and ultrastructural findings. Virchows Archiv Abteilung A 357: 199–212

Camera G, Dodero D, de Pascale S 1984 Prenatal diagnosis of thanatophoric dysplasia at 24 weeks. American Journal of Medical Genetics 18: 39–43

Cohen M M 1976 The clover leaf skull malformation. In: Bosma J F (ed) Symposium on development of the basicranium, Ch 21, pp 372–382

Comings D E 1965 The Kleeblattschaedel syndrome–a grotesque form of hydrocephalus. Journal of Pediatrics 67: 126–129

Connor J M, Connor R A C, Sweet E M et al 1985 Lethal neonatal chondroplasias in the west of Scotland 1970–1983 with a description of a thanatophoric dysplasialike, autosomal precessive disorder, Glasgow variant. American Journal of Medical Genetics 22: 243–253

David M, Hecan & Talairach 1947 (quoted by Montaut & Stricker 1977)

Eaton A P, Sommer A, Sayers M P 1975 The Kleeblattschaedel anomaly. Birth Defects 11: 238–246

Feingold M, O'Connor J F, Berkman M, Darling D B 1969 Kleeblattschaedel syndrome. American Journal of Diseases of Children 118: 589–594

Gathmann H A, Meyer R D 1977 Der Kleeblattschaedel. Ein Beitrag zur Morphogenese. Springer, Berlin

Giedion A 1968 Thanatophoric dwarsfism. Helvetica Paediatrica Acta 23: 175–183

Guzman R T 1976 Vide Cloverleaf Skull. In: Gorlin R J, Pindborg J J, Cohen M M (eds) Syndromes of the head and neck. McGraw Hill, New York

Hall B D, Smit D W, Sjiller J G 1972 Kleeblatt-schaedel (cloverleaf) syndrome: severe form of Crouzon's disease? Journal of Pediatrics 80: 526–528

Holtermuller K, Wiedemann H R 1960 Kleeblattschaedel-Syndrom. Medizinische Monatsschrift fur Pharmazenten 14: 439–446

Horton W A, Rimion D L, Hollister D W, Lachman R S 1979 Further heterogeneity within lethal neonatal short-limbed dwarfism. The platyspondylic types. Journal of Pediatrics 94: 736–742

Horton W A, Harrus D J, Collins D L 1983 Discordance for the Kleeblattschaedel anomaly in monozygotic twins with thanatophoric dysplasia. American Journal of Medical Genetics 15: 97–101

Iannacone G, Gerlinni G 1974 The so-called 'cloverleaf skull syndrome'. Pediatric Radiology 2: 175–184

Isaacson G, Blakemore K J, Chervenak F A 1983 Thanatophoric dysplasia with cloverleaf skull. American Journal of Diseases of Children 137: 876–898

Kokich V G, Moffet B C, Cohen M M Jr 1982 The cloverleaf skull anomaly. An anatomic and histologic study of two specimens. Cleft Palate Journal 19: 88–99

Kremens B, Kemperdick H, Borchert F, Liebert U G 1982 Thanatophoric dysplasia with cloverleaf skull: case report and review of the literature. European Journal of Pediatrics 139: 298–303

Langer L O Jr, Yang S S, Gilbert E F et al 1986 Thanatophoric dysplasia and cloverleaf skull. A report of nine cases and review of the literature. American Journal of Medical Genetics (in press)

Liebaldt G 1964 'Kleeblatt' Schaedel-Syndrom, als Beitrag zur formalen Genese der Entwicklungsstoerung des Schaedelsdaches. Ergeb Allg Pathol 45: 23–38

McCorquodale M, Erickson R P, Robinson M, Roszczipka K 1980 Kleeblattschaedel anomaly and partial trisomy for chromosome 13 (47 XY, + der(13),t(3,13)(q24 : q14) Clinical Genetics 17: 409–414

Moscatelli P, Gille G, Perfumo F 1968 Su un raro caso di synostosi intra-uterina delle suture coronarie e lambdoidee: Soui possibili rapporti con la sindrome di Holtermueller e Wiedemann. Clinical Pediatrics 50: 972–979

Muller P J, Hoffman J J 1975 Cloverleaf skull syndrome. Journal of Neurosurgery 43: 86–91

Nawalkha P L, Mangal H H 1970 Kleeblattschaedel deformity syndrome. Indian Journal of Pediatrics 37: 478–480

Ornoy A, Adomian G E, Ereson D J, Bergeson R E, Rimoin D L 1985 The role of mesenchyme-like tissue in the pathogenesis of thanatophoric dysplasia. American Journal of Medical Genetics 21: 613–630

Partington M W, Gonzales-Crussi F, Khakee S G 1971 Cloverleaf skull and thanatophoric dwarfism. Report of four cases, two in the sibship. Archives of Disease in Childhood 46: 656–664

Raffel L, Rogers D, Lachman R, Adomian G, Rimoin D L 1983 Thanatophoric dysplasia with and without Kleeblattschaedel: variability rather than heterogeneity. Proceedings of the American Society of Human Genetics 34, Oct 30–Nov 2

Schuch A, Pesch H J 1971 Beitrag zum Kleeblattschaedel-Syndrom. Zeitschrift fur Kinderheilkunde 109: 187–198

Sear H R 1937 Some notes on craniostenosis. British Journal of Radiology 10: 445–487

Serville F, Carles D, Maroteaux P 1984 Thanatophoric dysplasia of identical twins. Medical Genetics 17: 703–706

Vrolik W 1847 Tabulae ad Illustrandam Embryogenesin Hominis et Mammalium. Londonck, Amsterdam

Wollin D G, Binnington V I, Partington M W 1968 Cloverleaf skull. Journal of the Canadian Association of Radiology 19: 148–154

Craniofacial dysplasias with dyschondrosis

ACHONDROPLASIA

Bailey J A 1970 Orthopaedic aspects of achondroplasia. Journal of Bone and Joint Surgery 52: 1285

Cohen M E, Rosenthal A D, Matson D D 1967 Neurological abnormalities in achondroplastic children. Journal of Pediatrics 71: 367

Cohen M M Jr, Walker G F, Phillips C 1985 A morphometric analysis of the craniofacial configuration of achondroplasia. Journal of Craniofacial Genetics and Development Biology (suppl) 1: 139–165

Landauer W 1928 Ueber Wesen and Aetiologie der Chondrodystrophie. Klinische Wochenschrift 7: 2047

Maroteaux P, Lamy M 1964 Achondroplasia in man and animals. Clinical orthopaedics, no 33. Lippincott, Philadelphia

Mörch E T 1941 Chondrodystrophic dwarfs in Denmark. Munksgaard, Copenhagen

Parrot J 1878 Sur la malformation achondroplastique et le Dieu Ptah. Bulletin de la Société Anthropologique: 1–296

Rimoin D L, Hughes G N, Kaufman R L, Rosenthal R E, McAlister W H, Silberberg R 1970 Endochondral ossification in achondroplastic dwarfism. New England Journal of Medicine 283: 728

Vogl A 1962 The fate of the achondroplastic dwarf. Experimental Medicine and Surgery 20: 108

DIASTROPHIC DWARFISM

Kaplan M, Sauvegrain J, Hayem F et al 1961 Etude d'un nouveau cas de nanisme diastrophique. Archives Françaises de Pediatrie 18: 981

Lamy M, Maroteaux P 1960 Le nanisme diastrophique. Presse Medicale 68: 1977

Langer L O 1965 Diastrophic dwarfism in early infancy. American Journal of Roentgenology 93: 399

McKusick V A, Milch R A 1964 The clinical behaviour of genetic disease. Selected aspects. Clinics in Orthopedics 33: 22

Rubin P 1964 Dynamic classification of bone dysplasias. Year Book Medical Publishers, Chicago

Stover C N, Hayes J T, Holt J F 1963 Diastrophic dwarfism. American Journal of Roentgenology 89: 914

Taybi H 1963 Diastrophic dwarfsism. Radiology 80: 1

Wilson D W, Chrispin A R, Carter C O 1969 Diastrophic dwarfism. Archives of Disease in Childhood 44: 48

THANATOPHORIC DWARFISM

Giedion A 1968 Thanatophoric dwarfism. Helvetica Paediatrica Acta 23: 175

Harris R, Patton J T 1971 Achondroplasia and thanatophoric dwarfism in the newborn. Clinical Genetics 2: 61

Kaufman R L, Rimoin D L, McAlister W H, Kissane J M 1970 Thanatophoric dwarfism. American Journal of Diseases of Children 120: 53

Keats T E, Riddervold H O, Michaelis L L 1970 Thanatophoric dwarfism. American Journal of Roentgenology 108: 473

Kozlowski K, Prokop E, Zybaczynski J 1970 Thanatophoric dwarfism. British Journal of Radiology 43: 565

Langer L O, Spanger J W, Greinacher I, Herdman R C 1969 Thanatophoric dwarfism. Radiology 92: 285

Maroteaux P, Lamy M, Robert J M 1967 Le nanisme thanatophore. Presse Medicale 75: 2519

Maygrier C 1898 Fetus achondroplastique. Bulletin de la Société d'Obstétrique et Gynécologie 1: 248

Partington M W, Gonzales-Cruzzi F, Khakee S G, Wollin D G 1971 Cloverleaf skull and thanatophoric dwarfism. Archives of Disease in Childhood 46: 656

Rimoin D L, Hughes G N, Kaufman R L 1969 The chondrodystrophies. Journal of Laboratory and Clinical Medicine 74: 1002

Rimoin D L, Hughes G N, Kaufman R L et al 1970 Endochondral ossification in achondroplastic dwarfism. New England Journal of Medicine 283: 728

Zelweger H, Taylor B 1965 Genetic aspects of achondroplasia. Lancet i: 8

Craniofacial dysplasias with other origins

OSTEOPETROSIS

Albers-Schönberg H 1904 Roentgenbilder einer seltenen Knochenerkrankung. Munchener Medizinische Wochenschrift 51: 365

Allan W 1939 Relationship of hereditary pattern to clinical severity as illustrated by peroneal atrophy. Archives of Internal Medicine 63: 1123

Clifton W M, Frank A 1959 Osteopetrosis: marble bones. In McQuarrie I, Brennemann J (eds) Practice of Paediatrics, vol 4. Prior, Hagerstown, Md

Dent C E, Smellie J M, Watson L 1965 Studies in osteopetrosis. Archives of Disease of Childhood 40: 7

Enell H, Pehrson M 1958 Studies on osteopetrosis I. Clinical report of three cases with genetic considerations. Acta Paediatrica Scandinavica 47: 279

Hanhart E 1948 Uber die Genetik der einfachrezessiven Formen der Marmorknochenkrankheit und zwei entsprechende Stammbaume aus der Schweiz. Helvetica Paediatrica Acta 3: 113

Hasenhuttl K 1962 Osteopetrosis: review of the literature and comparative studies on a case with twenty-four year follow-up. Journal of Bone and Joint Surgery 44: 359

Higinbotham N L, Alexander S F 1941 Osteopetrosis: four cases in one family. American Journal of Surgery 53: 444

Johnstone C C, Lavy N, Vellios F, Merritt A D, Deiss W P 1968 Osteopetrosis. Medicine 47: 146

Karshner R G 1926 Osteopetrosis. American Journal of Roentgenology 16: 405

McCune D J, Bradley C 1934 Osteopetrosis (marble bones) in an infant: review of the literature and report of a case. American Journal of Diseases of Children 48: 949

Moe P J, Skaeveland A 1969 Therapeutic studies in osteopetrosis. Acta Paediatrica Scandinavica 58: 593

Pines B, Lederer M 1947 Osteopetrosis: Albers-Schonberg disease (marble bones). American Journal of Pathology 23: 755

Sjolin S 1959 Studies on osteopetrosis, II. Investigations concerning the nature of the anaemia. Acta paediatrica Scandinavica 48: 529

Smith D W 1970 Recognisable patterns of human malformation. Major problems in clinical paediatrics, vol VII. Saunders, Philadelphia

Turano A F, Fagan K A, Corbo P A 1954 Variations in clinical manifestations of osteopetrosis: report of two cases. Journal of Pediatrics 44: 688

Warkany J 1959 Osteopetrosis. In: Nelson W E (ed) Textbook of paediatrics. Saunders, Philadelphia. p 1240

Zetterstrom R 1957 Osteopetrosis (marble bone disease): clinical and pathological review. Modern Problems of Pediatrics 3: 488

CRANIOTUBULAR DYSPLASIA

Bakwin H, Krida A 1937 Familial metapyseal dysplasia. American Journal of Diseases of Children 53: 1521

Cohn M 1933 Konstitutionell Hyperspongiosierung des Skellets mit partiellem Riesenwuchs. Fortschritte der Rontgenstrahlen 47: 293

Gorlin R J, Cohen M M Jr 1969 Fronto metaphyseal dysplasia. American Journal of Diseases of Children 118: 487

Gorlin R J, Sedano H 1968 Cranio metaphyseal dysostosis and craniodiaphyseal dysostosis. Modern Medicine 36: 154

Gorlin R J, Spranger J, Koszalke M F 1969 Genetic craniotubular bone dysplasias and hyperostoses: a critical analysis. Birth Defects 5: 79

Gorlin R J, Koszalke M F, Spranger J 1970 Pyle's disease (familial metaphyseal dysplasia). Journal of Bone and Joint Surgery 52: 347

Guibad P, Hermier M 1973 La dysplasia craniometaphysaire. Pediatrie 28: 149

Halliday J 1949 A rare case of bone dystrophy. British Journal of Surgery 37: 52

Hunter J 1837 Experiments and observations on the growth of bones. The works of John Hunter, vol IV. Palmer, London. p 315

Komins C 1954 Familial metaphyseal dysplasia (Pyle's disease). British Journal of Surgery 27: 670

MacPherson R J 1974 Craniodiaphyseal dysplasia, a disease or group of diseases? Journal of the Canadian Association of Radiologists 25: 22

Melnick J C, Needles C F 1966 An undiagnosed bone dysplasia. American Journal of Roentgenology 97: 39

Millard D R, Maisels D O, Batstone J H 1967 Craniofacial surgery in craniometaphyseal dysplasia. American Journal of Surgery 113: 615

Mori P A, Holt J F 1956 Cranial manifestations of familial metaphyseal dysplasia. Neurology 66: 335

Neuhauser E B D 1953 Growth differentiation and disease. American Journal of Roentgenology 69: 723

Pyle E 1931 A case of unusual bone development. Journal of Bone and Joint Surgery 13: 874

Ross M W, Altman D H 1967 Familial metaphyseal dysplasia. Clinical Pediatrics 6: 143

Sauvegrain J, Lombard M, Garel M 1975 Dysplasie fronto-metapysaire. Annales de Radiologie, 10: 155

Stool S E, Caruso V G 1973 Cranio metaphyseal dysplasia — otolaryngologic aspects. Archives of Otolaryngology 97: 410

Taybi H 1962 Generalised skeletal dysplasia with multiple anomalies. American Journal of Roentgenology 88: 450

Vaandrager J M 1977 Cranio-tubular dysplasia. British Journal of Plastic Surgery 30: 127–133

FIBROUS DYSPLASIA

Derome P I, Viscot A 1982 Fibrous dysplasia of the skull. Neurochirurgie, vol 29, suppl I. Paris Masson

Jaffe H L, Lichtenstein L 1942 Fibrous dysplasia of bone; condition affecting one, several or many bones. Archives of Pathology 33: 777

Jaffe H L 1964 Tumors and tumorous conditions of the bones and joints. Kimpton, London. p 117–142

Ruppe Ch 1924 Osteite fibreuse des maxillaires. Thèse Médicale no 70, Paris

CUTANEOUS DYSPLASIA

Basan M 1965 Ektodermale dysplasie. Archiv fur Klinikale und Experimentell Dermatologie 222: 546

Chautard E A, Freire-Maia N 1970 Dermatoglyphic analysis in a highly mutilating syndrome. Acta Geneticae Medicae 19: 421

Christ J 1932 Uber die korrelationen der kongenitalen Defekte des Ektoderms untereinander mit besonderer Berucksichtigung ihrer Bezichungen zum Auge. Zentralblatt fur Haut und Gesundheit 40: 1

Clouston H R 1939 The major forms of hereditary ectodermal dysplasia. Canadian Medical Association Journal 40: 1

Costa O, Freire-Maia N 1972a Odontotrichomelic hypohidrotic dysplasia: a clinical reappraisal. Human Heredity, 22: 91

Costa O, Freire-Maia N 1972b A clinical reappraisal of a newly recognised ectodermal dysplasia. American Journal of Human Genetics 24: 598

Feinmesser M, Zelig S 1961 Congenital deafness with onychodystrophy. Archives of Otolaryngology 74: 507

Felsher Z 1944 Hereditary ectodermal dysplasia. Arch Derm Syph (Berlin) 49: 410

Freire-Maia N 1970 A newly recognised genetic syndrome of tetramelic deficiencies, ectodermal dysplasia, deformed ears and other abnormalities. American Journal of Human Genetics 22: 370

Friars J L, Smith D W 1968 Diminished sweat pores in hypohidrotic ectodermal dysplasia. Journal of Pediatrics 72: 606

Marshall D 1958 Ectodermal dysplasia. American Journal of Ophthalmology 45: 143

Reed W B, Lopez D A, Landing B 1970 Clinical spectrum of anhydrotic ectodermal dysplasia. Archives of Dermatology 102: 134

Robinson G C, Miller J R, Bensimon J R 1962 Familial ectodermal dysplasia with sensorineural deafness and other anomalies. Pediatrics 30: 797

Thurnan 1848 Two cases in which the skin, hair and teeth were very imperfectly developed. Médecine et Chirurgie Transactions 31: 71

NEUROCUTANEOUS DYSPLASIA

Binet E F, Kieffer S A, Martin S H et al 1969 Orbital dysplasia in neurofibromatosis. Radiology 93: 829

Bloem J J, Van der Meulen J C 1978 Neurofibromatosis in plastic surgery. British Journal of Plastic Surgery 31: 50

Brooks B, Lehman E P 1924 The bone changes in Recklinghausen's neurofibromatosis. Surgical Gynecology and Obstetrics 38: 587–595

Chutorian A M, Schwartz J F, Evans R A et al 1964 Optic gliomas in children. Neurology Minneap 14: 83–95

Davis W B, Edgerton M T, Hoffmeister S F 1954 Neurofibromatosis of the head and neck. Plastic and Reconstructive Surgery 14: 186

Francois J 1972 Ocular aspects of the phakomatoses. In: Vinken P J, Bruijn G W (eds) Handbook of Clinical Neurology, vol 14. pp 619–667

Grabb W C, Reed O, Dingman R M O et al 1980 Facial hamartomas in children: neurofibroma, lymphangioma, and hemangioma. Plastic and Reconstructive Surgery 66: 509

Harkin J C, Reed R J 1969 Tumors of the peripheral nervous system. In: Atlas of tumor pathology, second series, Fascicle 3. Armed Forces Institute of Pathology

Holt J F, Wright E M 1948 The radiologic features of neurofibromatosis. Radiology 51: 647–664

Jackson I T, Laws E R, Martin R D 1983 The surgical management of orbital neurofibromatosis. Plastic and Reconstructive Surgery 71: 751–758

Marchac D 1984 Intracranial enlargement of the orbital cavity and palpebral remodelling for orbitopalpebral neurofibromatosis. Plastic and Reconstructive Surgery 73: 534

Munro I R, Martin R D 1980 The management of gigantic benign craniofacial tumors: the reverse facial osteotomy. Plastic and Reconstructive Surgery 65: 777–785

Riccardi V M, Kleiner B, Lubs M L 1979 Neurofibromatosis: variable expression is not intrinsic to the mutant gene. Birth Defects: Original Article Series, 15: 283–289

Van der Meulen J C 1987 Orbital neurofibromatosis. Clinics in Plastic Surgery 123–135

Von Recklinghausen F D 1882 Über die multiplen Fibrome der Haut und ihre Beziehung zu den multiplen neuromen. Festschrift für Rudolph Virchow, Hirschwald, Berlin

NEUROMUSCULAR DYSPLASIA

Burston W R 1969 Mandibular retrognathia. In: Rickham P P, Johnston J H (eds) Neonatal surgery. Butterworths, London. p 137

Cohen M M 1976 The Robin anomalad: its non-specificity and associated syndromes. Journal of Oral Surgery 34: 587

Edwards J R G, Newall D R 1985 Cleft Palate Research Unit, University of Newcastle Upon Tyne. British Journal of Plastic Surgery 38: 339–342

Gorlin R J, Pindborg J J, Cohen M M Jr 1976 Syndromes of the head and neck, 2nd edn. McGraw Hill, New York

Geoffrey St Hilaire I 1832 Histoire générale et particulière des anomalies en l'organisation chez l'homme et les animaux . . . ou traite de teratologie. Baillière, Paris

Itoh T 1976 7 cases of Pierre Robin syndrome. Japanese Journal of Plastic and Reconstructive Surgery 19: 187–193 (Japanese)

Kipikasa A, Potocka E 1977 Pierre Robin Syndrome. Acta Chirurgia Plasticae 19: 3–4

Lannelongue M, Menard V 1891 Atrophie congénitale des maxillaires. In: Affections congénitales, vol I. Houzeau, Paris. p 418

Latham R A 1966 The pathogenesis of cleft palate associated with the P. Robin syndrome. An analysis of a seventeen-week human foetus. British Journal of Plastic Surgery 19: 205–214

Lenstrop E 1925 Hypoplasia of mandible of cause of choking fits in infancies. Acta Paediatrica 5: 554

Maisels D O, Strilwell J H 1980 The Pierre Robin syndrome associated with femoral dysgenesis. British Journal of Plastic Surgery 33: 237–241

Parsons R W, Smith D J 1980 A modified tongue–lip adhesion for Pierre Robin anomalad. Cleft Palate Journal 17: 144–147

Pinson L, Lassere J, 1967 Notre experience du syndrome de Pierre Robin. Ann Chir Inf 8: 127–134

Poswillo D E 1968 The aetiology and surgery of cleft palate with micrognathia. Annals of the Royal College of Surgeons of England 43: 61

Pruzansky S 1969 Not all dwarfed mandibles are alike. In: Bergsma D (ed) A clinical delineation of birth defects. Williams & Wilkins, Baltimore

Randall P, Krogman W M, Jahina S 1965 Pierre Robin and the syndrome that bears his name. Cleft Palate Journal 2: 237

Rintala A, Ranta R, Stegars T 1984 On the pathogenesis of cleft palate in the Pierre Robin syndrome. Scandinavian Journal of Plastic and Reconstructive Surgery 18: 237

Robin P 1929 La glossoptose. Un grave danger pour nos enfants. Doin, Paris

Rootledge R T 1960 The P. Robin Syndrome: a surgical emergency in the neonatal period. British Journal of Plastic Surgery 13: 204

Sanvenero-Rosselli G 1960 Microgenia e palatoschisi. Minerva Chirurgica 15: 956–964

Shukowski W P 1911 Zur Atiologie des Stridor Inspiratorius Congenitus. Jahr fur Kinderheilk 73: 459–474

Smith D W, Theiler K, Schachenmann G 1966 Rib gap defect with micrognathia malformed tracheal cartilages, and redundant skin: a new pattern of defective development. Journal of Pediatrics 69: 799–803

Smith J L, Stowe F C 1961 The P Robin syndrome. A review of thirty nine cases with emphasis on associated ocular lesions. Pediatrics 27: 128

Tandler J 1899 Zur Entwicklungsgeschichte des Uranoschisma. Wiener Klinische Wochenschrift 12: 153–156

Van der Kwast W A M 1975 Microgenia in young children. Nederlands Tijdschrift voor Geneeskunde 119: 225–228 (Dutch)

Warkany J 1971 Congenital malformation. Year book, Chicago. p 654

MUSCULAR DYSPLASIA

Alvarez G E 1976 The aglossia adactylia syndrome. British Journal of Plastic Surgery 29: 175

Bunnige M 1960 Angeborene Zungen-Munddach-Verwachsung. Annals of Pediatrics 195: 173

Burn J, Dezateux C, Hall C R, Baraitser M 1984 Orofaciodigital syndrome with mesomelic limb shortening. Journal of Medical Genetics 21: 189

Cayler G 1969 Cardio-facial syndrome. Archives of Disease in childhood 44: 69

Chicarilli Z N, Irving M P 1985 Oromandibular limb hypogenenis. Plastic and Reconstructive Surgery 76: 13

Christophorou M N, Nicolaidou P 1983 Median cleft lip, polydactyly, syndactlyly and toe anomalies in a non-Indian infant. British Journal of Plastic Surgery 36: 447

Cosack G 1952–1953 Die angeborene Zungen-Munddach-Verwacksung als Leitmotiv eines Komplexes von multiplen Abartungen (zur genes des Ankyloglossum Superius) Zeitschrift fur Kinderheilkunde 72: 240

de Jussieu M 1718 Observation sur la manière dont une fille sans langue s'acquitte des fonctions qui dependent de cet organe. Mémoires de l'Académie Royale de Science 6: 14

Farrington R K 1947 Aglossia congenita. North Carolina Medical Journal 8: 24

Fenton O M, Watt-Smith S R 1985 The spectrum of the oro-facial digital syndrome. British Journal of Plastic Surgery 38: 532–539

Freeman E A, Sheldon J H 1938 Cranio-carpo-tarsal dystrophy: an undescribed congenital malformation. Archives of Disease of Childhood 13: 277

Gopalakrishma A, Thatte R L 1982 Median cleft lip associated with bimanual hexadactyly and bilateral accessory toes: another case. British Journal of Plastic Surgery 35: 354

Gorlin R J 1969 Some facial syndromes. Birth Defects 5: 65

Gorlin R J, Psaume J 1962 Orofacial dysostosis: a new syndrome. A study of 22 cases. Journal of Pediatrics 61: 520

Hall B D 1971 Aglossia adactyly. Birth Defects 7: 233

Illera M D 1887 Congenital occlusion of the pharynx. Lancet i: 142

Kettner H 1907 Kongenitaler Zungendefekt Deutsche Medizinische Wochenschrift 33: 532

Khoo C T K, Saad M N 1980 Median cleft of the upper lip in association with bilateral hexadactyly and accessory toes. British Journal of Plastic Surgery 33: 407

Lannelongue O M, Menard V 1891 Affections congénitales. I. Tête et cou. Asselin & Houzeau, Paris

Marden P M 1966 The syndrome of ankyloglossia superior. Minnesota Medicine 49: 1223

Mobius P J 1888 Angeborene doppelseitiger Abducens-Facialis Lahmung. Munchener Medizinische Wochenschrift 35: 91

Mobius P J 1892 Uber infantilen Kernschwund. Munchener Medizinische Wochenschrift 39: 17, 41, 55

Mohr O L 1941 A hereditary sublethal syndrome in man. Avhandinger ugitt av det Norske Videnskaps-Akademi i Oslo. I. Matematisk Naturvidenskapelig Klasse 14: 3

Nervin N C, Kernahan D C, Ross A M 1980 Ankyloglossum superius syndrome. Oral Surgery 50: 254

Papillon-League, Psaume J 1954 Une malformation héréditaire de la mugueuse buccale, brides et friens anormaux. Revue de Stomatologie 55: 209

Petit P, Psaume J 1965 Fente Mediane de la lèvre inférieure. Annales de Chirurgie Plastique 10: 91

Pettersson G 1966 Aglossia congenito with bony fusion of the jaws. Acta Chirurgica Scandinavica 121: 93

Richards R N 1953 The Mobius syndrome. Journal of Bone and Joint Surgery 35: 437

Rimoin D L, Edgerton M T 1967 Genetic and clinical heterogeneity in the oral–facial–digital syndromes. Journal of Pediatrics 71: 94

Rosenthal R 1932 Aglossia congenita. American Journal of Diseases of Children 44: 383

Rucss A L, Pruzansky S, Lis E F, Patau K 1962 Oral–facial–digital syndrome: multiple congenital condition of females with associated chromosomal abnormalities. Pediatrics 29: 985

Shaw M, Gilkes J H, Nally F F 1981 Oral facial digital syndrome — case report and review of literature. British Journal of Oral Surgery 19: 142

Shukowski W P 1911 Zur Atiologie des Strider Inspiratorius Congenitus. Jahrbuch fur Kinderheilkunde 73: 459

Sinclair J G, McKay J 1915 Median harelip, cleft palate and glossal agenesis. Anatomical Review 91: 155

Snyman P G, Prinsloo J G 1966 Congenital fusion of the gums. American Journal of Diseases of Children 112: 593

Spivack J, Benett J E 1968 Glossopalatine ankylosis. Plastic and Reconstructive Surgery 42: 129

Sternberg N, Sagher U, Golan J et al 1983 Congenital fusion of the gums with bilateral fusion of the temperomandibular joints. Plastic and Reconstructive Surgery 72: 385

Tandler J 1899 Zur Entwicklungsgeschichte des Uranoschisma. Wiener Klinische Wochenschrift 7: 153

Thurston E D 1909 A case of median hare-lip associated with other malformations. Lancet ii: 996

Torpin R 1965 Amniochorionic mesoblastic fibrous strings and amnionic bands. American Journal of Obstetrics and Gynecology 91: 65

Touraine A 1937a L'état dysraphyque. Progrès Médical 6: 361

Touraine A 1937b Status dysraphicus. Angiomatose: meningée, imbecillitée. Bull Soc Franc Dermat et Syph 44: 123

Trelat U 1869 Sur un vice conformation très-rare de la lèvre inférieure. Journal de Médecine et Chirurgie Pratique 40: 442–445

Wehinger H 1970 Kiefermissbildung and peromelie. Zeitschrift fur Kinderheilkunde 108: 46

Wexler M R, Novark B W 1974 Hanhart's syndrome (case report). Plastic and Reconstructive Surgery 54: 99

Whelan D T, Feldman W, Dost I 1975 The oro-facial–digital syndrome. Clinical Genetics 8: 205

Wilson R A, Kliman M R, Hardymint A F 1963 Ankyloglossia superior (palato-glossal adhesion in the newborn infant). Pediatrics 31: 1051

Examination

10. Psychological aspects

P. Tridon

INTRODUCTION

There are some most important psychological considerations which must not be overlooked in children with craniofacial malformations before treatment is undertaken. One must strive to prevent psychological or psychiatric problems which may vitiate an anatomically satisfactory surgical result.

The parents of children born with malformations usually suffer some psychic trauma themselves and this is manifested in varying degrees: During pregnancy, the parents' fears of an abnormal child are understandable but one must assess the true parental reaction once the child is born. Many factors will influence the quality and the intensity of this reaction, such as the visible or invisible aspects of the malformation, its seriousness or the coexistence of other morphological abnormalities. A simple, minor craniosynostosis is unlikely to engender the same attitudes and feelings as a major acrocephalosyndactyly or a severe cleft of the lip and palate.

The gradual awareness of an abnormality which is less obvious will then give the parents more of a chance to adapt. Associated disorders which are not rare will also have a great impact. Visual and auditory disorders, psychomotor slowness, a prematurity entailing an early separation of the child from the mother, or the same malformation occurring in several children can arouse a feeling of guilt, which may be dealt with later. The strength and quality of the couple's personality, the attitudes of relatives or unkind words can all be expected to play a role.

THE MOTHER'S REACTION

Giving birth to a defective child, especially one with a facial deformity, may cause a psychic trauma in the mother. As Freud states in *Beyond the Principle of Pleasure*, a true reaction of fright and distress, linked with the effect of surprise, may develop and non-preparation and the inability to change this fear into anxiety may be significant. It will result in an uneasy mother–child relationship; the mother will have to overcome this and come to terms with the actual deformity and all the shame and guilt associated with it.

Over the last few years (Brazelton 1983) the importance of the communication between the infant and the mother during the first hours of infant life has been stressed. In addition the interrelation mediated by visual, auditory and motor activity of the newborn baby plays a part in the discovery of the mother.

The mother too will affect her child by her looks, words, physical contact and dreams. Mother and child 'create each other mutually' as Lebovici (1983) puts it. We can easily guess how ill at ease the mother may feel in the presence of this 'more or less monstrous' child. She may find it difficult to look at him, speak to him and she often cannot suckle him. The separation from the child to permit aftercare in the neonatal department may further disrupt the developing relationship and add well-known problems to the situation, especially in the case of premature babies.

The parents' reaction towards the birth of an abnormal child varies according to the case itself and with time. Drottar & Coll (1975) instituted a study of 20 children with serious facial malformations and followed them for several years (Fig. 10.1). Three different stages have been defined:

1. The initial state of shock, a real reaction of catastrophe, with a feeling of helplessness, as if life had stopped, leading sometimes to a denial of the truth.
2. A period of sadness, anxiety and anger usually follows, similar to a reaction of mourning. Aggression can be directed towards the child, the mother herself, the doctor or even the outside world.
3. Then comes a period of adaptation, leading to reorganization in which anxiety is better controlled, and mechanisms of defence settled. This permits a reorganization of life, new plans for the child, backed up by medical

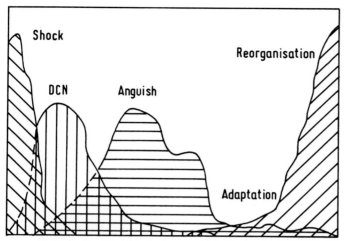

Fig. 10.1 Diagrammatic representation of the reaction and adjustment of parents to the birth of a malformed child (from Drottar & Coll 1975).

and surgical treatment, and a cathexis of the family and opportunities in socio-professional life. In many cases these mechanisms of defence and adaptation will fail, the state of initial shock will persist or the mother's durable anxiety will lead to harmful overprotection.

Finally a more or less hidden rejection is not exceptional. Guilt is often present, reactivated by the attitudes of relatives who try to find a culprit, by the hereditary character in certain forms, especially when they are cases transmitted by autosomic mechanisms, or sex-linked. The same applies when the malformation is caused by infection which occurred during the pregnancy or when medicines were taken during pregnancy (antiepileptics, for example). The parent's anxiety will be increased if they fear associated intellectual backwardness which could further worsen their child's future.

These reactions, ranging from stress to a relative balance, were compared to the reaction of mourning when a child dies (Solnit & Stark 1961) and to the reactions determined by other malformations, especially those affecting the limbs, as in thalidomide deformities (Roskies 1972).

THE MALFORMED CHILD

These different attitudes and reactions, which are far more varied and personalized in reality, will not be harmless for the child. The lack of early cathexis and interrelation may lead to a disharmonious personality, inducing an early psychosis.

Anxiety and overprotection may cause a delay in development. The same applies to rejection and aggression which may also cause character and behaviour disorders.

To these factors one may add repeated separation, including the well-known risks of hospitalization, which unfortunately are not uncommon. At this age, the repeated surgical operation on the head or mouth will also play an important part. Thus we can understand the frequent feeding difficulties encountered by these children. One may encounter anorexia or problems of mastication and deglutition that cannot be explained by the anatomical disorders which have been adequately corrected. The latter can be considered as relationship problems, increasing the mother's anxiety and worsening her narcissistic wound.

Another frequent difficulty can be with speech, whose disorders are often difficult to explain. These problems will be dealt with in another chapter, but it seems important to mention their associated relational dimension, whether it be a delay in speech and language, or a refusal to speak, approaching even dumbness.

One danger must be underlined: it consists of taxing many of these already dysmorphic children with psychointellectual backwardness because of their motor or verbal retardation, or of their inhibited, passive behaviour. But it is not a true retardation, only secondary to the factors we have mentioned. Real pathology, such as a motor handicap, epilepsy, sensory, visual or auditory disorders, will of course have a major effect on the future of these children.

The reactions that have been discussed so far affect the young child and should be given more prominence, because they will play an important part in further development and will actually be of significance throughout the child's life.

The consequences of these malformations in the older child cannot be ignored. There will be a frailty, a certain vulnerability and the child will have to face not only his family reactions but also those of his peers when he goes to school and when later he is integrated into society and work.

The actual experience of living with a malformation is not always easy or indeed harmless. This justifies an early and more aggressive surgical correction. Surgical correction is only part of the reparative process, good though it may be.

The child will have to face life with the knowledge that he is different from others; there will usually be some slight stigma which he cannot hide or disguise. The reactions of others are not always harmless. Jeers or more frequently pity from adults, and curiosity, may cause suffering. Nicknames are often quite commonly used and they may be cruel. This is perhaps a manifestation of the fear or alarm experienced by others who consider themselves normal. The reactions that follow can easily be imagined: they range from fear or shyness to defensive aggression.

Delinquency, antisocial behaviour or true rebellion are frequently thought to stem from the insecurity associated with major deformities. These disorders are usually expressed during adolescence when the image of the body assumes a great importance. A narcissistic crisis may develop in which the opinion and looks of others are important.

THE FAMILY

It is impossible to restrict the impact of such a malformation to the parents alone. The whole family is involved and one must stress the feelings of siblings, who are rarely the victims of the same abnormalities. They will be aware of the parents' worries and to some extent suffer from lack of attention caused by the parents' preoccupation with the abnormal child. Their feelings towards him are usually mixed; protection but also jealousy or even hatred may be the result of the situation. Grandparents also feel the wound and their attitude may help the parents if they are able to act with delicacy. They may aggravate the pain by clumsy interference, especially if they try to lay blame for the misfortune.

In the parents themselves, the birth of such a child can cause a cementing or strengthening of links in order to better face their misfortune together. It can also reveal defects and cause a rupture. One must be aware of narcissistic wounds felt by the father, whose pride is severely injured and who may escape from home to find shelter in his job. He may even reproach his wife for not paying him enough attention because she is so absorbed with her 'own' child.

Despite all these difficulties and mishaps in many cases, everything, however, does appear satisfactory. Parents usually overcome the initial trauma and the mother will accept her child. Love and care may awaken in her and a sound family relationship develop. If the child is not badly handicapped, he profits by all the care and attention bestowed on him from an early date. So one comes to the medical, or more particularly, the surgical attitude.

DOCTOR, SURGEON AND PSYCHOLOGICAL PROBLEMS

It is not only difficult for the parents of a handicapped child, but also for the medical specialists. Aetiological, clinical and therapeutic knowledge has improved considerably over the last few years. This has opened the door to earlier surgery so that function and appearance have been improved at a younger age.

These results, however, are usually obtained at the price of repeated interventions. The psychological phenomena associated with these malformations should not be allowed to interfere with or used as excuses for inadequate surgical correction.

At birth, once the diagnosis is made the family doctor and paediatrician are the specialists mainly involved. It is important that they should be aware of the family reactions. Such reactions as shock and denial, despair and anger, leading even to a wish for the child's demise, should be appreciated by the physicians.

Agression is frequently transferred to the doctor and the medical team and must be accepted. The revelation that the new baby is deformed must be made with tact to both parents. Apart from cases of extreme urgency, it is important for the mother to see and to nurse her child and establish early contact with him. If reality and the malformed child are not faced, fantasies may develop which can even exaggerate the deformity in the parents eyes. The parents must be reassured early on about the mental state and the therapeutic possibilities, especially those involving surgical correction. Photos and an outline of the surgical plan may help, as well as contact with families of children with similar deformities. Such contact can be of great importance during the first few months, when they may not have sufficient support from their own relatives or physicians.

Slowly, it is hoped the mother will develop a healthy relationship with her baby. But there is a need to overcome and understand the unkind words others use during the early days. Sensitive parents may suffer greatly at this time and the effect on them and the child may be long lasting.

Great faith is invested in the surgeon responsible for the correction of the abnormality. His relationship with the parents is most important. Hospitalization is always a traumatic experience for these children, who usually need many admissions. These must be carefully planned and reduced to a minimum. The mother's presence is naturally desirable.

Operations on the skull, because it is closely related to the brain, understandably cause more anxiety. Is there any need to involve a psychologist or a paedopsychiatrist? One cannot answer this question with a routine yes or no. Paediatricians and surgeons, thanks to their understanding, their sensitiveness and their experience of these problems are initially more suited to giving support and answering the family's questions.

In some cases, a specialist's intervention is necessary because of the seriousness of the parent's reactions, especially when a pathological interrelationship may seriously influence the child. It is always difficult and inadequate to direct families to a psychiatrist, because of the fear such a title engenders. It seems highly preferable, as Rufo (1983) advises, that the psychiatrist should be integrated into the management team. In this way he can observe the surgeon–family relationship and intervene as necessary once he fully understands the medical and psychological background.

REFERENCES

Brazelton T B, Cramer B, Kreisler L, Schapi R, Soule M 1983 La dynamique du nourrisson. Paris, E.S.F.
Drottar D, Baskiewicz A, Irvin N, Kennel J, Klaus M 1975 The adaptation of parents to the birth of an infant with a congenital malformation: a hypothetical model. Pediatrics 56: 710–717
Lebovici S 1983 Le bebe la mere et le psychanalyste. Paris, Le Centurion

Roskies E 1972 Abnormality and normality: the mothering of thalidomide children. New York, Cornell University Press
Rufo M 1983 Prevention de l'encopresie. Revue neuropsychologique infants 31: 205–208
Solnit A J, Stark M H 1961 Mourning and the birth of a defective child. Psychological Studies of Children 16: 523

11. Somatic aspects

M. Stricker, J. Van der Meulen, B. Raphael, R. Mazzola

PRENATAL EXAMINATION

In recent years a number of techniques have been developed for prenatal examination, such as amniocentesis, abdominal endoscopy and echoscopy. Amniocentesis permits the aspiration of amniotic fluid. Abdominal endoscopy entails the risk of an abortus in 5% of cases, the field of vision being reduced by the presence of a placenta.

Echoscopy is a new method. Its potential is the subject of many studies and some conclusions have been drawn.

The cephalic extremity can be distinguished at the end of the 6th–7th week, but cephalic contours can only be defined in the 11th or 12th week following ossification (Fig. 11.1).

The examination concerns alterations of anatomical landmarks. The profile is measured at the level of the orbits. A facial triangle may be distinguished between the 10th and 18th weeks. Below the anterior part of the cranial vault a face resembling that of an old man becomes visible between the 18th and 39th weeks (Fig. 11.2). The contours of a check may be defined in the 20th week. More precise information is not available at this stage but the prospects for this technique are certainly promising.

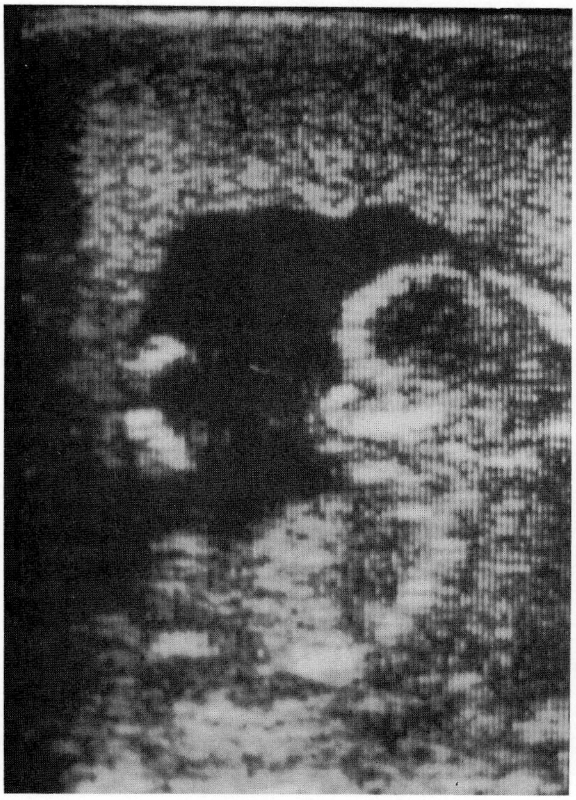

Fig. 11.1 Apparition of cephalic contours.

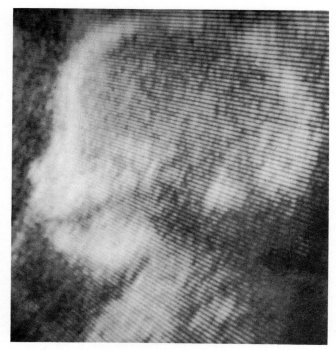

Fig. 11.2 Apparition of facial contours.

POSTNATAL EXAMINATION

The aim of the surgeon faced with a craniofacial malformation is to locate the abnormality within the framework of our classification. In this connection the normal approach, from the general to the particular, is reversed. The clinical picture emerges as a pattern of signs pointing to a topographical and nosological diagnosis.

The physical examination follows a rigid analytical procedure, regardless of the initial impression, and involves the physical characteristics of the abnormality as well as its dimensions.

Comparison with the contralateral side as regards symmetry is essential, as well as a study of the function of the affected region. If the patient's age and cooperation allow it, a search for associated abnormalities should also be made in the patient and in the family.

The examination follows a regional plan, structure by structure, starting with the skin and hair and ending in the bones, not forgetting the muscles and the glands. An assessment of sensory and motor neurological function should also be made. The logical sequence is inspection, followed by palpation and measurement (Fig. 11.3). A detailed family history is also desirable (Fig. 11.4).

Examination of different regions

The various anatomical and functional regions defined at the outset cannot all be examined in the same way, either clinically or paraclinically. Some parts can be almost wholly assessed by the normal methods of examination; an example is the median sagittal area, which is mainly external. Others are only partly available to observation by the clinician. The cranial sector is such a case, where only the vault is accessible to physical examination. Nevertheless one should adhere to the logical approach, that is to say one starts with the skin and soft parts and then moves on to the bones and an assessment of function.

THE SKULL: THE VAULT

This is most commonly the site of a malformation which is both visible and palpable. The vault may be partially or completely, and symmetrically or asymmetrically, affected. Deviation from the normal can be assessed by measuring the circumference of the skull and the sagittal and coronal diameters and then referring to standard tables.

Examination of soft parts

This includes the nature of the skin, its colour, its contours (cutis gyrata) and the characteristics of the hair, especially over the normally smooth forehead. Changes in the hairline, its pattern, and the presence of alopecia or skin tumours must be recorded. Skin dystrophy is even more important. Scarring indicative of a previous surgical operation should not be forgotten.

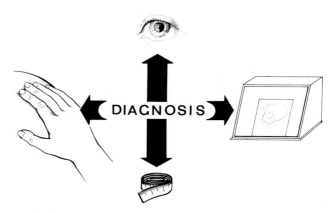

Fig. 11.3 Inspection, palpation, measurement and skeletal documentation.

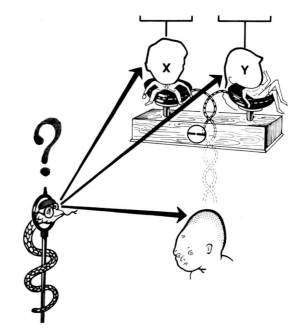

Fig. 11.4 Family history.

Examination of the bones

Here one is concerned with the relative mobility of the bony elements and the presence of gaps; these may be normal or abnormal and are related to age. Such gaps may permit herniation of the meninges or of the meninges and brain.

THE FACE

This must be examined with the greatest care, in view of its structural complexity.

The forehead

The anterior hairline above and laterally and the eyebrows below are a frequent source of specific information about the malformation. The forehead so delimited often has a particular appearance: it may be triangular or even Mephistophelian, especially when the hairline dips down centrally in the axis of the malformation — the so-called 'widow's peak'.

The vertical and transverse bifrontal dimensions are measured but particular attention is paid to the fronto-orbitonasal contour; these measurements may be given a numerical value if recorded with a goniometer. In practice, the measurements are made by teleradiography for reasons of convenience and reliability.

Symmetry of the sides is checked in a deflected view; The appearance of the frontal bases is noted and confirmed by palpation, which will reveal bony defects. Any abnormalities of contour will be obvious. The temporofrontal transition zone is the last feature to be studied.

Orbital Region

The eye is first examined, as the immediate orbital point of reference. Sometimes the striking feature consists not of the eyeball but of an associated deformity, such as ptosis or a coloboma. The eyebrow, too, is helpful in the assessment of the position and orientation of the orbital cavity, as it constitutes a perfect transitional structure between forehead and orbit.

Soft parts. The presence, dimensions and appearance of the eyeball are assessed; anophthalmia, microphthalmia, coloboma of iris, cataract and epibulbar dermoid, for example, may be observed. A note is made of the antero-posterior position of the globe on both sides, ranging from endophthalmos to exophthalmos. It may be calibrated with the Hertel exophthalmometer, despite the uncertainty of bony reference points involved in this examination. Sometimes there is a lateral displacement of the eyeball in the absence of any orbital dystopia (meningoencephalocele). The intrinsic and extrinsic motor functions of the eye are examined by the light reaction of the pupilla and voluntary eye movements, respectively.

Structures associated with the orbit are then examined. The palpebral fissures are examined for mongoloid and antimongoloid slant. Their transverse diameter (blepharophimosis), their vertical diameter (ptosis) and the presence of a medial epicanthal fold are recorded. The eyelids are studied for shortness, colobomas and for the form of the hairline. Finally, function during closure as well as during extreme upward and downward gaze is assessed. The patency of the tear ducts (when present) is verified by the injection of saline into one of the orifices; a fistulous tract may thus be revealed. Pressure on the eyeballs with the lids closed gives an indication of tension of the septum and the state of the intraorbital fat. The quality of the eyebrows, their position, continuity and orientation should also be studied.

Orbit. The spatial position of the orbits should be evaluated in three dimensions, both separately and in relation to one another. The interorbital diameter is measured, indicating hyper- or hypotelorism. The dimensions of each orbit can be approximately evaluated and then confirmed radiologically. The orbital bones, including the orbital margins, are palpated in order to demonstrate any loss of continuity, which is most common along the inferior border. The bony orbit must be studied radiologically. This is best achieved with the scanner.

The nasal pyramid, the nasal fossae and associated structures. The nasal pyramid is defined by its location, which may be ectopic (proboscis), by its direction, dimensions, shape and symmetry. It may be incomplete or, more rarely, totally absent. Midline or lateral cleft, either total or partial, should be noted. Sometimes one may discover a cleft on palpation of the dorsum, which gives a clue to bifidity. The height of the septum and its anterior projection are assessed. Examination of the soft parts may disclose fistulous remnants or dermoid cysts, normally situated in the midline; more rarely, folds of the dorsal integument or cutis gyrata may be encountered. The shape of the alae nasi determines the type of nasal orifice which in turn leads to the nasal cavities. Anterior rhinoscopy with a speculum demonstrates the nasal fossae and the state of the septum, the mucosa and the turbinates. Patency is checked with a soft catheter, which may reveal choanal obstruction. An intranasal mass may be evidence of a meningocele. Examination of the nasal cavities used to be by transillumination but is now essentially radiological, as is examination of the bony structures. Nasal ventilation is studied not only by exhalation on a mirror but also by active inspiration. The sense of smell should also be checked, but clinical evaluation may be very difficult.

LATERAL REGION

Soft parts

These form a lateral strip, meeting its contralateral counterpart to form a jugular (chin-strap) band in which fistulous openings may be embedded. These may be near the pinna and the midline of the neck. Cartilaginous skin inclusions which are vestiges of the developing pinna may also be encountered. One or both pinnae may be absent or may be abnormal in location, size or configuration. There may similarly be abnormalities of the lobule or tragus, which can be absent or cleft. The external auditory meatus may also be absent, narrowed, fissured or abnormally orientated.

The lateral contour is affected in different ways in relation to the posterior border of the mandibular stump. Anteriorly, the bones and the muscles of mastication are mainly affected, whereas posteriorly the parts effected are the parotid gland and the platysma. Most commonly the masseter muscle is absent or absorbed into a single temporomasseter muscle mass. The facies may reveal localized or global weakness or paralysis, which is usually more marked in the lower facial territory.

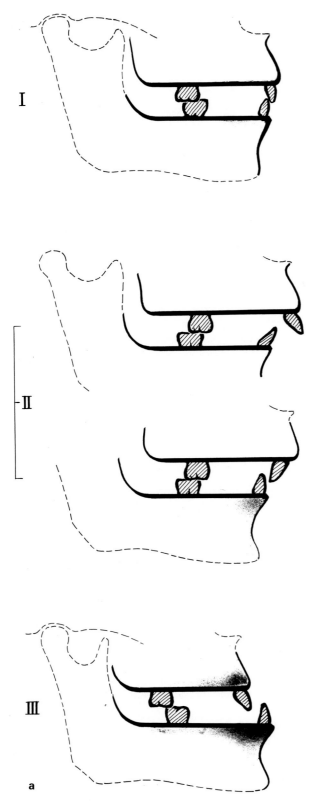

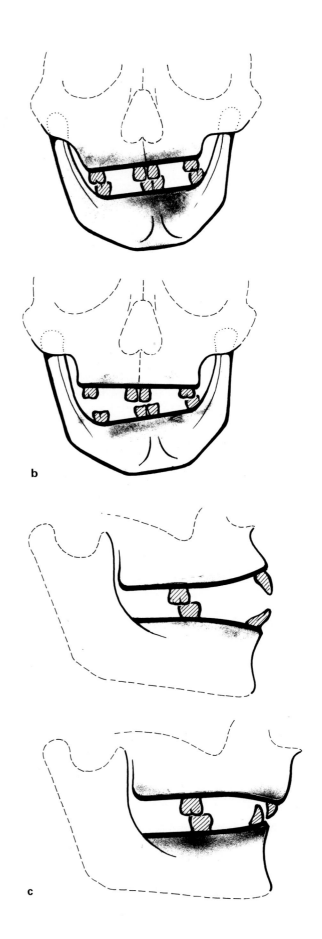

I

II

III

a

b

c

Fig. 11.5 The relationship between the jaws in three planes.
(a) sagittal plane, Angle's classification (I, II, III), (b) vertical plane
(top) patency, (bottom) overclusion, (c) horizontal plane (top)
asymmetry with an oblique plane of occlusion (bottom) laterognathia
with normal maxillary plane.

The bones

Above and anteriorly, the area borders on the orbit. At this level there may be a rounded depression, or an oblique cleft below and laterally, which is often an index of involvement of the malar bone in the lateral malformation. In fact the zygomatic arch is often absent, an abnormality which may coexist with a single temporomasseteric muscle. However, the term zygoma means not only the zygomatic arch but also a major part of the malar bone, which may very often be involved and reduced to a minor bony flake.

Palpation of any loss of continuity in the inferolateral part of the orbit usually extends directly downwards and outwards in the direction of the temporal bone.

The mandible is rarely affected in the body of the bone; however, the body may be the site of a midline defect usually associated with ankyloglossia. Sometimes there is a midline cervical vertical depression of the skin.

The ascending ramus may be abnormal in size, structure or in function, especially when it has lost contact with the pterygoid muscle masses. The mastoid process may be blunt or absent. These bony features are all best confirmed by X-rays. The hyoid bone is close to the thyroglossal tract and is usually involved in malformations of the latter.

BUCCAL REGION

The lips, the alveolodental region and the oral cavity constitute an autonomous transitional system. The shape and outline of the lips, particularly of the upper lip at the philtrum, are studied.

The continuity of the buccal orifice is most commonly interrupted in the upper lip by labiomaxillary clefts; more rarely it may be widened transversely by a horizontal cleft which produces a macrostomia; clefts of the lower lip which may extend to the mandible are rare.

The presence of inferior fistulas and of cysts is immediately apparent on examination. The lips must be everted in order to inspect the frenum, which may be double, hypertrophied, short or the site of fistulas. Labial competence (the two lips in contact at rest) is a major element in orofacial comportment.

It should be remembered that the philtrum, which is apparently a labial structure, is in fact a structure of nasal origin and it may be involved in malformations of the pyramid.

The examination of the oral cavity explores the alveolodental region, the tongue, the palate and pharynx and defines the types of occlusion as well as the depression of the mandible. The opening of the mouth is measured by the interincisive distance.

The number, shape, dimensions, location and characteristics of the teeth must be defined. The incisors,

together with gingival notches, supernumerary frenums or clefts, are of particular interest.

The position of the tongue, its size and shape and clefting are observed. Tongue movements must be determined and may be limited by a short frenum. The tongue may be centrally enlarged owing, most often, to a dermoid cyst. Examination of the palate and pharynx involves the shape and dimensions of the palate (palate arch) as well as the presence of a complete or partial or submucous cleft. In certain malformations there may be extreme fibromucous hypertrophy of the palate (Apert), which may give a false impression of a cleft palate. Examination of the dental articulation discloses the type of occlusion and thus the maxillomandibular relationship.

The examination should include an assessment of the mobility of the soft palate and of the pharynx. By asking the patient to say 'ah' an impression of palatopharyngeal competence can also be obtained at this stage. The tonsils and the adenoids are examined and signs of infection of the nose and pharynx are noted.

The relationship of the jaws are studied in three directions: anteroposteriorly (angle I, II, III) (Fig. 11.5); vertically — patency or overocclusion may be present; transversely — laterognathia which may be associated with an oblique plane of occlusion is sometimes seen.

OCCIPITOVERTEBRAL REGION

The clinical examination is limited in view of the reduced skin territory which is accessible. It is possible to study the length of the neck, lateral deviation, the presence of a pterygium colli, and to palpate the spinous processes and the paravertebral muscle masses. The essential part of the examination is a lateral X-ray of the neck.

In the presence of specific organ abnormalities a specialist should be consulted: the ophthalmologist will assess visual and oculomotor function and give a prognosis; the otorhinolaryngologist assesses respiratory, olfactory and auditory function; the neurologist can specify the psychomotor status; the orthodontist assesses the type of dental occlusion and will outline the possibilities for treatment.

Finally, the clinical examination should not be restricted to the patient alone, but should include a study of the family and a genetic enquiry.

REFERENCES

Angle E H 1907 Malocclusion of the teeth. White Dental Manufacturing Co.
Aubry M C, Dumez Y, Gillet J Y 1983 Diagnostile antenatal de malformations foetals par l'echographie Vigot, Paris
Tortil J M 1986 Etude de la croissance faciale chez le foetus in utero an moyen de l'echographie. Thèse medical, Nancy

12. Ophthalmological aspects

A. Th. M. van Balen

INTRODUCTION

In the context of this book a short description of the ophthalmological examination and of the symptoms and signs that can be found may serve three ends:

1. to contribute to the diagnosis;
2. to assess the preoperative state in order to evaluate the effects of craniofacial reconstructive surgery on eye function;
3. to designate malformations in which eye function may be improved by craniofacial surgery.

ANAMNESIS

An ophthalmological anomaly found in patients with craniofacial anomalies is not necessarily part of a syndrome. For instance, strabismus can be a family trait and not a sign of dyscephaly. The anamnesis of the family and the history of the patient himself has to be taken regarding eye diseases and anomalies.

EXAMINATION

Eye exposure

Exorbitism can be found in patients with shallow orbits (e.g. Apert, Crouzon). Its severity can be established with the instrument of Hertel, in which the distance between the lateral orbital rim and the top of the cornea is measured by way of two mirrors. The instrument can be adapted to the width of the skull and has to rest on the lateral orbital rim. In Figure 12.1 it is shown how the observer sees the profile of the cornea in the upper small mirror and the scale in the lower mirror. The observer has to place his head between the two observed eyes to keep his viewing line parallel to the sagittal plane of the patient's head. In extreme proptosis the possibility of exposure keratopathy, because of the defective lid closure, ectropion

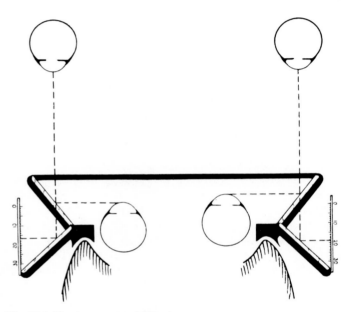

Fig. 12.1 The instrument of Hertel.

of the eyelids and even luxation of the globes have to be considered.

Position and movements of the eyes

The position of the eyes is partly determined by the configuration of the orbits. Although the anatomy of the orbits is described elsewhere in this book, some remarks are appropriate.

ANATOMY

It is particularly important to note that the orbital rims or margins are not placed horizontally to the side of the nose but tend to dip down and out so that the longer axes, if prolonged, would meet well above the root of the nose.

Of even greater importance is the angle formed by the vertical planes or bases of the orbits. Measurements vary from 130°– 150°. It is also essential to bear in mind that the outer rim of the orbital cavity is on a plane considerably farther back than the median rim.

The angle formed by the medial and external walls is from 46°–48° (the two medial walls are rarely exactly parallel). In most instances the distance between the posterior part of the medial walls is several millimetres greater than the distance between the anterior ends (Fig. 12.2). In hypertelorism or telorbitism the distance between the bases of the orbit can be enormously increased, while the apices of the orbits have a normal distance. Tessier was the first to show that the bony orbits can be moved substantially towards the midline of the face without damaging the optic nerves. Jöhr (1953) gave us normal values for the distance of the medial canthi, the lateral canthi and the nasal limbi of the corneas in the different age groups. The last criterion is the interpupillary distance minus the corneal diameter (Fig. 12.3).

The definition of hypertelorism is discussed elsewhere in this book. With the sagittal axis of the skull the axis of the orbit forms an angle of approximately 23° according to different authorities. If prolonged backwards the two axes should meet slightly posterior to the posterior wall of the sella turcica. It is of interest to note that while the anterior posterior axis of the orbit forms an angle of approximately 23° with the optic axis it practically coincides with the muscle plane of the superior and inferior rectus muscle (Fig. 12.4). The ocular muscles, with the exception of the inferior oblique, arise from the back of the orbit and run forward to attach to the globe by means of tendinous expansions. The four recti attach in front of the equator, while the superior oblique tendon, after passing through the trochlea, turns backwards to attach to the sclera behind the equator, and the inferior oblique, arising from the nasal aspect of the orbit just inside its

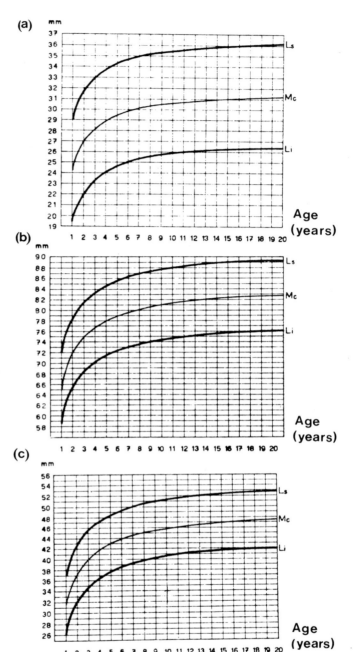

Fig. 12.3 Normal values of distance of (a) the canthi interni (b) canthi externi and (c) distance of the nasal limbi in different age groups.

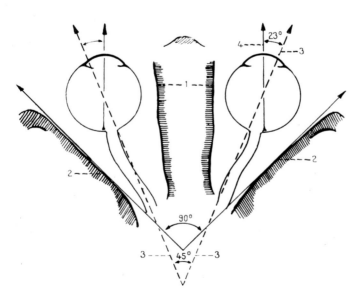

Fig. 12.2 Schematic representation of the orbital region.

rims, also passes backwards to insert on the globe behind the equator. The ocular muscles are paired, each pair having a common muscle plane, which is formed by joining the central point of the origin of the muscles with the central point of their tendinous insertions.

These four points determine a plane running through the long axis of each of the muscles. The angle formed by this plane with the direction of vision or line of fixation depends on the position of the globe. When the line of

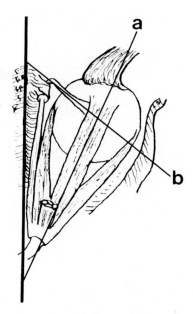

Fig. 12.4 Muscle planes of vertical recti (a) and obliqui (b).

fixation runs through the muscle plane, the angle is zero. The medial and lateral recti have a common muscle plane lying in the horizontal plane of the globe. The superior and inferior recti lie in a common vertical plane ($\pm$ anteroposterior axis) which forms an angle of 23° with the line of fixation, when the eyes are directed straight ahead, i.e. in the primary position. The superior and inferior oblique muscles also lie in a common plane and this plane forms an angle of approximately 51° with the line of fixation when the eyes are in the primary position (Fig. 12.4).

There is, of course, more to be said about the contents of the orbit but the above-mentioned measurements and topical relations are important in case of displacement of the orbital bones.

Six pairs of eye muscles work together to keep bifoveal fixation in all directions of gaze (versions) and at all distances (vergences). To achieve this the muscles act according to two laws:

1. Sherrington's law — contraction of an extraocular muscle is always accompanied by relaxation of its antagonist.
2. Hering's law — equal and simultaneous flow of impulses is directed to both contralateral synergists concerned with the desired direction of gaze.

ASSESSMENT

The examination methods are relatively simple. As the normal position of the eyes is the position of bifoveal fixation the corneal reflexes of a penlight held before the eyes are bilaterally in the centre of the cornea, irrespective of the distance of that penlight. More accurately the

corneal reflexes are slightly nasal to the centre owing to the small angle (κ) between the optical or anatomical axis of the eye and the fixation line (Fig. 12.5). Convergent squint or strabismus convergens is found when the corneal reflex is more nasal. Vertical displacement of the corneal reflex leads to the diagnosis of vertical strabismus, which needs the specification right over left or left over right.

The diagnosis of strabismus can be refined by the so-called cover test. In the normal situation of bifoveal fixation the covering of one eye will not alter the position of the non-covered eye, but in strabismus the covering of the fixing eye will cause a fixation movement of the previously non-fixing squinting eye. When the non-covered eye is seen moving from nasal to temporal position this means that the eye was convergent and movement in the other direction indicates divergent strabismus. When the non-covered eye moves insufficiently or makes roving movements this indicates low vision, usually on the basis of amblyopia but sometimes on the basis of an organic lesion. The second part of the cover test is aimed at the position of the covered eye (phoria). This test can also be called the cover–uncover test. It detects deviations that are kept under control by the fusion mechanism, as long as both eyes are open. However, when fusion is disrupted by covering one eye, a deviation of the covered eye occurs when latent strabismus or heterophoria is present. The occluder or covering hand is quickly removed and the examiner notes whether or not the just uncovered eye is moving, indicating refixation from a deviated position under cover. Cyclo, hyper, hypo, exo and esophoria may thus be detected and differentiated. Minor forms of hypertelorism, for instance, can show latent divergent squint. The existence of fusion is a guarantee for binocular vision after surgical intervention.

Once the diagnosis of strabismus is established the differentiation of non-paralytic or concomitant strabismus

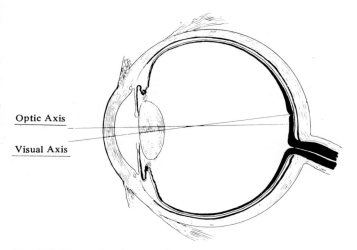

Fig. 12.5 The angle κ between the anatomical axis and the fixation line.

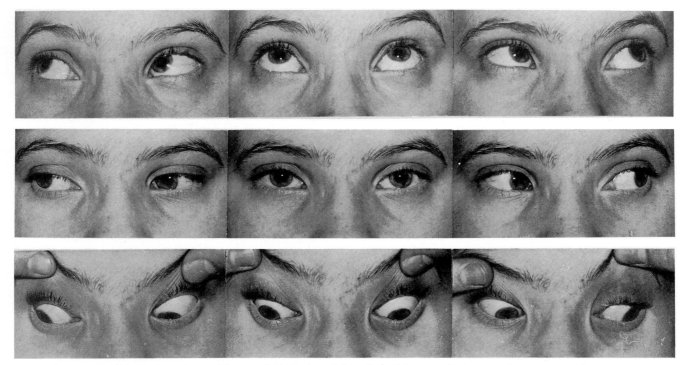

Fig. 12.6 Nine gaze directions of a patient with mongoloid slanting of the palpebral fissures and A-pattern incompetence of eye movements (personal observation).

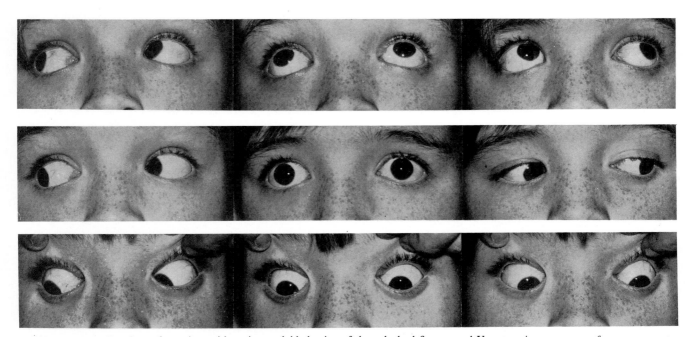

Fig. 12.7 Nine gaze directions of a patient with antimongoloid slanting of the palpebral fissures and V-pattern incompetence of eye movements (personal observation).

with a fairly constant angular relation between the visual axes, whatever the position of the eye, and paralytic or incomitant strabismus in which the angular relation between the visual axes is not maintained, has to be made. This can be done by the examination of the motility of the eyes. By following a fixation object (preferably a penlight) the eyes move from the primary position (straight ahead) to eight extreme positions (Figs. 12.6 and 12.7).

From the direction in which one of the eyes does not follow one reads the muscle that is involved. This is very simple in the case of paralysis of one of the horizontal eye muscles. In the case of vertical eye muscle paralysis a procedure of examination is recommended according to the scheme of Figure 12.8.

Exotropia, manifest deviation of the visual axes resulting in hypertropia and rarely esotropia are seen in a great number of craniofacial malformations and may be attributed to several causes:

1. an abnormal position of the eyeballs in relation to the orbits;
2. a muscular deficit related to the deformation of the orbital cavities;

3. fibrosis or absence of eye muscles;
4. an injury of the oculomotor nerves;
5. disruption of binocular vision.

Exotropia is frequently associated with orbital hypertelorism. In 27 teleorbitism patients of Morax, exotropia was found in 14 cases. The exotropia deviation is thought to result from the abnormally increased interorbital distance, which changes the angle between the axis of the orbit and the axis of the eye, which is normally 23° and can become 40°. This influences also the angle between the direction of the eye muscles and the axis of the eye (Morax 1982a,b).

Esotropia is much less frequent in teleorbitism and craniofacial stenoses and can sometimes be ascribed to paralysis or anatomic lesion.

Vertical imbalance is more frequent than horizontal imbalance.

The V-syndrome is the most frequent vertical deviation. It may be observed in cases with zygomaxillary hypoplasia such as the Franceschetti Zwahlen or Treacher Collins syndromes and in many cases of craniostenosis, especially Crouzon and Apert. In the V-syndrome the position of the eyes is more convergent in downgaze and in right and left gaze the adducted eye moves upward (Fig. 12.7). According to Gobin (1969) this is probably caused by a discrepancy between the angles formed by the obliquus superior and inferior with the axes of the eyeballs. In the case of antimongoloid palpebral fissures the orbits are extorted and the external eye muscles cause rotation of the eyes. In fundoscopy rotation of the eye manifests itself as pseudo-ectopia of the macula (Morax & Pascal 1982).

The A-pattern disturbance of the eye movements is much less frequent than the V-pattern (Fig. 12.6).

Restriction of eye movements is not always caused by paralysis of one of the eye muscles but can also be the result of mechanical obstruction, e.g. scar formation in the conjunctiva or in Tenon's capsule, congenital absence of external eye muscle, as for instance the absence of the rectus superior in Apert's syndrome (Morax & Pascal 1982) or the presence of fibrous bands instead of muscles. In plagiocephaly the eye on the side of the synostosis can be turned upwards, although the eyeball and the orbit are low-set. In 15 of 21 cases of plagiocephaly a hyperactivity of the obliquus inferior was found. Incarceration of Tenon's capsule and muscles may occur following surgical movement of the orbits, although the forces active in blow-out fracture are not present. The diagnosis of mechanical obstruction of eye movements is made by use of the so-called forced duction test. Congenital forms of paralytic or mechanical obstruction strabismus lack the symptom of diplopia but can be accompanied by torticollis or head tilt. Concomitant squint secondary to orbital operations can cause diplopia. As stated before, the existence of fusion is very important for the prognosis of binocular vision after surgical movements of the orbits.

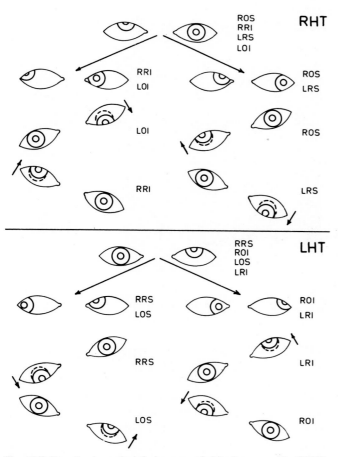

Fig. 12.8 Examination schedule in cases of right hypertrophia (RHT) and left hypertrophia (LHT).

The surgical errors of vertical positioning produce disturbances in the binocular cooperation much more easily than would a comparable error, as the result of correcting horizontal dystopia. That is because the motoric fusion in the horizontal plane is more than ten times the motoric fusion in the vertical plane. Small errors in rotation of the orbit–eye unit around the visual axis also cause few postoperative visual symptoms because of the ability of human eyes to fuse images with a rotational disparity of 44°.

Early strabismus surgery is advantageous (Diamond & Whitaker 1984) because:

1. earlier surgery is more likely to result in binocular vision;
2. motility surgery after orbital manipulation is technically less ideal, since haemorrhage is more profuse and soft tissues are more friable:

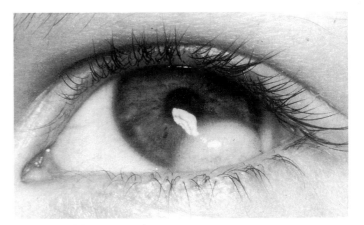

Fig. 12.9 Epibulbar dermoid in a case of Goldenhar's syndrome (personal observation).

According to Limon de Brown et al (1979) the surgical reduction of the interpupillary distance can result in decrease of exotropia, sometimes even producing esotropia. It is not yet possible to predict the effect of the correction of the interpupillary distance on the angle of squint.

Concomitant convergent strabismus in combination with pendular nystagmus is a feature of low visual acuity in, for instance, congenital cataract. These signs of low visual acuity and the low visual acuity itself persist after successful operation of the cataracts because of the so-called deprivation amblyopia. After much experimental evidence some clinical evidence has recently become available that low visual acuity and pendular nystagmus could be prevented by operating on the cataracts as early as possible in the first half year of life. In general pendular nystagmus has to be considered a sign of severe visual handicap until proven otherwise.

Conjunctiva and cornea and anterior chamber

The conjunctiva and cornea have to be examined with incident light and a magnifying loupe. The most conspicuous abnormality is the epibulbar dermoid (Fig. 12.9), found in Goldenhar's syndrome, sometimes associated with a coloboma of the upper eyelid.

Lipodermoids of the conjunctiva are usually less conspicuous because they are partially covered by the eyelids in the temporal upper part of the conjunctiva. The cornea can be small, less than 11 mm in diameter indicating microphthalmia, which can be found eventually in several craniofacial malformations, but is obligatory in the Hallerman Streiff syndrome (Fig. 12.10). In exorbitism the cornea has to be examined carefully because insufficient closure of the eyelids (lagophthalmus) may have caused a keratopathy, i.e. desiccation of the corneal surface with resulting ulceration. The anterior chamber can be studied

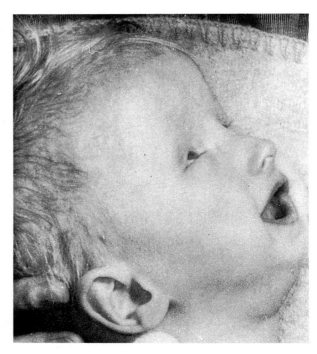

Fig. 12.10 Microphthalmos in a case of Hallerman Streiff syndrome (personal observation).

sufficiently only by use of the slitlamp cornea microscope and gonioscope. Anterior chamber malformation in the sense of the 'cleavage syndrome' can be found in every microphthalmic eye but the full 'anterior chamber cleavage syndrome' is found in the so-called Rieger's syndrome, which is mentioned here because it is frequently accompanied by slight hypertelorism, although never so disfiguring that reconstructive surgery is necessary (Fig. 12.11).

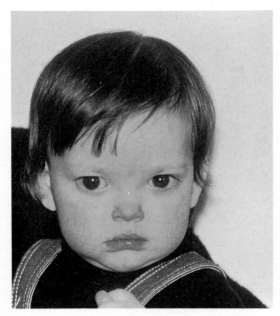

Fig. 12.11 Hypertelorism and buphthalmos due to disturbances of the anterior chamber cleavage in a child with Rieger's syndrome (personal observation).

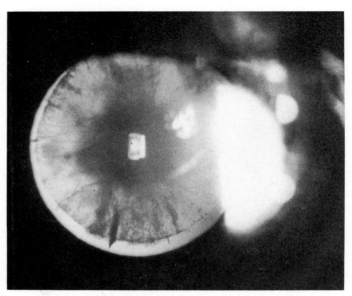

Fig. 12.12 The appearance of cataract against the (red) fundus reflex in the examination with coaxial light.

Pupil

Normally the pupils are round and symmetrical in the centre of the iris. A coloboma of the iris can be a sign of an early disturbance of development of the eye and is sometimes combined with microphthalmia (for instance in the Hallerman Streiff syndrome). In the developmental anomalies of the anterior chamber the pupil can be eccentric and elliptical.

The pupillary reflex on light is an important objective sign of the function of the eye. Directly positive is the reflex when the pupil of the eye on which the light falls constricts — indirectly positive when the pupil of the other eye constricts. Because of the indirect or consensual pupil constriction normally there is no change when one moves the light from one pupil to the other. In case of low sensitivity of one eye, the movement of the light from the good eye to the eye with low sensitivity will cause increase of both pupils (Marcus Gunn phenomenon). This can be a sign of involvement of the optic nerve.

The next feature to be examined is the colour of the pupil. Normally the pupil is black, because of the camera obscura effect, but in cases of opacification of the lens (cataract) the colour of the pupil is grey or white (leucocoria). When the opacification of the lens is not total, it is best detected by the examination of the fundus reflex with a funduscope. The cataract will then show as black configuration against the red fundus reflex (Fig. 12.12).

Cataract is found in various craniofacial malformations but it is almost obligatory in the Hallerman Streiff syndrome (van Balen 1961). The necessity to diagnose cataract as early as possible in all congenital syndromes has already been mentioned above. The possibility of preventing deprivation amblyopia and pendular nystagmus by early operation is not yet common knowledge. In practice the child with congenital cataract is seen much later by the ophthalmologist because observation and treatment of other congenital defects has taken much time and the pendular nystagmus has been considered a neurological sign with no therapeutical consequence. Spontaneous resorption is seen, specifically in the cataract of the Hallerman Streiff syndrome. The examination of the fundus reflex is of course enhanced by dilatation of the pupil but it needs mentioning here that before the administration of mydriatics the pupillary reflex on light should be examined because in children this can be the only means to ascertain visual function.

Fundus

When the lens and vitreous are clear, funduscopy is possible. The papilla nerve optici can show congenital deformation.

A coloboma of the pupil or 'morning glory pupil' can be found in midfacial deformities, e.g. transsphenoidal encephalocele with hypertelorism (Fig. 12.13).

Atrophy of the pupil can be found as a consequence of a narrow optic canal in craniostenoses and craniometaphyseal dysplasia (Puliafilo et al 1981), but usually appears as a primary one. To some authors atrophy secondary to papiloedema seems to be excluded or at least very rare, but others say that optic atrophy in the syndromes of Apert, Crouzon and Greig can develop from increased intracranial pressure and therefore is not a primary defect. Careful

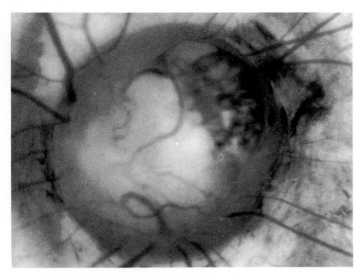

Fig. 12.13 Colobomatous optic nerve head in a patient with hypertelorism.

autopsy studies showed that in somes cases stretch on the optic nerve is the only cause of the atrophy (Gross 1956).

Stretching of the nerve is due to the increased flexion of the cerebral hemisphere. A nicking of the optic nerves by pressure of the internal carotid against the roof of the foramen has also been assumed to be a factor in producing optic atrophy.

Visual acuity

In children up to about 3 years old visual acuity is very difficult to measure but one can always estimate the relative visual acuity by alternate occlusion of the eyes and comparison of the behaviour of the child in either condition. From 3 years on the visual acuity can be measured by the use of any kind of optotypes. This depends of course on the level of mental development. When the measurement of visual acuity is possible, the differentiation of refraction anomalies is called for.

Subjective and objective methods of refraction can be carried out by an ophthalmologist, but screening is easily done by using a stenopeic hole. In the case of low visual acuity caused by refraction anomaly the stenopeic hole will improve the visual acuity, whereas low visual acuity of other origin will be the same or even less. Low visual acuity of one eye can be an indication of a structural anomaly but also of amblyopia, i.e. functional disturbance of visual acuity. In the case of low visual acuity of both eyes on account of congenital cataract or opticus atrophy the eyes will show pendular nystagmus or searching eye movements. The diagnosis of blindness in young children is not easily made, but is certainly asked for when the indication of extensive craniofacial surgery is discussed. The pupillary reflex on light (direct and indirect) is a sign of the function of the afferent pathway up to the lateral geniculate body and the colliculi superiores. In the case of absence of the pupillary reflex on light, it is advisable to examine the electroretinogram in order to differentiate between a retinal defect and an optic nerve defect. The electroretinogram can be made under general anaesthesia because it is not seriously influenced by narcotics.

In the case of positive pupil reflex on light, the visual evoked response has to be registered to exclude or confirm the diagnosis of cortical blindness. The visual evoked response has to be examined without general anaesthesia because narcotics seriously influence the cortical evoked potential (Regensburg & Van Balen 1975).

CONCLUSION

There are two reasons to request early ophthalmological examination in cases of craniofacial malformation.

Table 12.1 Ophthalmological signs in craniofacial malformations

	Oculovertebral dysplasia	Mandibulofacial dystosis	Hemifacial microsomia	Hallerman Steriff	Hypertelorism	Craniostenosis
Eyebrow, absence of external third		+				
Exophthalmos						+
Exotropia					+ +	+ +
Upper lid coloboma	+ + +					
Lower lid coloboma		+ + + +				
Antimongoloid lid obliquity	+ +	+ + + +	+			
Canaliculi lacrimalis		+ +				
Epibulbar dermoids	+ + + +					
Dermolipoma	+ + +					
Iris and/or choroid coloboma	+		+			
Cataract				+		
Microphthalmia	+		+	+ + +	+	
Optic atrophy					+	+ +

Combination of data from the publications of Blodi (1957), Feingold & Gellis (1968) and Rougier (1977).

1. Cataract has to be operated in the first 6 months of life in order to prevent deprivation amblyopia.
2. Strabismus has to be managed in the first 4 years of life in order to prevent strabismus amblyopia and/or abnormal correspondence and to restore normal binocular vision.

Diamond et al (1980) did not find any alteration of ocular alignment by orbital manipulation, whereas Converse & McCarthy (1981) did find a definite trend towards esotropia following medical translocation of the orbits. Certainly binocular cooperating eyes are much less liable to alteration of alignment and therefore strabismus surgery should not be deferred until after major craniofacial surgery.

REFERENCES AND BIBLIOGRAPHY

Bagolini B, Campos E C, Chiesi E 1982 Plagiocephaly causing superior oblique deficiency and ocular torticollis. Archives of Ophthalmology 100: 1093–1096

Blodi F D 1957 Developmental anomalies of the skull affecting the eye. Archives of Ophthalmology 57: 593–610

Converse J M, McCarthy J G 1981 Orbital hypertelorism. Scandinavian Journal of Plastic and Reconstructive Surgery 15: 265–276

Diamond G R, Whitaker L A 1984 Ocular motility in craniofacial reconstruction. Plastic Reconstructive Surgery 73: 31–37

Diamond G R, Katowitz J A, Whitaker L H, Quinn G E, Schaffer D B 1984 Ocular alignment after craniofacial reconstruction. American Journal of Ophthalmology 90: 248–250

Feingold M, Gellis S 1968 Ocular abnormalities associated with first and second arch syndromes. Survey of Ophthalmology 14: 30–42

Gobin M H 1969 Cyclotropia and squint. Thesis, Krol & Courtin, Antwerp

Gross H 1956 Zur Pathogenese der Sehnerven Atrophie bei den turrizephalen Schädeldysostose. A. Von Graefes Archiv für Klinische und Experimentelle Ophthalmologie 157: 225–236

Jöhr P 1953 Valeurs moyennes et limites normales en fonction de l'âge de quelques mesures de la tête et de la région orbitaire. Journal de Génétique Humaine 2: 247–282

Limon de Brown E, Ortiz Monasterio F, Barrera Padilla G 1979 Estrabismo en hiperteleorbitismo. Cirurgia Plastica Ibero-Latinoamerica, numero especial extra monografico cirurgia craneofacial: 153–178

Morax S, Pascal D 1982a Absence du muscle droit supérieur dans le syndrome d'Apert. Journal Français d'Ophthalmologie 5: 323–326

Morax S, Pascal D 1982b Syndrome de torsion au cours des malformations crânio-faciales. Bulletin de la Société d'Ophthalmologie 810–814

Nelson L B, Ingoglia S, Breinin G M 1981 Sensorimotor disturbances in craniostenosis. Journal of Pediatric Ophthalmology and Strabismus 18: 323–340

Puliafilo C A, Wray S H, Murray J E, Boger W P III 1981 Optic atrophy and visual loss in craniometaphyseal dysplasia. American Journal of Ophthalmology 92: 701.

Regensburg N I, van Balen A Th M 1975 Electro-ophthalmological diagnosis in children with defective vision. In: Maione M, Orsoni J G (eds) Simposio Internazionale d'Oftalmologica Pediatrica, Parma. pp 83–89

Rougier J 1977 Chirurgie plastique orbito palpebrale. Rapport SFO, Paris

Urrets-Zavalia A, Solares-Zamora J, Olmos H R 1961 Anthropological studies on the nature of cyclovertical squint. British Journal of Ophthalmology 45: 578–596

van Balen A Th M 1961 Dyscephaly with microphthalmos cataract and hypoplasia of the mandible. Ophthalmologica 141: 53–63

Weinstock F J, Hardesty H 1965 Absence of superior recti in craniofacial dysostosis. Archives of Ophthalmology 74: 152–153

13. Otological aspects

E. H. Huizing

INTRODUCTION

Craniofacial anomalies are associated with ear deformities in the majority of cases. The otologic malformations almost always concern the auricle, the external ear canal and the middle ear. The inner ear and the vestibular organ are rarely involved.

This is understandable from our knowledge of the embryological origin of the various parts of the auditory organ. The external ear and the middle ear are both derived from the first and second branchial arches and clefts, whereas the inner ear and the vestibular organ originate from the ectoderm.

Tragus and crus helicis of the auricle are derived from the first arch, whereas the remaining part of the concha comes from second arch material. The ectodermal and entodermal part of the first cleft give rise to the external meatus and the middle ear, the entodermal part to the Eustachian tube.

The ossicles are formed from first and second branch tissue. The cranial part of the malleus (head) and of the incus (body and short process) are made from first branch material. The caudal parts of the malleus (handle), incus (long process) and the stapes are derived from the second branch.

The primordium of the inner ear is an epithelial thickening (placode) of the primitive ectoderm which is transformed into a pit and then into the so-called otic vesicle. This vesicle becomes later divided into the vestibular and cochlear part of the labyrinth.

INCIDENCE

In Table 13.1 the incidence of the various otological anomalies is given as observed in the most frequent craniofacial and head and neck syndromes. Because of the difficulties in diagnosis and their relative rarity, data in this respect are still scarce.

MANIFESTATIONS

Otological manifestations in craniofacial malformations are numerous. Almost each case is unique, but in spite of the infinite scale of possibilities some general rules are apparent: deformities of the external and the middle ear are usually combined; deformities of the external and the middle ear are rarely associated with inner ear disorders; in major anomalies a combination of microtia, meatal atresia and ossicular anomalies is found; in moderate and minor malformations discrepancies in the degree of involvement of the various parts of the ear are common, e.g. a normal auricle, meatus and tympanic membrane do not exclude an ossicular anomaly with conductive hearing loss of 50–60 dB.

EXTERNAL EAR

Auricle All degrees of concha dysplasia are possible, from a minor variation of the conchal configuration to a complete absence of the ear lobe. The chances of hearing loss are greater in patients with major malformations. However, as mentioned before a minor deformity and even a normal auricle can be associated with a maximal (50 dB) conductive hearing loss.

Preauricular fistula or sinus may be present as a single manifestation. It may also occur as a part of a syndrome, e.g. the branchio-oto-renal or BOR syndrome.

External ear canal All grades of developmental anomaly, ranging from a slight narrowing to a complete absence of the external meatus, may occur. The most frequent deformities are: (1) a funnel-shaped meatus; (2) a normal ear canal with a bony occlusion plate at the level of the tympanic membrane (Fig. 13.1); (3) a short, blindly ending meatus; and (4) a complete atresia (Figs. 13.2, 13.3b).

As long as the ear canal is open sound stimuli will reach the eardrum undisturbed, no matter how small the diameter of the opening.

Table 13.1 Incidence of the otological malformations in some of the most frequent craniofacial and head and neck syndromes

Syndrome	External ear	Middle ear	Inner ear	Hearing loss	Other anomalies
Skull					
1. Dysostosis craniofacialis (Crouzon)					
	30%	30%	Rare	30% Conductive	
2. Acrocephalosyndactyly (Apert)					
		Ossicle dysplasia	Rare	Conductive or mixed	Oligophrenia
Branchial					
1. Dysostosis mandibulofacialis (Treacher Collins)					
Auricle	75%	50%	Rare	50%	Fistula neck;
Atresia	25%			Conductive	renal dysplasia
2. Branchio-oto-renal syndrome					
Fistula	70%	50%	Rare	Conductive; mixed	
Other					
1. Oculo-auriculo-vertebral dysplasia (Goldenhar; hemifacial microsomia)					
	Frequently involved	Frequently involved	Maybe involved	Conductive or mixed	Macrostomia Mandibular hypoplasia Vertebral anomalies
2. Cervico-oculoacusticus syndrome (Wildervanck)					
	Frequently involved	Frequently involved	Dysplasia	Total deafness or severe mixed loss	Klippel–Feil anomaly; abducens paralysis
3. Otopalatodigital syndrome					
	Normal	Ossicular dysplasia	Normal	Conductive	Hypertelorism; cleft palate; hand/foot malformation

Compiled from data by Konigsmark & Gorlin (1976) and Cremers et al (1982).

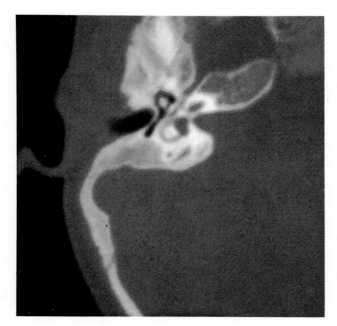

Fig. 13.1 Partial meatal atresia, bony occlusion plate at eardrum level and severely underdeveloped tympanic cavity with ossicular malformation in a child with Treacher Collins' syndrome. Transverse plane.

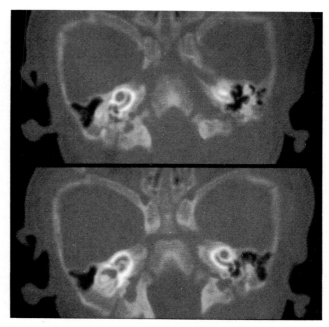

Fig. 13.2 Bilateral microtia, atresia of external meatus, severe middle ear and ossicular chain anomaly and normal cochlea in a child with Apert's syndrome. Transverse plane.

MIDDLE EAR

Eardrum The tympanic membrane may be completely or partially lacking. A bony plate may be present instead. It may also be partially missing. The anterior part can be non-developed and the malleus may be fixed to the anterior bony wall.

The middle ear cavity is smaller in most cases, but always present in some form (Figs. 13.1, 13.2, 13.3b). The middle ear may be filled with mucus because of a non-functioning Eustachian tube. Sometimes it consists of several compartments as a result of an incomplete resolution of the primordial connective tissue.

The Eustachian tube is usually non- or malfunctioning. Very little is known about its anatomical malformation.

INNER EAR

Cochlea and vestibular organ In most patients we find a normally developed and functioning inner ear and vestibular apparatus (Figs. 13.2, 13.3). Severe sensorineural loss or total deafness has nevertheless been observed. Mixed hearing loss has been reported to occur in various syndromes. It is not certain, however, to what extent the bone conduction losses found in these patients represent a true sensorineural impairment. They may partially result from the middle ear deformity.

Facial nerve In the more severe cases the facial nerve may run an abnormal course through the temporal bone and its bony canal may be partially lacking.

The mastoid is usually underdeveloped and poorly or non-pneumatized. An antral cell can nearly always be found.

DIAGNOSIS

The diagnosis of congenital ear anomalies is difficult and full of pitfalls. The most common error is that from a normal appearance on inspection a normal function is concluded. Function can only be established by hearing examination.

Inspection

A careful examination of the auricle, external meatus and eardrum should be performed in the first month after birth. The configuration of both auricles has to be compared. If a membrane can be seen and palpated at the end of the ear canal we cannot be sure that we are dealing with a tympanic membrane. Sometimes a cushion of connective tissue is present.

Hearing assessment

Audiometry is the most important part of the examination. Hearing is essential for normal intellectual, psychological and speech development of the young child. The choice of hearing test to be carried out depends on the age and the developmental level of the child (Table 13.2).

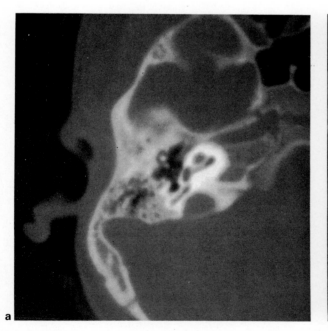 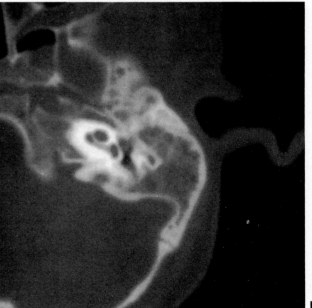

a   b

Fig. 13.3 Hemifacial microtia: (a) transverse plane, normal right ear; (b) transverse plane, left ear: microtia, complete meatal atresia, rudimentary middle ear, normal cochlea.

Table 13.2 Type of hearing test in relation to the age (and the developmental level) of the child

Test	Age (years)		
	0–1	1–5	>5
Electroaudiometry (BERA, ECoG)	+	+	+
Reflex audiometry (Ewing test, eyeblink, arousal)	+		
Free-field audiometry	+	+	+*
Standard octave audiometry (headphones)	–	–	+

* In the mentally retarded child.

STANDARD AUDIOMETRY

Using headphones, this cannot generally be carried out before the age of 4–5 years. It provides quantitative information on both ears separately. As soon as masking (eliminating the other ear during testing) can be applied a distinction between conductive and sensorineural hearing loss becomes possible. Young children are conditioned to respond by pressing a button for a picture or moving a toy. It sometimes requires several sessions to obtain sufficiently reliable results.

FREE-FIELD AUDIOMETRY

This will be the method of choice in younger children and in children with mental retardation. Sound stimuli are presented in a free-field situation and the child is requested to respond by some kind of conditioning method. It is clear that in this way only a rough estimation of the hearing acuity can be obtained.

REFLEX AUDIOMETRY

This is used in babies and young infants. Quantitative sound stimuli that are familiar to the child, such as that of a rattle, a whistle, a spoon on a plate, etc., are offered in a free-field situation (Ewing test). This test is based on the reflex turning of the head towards the origin of the sound stimulus. In the normally developed and hearing child this test is positive from the 6th to 9th month onwards.

Instead of the head-turning reflex the eyeblink reflex or the arousal reflex is used in some centres. These reflexes are already positive at an earlier age but are less reliable.

ELECTROAUDIOMETRY

In all children in whom normal hearing could not definitely be established by one of the methods described above electroaudiometry has to be performed. Two methods are available, as described below.

Brainstem audiometry (BERA) The electrical response elicited by repeated sound stimuli is recorded by means of electrodes on the forehead, mastoid and neck. The technique requires a quiet child. Infants usually need some sedation, whereas sometimes general anaesthesia may be necessary. Brainstem audiometry is more difficult to interpret in the first years of life as the results are dependent on the maturation of the nervous system.

Electrocochleography (ECoG) With this technique the electrical responses are recorded by a transtympanic electrode on the promontory. ECoG gives more reliable results than BERA as it directly registers cochlear activity. This type of electroaudiometry requires general anaesthesia in all children. It is evident that it cannot be used in patients with a meatal atresia.

TYMPANOMETRY

This gives information about the mobility of the eardrum and the contents of the middle ear (fluid or air). The method is simple, objective and reliable and can be carried out at young age. It can, however, only be used when the external meatus has been developed.

X-ray examination (computerized tomography)

Standard otological X-ray examination in the Schüller and Stenvers position only gives rough information about the mastoid, middle ear and petrous bone. By computerized tomography it is possible to visualize all anatomical structures in much greater detail.

The external meatus and the ossicles can best be visualized in the transverse and the semi-axial plane, the labyrinth in the transversal and the semi-longitudinal plane.

For the preferred plane of investigation of the various structures the reader is referred to the visualization matrix presented in Table 13.3.

Examples of some of the most characteristic findings in craniofacial anomalies are given in Figures 13.1–13.3.

Table 13.3 Preferable planes of CT imaging of the most important anatomical structures in the diagnosis of the congenital anomalies of the ear (de Groot & Huizing (1987), Zonneveld (1987))

Anatomical structure	Radiological planes
External ear canal	Transverse and coronal
Middle ear cavity and ossicles	Transverse and axial
Cochlea	Transverse and semilongitudinal
Oval window	Transverse and semiaxial (or semilongitudinal)
Vestibular labyrinth	Transverse and semilongitudinal
Facial nerve	Transverse and sagittal
Internal auditory meatus	Transverse and coronal

TREATMENT

Our main concern in treating congenital otological malformations is the restoration of hearing. Hearing is essential for speech and language development and also for the intellectual and physical evolution of the child. The cosmetic correction of earlobe deformities is of secondary importance, although the parents of the child often give it priority.

Hearing restoration can be achieved in two different ways: by means of surgery or by fitting a hearing aid. The spectacular successes of microscopic middle ear surgery in otosclerosis and otitis media have induced hope for similar results in congenital ear defects. However, the otological surgeon has to admit that the best (immediate) results in congenital ear anomalies are still obtained by hearing aids. They can almost completely compensate the hearing deficit and they are safe and reliable. From this statement one should not conclude that there is no place for surgery in the treatment of congenital ear disorders. Particularly in patients in whom only one structure of the sound conductive apparatus is affected (occlusion of the ear canal by a bony plate or anomalies of the ossicles) hearing can be considerably improved by surgery. However, in the more complicated cases where both an ear canal and eardrum have to be created and an ossicular defect has to be reconstructed, satisfying results are difficult to obtain. In most cases patient and surgeon will have to be content with a hearing improvement of 20–30 dB. This implies that in many cases a hearing aid remains necessary.

Surgery

As to surgical treatment there are always two questions to be answered: yes or no, and when? The answers depend on a number of factors, that will have to be answered separately in every case. The following should be taken into account:

The type and the degree of hearing loss. Only a conductive hearing loss can be treated by surgery.

Unilateral or bilateral hearing loss. When one ear is functioning normally, the child has no significant hearing problems. Speech development will be unimpaired and consequently there is no immediate indication for surgery. An operation can be carried out at a later stage.

Type and degree of the anomaly. The fewer the number of structures involved, the better the chances for a hearing improvement. The best results are generally obtained in cases with an ossicular discontinuity and a normal functioning ear canal and tympanic membrane. Moderate results can usually be achieved in patients with an atretic ear canal, no eardrum, but a normal ossicular chain.

Age. Age plays a role in several ways. In grown-up children the technical difficulties are usually smaller, the chances for intercurrent infections diminish and the essential aftercare of the newly created ear canal and eardrum is easier.

Hearing aids

Remarkably enough most textbooks and chapters on congenital atresia and middle ear anomalies dwell only superficially on the subject of hearing aids, although the greater percentage of patients have to be equipped with some kind of hearing device. The following types have to be considered.

BEHIND-THE-EAR HEARING AID

This type is most commonly used as it gives sufficient amplification in almost all cases. The only requirement is the presence of an earlobe and a meatus of at least 0.5 cm in length. In cases with an insufficient meatal length one might consider creating a longer canal by surgery. This can successfully be performed in young children.

IN-THE-EAR HEARING AID (CANAL AID)

Amplification is less and, in the majority of children with middle ear malformation, insufficient. Fitting may be technically more difficult when the auricle is abnormal. On the other hand the in-the-ear hearing aid may be advantageous in maintaining and modelling a freshly surgically created ear canal.

BONE CONDUCTION VIBRATOR

This aid has to be applied in all cases of bilateral atresia and severe microtia, when a behind-the-ear apparatus cannot be used. The acoustic quality of this type of bone-conduction hearing aid is inferior to that of air-conduction devices. In addition there is the psychological effect of this less elegant solution to the problem. The otologist might therefore choose to operate earlier in children who are obliged to wear a bone conduction vibrator in order to create an external ear canal.

COCHLEAR IMPLANT

At present a cochlear implant can only be taken into consideration in patients with bilateral total deafness. The results of this newly developed device do not justify its use when usable hearing remnants are present.

BONE ANCHORD HEARING AID

Recently a so-called 'bone anchord hearing aid' has become available. A special titanium screw is subcutaneously implanted into the mastoid bone. The electrical signal from the hearing aid is transmitted to the skin by an external coil which is magnetically kept in place opposite the internal screw. This device is only indicated in cases with normal cochlear en retrocochlear function, i.e. conductive deafness and moderate mixed deafness when an external ear canal is lacking. The experience with this new technique in children is still very scarce.

SURGICAL TECHNIQUE

Reconstruction of the external ear canal

An external meatus is created by resecting the connective tissue from the fissure between the temporomandibular joint and the mastoid and by drilling a canal in the rudimentary mastoid and the squama temporalis. It is advisable to create a canal of at least 7–8 mm diameter to reduce the chances of stenosis during the healing process. The new meatus is then carefully covered by small pieces of split skin. Intensive postoperative care until complete epithelialization of the new ear canal has taken place is essential for a good result.

Reconstruction of the eardrum and the ossicular chain

In minor deformities the middle ear cavity can be identified without difficulty. In major deformities, however, the lateral semicircular canal, cochlea and facial nerve are identified before any attempt at reconstruction is made.

The underdeveloped tympanic cavity is opened as widely as possible and the ossicular chain, the inner ear windows and the Eustachian tube are inspected.

Defects of the malleus and/or incus are corrected using an allogeneic incus (or malleus). Malformations of the stapes are treated by using a non-biological prosthesis. A tympanic membrane is constructed from membranous connective material such as a fascia, pericardium or dura.

The main risks of the operation are facial nerve damage and lesion of the labyrinth with deafness and vestibular impairment. Infection of the created open mastoid cavity may constitute a problem after the operation and require long aftercare. For these reasons surgery of congenital ear anomalies should only be carried out by a limited number of experienced otological surgeons.

CONCLUSIONS

1. In all children with craniofacial anomalies a hearing examination has to be carried out as early as possible.
2. Hearing can be measured at all ages. When subjective methods fail electroaudiometry (brainstem audiometry or electrocochleography) should be performed.
3. The presence of a normal auricle, ear canal and eardrum does not exclude an ossicular anomaly and a 50-dB conductive hearing loss.
4. Deformities of the external and middle ear are common in craniofacial anomalies, whereas inner ear defects are extremely rare.
5. In bilateral congenital hearing loss hearing rehabilitation should start as early as possible to prevent retardation in speech, language and intellectual development. A hearing aid should be fitted before the end of the first year.
6. In bilateral malformation involving all structures (microtia, atresia, middle ear dysfunction) surgery can best be postponed to school age. In children who have to use a bone conduction receiver an external ear canal might be created at an earlier stage.
7. In unilateral malformation involving all structures surgery is usually not indicated. The improvement that can be obtained is usually of no practical significance for the patient since his other ear is hearing normally.
8. In unilateral malformation involving only one structure, i.e. ossicular malformation in an otherwise normal ear, surgery is generally advisable.
9. Otological surgery should precede earlobe correction.

REFERENCES

Bellucci R J 1981 Congenital aural malformation: diagnosis and treatment. Otolaryngologic Clinics of North America 14: 95–124 1981
Cremers C W R J, Hageman M J, Huizing E H 1982 Erfelijke doofheid en slechthorendheid. Bohn, Scheltema, Holkema, Utrecht
de Groot J A M, Huizing E H 1987 Computed tomography of the temporal bone. Acta Otolaryngologica (Stockholm) Suppl 434 pt I

Huizing E H 1980 Frühkindliche Schwerhörigkeit. Ch 44, Band 6. Hals-Nasen-Ohrenheilkunde. Thieme, Stuttgart
Konigsmark B W, Gorlin R J 1976 Genetic and metabolic deafness. Saunders, Philadelphia
Zonneveld F W 1987 Computed tomography of the temporal bone and orbit. Urban and Schwarzenberg, Munich and Baltimore

14. Phonation

A. R. Chancholle

INTRODUCTION

Any craniofacial malformation does not inevitably carry with it a disorder of phonation; however, numerous arguments militate in favour of a systematic investigation.

The phonation organs can be altered by the craniofacial malformation, but rarely at the larynx level. The velopharyngeal and buccolabial groups are often interrupted or modified.

We can distinguish two types of voice: the first is the 'useful' voice, close to the fundamental sound, the result of the laryngeal vibration carried by the expiration, then modulated by the articulation zones (velopharynx, tongue, palate, teeth and lips.)

The second type of voice is the 'social' voice, characteristic of the individual, in conversation and communication with others, which has as its originality and as its quality *the vocal space*. This vocal space is represented by all the hollow structures of the face: oro-nasopharyngeal cavities and facial–paranasal pneumatization. This vocal space is generally modified by the malformation. The patient is dependent on these two parts of phonation: (1) the necessity to be understood when he expresses himself; and (2) sophistication: to handle with ease and harmony the nuances of speech, which naturally presupposes a normal intelligence quotient.

The verbal communication disorder of the malformed child has sometimes a neurological origin, without direct relation to the malformation. There is an important risk of confusing the origin of the disorder and attributing it to the craniofacial malformation. An efficient therapeutic approach becomes feasible only after an accurate diagnosis.

Language, speech and phonation retardation are indiscriminately employed and confused one with another, because confusion persists in the employed terms to designate the verbal communication disorders. To specify the meaning of these terms, their frontiers and their connections, is one of the subjects of the present study. To distinguish them enables us to understand them and to treat them.

DEFINITIONS

First of all it is convenient to define the terms employed. The words and the relations that organize them according to the rules of syntax and grammar, which apply to objects or conceptions, constitute the *language*, that appears in different forms. This depends on each human group which expresses itself in its own proper language. *Verbal communication* is the relation established between two or more persons by the use of words of the same language.

Speech is the group of sounds produced by the pronunciation of the letters. These sounds are called phonemes. The phonemes are the result of voice production: laryngeal emission which is moulded by the articulation, or articulation points (anatomical zone of the pronunciation of the phonemes, for example linguodental). It is a more accurate term than 'pronunciation', for which the same phoneme is variable with the employed languages; this term will not be kept in an anatomophysiological study. Secondly, it is influenced by the naso-oropharyngeal resonance spaces.

Phonation is the function of talking, and the term has a wide meaning including the voice, speech and language. *Orthophony* is the re-education of the phonation taken in a still wider meaning of oral and written expressions. The normal functions are upset by malformation and the injured level concerns one of the phonation circuits.

The phonation circuits

The circuits of language have been described and schematized in multiple and different ways according to the concerned discipline: elaboration of the idea (psychology), codification and verbal realization by the cerebral motor areas (neurology), production of speech (the peripheral effectors concern the different clinical disciplines of the face), sound transmission (physical study of sound vibration), reception of the message from audition to interpretation (return chain with its links — otology, neurology and psychology).

The model has been clearly explained by Paule Aimard (1974): *a peripheral hemicircuit* — the action of talking and hearing (from mouth to ear) — and *a central hemicircuit*: afferent ducts of audition and efferent ducts of phonation, which exclude 'any idea of compartmentalization or of accurate limit of these different steps'.

While using these ideas our scheme will be different and will follow that based on observation of the phonatory function in relation to the age of the subject.

Observation has to begin as early as possible, but cannot totally precede the appearance of the disorder. Treatment has to take place before school age, but in certain cases the child is understood within the family circle and detection is late — after the child has started school.

Observation can anticipate the disorder at the level of the peripheral hemicircuit, as from birth: (1) by the direct observation at birth of the speech structures — larynx, pharynx and all the structures of the naso-buccal cavity; (2) shortly after birth by hearing tests.

Observation cannot always anticipate and can often only diagnose the disorder at the level of the central hemicircuit when it will produce itself. It concerns the interpretation of the heard message and the elaboration of the answer, employing all the possibilities of orthophony. One must be aware of all stages of phonation from birth and be able to observe them.

Verbal communication brings together a subject who talks and a subject who listens and who will answer. These two activities are indissociable and alternated and the phonation disorder will always come within the scope of this duality. Parents ask us if their child, suffering from craniofacial malformation, will talk. The answer will always have to take into account not only the child's own factors of phonation, but also the factors linked to the circle who will listen to him. We can answer the parents when we can reassure them about the normality of the organic speaking structures of the child.

It must not be forgotten that at the opportune moment of the observation the different parameters will appear only successively; dates when the norms are postulated vary from one child to another. Also the child will understand until 6 years of age only the spoken language, with its faults and individual characteristics of the family and social circle where he lives.

For a long time, the investigation relies on a subjective approximation based on numbers that quantify and describe the situation poorly. One factor influencing the examination is the medical examination itself and the child may be ill at ease in the doctor's room.

THE LESIONS AND THEIR FRONTIERS: THE INJURED AREAS

The observation that allows one to say that the phonation will be normal or to predict defects has to focus on all the links of the phonatory circuit:

1. The peripheral hemicircuit:
   (a) auditive — external ear and middle ear
   (b) phonatory — larynx; velopharynx and nasal cavity; buccal cavity
2. The central hemi-circuit: the central nervous system of audition — internal ear, thought, phonation.

It should be possible to distinguish organic lesions from functional lesions.

INVESTIGATION OF THE PERIPHERAL HEMICIRCUIT

The peripheral lesions do not go together with a central lesion, at least in the typical cases. It is also possible to assume that the child will understand and that he will try to express himself, but can be prevented from doing so by a deficient effector.

The direct and prompt observation of these effectors will allow one to diagnose the lesion and to predict the future phonatory disorder. The correct treatment of the lesion, when treatment is possible, will prevent the appearance of the phonation disorders. If the lesion cannot be usefully corrected, it will at least be possible to institute an early palliative re-education.

Peripheral lesions of the ear: hearing disorders

These are the transmission defects in which the osseous conduction is normal. The lesion is situated at the level of the external and/or middle ear. There may be associated lesions, the most frequent example being microtia. The lesions lead to a serious defect only when they are bilateral. By clinical observation we recognize two problems from birth: the surgical reconstruction of the ear, which will be postponed until the age of 10 years; and the reconstruction of the middle ear. This may be possible but should be discussed in unilateral cases. In bilateral cases it is usually attempted.

An early audiogram can be made but the surgical decision on the middle ear is not made until X-rays are possible. A lesion of the peripheral effectors of hearing will never have any repercussion on phonation when the lesion is unilateral and will only rarely have a phonatory repercussion in bilateral lesions, because the integrity of the osseous conduction allows either a surgical correction or a prosthetic appliance. We are thus confident that the child will be able to talk.

Peripheral lesions of phonation: speech disorders

These lesions do not disorganize language but upset speech

emission. The anomalies of the speaking organs can be studied in an analytical way at the level of the labial, lingual, dental and palatal articulation (the larynx is not the seat of malformations compatible with life).

As in the first investigation, we can observe the following malformations:

1. Labial or labioalveolar clefts.
2. Macroglossia: hypotonic tongue that occupies the whole buccal cavity and interposes itself between the gums.
3. Ankyloglossia — very short frenum lingulae inserted at the tip of the tongue, or complete synechia of the ventral surface of the tongue.
4. Anomalies of maxillomandibulary proportions — small mandible.
5. Palatovelar malformations — complete or submucosal cleft, congenital short soft palate.
6. (1) + (5) — labiopalatine clefts (Chancholle 1980, Launay & Borel-Maisonny 1972).

The labial or labioalveolar cleft causes a minor articulatory disorder which disturbs the bilabials. Isolated macroglossia will not disturb phonation, but may upset occlusion or cause sigmatism. Orthodontic treatments and partial glossectomy are usually indicated, later.

Macroglossia with trisomy 21 will not directly affect phonation, since the phonatory disorder is situated at the level of language organization. Early treatment is not indicated, but eventually a partial glossectomy may be helpful. Treatment is delayed until 4 years, when speech can be compared with normal patterns.

Tight ankyloglossia is best corrected surgically as early as possible. Its effect on the maxillo-mandibulodental growth and phonation is significant.

Total cleft palate is easily recognized. Submucous cleft palate, on the other hand, is often unrecognized. The signs are: pellucid, bluish aspect of the median line of the soft palate; bifid uvula (which on the other hand can be isolated and without functional consequence on speech); on inducing the nausea reflex one sees two vertical laterally bulbing on the palate, which are the lateral muscular masses, not fused in the median line.

The palatine cleft blocks the variable compartmentalization of the pharynx and bucconasal resonator. The direct consequence will be open rhinolalia, but we must also consider the repercussion of the cleft on the anatomophysiological group constituted by the velopharynx. Velo-pharyngofacial incompetence is present in isolated palatal cleft. It is increased in cases of cleft lip. A palatal plate used as early as possible will help to normalize lingual function.

Facial diplegia (Möbius' syndrome) will always cause speech disorders owing to the secondary effect of the facial muscles.

INVESTIGATION OF THE CENTRAL HEMICIRCUIT

Lesions of the peripheral hemicircuit of phonation are obvious during early clinical observations. Lesions of the central hemicircuit are very different. The craniofacial malformation suggests a brain abnormality. Early recognition is important lest abnormalities are confused with psychological disturbances later in life. We will here consider:

1. Organic or functional encephalic lesions which can disturb the central hemicircuit of phonation.
2. Immediate or precocious detection and diagnosis.

The central hemicircuit of phonation can be injured: at the auditory level — internal ear and auditory ducts; in the nervous tissue — the efferent ducts of phonation; at the psychological level.

Central auditory lesions

These are: genetic, hereditary; acquired — the most frequent is rubella, which injures the organ of Corti between the seventh and tenth weeks of pregnancy; toxicity — thalidomide or streptomycin; at birth — neonatal hypoxia and prematurity (toxic role of bilirubin).

Diagnosis is made by a systematic investigation of the auditory system as early as possible. The result is expressed in decibels and this gives an idea of the severity of speech disorders to be excepted.

1. The *bad hearer* has a defect inferior to 40 dB, which will cause articulatory disorders. The child will talk, however.
2. The *half deaf*. Here the defect is situated between 40 and 60 dB. Speech and articulation disorders will develop.
3. The *severely half deaf*. The defect is situated between 60 and 85 dB. No spontaneous language develops and sounds such as those from the vowels and to a lesser extent consonants may be heard.
4. *Cophosis* — the defect is over 85 dB. The voice is altered in all its characters, and speech in all its articulatory forms. Mutism may develop owing to incomprehension and the impossibility of spontaneous expression.

The re-education of these two last forms must be undertaken as early as possible. The audiometric investigation done during the first days of life allows an early diagnosis.

The central lesions of the phonation

The central effectors of phonation can be injured at three

different levels: (1) cortical and subcortical — aphasia; (2) the whole effector duct — cerebral motor infirmity (CMI), or cerebral palsy; (3) global attack — encephalopathies.

1. Here *aphasia* develops after the constitution of language. The only type to be considered as a true aphasia does not concern the newborn. The congenital aphasia (Broadbent–Cohen) or 'audimutité' of De Ajuriaguerra or verbal surdity of Wild is related to the actual structure of the personality and is caused by psychological disorders: they do not concern this group.

2. Cerebral motor infirmity (CMI) develops during pregnancy, at birth or before talking and speech establishment. It does not seriously affect intelligence and can be treated. Corticosubcortical lesions upset language elaboration. Dystonia and dyspraxia of the articulatory muscles disturb speech. Eighty per cent of CMI disorders present abnormalities of phonation and require orthophonic treatment. Diagnosis, before speech develops, is made while observing peripheral motor disorders such as infantile hemiplegia: clumsiness of a hemibody, elbow or wrist flexion, hyperextension of the neck or knee. Spastic palsy (Little) often affects the voice articulation.

These signs are present during the neonatal period and if the parents and the doctor have not been alerted by an abnormal pregnancy or by an obstetrical incident, the diagnosis will be difficult. The tests for the general capacity of the child are not satisfactory before the age of 2 years. The sucking of the child gives some idea of movements.

An instrument for measuring sucking (Kron 1970) shows the curve of rhythm, frequency and regularity of the pressure variations in the feeding-bottle. The test may be a helpful guide to the development of speech. This was applied by Kron for the detection of minimal brain dysfunction. We are at present trying to establish more precisely the correlation of sucking with the quality of later phonation.

3. Encephalopathy: the lesion concerns the encephalic group attacked during pregnancy, at birth or during the first months of life. The lesion is diffuse and is related to the motor lesions of the CMI and major intelligence disorders. The seriousness of the lesions is also due to their bilaterality, which affects auditory function, the articulatory sphere and the elaboration areas of language. The phonation disorder in these cases is complete and major.

Phonation and thought disorders: the disorders of language

The central hemicircuit of phonation can be organically normal. No physical lesion (haemorrhage, infection, toxicosis) of the auditive ducts or of the effector ducts is present, but speech is poor or absent. At birth, only an organic lesion can be diagnosed but the cerebral function cannot be assessed. There is often an indistinct borderline between the two.

The paediatric psychiatrist will be able to diagnose some problems clinically: mental retardation; endogenous — a very low level of intelligence is present; exogenous chromosomal anomalies or disorders of cerebral metabolism; the infantile psychoses, of which autism is seen earliest.

A second group is more difficult to diagnose: the dysphasias; retarded speech or auditory mutism, familial defects, psycho-affective deficiencies due to hospitalization, poorly developed language (in the family), but one must be able to observe abnormalities and be aware of milestones in development.

GROWTH OF NORMAL PHONATION: CHRONOLOGICAL EVOLUTION OF GESTURAL AND PHONIC SIGNS

The growth of speech is only one aspect of the general growth and comes within the scope of a psychomotor whole. It is therefore necessary to observe the development of the phonemes, of words, of phrases and their general meaning. The normal crying sound and pattern should be studied.

At about 1–2 months, suction movements occur. Sudden loss of contact of the tongue with the palate may be important. At about 2–3 until 4 months, chattering and babbling 'a', then 'r', appear. The sound is formed in the back of the throat by the tongue.

With chatter, the child explores all the possibilities of emitted sound: Jakobson says 'all the imaginable sounds' and Aimard (1974) states: 'he constitutes himself a stock of ulterior sonorous forms'. During the same period, he plays with his fingers (3 months), then with his feet (6 months). The chatter leads to an answer from the parents: at first it is a non-intentional articulatory exchange, leading slowly to full speech. From 3.5 months to 4.5 months modifications of articulation appear.

The dental crisis (Tronchere 1978)

The gingival submucosal space is then the seat of intense activity. The beginning of dental emergence modifies the gingival space ('the child doubles his gums') and exacerbates their sensibility. Salivation becomes intense. The sensible and sensorial attention of the child is drawn forwards where the lingual motor activity is now transferred. The tongue searches out the place that hurts: — Italian people say: 'la lingua batte dove il dente duole'. At this moment, the articulation will anteriorize and it is a normal and primitive development. To say that a child posteriorizes his tongue because he has a palatine fissure is to misjudge the fundamental biology of the species. The only problem that exists for the child who has a total cleft is irregular tongue movement and location, due to the cleft anatomy, which can disturb the speech. When lingual anteriorization has succeeded, the bilabials ('p', 'b' and 'm') appear around 15–20 days after the first gingivodental modifications. Anteriorization will then modify the vowel emission; 'a' and 'e' are posterior, while 'eu' and 'on' are anterior.

During this period, the child begins to lie prone and this assists lingual anteriorization. At the same time, the tonic neck reflex in extension becomes established and this indicates that before this period the child must be laid on his back or on his side. From 6 to 9 months the dentals 't', 'd' and 'n' appear, associated with a posterior vowel 'a'. The lingual movement adapts to the change of position. This corresponds to the upper gingival distension and to teething.

Occasionally 'papa' is formed but it is not intentional, because this is the period of the reduplication: 'ta ta ta . . . ' etc. During the same period, the child begins to sit and starts to suck its thumb. Sounds are of no significance as they are part of a sensorimotor game, but the child has begun to communicate already.

SIGNS OF COMPREHENSION: THE INTENTION TO COMMUNICATE

At about 11 months the child starts to ask for help, tries to catch objects, to climb and to crawl. Slowly his movements have a purpose (lifting his leg on getting into a bath). This is an expression of intention, appearing about 12–13 months of age. A gesture will be answered in the same way at about 14 months. This is what Marcel Cohen (in Tronchere 1978) calls 'gesture-communication' (gestcom) and when the gesture is underlined by a noise, 'groaning-communication' (grocom). It is usually a call for help that indicates the absolute necessity for a quick reaction of the environment. The attention and confidence of the child would otherwise be in danger.

During this period, intonation will precede the word. The reproduction of the intonation at about 10–13 months, then the repetition of intonation, is the first sign of a syntaxed language: affirmation, demand, surprise. This constitutes an amazing performance, combining audition, memory and vocal skill.

During this period, individual differences appear. From 14 to 20 months, the child emits from three to several syllables in a speech lasting several minutes. One must judge the articulatory perfection with lenience as articulatory error has no pathological significance. This period is that of immediate repetition (echolalia), for practising better articulation. It will quickly lead to the emission of real phrases.

The phrase

Long before the grammatically organized phrase develops the gestural and linguistic expression of the child can be seen as 'phrase'.

LOCUTIVE OR COMPOSITE PHRASE

Guiraud says that a word employed with a particular intonation can have a precise meaning and deserves therefore the term 'locutive phrase'. This frequent and current experience of the adult is different in the child. A gesture is associated with a noise or a word and when grouped together are seen as a will of the child to express himself. This is why we prefer the term 'composite phrase' (Tronchere 1978).

The intonation at 18 months will be reduced but more active than during the period 10–12 months and will improve until 24–30 months of age. Gesture will more or less persist (according to the character) but words will be more often used so that the composite phrase will quickly become a real spoken phrase between 18 and 21 months.

Sudden quantitative changes will appear: acquisition of new words (stock triples at about 18 months) and will very clearly increase from 24 to 26 months and again from 36 to 39 months.

PREDICATIVE PHRASE

The subject is the 'predicate': either an attribute with a verb of state, or a complement with a verb of action. Syntax, without directed teaching, will develop at 24 months. The first syntactic form is the imperative, no doubt because the child requires help. The indicative appears at about 28–30 months, at the same time as articles ('the' and 'a'). Then very quickly intonation, changed in the affirmative phrase, will give way to the interrogative form. During this same period manual skills will improve.

The child and time

When the child is about 30 months old, he knows that the present is different from vague past and future. Everything that is done is 'yesterday' and everything that will be done is 'tomorrow'. Temporal comparison develops at about 31 or 32 months.

The last rules: perfection

Language is formed at $2\frac{1}{2}$ years and the 'speech bath' is very important. The desire to talk and to talk quickly means articulatory errors will appear. Reduction to two syllables (e.g. 'cine' for 'cinema') has no pathological significance.

During the second year, words correspond to an

abstract significance that can be employed by the child by choice: the term 'cluck-cluck', which is applied to a bird, will be immediately rejected for a rabbit (Tronchere 1978). Here it is necessary to understand that the acquisition of syntactic forms is not conscious. As Jakobson notes 'the most fascinating, most amazing phenomenon in linguistics is the fact that there is a very logical, very complex system, but that this system stays unconscious for the talking subject'. The logic of the syntax necessarily allows multiple exceptions: for example (in French) the verb 'aller' will give: 'j'allais, je vais, j'irai', and these exceptions are difficult for the logic present in the child's brain. The child will therefore come up against exceptions that will constitute spontaneous errors. He has been told 'voulu' (from 'vouloir') and 'couru' (from 'courir') and he will say 'peindu' (from 'peindre') instead of 'peint'. This is normal and the period of adaptative syntactic irregularities will last from 3 to 4 years. Its persistence later is a sign of a defect.

The variations

The appearance date of acquisitions made before 6–10 months can vary by about 15 days. The appearance date of acquisitions after 10 months and until 2 years can vary by 3–4 months. Girls are more precocious and the child's character plays an important role.

The prognosis of a newborn's phonation in the presence of a craniofacial malformation can be seen as facial malformations attacking the peripheral hemicircuit of phonation, or as cerebral lesions attacking organically the central hemicircuit of phonation. If a child presents no organic sign of a lesion in the phonatory circuit, the growth of the phonation must be followed clinically.

We ask the parents to establish a 'phonation calendar', writing down in an exercise book:

1. Stages of speech: posterior articulation — 'a', 'r'; lingual anteriorization — bilabials and dentals; antero-posterior swinging of the lingual play — association of dentals to a posterior vowel 'a'; appearance of the intonation and appearance of the composite phrase.
2. Appreciation of comprehension: gestcom and grocom.
3. Gestures involving the head, the upper and lower limbs and the orientation of the body in space, e.g. steps, crawling, walking and balance.

This observation can be made by any parent, because a mother is always attentive. A mother who is patiently educated by a doctor who takes his time, and who is persuaded of the use of what he demands, understands and realizes the value of a comprehension calendar.

It can be an indispensable tool, either to alert the doctor about some anomaly, or as the basis of the observations of the speech therapist.

Speech evaluation can be made at any time as an indication of speech development. Parents of children suffering from clefts are contacted as soon as possible after birth and the observations, re-education and performance of the parent–child–surgeon–speech therapist team are unlimited.

REFERENCES

Aimard P 1974 L'enfant et son language, Simep-Editions, France
Chancholle A R 1980 Anatomie et physiologie pathologiques de la fente palatine; l'incompetence velo-pharyngo-faciale. Annales de Chirurgie Plastique 25: 205–211
Guiraud P. La syntaxe du Français. PUF
Kron R E 1970 In Bosma J F (ed) Second symposium on oral sensation and perception. Thomas, Springfield, Ill. pp 362–374
Launay C, Borel-Maisonny S 1972 Les troubles du language, de la parole et de la voix chez l'enfant. Masson, Paris
Tronchere J 1978 L'enfant qui va parler, collection d'orthophonie. Masson, Paris

15. Radiology

L. Picard, P. Forlodou, C. Moret, S. Bracard

INTRODUCTION

The role of the radiologist in cranio-orbitofacial malformations is to provide a precise diagnosis of the malformative lesions as well as their eventual repercussions on neighbouring structures. This requires a study of the skeletal elements of the base of the skull, the cranial vault and the surrounding soft tissues. In addition the eventual consequences of the malformations on underlying organs (brain, eyes, etc.) must be appreciated, as well as the possibility of associated malformations.

The so-called 'simple' malformations involving purely skeletal structural or geometric anomalies can be opposed to the 'complex' malformations. The former involve the structure of a bone or alterations in the organization of the different bones which make up the skull. In the latter major cranial, orbital, facial and encephalic malformations are included as, for example, in holoprosencephaly or fronto-ethmoidonasal encephaloceles.

Even though it has long been common knowledge, repercussions on the vascular system are rare. It is only in the presence of precise clinical and paraclinical data that a diagnosis aimed at finding such vascular malformations will be indicated.

RADIOLOGICAL TECHNIQUES

An early diagnosis of cranio-orbitofacial malformations should be established to allow surgery to be performed before its consequences on the brain are irreversible. Several radiological methods are available: standard radiography, computerized tomography (CT scan) magnetic resonance imaging (MRI) and various types of angiography. Before considering each of these individually, a discussion of some of the general considerations pertaining to neuroradiology and the newborn, premature and older child is in order.

Technical variations depending on the child's age

THE NEWBORN AND THE PREMATURE PATIENT

The early diagnosis of craniosynostosis is most important in this age group. The tendency at this time is to operate on these infants as early as is possible. In general, these newborn and premature infants are kept in incubators. Under normal circumstances, the necessary complementary investigations tend to be contraindicated. However, experience has shown that there are no major risks if these newborns are removed from their incubators for a short time, as long as they remain correctly wrapped. If needed, an infrared lamp can be used to assure that a warm enough room temperature is maintained.

Various solutions are available for keeping the child immobilized and properly positioned. These depend on the child and the examination to be performed. Manual positioning is used most often for standard roentgenograms; however, frames (Sauvegrain) can be of use. It is noteworthy that many neuroradiologists rely on more or less 'home-made' equipment for immobilizing paediatric patients. CT scanography usually requires prolonged immobilization. Some patients respond positively to 'forced feeding', whereas others require sedation (diazepam given rectally) or in the most extreme cases general anaesthesia.

The plasticity of the craniofacial complex in the very young child should be underlined. It is responsible for the notable positional deformations found on examination of the base and vault of the skull. These deformations occur when the position of the head is not regularly modified by health care personnel during the day. These positional deformities must be included in the possible differential diagnosis of cranio-orbitofacial dysmorphism (Fig. 15.1).

OLDER CHILDREN

In these patients, the problems created by these investigations are more often psychological than organic. In fact,

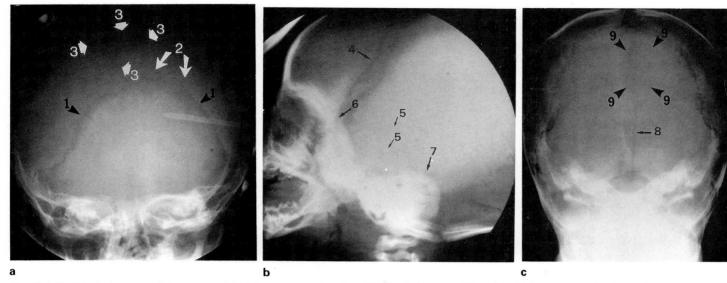

a   b   c

Fig. 15.1 Radiological aspects of the sutures: (a) high anteroposterior view. The lomboid suture (1), amid which many wormian bones (2) are distinguished, is seen. The edges of the bregmatic fontanelle (3) are fuzzy; (b) lateral view. The edges of the coronal suture (4) are completely free of identations. The two squamous sutures (5) appear narrower than the coronal suture. Because of their superposition the anterolateral (pterion) (6) and the posterolateral (asterion) (7) fontanelles are difficult to distinguish; (c) frontal-suboccipital (anteroposterior) view. The metopic suture (8) appears fine and linear. Its projection is often paramedial. The edges of the posterior fontanelles (9) are uniformly fuzzy.

because of the relative frequency of psychomotor retardation, which is sometimes associated with slight debility, it is often impossible to achieve the immobilization required in these children. Often these problems can be aggravated by the family. Parents do not always understand the need for numerous preoperative radiological investigations. If persuasion and prescription of minor sedatives are ineffective in these patients, general anaesthesia is indicated. It should be noted that in another context this anaesthesia would certainly not be indicated at this age.

Quantimetric problems

In the infant and young child bone structures are small and quite thin. This requires short exposure time and relatively high amperage. Kilovoltage should be as low as possible (approximately 50 kV).

In the case of repeated comparative examinations the dose of radiation secondary to the different investigations must be precisely taken into account. A diagnostic strategy based on protocols which minimize irradiation should be established. Radiation can be further reduced using the classic means of protection (adequate filters, efficient collimation, protection of the more sensitive tissues: eye lens, gonads, epiphysis).

Examination techniques

Diagnosis of cranio-orbitofacial malformations requires standard radiography and scanography. Teleroentgenography, which increases the amount of radiation, has limited indications. These are given in more detail in the section dealing with this technique. Xeroradiography, which also requires a high dose of radiation for the information it provides, is practised less and less.

The use of radioisotopes, which may prove useful, is not systematic in the diagnosis of craniosynostosis. Radioisotopic scintigraphy indicates the metabolic activity of the sutures. In cases where standard radiography fails to confirm craniosynostosis, radioisotopic investigations can show the hyperactivity of the suture or the sutures. This hyperactivity signals the evolution towards premature fusion. This was previously investigated by Montaut & Stricker (1977) and was recently confirmed by Tait et al (1979).

Although it is relatively recent, there is no doubt that MR imaging will be the method of choice in the radiological diagnosis of these malformations in the near future. This method has the major advantage of producing the three fundamental views required for three-dimensional reconstruction. It does not rely on ionizing radiation and it shows the relation between the surrounding soft tissues and the bone structures remarkably.

MR imaging aside, the diagnostic work-up for craniofacial malformations must include clinical photographs, standard roentgenograms and CT scan. Cerebral angiography is only indicated in precise clinical situations.

DIAGNOSTIC PROTOCOL

Standard roentgenograms

The interest of teleroentgenograms, which provide bone images without magnification, allowing precise craniometry, has already been indicated. Standard roentgenograms include the five usual views: the high anteroposterior view shows the sutures of the cranial vault; the two lateral views show the bregmatic suture; the frontal suboccipital view shows the lambdoid suture and the foramen magnum; Hirtz's (axial) view shows the metopic suture.

Because craniosynostoses are often associated with facial and orbital malformations, Blondeau and Water's view is often associated. With the advent of CT scan Hartmann's view of the optic canals has just about ceased to be of interest. An orthopantomogram is necessary but is all but impossible to perform in the young child or infant.

CT scan

CT scan performed without injection of contrast using axial and frontal views allows the study of the bone structures of the cranial vault, base, the face, the orbits, the brain and the extracranial soft tissues. Once the fundamental axial and frontal sections have been made, reconstruction along a medial sagittal or paramedial plane is possible. Three-dimensional reconstruction is also possible. Reconstruction using scanography brings out the details of anatomical structures which often go unnoticed on standard roetgenograms. It also helps the surgeon to plan his surgical strategy and it allows a precise appreciation of the benefits of surgery.

Pneumoencephalography and venticulography have been definitely replaced by CT scan. The need for an intravenously or intrathecally injected contrast substance should be determined. Intravenously injected contrast substance is used for demonstrating lesions of the blood–brain barriers and for visualizing abnormal blood vessels, be they venous or certain arterial ectasias. The systemic indication for intravenously injecting a contrast substance in the study of craniofacial malformations is of little use.

As for the intrathecal injection of a contrast substance, whether by a lumbar or lateral cervical approach, we also feel that it has little or no use. It allows a more detailed study of the subarachnoid spaces as well as their contents. Finally, it should be noted that the intrathecal injection of a contrast substance is not without risk and some cases of blindness attributable to it have been reported (Cabanis et al 1986).

Cerebral angiography

Its indication is exceptional. It should only be retained if there is doubt due to clinical manifestations or an abnormal CT scan indicating the existence of vascular anomalies.

When practised it shows the indirect signs which are secondary to the malformation analysed. Ventricular dilation is translated by an unwinding aspect of the pericallosal arteries as well as straightening of the internal cerebral vein. Stretching of the intracavernous carotid as well as the deformation of the ophthalmic arteries can be appreciated at the base of the skull and the orbits.

Angiography is sometimes indicated for studying the cervical vessels and certain branches of the external carotids. These are often required for preparing the vascularized flaps used for surgical repair of certain facial malformations.

RESULTS

Normal radiological semeiology (Harwood-Nash & Fitz 1976, Hassan 1982, Taveras & Wood 1977, Virapongse et al 1985a)

Semeiological analysis includes: the sutures and synchondroses; the fontanelles; the cranial vault (calvaria); the cranial base and the facial skeleton.

SUTURES AND SYNCHONDROSES

The sutures (Hassan 1982)

The skull of the child presents two kinds of permanent sutures. The fontanelles and accessory sutures are often attached to these. The main permanent sutures are the coronal, sagittal, lambdoid and metopic sutures. The mendosal, the parieto-occipital mastoid, the frontoethmoidal and the zygomatic sutures are added to these main sutures.

The accessory sutures are not constant. Some are rather rare: these include the accessory parietal and occipital sutures. Wormian bones — small ossicles located mainly in the lambdoid suture — are a relatively common finding (Fig. 15.1).

Radiologically the normal suture in the newborn appears as a darkened zone with fuzzy edges lacking interdigitations. Their width varies from 2 to 12 mm. In the older child interdigitations appear. They are located on the outer table. The bone which borders them on each side has a denser aspect. The inner table is seen as a fine line and may be mistaken for a fracture. Some are quite visible, including the squamous and coronal sutures seen on a lateral view or the lambdoid sutures and the metopic suture, when present. The sagittal suture, on the contrary, is not visible.

All the sutures are seen on CT scan sections. They are bevelled, which is their classic aspect. They are seen as an interruption between two bones (Fig. 15.2).

The synchondroses (Cabanis et al 1986, Montaut & Stricker 1977, Tait et al 1979)

The synchondroses are of cartilaginous origin. They are unossified zones which separate the bones of the base of

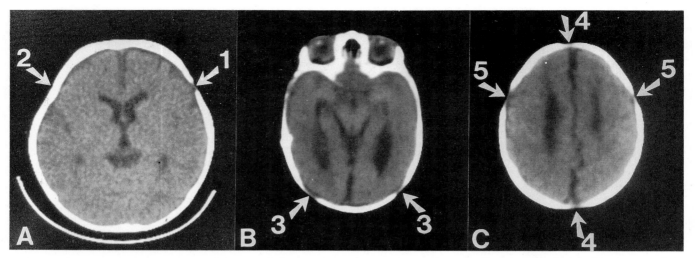

Fig. 15.2 CT scan aspect of the sutures: (a) 19-month-old infant. The coronal suture is evolving towards fusion. On the left side, the coronal suture (1) is still visible with its bevelled aspect, which is classic in the newborn. A veritable interruption between the frontal and parietal bones exists. On the contrary, on the right the evolution of this suture (2) is more advanced and is no longer visible; (b) lamboid suture (3); (c) sagittal (4) and coronal (5) sutures.

the skull from each other and attach some bones of the base to the cranial vault (Fig. 15.3). They are particularly common in the occipital region. Ordinarily they evolve towards ossification before adult life.

The spheno-occipital synchondrosis is visible in the newborn and the child. It usually disappears at the age of 19–20 years old. Its persistence, however, is not pathological.

On the other hand, the intersphenoidal synchondrosis

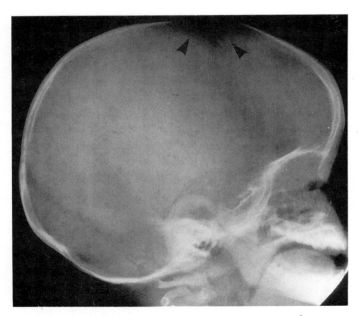

Fig. 15.3 The bregmatic fontanelle seen on a standard lateral view of a newborn. The edges of this fontanelle (arrows) appear fuzzy and unindented. The remaining fontanelles have already closed.

is normally only visible during the neonatal period. It is rapidly replaced by a dense line which subsequently disappears.

THE FONTANELLES

The fontanelles, or soft spots, are the large membranous areas found between the cranial vault bones of the newborn (Figs. 15.1, 15.4). There are six fontanelles: two are unpaired and medial whereas there are two pairs of symmetrical lateral fontanelles.

The largest of these is the anterior or bregmatic fontanelle. It is located at the junction of the coronal and sagittal sutures at the point where the two parietal bones and the two frontal bones meet. It is the last to ossify, doing so during the third year.

The posterior or lambdoid fontanelle is located on the posterior portion of the medial line. It has the shape of a small triangle and is found at the meeting point of the parietal bones and the occipital bone.

The lateral fontanelles are smaller and include the anterolateral fontanelle or pterion and the posterolateral fontanelle or asterion. The former is located at the meeting point of the frontal, parietal and temporal bones, and the greater wing of the sphenoid bone; the latter is located at the meeting point of the occipital bone and the mastoid portion of the temporal bone.

Other less constant accessory fontanelles have also been described. Among these is Gerdy's fontanelle, which occasionally occurs in the sagittal suture between the parietal bones. On standard roentgenograms and CT scan sections, the fontanelles appear as defects in the cranial vault. In the newborn they are seen quite clearly.

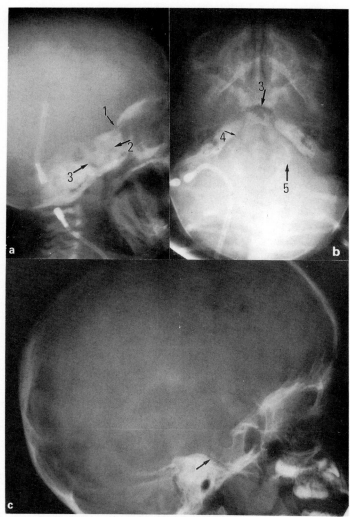

Fig. 15.4 Radiological aspects of several synchondrosis: (a) standard lateral view and Hirtz's axial view (b) of a newborn's skull. (1) Sphenoethmoidal synchondrosis, (2) intersphenoidal synchondrosis, (3) spheno-occipital synchondrosis, (4) anterior occipital synchondrosis, (5) posterior occipital synchondrosis; (c) standard lateral view of a 1-year-old infant's skull. The sphenoethmoidal and intersphenoidal synchondrosis have disappeared. Persistence of the spheno-occipital synchondrosis is shown by the arrow.

THE CRANIAL VAULT

This is made up of several flat bones. They include the frontal and two parietal bones, the temporal squama and the occipital squama. Several elements are seen on the vault, including vascular markings, orifices and convolutional impressions (digital impressions). Vascular markings indicate the presence of the venous sinuses of the dura mater, the emissary veins and the meningeal blood vessels.

The venous sinuses of the dura mater mark the inner table of the cranial vault. They are easily distinguished after 3 years of life. Their depth can vary in a given child. The most notable of these is the transverse (occipital) sinus of the dura mater. It extends from the occipital squama to the temporal squama. Its different parts are easily iden-

tified. It should be noted that the absence of sinus markings does not necessarily mean that there is agenesis of this sinus (Harwood-Nash & Fitz 1976). This sinus is visible in lateral view and frontal suboccipital views. The markings of the sagittal sinus are visible in an anterioposterior view. It terminates distally at the torcular Herophili (internal occipital protuberance) or in one of the two portions of the transverse sinus.

The diploic veins are readily visible in the small child. They usually disappear during growth. Classically, they are known as Breschet's veins. They are mostly found in the anterior frontoparietal region. On scintigraphs they have a tortuous and dark appearance, resembling a vermiculous network.

The emissary veins unite the intracranial sinuses with the external veins. They are most often located behind the mastoid process. Depending on the view they appear either as a defect or as tortuous, winding vessels.

The meningeal arteries are usually not visible in subjects younger than 12 years old. There are major variations in their distribution and location as well as in the importance of their markings on the inner table of the vault.

Convolutional impressions are only visible on standard roentgenograms (Fig. 15.5). They are mainly seen anteriorly on the frontal and parietal bones. Normally they are not very intense and appear as rounded clear zones grouped together. They are usually only visible between 18 months and 5 years. They indicate the intracranial pressure, in other words the normal growth of the brain. If intracranial hypertension is present these impressions are intensified ('beaten silver' appearance) and they can appear over the entire cranial vault. However, if isolated their radiological sign is not of value. On the other hand, if convolutional impressions are absent after 1 year, the diagnosis of insufficient brain growth, which bears a poor prognosis, may be made.

The fissures of the cranial vault extend from sutures and are free of interdigitations. They are distinguishable from fractures by their slightly wider size. They are present in the newborn and disappear within a month.

THE BASE OF THE SKULL AND THE ORBITS (Tessier 1971, Virapongse et al 1985a,b)

The sphenoid bone

The sphenoid bone represents the 'keystone' of the architecture of the base of the skull. This medial bone is normally perfectly symmetrical. This symmetry is such that any asymmetry in the shape or form of its different parts has major semeiological implications. These implications are only valid in the event that the axial and frontal CT scan sections have themselves been perfectly oriented (Fig. 15.6).

The lesser wings of the sphenoid extend laterally from

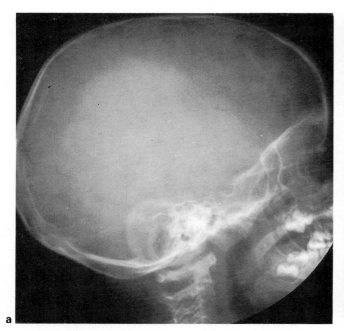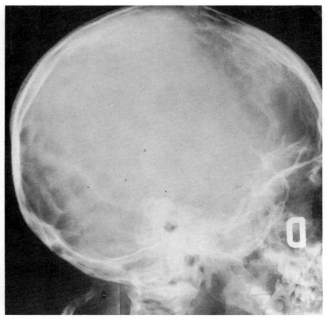

a   b

Fig. 15.5 Convolutional impressions: (a) normal aspect. The impressions appear as greyish areas having a rounded form. They are predominantly located at the frontal and the parieto-occipital regions; (b) pathological aspect. Intracranial hypertension with craniosynostosis. There is a notable increase (beaten silver appearence) in the frontal as well as the parieto-occipital regions.

the superior and anterior portions of the sphenoid to form the upper margin of the superior orbital fissures. At the same time, they contribute to the formation of the optic canal.

The optic canals are symmetrical and form an angle of 25° ± 5° with the sagittal plane (Fig. 15.7). Since they contain the optic nerve and the ophthalmic artery their measurement is important. Their mean diameter is 4 mm in the newborn, 5 mm in the 6-month-old infant to reach a maximum of 6–7 mm in the 6-year-old. Analysis of the optic canal is no longer performed using standard radiography. Axial and frontal CT scan sections ensure precise measurement. In the presence of multiple malformations, enlargement of one or both of the optic canals indicates bone dysplasia, which is usually associated with or secondary to the malformation rather than to a tumoral process.

The morphology of the sella turcica is often variable. This variability depends on the degree of ossification of the elements which limit the sella turcica. These include the sphenoidal planum, the optic groove, the tuberculum sellae, the sellar floor, the dorsum sellae and the posterior clinoids. The varying depth of the chiasmatic groove explains the classic aspect of omega (ω) seen in the child on the lateral view (Fig. 15.8).

The greater wings of the sphenoid contribute to the formation of the lower margin of the superior orbital fissure and the greater part of the posterolateral walls of the orbit, as well as the apex and the floor of the middle cerebral fossa. It is, in fact, the role of the sphenoid as the 'keystone' of the base of the skull which explains the deformities and asymmetry noted during malformative processes with repercussions on the entire skull base. On lateral view the overall morphology can be appreciated using Welcker's sphenoidal angle (normal basal angle). This angle is formed by drawing a line from the nasion to the centre of the sella turcica and joining it to a line drawn on the plane extending from the anterior lip of the foramen magnum to the tuberculum sellae. Its normal value is about 130°.

The orbits

Analysis of the orbital cavities must be done to establish the function of their walls, contents and morphology; this includes dimensional as well as volume variants (Cabanis et al 1986, Tessier 1971). In general the roof of the orbits is formed anteriorly by the orbital plate of the frontal bone. The lateral wall is made up of the zygomatic bone and the greater sphenoidal wing. The medial wall includes the orbital process of the frontal bone, the lacrimal bone, the orbital process of the palatine and the inferior part of the maxilla.

Despite their complexity, the contents (eyeball, optic nerve, vascular structures, muscles, fat tissue and lacrimal gland) can readily be analysed using CT scan or MR imaging. This is because of the large variations in density and contrast of these structures compared to the

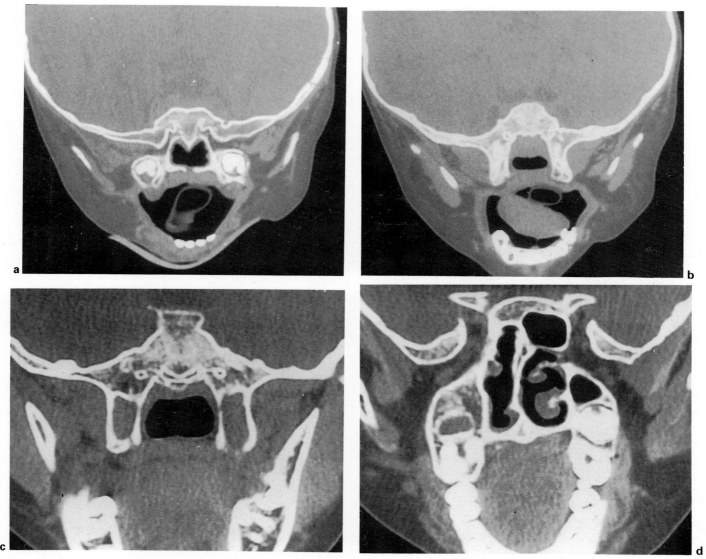

Fig. 15.6 CT scan of the sphenoid bone (frontal view): (a, b) 1-year-old child. The sphenoidal wings and the pterygoid processes are perfectly symmetrical. The presence of perfectly symmetrical muscular masses as well as connective and fatty tissue compartments should be underlined; (c) 7-year-old child, normal symmetrical development. This is appreciated at the pterygoid processes and the two foramen rotundum; (d) 7-year-old child. The harmony of the development explains the normal aspect of the sphenomaxillary fissures. The asymmetry of the sphenoidal sinus is a normal anatomic variant.

orbital fat. The morphological aspect is important and, for example, conditions the differential diagnosis between exorbitism and exophthalmos.

Several indices have been proposed for appreciating the presence and the importance of exophthalmos. Most often the exophthalmic index (also known as the 'oculo-orbital' index) is used. This index is calculated by tracing the lateral bicanthal line and then tracing a line perpendicular to it, passing through the most anterior point of each eyeball. The distance separating the most anterior point of the eye from this lateral bicanthal line is divided by the greatest anteroposterior distance of the corresponding

eyeball. The index is normally between 0.60 and 0.75. Above the latter value exophthalmos can be affirmed. The first degree of exophthalmos is between 0.75 and 1.0. The second degree is around 1.0 and the third degree is at values considerably more than 1.0 (Fig. 15.9).

Pathological radiological semeiology (Braun & Tournade 1982, Cabanis et al 1986, Faerber & Swartz 1985, Fields et al 1978, Montaut & Stricker 1977, Tessier 1971)

Following clinical examination, radiology confirms

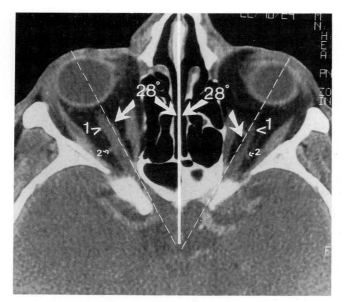

Fig. 15.7 Axial CT scan section of the optic canal: normal aspect. The angle formed by the axis of the optic canals with the sagittal plane equals 28° on both sides. The optic nerves (1) as well as the ophthalmic arteries (2) are readily seen.

craniofacial dysmorphism. It allows a study of the sutures of the cranial vault, the base of the skull and its components, the orbits and the face.

THE SUTURES

Regardless of the type of craniosynostosis and its degree of tolerance, the aspect of the synostosis is characteristic. On standard roetgenograms it is indicated by a loss of its physiological indentations. This loss can be complete or partial and it is predominant on the outer table of the

cranial vault. At times condensation of the suture edges may be associated. This may provoke a false impression of widening, on the one hand, or thinning with bony bridges uniting the suture's edges, on the other.

CT scan shows only one element: the complete or partial disappearance of the suture's normal aspect. In order to see this anomaly CT scan sections must be made in a plane perpendicular to the involved suture.

The major contribution of three-dimensional imaging (three-dimensional reconstruction) has been the possibility of reproducing an exact image of the 'dry pathological bone'. These precise images can be made without taking multiple views. Because of the advantages of three-dimensional imaging it is possible to turn the image and therefore a better appreciation of the deformation as well as the strategies to correct it can be obtained.

THE CRANIAL VAULT

This presents considerable alterations. These include the presence of thinned zones which alternate with thickened zones. The convolutional impressions which are, at times, physiological become pathological if they are diffuse and intense. On standard roetgenograms they are characterized by their clear and round appearance, separated by opaque lines (Fig. 15.10a). On CT scan sections they appear on their inner table of the cranial vault as a thinned zone presenting an endocranial concavity. These zones are separated by crests which correspond to the opaque zones seen on standard roentgenograms.

THE BASE OF THE SKULL (Virapongse et al 1985a,b)

The analysis and appreciation of the deformities is performed using the three planes of space. Each plane

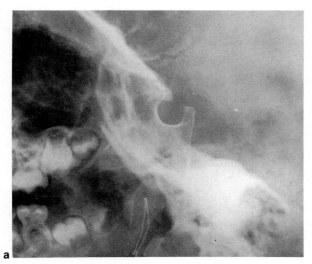
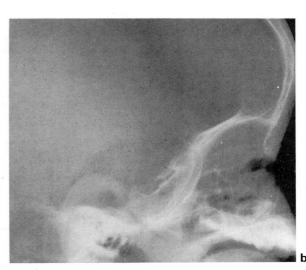

Fig. 15.8 Sella turcica. The classic aspect of the sella turcica (a) can be compared to the less classic denomination of ω seen in normal infant (b). This is due to the depth of the optic groove.

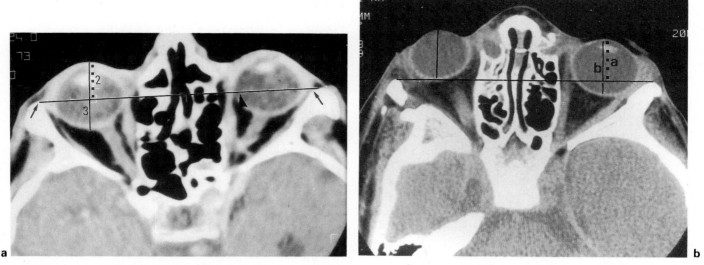

Fig. 15.9 Exophthalmic index: (a) normal aspect. The ratio between the length of the perpendicular drawn (2) from the most anterior point of the eyeball to the bicanthal lateral line (arrows) and the anteroposterior dimension of the corresponding eyeball (3) equals 0.60; (b) pathological aspect. True asymmetrical exophthalmos predominating on the right. On the right, both distances are equal. The exophthalmic index therefore equals 1, which corresponds to second-degree exophthalmos. The entire eyeball is projected in front of the lateral bicanthal line. On the left, a/b = 19/20 = 0.95. This corresponds to first-degree exophthalmos.

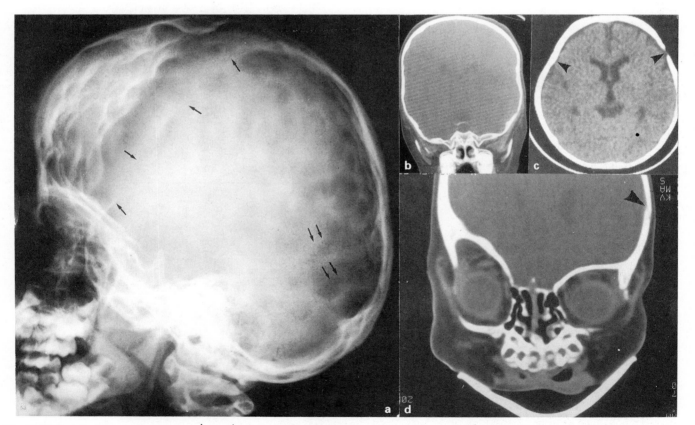

Fig. 15.10 Radiological aspect of synostosis: (a) brachycephaly. The coronal suture has completely disappeared. Its theoretical location is marked by a slight condensation (single arrows). Several deepened convolutional impressions, especially at the frontal region, can be noted. The parieto-occipital sutures (double arrows) are normal; (b) turricephaly (turret head). All the sutures on this frontal section have completely disappeared; (c) trigonocephaly, axial CT scan section, asymmetrical synostosis. The coronal suture is clearly visible on the left but has completely disappeared on the right side (arrows); (d) plagiocephaly, frontal CT scan section. In this synostosis, which is by definition asymmetrical, the left coronal suture (arrow) is visible and is normally oblique. On the right, the suture has disappeared and the cranial vault is thickened.

shows the extent to which the skeletal parts are completely or partially affected, as well as the consequences on neighbouring bones.

The sagittal plane

Whether studied on a standard roentgenogram, a lateral tomograph, a direct sagittal CT scan section or MR imaging, this view shows the more or less major changes of Welker's angle as well as the shortening of the anterior fossa. This angle tends to open and at its extreme platybasia is presented. At times the platybasia may be associated with malformation of the atlanto-occipital articulation, which is represented essentially by basilar impression (Fig. 15.11). The shortness of the anterior fossa is best appreciated on axial CT scan section since each part of this fossa can be analysed separately.

The axial plane

Figure 15.12 shows the deformities of the three parts of the skull base. The size of the anterior fossa is reduced. The endocranial orbital plate of the frontal bone is dysplastic and the cribriform plate of the ethmoid bone is hypoplastic. Usually, the wings of the sphenoid bone present a torsion of their transversal axis. This leads to the disorganization of the optic canals and the superior optic fissure as well. The axis of the canals is modified in all the planes of space. The associated alterations of the orbits will be discussed later.

At the middle fossa, torsion and hypoplasia of the greater wing of the sphenoid bone are often encountered. The petrous bones are asymmetrical. This is responsible for a modification in the geometry of the Fallopian canal which, at most, can lose its natural curvature (dystopia). In addition the asymmetry of the temporal bones is also

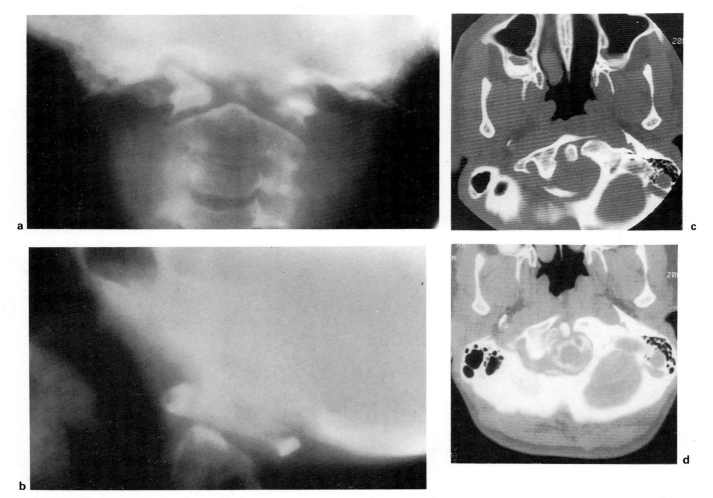

Fig. 15.11 (a, b) Coronal and sagittal tomographies of the craniovertebral region. Important basilar invagination with hypoplasia of odontoid process; (c, d) CT scan axial cuts of craniovertebral region. The asymmetry explains the difficulties in studying such malformations. After intrathecal injection of contrast medium, the vertebral arteries are well seen; the situation of the tonsils proves Chiari's malformation.

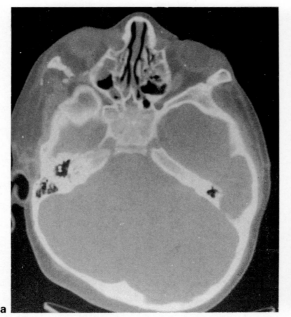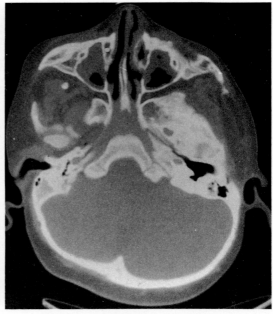

Fig. 15.12 Use of axial sections in the study of the modifications of the base of the skull: (a) the orbits are considerably deformed, with exorbitism on the right. The medial walls of the two orbit cavities are modified. The asymmetry of the greater wings of the sphenoid as well as the petrosal portions of the temporal bone is clearly visible. This explains the variations in the size of the temporal fossa. The posterior fossa also participate in the malformation — hemiatrophy on the right is evident; (b) the inferior section shows the right hemiatrophy, explaining the 'pseudo-ascension' of the right mandibular condyle. On the left side the section passes through the petrosal pyramid of the temporal. This is accompanied by a dextroconvex scoliosis of the medial line.

responsible for important modifications of the temporo-mandibular joint. The glenoid fossa may be more or less obliterated, with associated hypoplasia of the mandibular condyles.

The frontal plane

Three major elements are studied (Fig. 15.13): these include the middle fossa of the base of the skull and the pterygoid processes of the sphenoid; the cribriform plate of the ethmoid; and the frontal sinuses.

Just as in the axial plane the asymmetric development of the petrous bones as well as their positional modifications are clearly analysable. An example includes the raising or lowering of one petrous bone compared to the other. The modifications of the temporomandibular joint require careful study. In this case one may find hypoplasia of the glenoid fossa and the condyles, with obliteration of the articular interline. The temporal fossae are also asymmetrical. In particular they are unequally deep and this has progressive consequences on the brain. The pterygoid processes are also asymmetrical. They present a lateral displacement which can be more or less important. This displacement affects the muscles associated with the pharynx and the mandible.

Frequently, the cribriform plate of the ethmoid, normally located at the union of the superior third with the inferior two-thirds of the orbits, is lowered. Its structure may be modified, in which case it tends to take on a grooved aspect. In some cases the cribriform plate may be raised, in which case it juts between the orbital relief. In cases presenting a lowering of the ethmoidal cribriform plate, dehiscence, resulting in an ethmoidal meningocele or, if the process extends posteriorly and/or anteriorly, an ethmoidofrontal or ethmoidosphenoidal meningocele, is often associated.

Frontal sinus hypertrophy may be present at onset. In some cases frontal hypertrophy may evolve, resulting in pneumosinus dilatans. On the other hand, sinus hypotrophy or even the complete absence of pneumatization is not a rare finding.

THE ORBITS

The orbits may be conceived of as the meeting point of the various resultants of the alterations of the base, vault and face (Fig. 15.14). Their modification results from the sutural alterations which are a consequence of the craniosynostosis. Their position, contents and volume are likewise modified. In other words there are problems of a container and its contents.

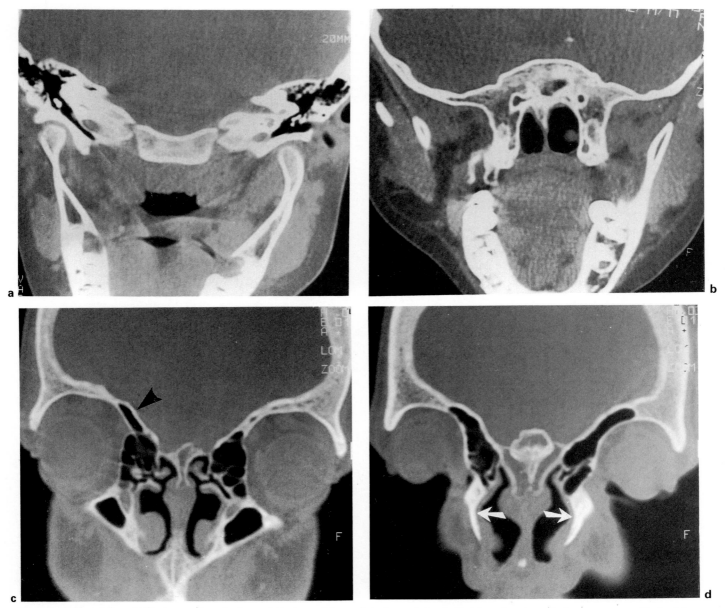

Fig. 15.13 Use of frontal CT scan sections in the analytical semeiology of the base of the skull: (a) section through the temporomandibular joints. The orientation of the mandibular fossae is asymmetrical, the form of the mandibular condyles is modified, the position of the temporal petrous is asymmetrical and the different muscular groups are asymmetrically developed; (b) section through the pterygoid processes. The pterygoid processes are sensibly symmetric, which confirms that the plane of the section is correctly oriented. This allows an appreciation of the asymmetry of the greater sphenoidal wings, affecting the temporal fossae as well as, by way of consequence, mandibular asymmetry; (c) section through the posterior part of the orbits. Lowering of the cribiform plate of the ethmoid with transversal enlargement of the nasal fossae and hypertelorism. Abnormal pneumatization of the orbital plates of the frontal bones is seen on the right (arrow); (d) frontal CT scan section through the anterior part of the orbits. Besides the extreme hypertelorism, the importance of the deviation of the nasal bones should be underlined.

The most severe malformation is anorbitism, in which the eye, ocular muscles and the optic nerve are absent.

Hypo-orbitism results in a small orbital cavity containing a small hypoplastic eye.

Cyclopia, in which the eye is unique, is always associated with a cerebral malformation. This malformation involves the forebrain and is of the holoprosencephalic type. It is most often lethal at birth.

Exorbitism corresponds to the reduction in the size of the orbit in the sagittal plane, with the eyeball having a normal size and structure. The neighbouring anatomic elements (nerves, muscles, fat and aponevroses) are normal. Exophthalmos, on the other hand, corresponds to an increase in the volume of the contents of the orbit without modification of the bone envelope.

The cranial vault malformations, particularly those of

the frontal bones (sinus hypertrophy, shortening of the orbital plates), have important repercussions on the superior portions of the orbital cavity. This secondary deformity is severe in cases of brachycephaly or partial in cases of plagiocephaly (deformity of the lateral portion of the orbit) and trigonocephaly (deformity of the medial portion of the orbit).

Variations in the ethmoid also affect the structure of the orbit since its lateral masses form the medial walls of the orbit. Malformations of the face (facial and maxillary retrusion) can provoke deformities of the lower portion of the orbit with a loss of the harmony of its structures, resulting in oval deformation of the orbit.

THE MANDIBLE, THE MASTICATOR MUSCLES AND THE PTERYGOID MUSCLES

The malformations of the mandible and its annexes are studied in the context of auromandibular dysotosis. This is a congenital malformation of the face. It develops at the expense of the first two branchial arches, the first pharyngeal pouch, the first brachial groove and the temporal bone. Numerous variants, depending on the participation of the brachial arches, have been described. The most classic concern those related to the first arch. These include the Francheschetti–Zweller syndrome, Goldenhar's syndrome or the Ogston syndrome.

The mandibular condyles are also the site of hypo- or hyperplastic malformations. Hyperplasia is responsible for prognathism and meniscal lesions contralateral to this hypertrophy. Hypoplasia affects the condyle and mandibular neck unilaterally or bilaterally. Muscular lesions, presenting short, hypotrophic and hypoplastic muscles, are associated with these skeletal malformations. The lesions are most often unilateral but in some cases, such as in Franschetti's or Goldenhar's syndrome, they are bilateral.

THE SURROUNDING SOFT TISSUES AND THE ZYGOMATIC PROCESSES

For studying the 'peripheral structures' of the face and skull we rely on CT scans, xerography, whose indications are of interest for studying these structures, and MR imaging. The CT scans are realized axially using adapted windows. They show the anomalies of the zygomatic processes and masseter hypoplasia, and they allow the line of the largest contour passing through the plane of the zygomatic processes to be analysed. In this way a study of the relation of the skin, the subcutaneous fat and the underlying muscle is possible.

CONCLUSIONS

The main semeiological parameters in regard to their normal and pathological radiological aspects have been analysed. By associating and synthesizing the elements which are discussed it is possible, on the one hand, to diagnose the principal syndromes and, on the other, to understand the elements required for choosing a therapeutic indication.

In order to avoid needless repetition, the specific neuroradiological semeiology of these syndromes is described in the chapters dealing with the different pathological entities.

REFERENCES AND BIBLIOGRAPHY

Braun J P, Tournade A 1982 La porencéphalie. Journal of Neuroradiology 9: 161–178
Cabanis E A, Iba-Zizen M T, Lopez A 1986 Le syndrome malformatif du massif facial. Radiologie 6: 231–242
Faerber E N, Swartz J D 1985 Congenital malformations of the external and middle ear: high resolution CT findings of surgical import. Americal Journal of Neuroradiology 6: 71–76
Fields H W Jr, Metzner L, Garol J D, Kokich V G 1978 The craniofacial skeleton in anencephalic human fetuses. 1. Cranial floor. Teratology 17: 57–66
Harwood-Nash D C, Fitz C 1976 Neuroradiology in infants and children, vol 1. Mosby Cie, St Louis. 1–214
Hassan M 1982 Semiologie radiologique du crâne du nouveau-né et de l'enfant. Aspects normaux et pièges. EMC Paris, Radiodiagnostic II, 31620-A.10, 5
Montaut J, Stricker M 1977 Dysmorphies cranio-faciales. Les synostoses prématurées (crâniosténoses et facio-sténoses). Neurochirurgie 23: Suppl 2

Salamon G, Raybaud C, Choux M 1982 Les troubles de la gyration. Journal of Neuroradiology 9: 91–96
Tait M V, Gilday D L, Ash J M et al 1979 Craniosynostosis: correlation of bone scans, radiographic and surgical findings. Radiology 133: 615–621
Taveras J M, Wood E H 1977 Diagnostic neuroradiology, vol 1. Williams & Wilkins, Baltimore. pp 1–230
Tessier P 1971 Relationship of craniostenoses to craniofacial synostoses and to faciostenoses. Plastic and Reconstructive Surgery 48: 224–237
Virapongse C, Shapiro R, Sarwar M, Bhimani S, Crelin E S 1985a Computed tomography in the study of the development of the skull base. 1. Normal morphology. Journal of Computer Assisted Tomography, 9: 85–94
Virapongse C, Sarwar M, Ghimani S, Crelin E S 1985b Computed tomography in the study of the development of the skull base. 2. Anencephaly, the aberrant skull form. Journal of Computer Assisted Tomography 9: 95–102

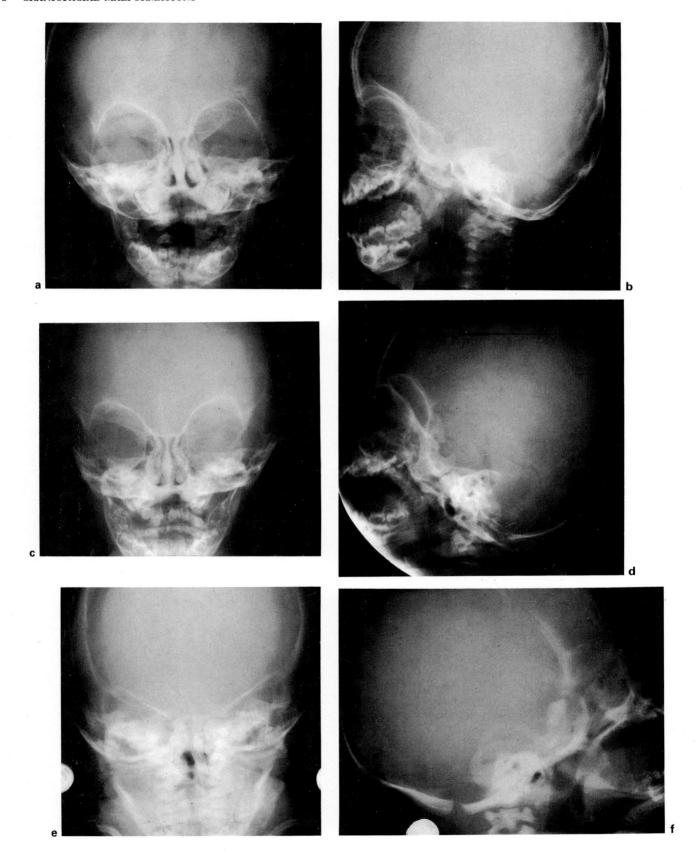

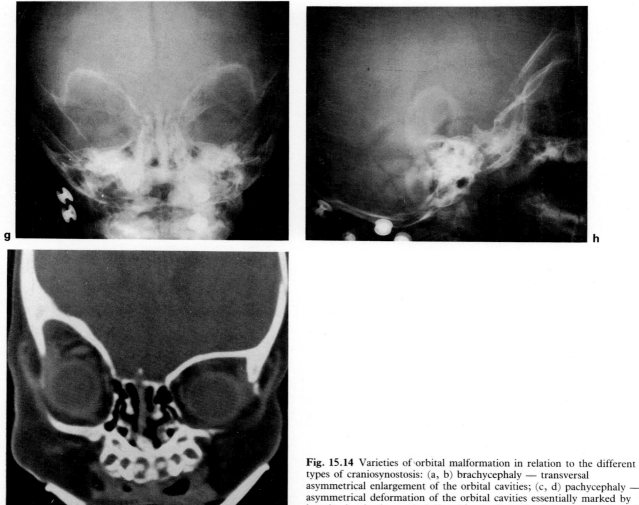

Fig. 15.14 Varieties of orbital malformation in relation to the different types of craniosynostosis: (a, b) brachycephaly — transversal asymmetrical enlargement of the orbital cavities; (c, d) pachycephaly — asymmetrical deformation of the orbital cavities essentially marked by lengthening in the vertical direction; (e, f) turricephaly — flattening of the roofs of the orbital cavities and the lateral angulation of their greater axis; (g–i) plagiocephaly — the asymmetry of the size of the orbital cavities is clearly visible on the lateral view and especially on the frontal CT scan section.

16. Teleradiography

B. Raphael, M. Stricker, J. Van der Meulen, R. Mazzola

INTRODUCTION

Teleradiography is essential in craniofacial surgery, despite its rigorous requirements and despite its apparent complexity for the non-specialist and the disappointments awaiting those seeking to penetrate its subtleties.

Cephalometry was initially used for orthodontic diagnosis, with its essential aim the detection and assessment of alveolodental disorders. It then progressed beyond the mere study of occlusion to consider the proportions and architectural arrangements of the skull and face, replacing linear measurements by volumetric ratios.

The most recent cephalometric recordings provide a sufficiently precise insight into both the skeletal structures and the soft parts enabling one: to assess the balance of relationship between the different sectors in a given subject, at any given time and in relation to the normal; to predict changes in this relationship during growth; and, finally, to decide on what restorative steps to take where there is facial imbalance.

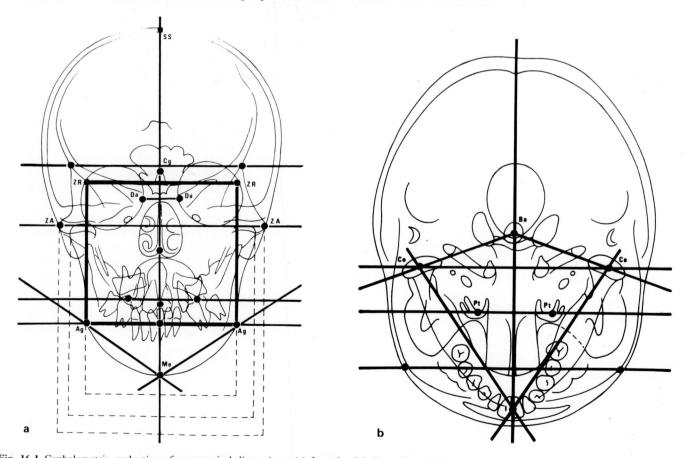

Fig. 16.1 Cephalometric evaluation of symmetrical dimensions: (a) frontal axial view; (b) axial view.

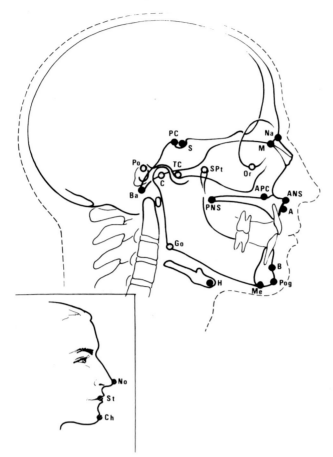

Fig. 16.2 The standard reference points; median, lateral, constructed and cutaneous (see inset).

TECHNIQUE

At the beginning of the century, Carrea & Atkinson adapted X-rays for the purposes of cephalometry. Image deformation is minimized by increasing the tube-patient distance, which must be not less than 4 m. Reliable reproduction of the films, which is essential for the comparability of records, stems from the tucked-in position of the head in a cephalostat in dental occlusion, with the lips at rest and the Frankfort plane horizontal.

The lateral view is the one most commonly used. It shows the vertical proportions and anteroposterior dimensions, which suffice to define the craniofacial typology. However, in cases of asymmetry a three-dimensional study is needed, using two supplementary views: axial (Hirtz teleradiography) and frontal (facial teleradiography) (Fig. 16.1). Study of the soft parts and particularly of the skin profile, formerly outlined by a metal wire, is now done by interposition of a filter.

REFERENCE POINTS AND LINES

Teleradiographic analysis, when employed in orthodontic practice, uses a large number of dental references, whereas its use in surgery requires tracings of all the structures, including the teeth. The reference points are classic and unvarying, but the resultant analysis varies from author to author.

First, the principal points, lines and angles commonly used will be described. Then a few selected analyses will be considered, because of either their surgical interest or their usefulness in predicting growth.

Standard points

These mostly correspond to anthropometric references, but their localization in a teleradiographic record is not always obvious. It requires care and unerring anatomical assessment. The points most used are classified by Chateau (1975) as median, lateral and 'constructed' (Fig. 16.2).

MEDIAN POINTS

Ba = basion: inferior point of the anterior border of occipital foramen at the junction of the spheno-occipital groove and the external surface of the occipital bone

S = sella: centre of sella turcica

PCP = posterior clinoid process

N = nasion: nasofrontal suture

M = (Enlow 1968, Delaire 1978) naso-frontomaxillary suture

ANS = anterior peak of anterior nasal spine

PNS = posterior nasal spine

APC = anterior palatine canal (its localization defines the primary palate or incisive bone, anteriorly, and the secondary palate posteriorly)

A = (Downs 1952): the most posterior part of the concavity of the superior alveolar process

B = homologous point of the mandible

Pg = most anterior point of the dental symphysis

Me = most inferior point of the symphysis

H = median point of the body of the hyoid bone

LATERAL POINTS

Po = Porion: superior edge of the external auditory canal

Or = orbital (or inferior orbital): steepest point of the orbital ring (not to be confused with the infraorbital point)

TC = temporal condyle: posteroinferior part of the temporal condyle, normally opposite the center of the mandibular condyle

C = capitular (Bimler 1969) centre of mandibular condyle

Go = gonion: middle of the curve of the gonial angle

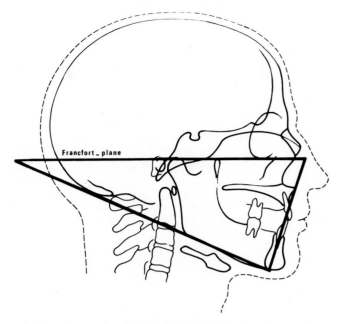

Fig. 16.3 Tweed's triangle. FMA, Frankfort mandibular plane angle; IMPA, inferior incisive mandibular plane angle; FMIA, inferior incisive Frankfort plane angle.

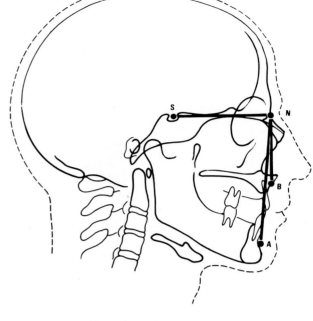

Fig. 16.4 SNA and SNB angles of Downs.

CONSTRUCTED POINTS

SPt = superior pterygoid (Enlow 1968, Ricketts 1957, Delaire 1978): a point of the greatest importance, through' which passes the facial axis of Ricketts. According to Delaire, it represents the boundary between the maxillary and mandibular zones and is situated at the junction of the anterior border of the pterygoid with the base of the skull, at the foramen magnum. Its localization is often blurred by superimposition of the ethmoid cells but it can be defined by locating the sphenopalatine foramen (Vion 1984), whose image is always protected immediately above the tail of the middle concha.

ST = stomion: essential reference point in defining the soft parts. It is situated at the point of contact of upper and lower lips. Its visualization is crucial in locating the position of the free border of the upper lip in relation to the superior incisive border.

When studying the skin profile it may also be useful to indicate the projection of the point of the nose (No) and of the chin (Ch) on the tracing of the soft parts.

Lines, planes and angles

On the basis of a number of the reference points previously described, tracings are made using modalities appropiate to the concepts of the various authors. Every method of analysis thus defines lines and planes whose orientation and relationships are assessed by angular measurements.

The reference plane which is still widely used, if only to orientate the film, is the Frankfort plane, joining the porion (Po) and the inferior orbital point (Or). Tweed (1954) constructs a triangle on the basis of the Frankfort plane and of the base of the mandible. It has, in his view, prognostic value in the treatment of mandibular retrognathism (Fig. 16.3).

The SN line, still commonly used, lies at an angle of 6° to the Frankfort plane. With NA and NB it defines the SNA and SNB angles of Downs; these references are unreliable, being unduly influenced by the position of the nasion (Fig. 16.4).

Many authors, following Enlow and Delaire, refer to more stable lines, for example:

the superior line of the base of the skull — this joins point M to point PCP (posterior clinoid process);
  the basal craniofacial line, which links M, SPt and Tc;
the bispinous (or palatine) plane, joining ANS and PNS. This line may be interrupted at the level of the APC, thus indicating the premaxillary portion of the maxillary;
the occlusive plane — this is the most difficult to plot, since the only points of reference are dental and rarely situated on a straight line but most often on a curve — that of Spee;
the mandibular plane: classically in contact with the lower mandibular border, it must be plotted more precisely according to Bimler (1969) with the help of a tangent to the occipital squama. It runs from the point of the chin (Me) and traverses the mandible at its preangular notch (Bimler notch) to reach the squama at the occipito-manducatory point Om). This plot gives a better picture of the tilt of the body of the mandible.

These principal craniofacial planes, whether parallel or convergent at the lower part of the occiput (Chateau 1975) are crossed frontally by lines (Bimler 1969, Ricketts 1981, Delaire 1978) or by curves (Sassouni & Nanda 1964) and they thus define the anteroposterior balance of the craniofacial structures. Three lines are normally used:

the anterior line, which defines the fronto-maxillomandibular relationship;
the middle or pterygomaxillary line, which defines the facial axis of Ricketts and, according to Delaire, demarcates the maxillary or mandibular zones;
the posterior line defines the relation of the ramus to the sphenoidal region and the cervical spine.

Finally, the following must be noted in connection with the mandible:

the orientation of the condyle,
the position of the spine of Spix,
the curve of the dental canal,

these being features which predict the type of rotation during growth of the mandible (Björk 1969).

The tracings

The impressive number of tracings in current use bears witness to their inadequacies and only those three will be retained which contribute to the analysis, treatment and monitoring of craniofacial deformities.

DIAGNOSTIC STAGE

The architectural analysis of Sassouni & Nanda (1964) provides a very convenient classification of the skeletal bases into class II and class III, open-bite and deep-bite (Fig. 16.5).

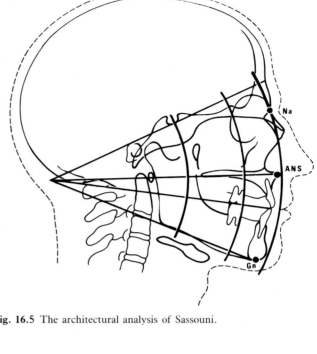

Fig. 16.5 The architectural analysis of Sassouni.

THE RICKETTS ANALYSIS

This aims to produce a predictive study of growth, by extrapolating a number of cephalometric indices. This objective has been the concern of many authors. Tweed (1954) based the prognosis of malocclusion on the direction of growth made visible by the alterations in the angle ANB after a one-year interval. Björk (1969) assesses the type of rotation from a number of mandibular criteria, such as the orientations of the condyle, the curve of the dental canal and the shape of the mandibular border (Fig. 16.6). The method of Ricketts (1981), where it applies, appears to be the most reliable. It refers to the base of the skull, taking account of mandibular rotation. After evaluating the rate

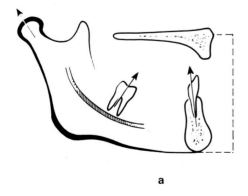 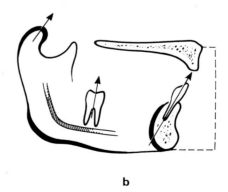

a   b

Fig. 16.6 Cephalometric characteristics allowing the definition of two types of rotation; according to Björk: (a) anteriorly; (b) posteriorly.

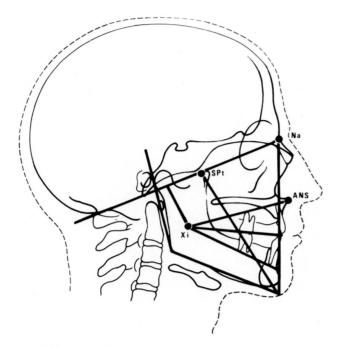

Fig. 16.7 Ricketts analysis.

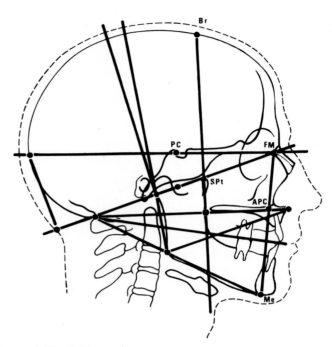

Fig. 16.8 The Delaire tracing.

of growth, it reconstitutes the bone structures and soft parts, sector by sector and from above down, using a strict methodology (Fig. 16.7).

THE DELAIRE TRACING

The author refers to it as an architectural analysis and it is undoubtedly the most suitable for craniofacial surgery. It is derived from the principles of Enlow (1968) and the Bimler (1969) tracing. It combines an architectural analysis of the cephalic components, in relation to an ideally balanced subject, with a structural analysis of each bony element and of the soft parts (Fig. 16.8).

This procedure envisages an alveolodental equilibrium within a craniofacial equilibrium, while providing the constitutional and morphofunctional causes of the dysmorphism.

The notion of proportionality between the different sectors introduced by this procedure allows the surgeon to establish a preoperative set-up and to simulate, with some accuracy, the displacements to be produced in order to secure an ideal balance.

REFERENCES AND BIBLIOGRAPHY

Bimler H P 1969 The Bimler cephalometric analysis. Printed privately
Björk A 1969 Prediction of mandibular growth rotation. American Journal of Orthodontics 55: 109–123
Chateau M 1975 Orthopédie dento-faciale. Tome II. Prelat, Paris. pp 73–109
Coccaro P J 1984 Pediatric cephalometrics. In: Serafin D Georgiade N G (eds) Pediatric plastic surgery, vol 1. Mosby, St Louis pp 230–245
Delaire J 1978 L'analyse architecturale et structurale crânio-faciale (de profil). Principle théorique. Quelques exemples d'emploi en chirurgie maxillo-faciale. Revue de Stomatologie 79: 1–33
Downs W B 1952 The role of cephalometrics in orthodontic cases. Analysis and treatment planning. American Journal of Orthodontics 38: 162–182
Enlow D H 1968 The human face. Harper & Row, New York
Muller L 1962 Cephalmétrie et orthodontie. Société des publications médicales et dentaires, Paris

Ricketts R M, Palisades P 1960 A foundation for cephalometric communication. Journal of Orthodontics American 1981 46: 330–357
Ricketts R M 1981 Perspectives in the clinical application of cephalometrics. Angle Orthodontist 51: 115–150
Sassouni V, Nanda S 1964 Analysis of dento-facial vertical proportions. American Journal of Orthodontics 50: 801–823
Sassouni V 1969 Classification of skeletal types. American Journal of Orthodontics 55: 109–123
Sassouni V 1971 Orthodontics in dental practice. Mosby, St Louis
Tweed C H 1954 The Frankfort mandibular plane angle in orthodontic diagnosis, classification, treatment planning and prognosis. Angle Orthodontic 24: 121–169
Vion P E 1984 Anatomie céphalométrique. La bibliothéque d'orthodontie. S I D, Vanves

17. Three-dimensional imaging from CT scans for evaluation of patients with craniofacial anomalies

J. L. Marsh, M. W. Vannier

Two-dimensional conventional X-ray and computerized tomographic imaging systems contribute to the diagnosis, surgical planning and postoperative follow-up of patients with craniofacial malformations. The recently developed ability (Vannier et al 1983, 1984, Herman & Lie 1979, Dev et al 1983) to reformat CT scans into three-dimensional osseous or soft tissue surface images has significant implications in the management of craniofacial malformations. Although CT scan images discriminate hard and soft tissues well, the number of images produced from a single malformed skull and their slice format makes 3-D spatial integration and understanding difficult. This is especially true for patients with bony clefts, e.g. mandibulofacial dysostosis (Marsh et al 1986). While paraxial reformations, i.e. coronal, sagittal, longitudinal orbital (Marsh & Gado 1983), suggest the relationships of regional anatomy from several viewing planes, the whole remains a product of the viewer's imagination. Three-dimensional surface reconstructions from CT scans present an integrated image which can be viewed from any desired vantage point. The osseous 3-D images resemble photographs of prepared skulls (Fig. 17.1). As such, they are readily comprehended by non-radiologist physicians, patients and parents. These reconstructions, in combination with the original axial and reformatted paraxial scan images, allow the student of craniofacial malformations to arrive sooner at a more complete understanding of the dysmorphic anatomy (Marsh & Vannier 1985).

Effective use of 3-D surface reconstruction software requires dedicated personnel within a medical imaging section (Marsh et al 1985a). We obtain the axial CT scans with a predefined protocol: high resolution, thin (2 mm) slice scans oriented along the orbitomeatal line obtained in anatomical sequence. Parenteral sedation (Nembutal 6 mg/kg for infants under 15 kg, Nembutal 5 mg/kg for children over 15 kg) is necessary for infants and small children. Oral sedation (chloral hydrate 50 mg/kg up to a 2-g dose) is used for anxious older children and adults. Patients with unstable airways, e.g. microretrognathia,

require general anaesthesia with endotracheal intubation to maintain a secure airway.

The scans are then processed with specially developed 3-D software according to the specifications of the requesting physician by a specially trained radiological technologist. This individual performs selected tasks appropriate to the imaging study. Recently, several software tools have been added to improve the utility of 3-D surface imaging in our centre. These include cranial suture enhancement, globe opacification, brain extraction and mandible disarticulation. The results of the 3-D software postprocessing can then be evaluated on a CRT screen, as transparent film hard copy, as photographic prints, or as a life-size space-filling model (Marsh et al 1985b).

Cranial suture enhancement (Fig. 17.2) software was created to delineate patent sutures seen on the original 2-D CT scan slices. In the past, these sutural markings were frequently obliterated by the smoothing programs used in production of 3-D images. Sutural enhancement has been useful in the diagnosis of craniosynostosis and the monitoring of sutural status over time.

Globe opacification (Fig. 17.3) software has been developed to retain the outline of the ocular globes in osseous 3-D skull reconstructions. This permits study of the anatomy of dysmorphic orbits and their contents as well as of the effect of orbital translocations. These data should provide better quantitative surgical 'blue-prints' to normalize globe position as well as orbital configuration.

Mandible disarticulation (Fig. 17.4) exposes the exocranial base, including the glenoid fossae, for examination. In addition, the isolated mandible can be viewed from any desired vantage point, including the top view, which exposes the articular surface of the mandibular condyles. This imaging is especially useful in the evaluation of patients with craniofacial microsomia when deciding whether to perform a ramus osteotomy or a condylar reconstruction for mandibular lengthening.

Beyond the initial enthusiasm for 3-D images which their familiarity and ease of comprehension engenders

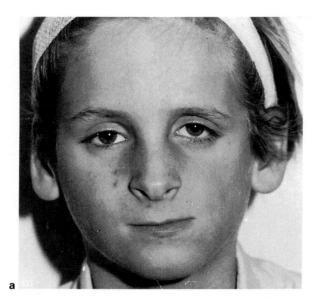

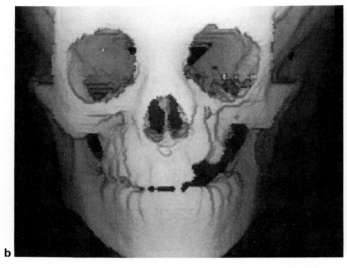
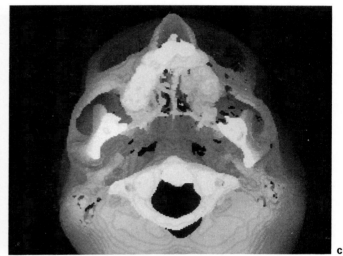

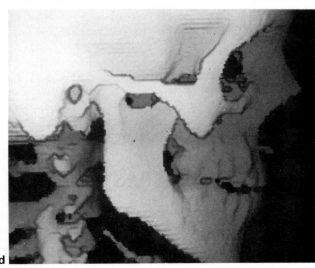
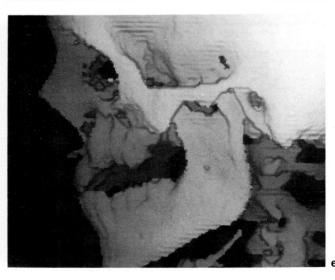

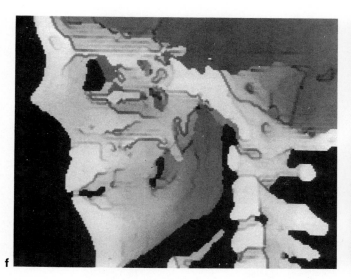 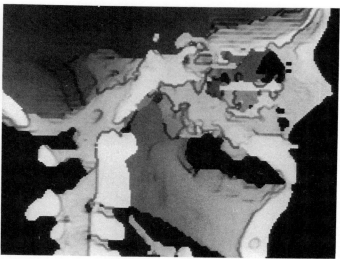

f   g

Fig. 17.1 (a) 11-year-old boy with hypoplastic left midface of unknown aetiology; (b) frontal 3-D osseous surface CT reconstruction. The left maxilla is severely hypoplastic; (c) bottom 3-D osseous surface CT reconstruction (mandible removed at the angle). The left maxillary dentoalveolar segment is smaller than the right and elevated (the brightest white is closest to the viewer). The posterior palate (horizontal process of the palatine bone) is normal appearing and right–left symmetrical, as are the pterygoid plates. The anterior wall of the left maxilla is concave. The left malar block is hypoplastic and the temporal process of the zygoma is displaced dorsally; (d) right lateral 3-D osseous surface CT reconstruction. The patient's unaffected side demonstrates normal anatomy; (e) left lateral 3-D osseous surface CT reconstruction. There is hypoplasia of the maxilla and body of the zygoma. There is mild deformity of the neck of the mandibular condyle; (f) midsagittal 3-D osseous surface CT reconstruction (viewer looking into the right hemicranium). The nasal conchae and pterygoid plates are prominent in the midface region. The patient's unaffected side demonstrates the normal anatomy of this vantage point; (g) midsagittal 3-D osseous surface CT reconstruction (viewer looking into the left hemicranium). There is hypoplasia of the maxillary dentoalveolar segment, the hamulus and medial pterygoid plate, and the inferior concha.

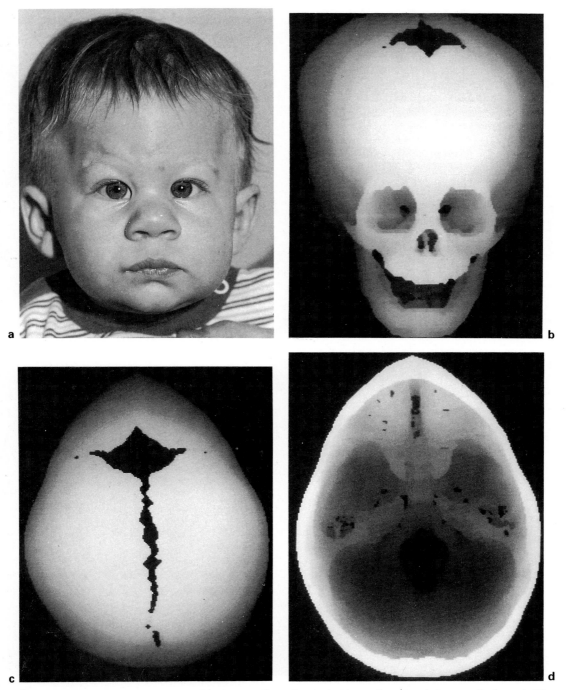

Fig. 17.2 (a) 3-month-old boy with metopic synostosis. The interpupillary distance is 32 mm (less than 3rd percentile for age). The ophthalmological and neurological examinations were otherwise normal; (b) frontal 3-D osseous surface CT reconstruction. The metopic suture is not visualized. The anterior fontanelle is patent. There is orbital hypotelorism (bony interorbital distance = 11 mm); (c) top 3-D osseous surface CT reconstruction. The sagittal suture and anterior fontanelle are clearly patent. While the coronal sutures are moderately opacified on this image, they are patent on the original CT scans. The metopic suture is not visualized; (d) intracranial base osseous surface CT reconstruction. Triangular compression of the anterior fossa is evident. The cribriform plate is narrow and deep, relative to the roof of the orbits.

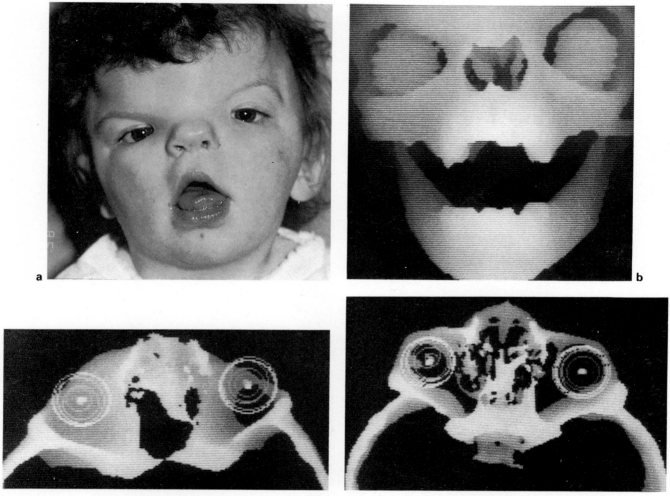

Fig. 17.3 (a) 2-year-old girl with frontonasal dysplasia, left unicoronal synostosis and orbital hypertelorism. She underwent extended bilateral coronal craniectomies and superolateral orbital advancements at 3 months of age. Her interpupillary distance is 65 mm (greater than 97th percentile for age). Vision is intact in both eyes with ocular motility disorder. Neurological development is intact; (b) frontal 3-D osseous surface CT reconstruction with globe opacification. The bony interorbital distance is 31 mm; the distance between the centroids of the globes is 57 mm. The superior rim of the left orbit is more cephalad than the right. Both orbits are maloriented with inferolateral angulation of their horizontal axes; (c) 'split-orbit' 3-D osseous surface CT reconstruction with globe opacification (viewer looking cephalad toward the roofs of the orbits). Lateral splaying of both the nasal bones and the greater wings of the sphenoids is present. The left globe projects ventrally to the superior orbital rim (proptosis). In this patient, this is the result of brow recession due to left unicoronal synostosis; (d) 'split-orbit' 3-D osseous surface CT reconstruction with globe opacification (viewer looking caudally towards the floors of the orbits). The ethmoid air cells occupy the widened interorbital space. The relationship of the globes to the inferior orbital rims is symmetrical.

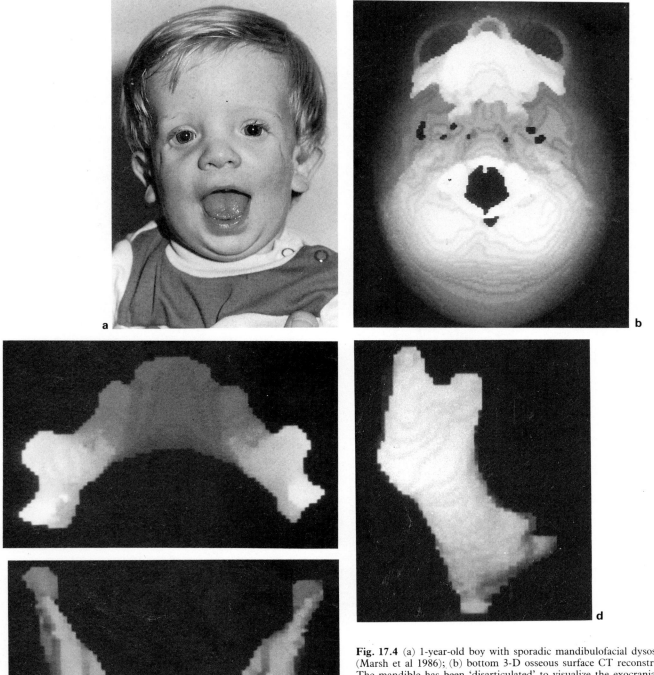

Fig. 17.4 (a) 1-year-old boy with sporadic mandibulofacial dysostosis (Marsh et al 1986); (b) bottom 3-D osseous surface CT reconstruction. The mandible has been 'disarticulated' to visualize the exocranial base. The zygomatic arches are incomplete owing to aplasia of the zygomatic processes of the temporal bones and marked hypoplasia of the temporal processes of the zygomas; (c) top 3-D osseous surface CT reconstruction of isolated mandible. Asymmetry of the condyles is present. The inferior alveolar foramina are visible; (d) right lateral 3-D osseous surface CT reconstruction of isolated mandible. The gonial angle is excessively obtuse with verticalization of the body and caudal direction of the chin; (e) frontal 3-D osseous surface CT reconstruction of isolated mandible. Asymmetry of the angulation of the ascending rami and the orientation of the condylar heads is present.

remain significant imaging problems. These include sequential degradation of data in processing, pseudoforamina, motion artifacts, inability to re-register skull arbitrarily in three-dimensions, and the absence of a normative database.

Three-dimensional surface reconstructions from CT scans is a new technology undergoing rapid evolution. It has already been of clinical and research use for those students of craniofacial malformations who have access to it. (Marsh et al 1986, Marsh & Vannier 1986, 1987). New software and hardware should result in better, more widely available imaging tools. Three-dimensional reconstructions are not an end in themselves, but rather a means to improved patient care.

REFERENCES

Dev P, Wood S, White D, Young S, Duncan J P 1983 An interactive graphics system for planning reconstructive surgery. Proceedings of the National Computer Graphics Association, Chicago. pp 130–135

Herman G T, Lie H K 1979 Three-dimensional display of human organs from computer tomograms. Computer Graphics Image Processing 9: 1

Marsh J L, Gado M 1983 The longitudinal orbital CT projection: a versatile image for orbital assessment. Plastic and Reconstructive Surgery 71: 308

Marsh J L, Vannier M W 1985 Comprehensive care for craniofacial deformities. Mosby, St Louis

Marsh J L, Vannier M W 1986 Cranial base change following surgical treatment of craniosynostosis. Cleft Palate Journal (suppl) 23: 9–18

Marsh J L, Vannier M W 1987 The anatomy of the cranio-orbital deformities of craniosynostosis: insights from 3-D images of CT scans. Clinics in Plastic Surgery 14: 49

Marsh J L, Vannier M W, Knapp R H 1985a Computer assisted surface imaging for craniofacial deformities. In: Habal M (ed) Advances in plastic and reconstructive surgery, vol 2. Yearbook, Chicago

Marsh J L, Vannier M W, Stevens W G et al 1985b Computerized imaging for soft tissue and osseous reconstruction in the head and neck. Plastic Surgery Clinics of North America 12: 279–291

Marsh J L, Celin S E, Vannier M W, Gado M H 1986 The skeletal anatomy of mandibulofacial dysostosis (Treacher Collins syndrome). Plastic and Reconstructive Surgery 78: 460

Vannier M W, Marsh J L, Warren J O 1983 Three dimensional computer graphics for craniofacial surgical planning and evaluation. Computer Graphics 17: 263

Vannier M W, Marsh J L, Warren J O 1984 Three dimensional CT reconstruction images for craniofacial surgical planning and evaluation. Radiology 150: 179–184

Treatment

18. Orthodontics and orthopaedics

B. Raphael, M. Stricker, J. Van der Meulen, R. Mazzola

INTRODUCTION

If the treatment of craniofacial malformations has benefited from the progress of surgery in the last years, there is no question that the quality of the achieved results, particularly at the maxillary level, is mainly due to a better knowledge of the relation between facial and occlusal balance. Indeed, an important characteristic of craniofacial architecture is represented by the position of the maxillary parts, which is subject to two references: the cranial base above and the occlusal plane below, the latter defining the maxillomandibular relationship.

This approach, new to the plastic surgeon, who will now have to adjust to the imperatives of occlusion, becomes manifest in many protocols in which the operation is associated with preoperative orthodontics or postoperative orthopaedic care.

The role and efficacy of orthodontic and orthopaedic techniques in the treatment of craniofacial malformations depend mainly on the type of the deformity, considering in particular the growth potential. Therefore, while orthodontic and orthopaedic treatment may be justified in clefting (Fig. 18.1a,b), it will be a waste of time in the majority of patients with severe dysostosis. Any attempt at orthodontic or orthopaedic correction in severe dysostosis is ineffective in the long run and orthodontic treatment should only be applied to support the surgical procedure. In contrast, the treatment of synostosis may well benefit from these techniques. They may help to improve the efficacy of the operation which in itself may momentarily release an intrinsic growth potential in related bony parts.

THE MEANS AND THEIR CLINICAL APPLICATIONS

The terms orthodontics and orthopaedics define two techniques, which are basically different in their means and goals.

Orthodontics

Orthodontics represents a combination of techniques capable of moving the teeth through the alveolar bone. Its goal consists of correcting dental malocclusions in order to harmonize and realign the dental arches. Orthodontics reveals its potential in its aid prior to the surgery of craniofacial malformations. In fact, each time the mobilization of a skeletal part includes the alveolar process, the final location of the osteotomized bony piece is determined by the occlusal relation.

The quality of this relation is, in our opinion, of paramount importance. It determines the stability and the permanency of the restored facial balance and justifies a meticulous orthodontic preparation prior to surgery. This orthodontic step usually requires the use of fixed appliances. Extremely effective, it makes it possible in most instances to obtain harmonization of the arches by treatment during 18–24 months (Fig. 18.1c). This treatment follows a rigid protocol, which is planned through discussion between the orthodontist and the surgeon.

It is based on a cephalometric analysis and dental case analyses. It is also based on the simulation of the surgical skeletal movements necessary to restore craniofacial balance. The orthodontist is then able to predict the necessary dental movements and adapt these not only to the planned osteotomy sites, but also to the future skeletal position.

Preoperative orthopaedic treatment may be applied:

to correct crowding in a dental arch after dental extraction of premolars or molars;
to correct dental rotations;
to close diastemas;
to level the dental arches, in particular by horizontalization of the curve of Spee.

The result of this treatment is controlled with dental plaster casts (or orthognathic set-up). Skeletal movements by surgery can then be simulated by gypsotomy. This

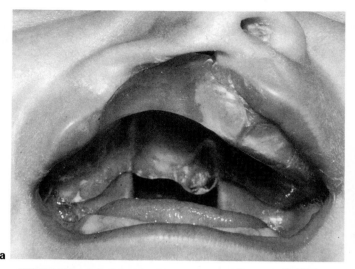

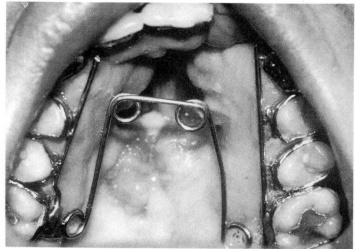

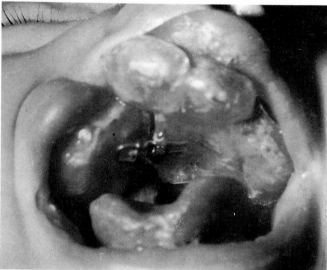

Fig. 18.1 Three orthopaedic modalities in the treatment of clefts: (a) the acrylic plate used in the newborn; (b) the expansion plate following closure of one side in a bilateral cleft; (c) combination of orthodontic and orthopaedic treatment in permanent dentition.

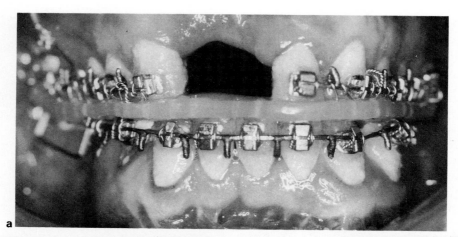

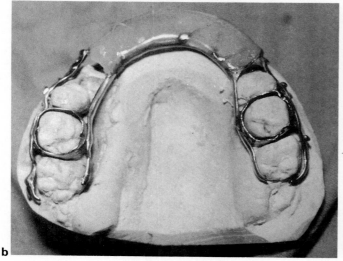

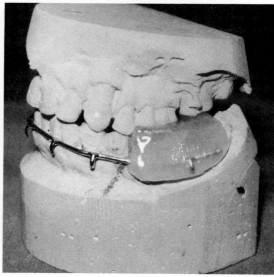

Fig. 18.2 The orthodontic bands and intercuspidation: (a) acrylic plates which will be used at the time of the intermaxillary fixation; (b, c) surgical arch.

study, carried out in an articulator, allows for accurate calculation of the necessary displacement and the definition of a new occlusion which can be fixed by a splint or wafer.

These devices are used for reference and immobilization at the time of the intermaxillary fixation (Fig. 18.2a). The orthodontic appliance can generally be maintained and used for intermaxillary fixation. A few days prior to surgery an arch wire with interdental stops is ligated in both dental arches. The orthodontic brackets usually cemented to the vestibular surface of the teeth cannot resist strong traction, especially in a vertical direction. When strong intra- or extraoral forces are expected pre- or postoperatively, it is advisable to add a bar, secured to each tooth by means of stainless steel wire (Fig. 18.2b,c).

The intermaxillary fixation which preserves the new occlusion at the end of the operation will be removed in 6–8 weeks. It is, however, essential that this removal is immediately followed by a period of retention or further orthodontic treatment.

While the control of tooth movements can be secured by an orthodontic appliance, this is not possible with the skeletal stability, which is subject to muscular dysfunction and soft tissue retraction. With skeletal relapse follows the necessity for correction of the then established malocclusion. It necessitates the use of intra- or extraelastic forces. The orthopaedic measures form a precious ally in the work of the craniofacial surgeon.

Orthopaedics

Orthopaedics, more ambitious in its goals, aims to modify the position, size and shape of dentofacial parts. The tooth serves as an anchor through which orthopaedic forces can be exerted.

The effect of an intermaxillary or extraoral force on an osteotomized bony piece is incontestable, but it is not certain whether the same effect may be obtained by this procedure when applied to an intact skeleton.

It is not our aim to enter the polemic on the real efficacy of orthopaedic forces applied in infancy, but one cannot deny that good results are achieved by palatal-splitting devices, by expansion devices for the upper jaw and by forward traction of the upper jaw produced by forehead–chin appliances (Delaire et al 1975, 1979) (Fig. 18.3). Using extraoral forces applied on mobilized

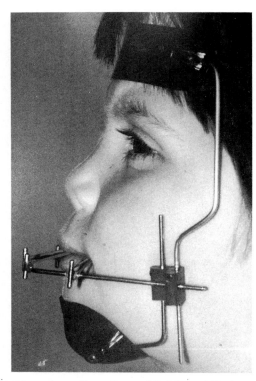

Fig. 18.3 The orthopaedic appliance of Delaire and Verdon.

segments and opposing the retraction of soft tissues brutally dislocated by the surgical displacement of the bony pieces, orthopaedics can constitute a most valuable aid (Fig. 18.4). Maintained during the period of consolidation it assures a retention under slight tension and favours bony remodelling in children (Fig. 18.4b).

In order to be effective, the applied forces must be relative strong and applied regularly, preferably at night. The usual length of treatment is three months. It may be repeated after a pause of three weeks. Application of these orthopaedic methods in young children can be difficult owing to deficiency or absence of teeth. A palatal splint firmly suspended to the zygomatic arch can, however, be used instead.

It is finally in this sense that cavital conformers (nasal or orbital) are commonly used. Their efficacy is unquestionable if applied over a period of three to six months (Fig. 18.5).

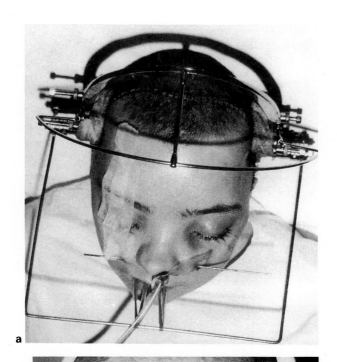

Fig. 18.4 Postoperative orthopaedic treatment by extraoral forces: (a) traction applied on the superior arch following the Le Fort III procedure; (b) traction applied on the inferior arch following mandibular lengthening; (c)traction applied on a transfacial wire following a Le Fort IV or monoblock procedure.

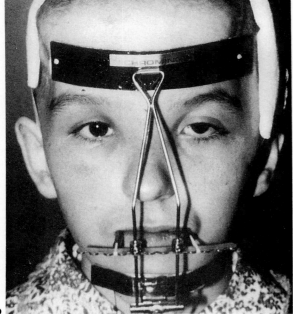

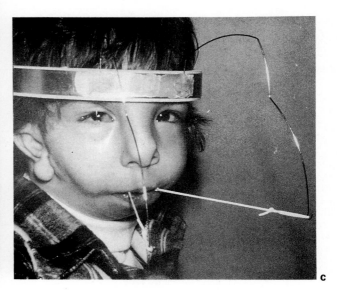

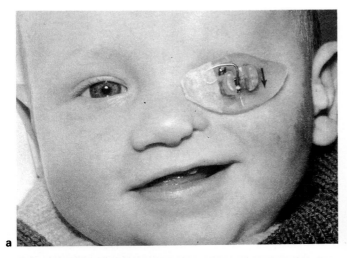

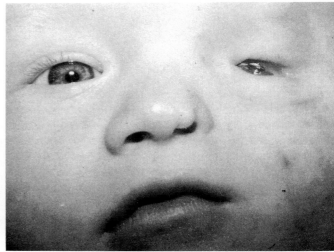

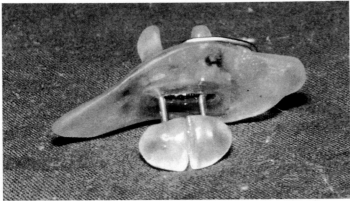

Fig. 18.5 Technique of orbital expansion in a patient with microorbitism due to anophthalmia.

REFERENCES AND BIBLIOGRAPHY

Coccaro P J 1984 Orthodontic treatment in cranio-facial anomalies. In Serafin D, Georgiade N G Pediatric plastic surgery, Vol 1. Mosby, St Louis pp 379–389

Cugny Ph 1979a Le traitement des malformations faciales par les moyens orthodontiques et chirurgicaux. Revue d'Orthopedie Dento-Faciale 13: 479–496

Cugny Ph 1979b Contribution orthodontique au traitement des crânio-facio-sténoses. Actualites Odonto-Stomatologiques 128: 681–695

Delaire J, Verain P, Flour J 1975 Buts et résultats des tractions extra-orales postéro-antérieures sur masque orthopédique dans le traitement des rétrognathies et brachygnathies maxillaires. Fortschritte der Kieferorthopadie 37: 247

Delaire J, Verdon P, Salagnac J M, Felpetto Y, Zayat S 1979 Bases physiologiques de l'équilibre du maxillaire supérieur. Incidences en ce qui concerne le mode d'action des forces lourdes extra-orales. Actualités Odonto-stomatologiques 128: 611–644

McCarthy J G, Grayson B, Zide B 1982 The relationship between the surgeon and the orthodontist in orthognathic surgery. Clinics in Plastic Surgery 9: 423–442

Raphael B, Labboz P, Lebeau J 1980 L'étape orthopédique dans le traitement primaire des fentes labio-maxillo-palatines. Annales de Chirurgie Plastique 25: 217–224

Ricketts R M 1960 The influence of orthodontic treatment on facial growth and development. Angle Orthodontist 30: 103–133

19. Anaesthesiology

M. Jupa, N. M. Hilgevoord

INTRODUCTION

This chapter has been written to assist the surgeon in understanding the problems and complications associated with anaesthesia for the rapidly developing domain of plastic and reconstructive surgery. The authors have attempted to avoid controversy and present the more practical aspect of the speciality.

GENERAL REMARKS

The extensive and prolonged duration of the surgical procedures and protracted recovery period demands close teamwork between the various specialists: plastic surgeon, neurosurgeon, oromaxillary surgeon, otorhinolaryngologist and anaesthesiologist (Whitaker et al 1980). It is the aim of the anaesthesiologist to concern himself with the special problems of these patients which merit his skill in achieving a successful outcome of the operation.

PREOPERATIVE CONFERENCE

A meeting of specialists concerned in the management of the patient should take place several days beforehand. The anaesthesiologist requires general information about the planned procedures of the other specialists. He can then summarize their requirements and plan the anaesthesia most suitable for the patient and operation. Depending upon examination of the anatomy of the airway and the requirements of the surgeon, the anaesthesiologist decides whether to intubate orally or nasotracheally and which induction method will suit best (Delèque et al 1985, Handler et al 1978).

It is important to ascertain whether preoperative tracheostomy should be carried out or not. Should this be necessary, it should be done 24–48 hours before the main operation, because of the complications resulting from a fresh tracheostomy. Personal experience and complications of insertion of tracheal cannulae in freshly tracheotomized patients should be a warning to others.

PREOPERATIVE VISIT

An adequate preoperative evaluation must be made of the patient and his ability to withstand the planned procedure. One should never neglect the patient's history. Certain diseases such as allergies and epilepsy are treated with a variety of drugs (mydriatics, miotics, tranquillizers, anticonvulsants), which have a pharmacological interaction with certain anaesthetics and can produce a modification of their therapeutic effect (Stark 1974). An even greater danger lies in the lack of knowledge of the prescription of a drug. Let us stress two diseases, whose evaluation must never be omitted: allergic disease and epilepsy.

Allergic disease

Patients with asthma and/or hay fever react badly to the histamine release associated with some drugs used in anaesthesia (curare, atropine); furthermore, many of these patients have been prescribed steroids for a long time.

Epilepsy

Other patients may have a history of epilepsy and use anticonvulsants. These drugs should be continued up to and including the day of surgery and a parenteral form should be available on that day. Their administration must not be omitted, in spite of the fact that general anaesthetics are anticonvulsants. Variations in pH and pCO_2, hypoxia and hypercarbia per- and postoperatively may induce epileptic seizures in the susceptible patient. Inspection of the patient's dentition should be carried out. Loose teeth, periodontal disease, inability to protrude the mandible, limited mobility of the temporomandibular joint and reduced flexion and extension of the cervical spine could result in difficulties in intubation. Special attention should be paid to evaluation of the psychic state of the patient. The majority of patients undergoing the operation are young people between 6 months and 15 years of age. Many of them have normal intellectual function. However, due to congenital malformations of the face, epileptic seizures or weakness of eyesight, they may be living in social isolation. The patient should be informed about the impression obtained during the preoperative examination, of the proposed method of anaesthesia and of the expected effect of premedication.

A dialogue with the patient and the parents should prepare them to withstand better the prolonged postoperative period and to gain an understanding of the stay in the intensive care unit.

Attention to patient education in the use of respiratory support is of great benefit. Most of the older patients look forward hopefully to the result of the operation. Immeasurable confidence can be created by the anaesthesiologist during this preoperative visit.

ANAESTHETIC MANAGEMENT

Premedication

This must be selected with regard to the psychic and somatic state of the patient, the intended anaesthetic techniques, the length of the operation and the anaesthesiologist's preference. We tend to give drugs with sedative or tranquilizing effects in combination with an antisialogogue.

It is difficult to recommend a particular drug, because there exist between anaesthesiologists personal preferences which should be respected.

Intubation and anaesthesia

After the mode of intubation has been decided, the correct form of tube must be selected. In older patients a tube with a high-volume, low-pressure cuff is chosen when prolonged ventilation in the intensive care unit is contemplated. We use a flexometallic, siliconized, non-kinking tube for naso- and orotracheal intubation in adults, and normal RAE tubes in children. The tube should be supported by a pharyngeal pack placed round the tube for the prevention of aspiration. It should be borne in mind that the length of operating time varies between three and twelve hours, depending on the extent of the procedure performed and the experience of the surgical team. A gastric tube should be inserted for feeding after the operation. This should be eliminated as soon as gastric motility is established. When a difficult intubation is expected and no decision for an elective tracheostomy has been made, inhalational induction is preferable to an intravenous induction.

The flexible laryngoscope may be of assistance if difficulties in intubation occur, but this requires adequate training. There is no special preference for the anaesthetic technique used for this kind of operation; the anaesthetist's experience and preference are the determining factors. However, anaesthetics preserving the cardiovascular stability and with minimal influence on cardial metabolism should be used (Wilton & Cochrane 1980). The use of barbiturates in combination with high dosage of analgesics and non-depolarizing relaxants is an alternative to neuroleptanalgesia. Volatile anaesthetics should be avoided; if inevitable, Isoflorane in concentrations as low as possible is the best choice (Artru 1987). Satisfactory ventilation during operation can be guaranteed by intermittent positive pressure ventilation (IPPV).

MONITORING

The patient's state, anticipated surgical intervention and postoperative course are the factors determining the degree of monitoring. Progress in electronics and invasive methods of monitoring only serve to complete the information obtained by careful observation and clinical judgement. The parameters monitored are:

Heart and haemodynamics (ECG, blood pressure, CVP)
Respiratory functions
Blood gas and electrolyte analysis
Urine output
Temperature
Blood loss

Heart and haemodynamics

Three important types of information from the ECG are derived: heart rate, arrhythmias and ischaemic changes.

ECG monitoring is performed with standard leads.

Arterial blood pressure monitoring using the sphygmomanometric method is not suitable for this kind of intervention. A direct intra-arterial blood pressure measurement is preferred via cannulation of the radial artery. This is also important in monitoring blood gases and in some situations for a qualitative evaluation of the blood pressure tracing, as well as facilitating sampling for haemoglobin, acid–base status, etc.

Central venous pressure monitoring. There is little ventricular disparity with normal cardiopulmonary functions, so that measurements of right atrial pressure provide sufficient information about the intravascular volume and myocardial performance.

Respiratory functions

In practice most anaesthesia-related accidents involve those of ventilation. Ventilators with incorporated controlled systems of gas flow, inspiratory pressure, minute volume, oxygen concentration and end-expiratory carbon dioxide measurements belong to the current anaesthetic equipment.

Haemoglobin, blood gas and electrolyte analysis

The determinations of pH, pCO_2, pO_2 and bicarbonate concentration are necessary in all patients ventilated during lengthy procedures. The frequency of sampling depends upon the clinical status; we carry out hourly determinations and correct any deviation immediately. Where massive fluid and blood restitutions are carried out, a knowledge of haemoglobin and plasma electrolytes (Na, K) are of value. Massive blood transfusions are not uncommonly complicated by defects in the blood-coagulating mechanism, so that an analysis of the nature of the clotting defect at the end of the operation should be performed.

Urine output

This reflects the patient's circulatory state, adequacy of renal perfusion and the status of the intravascular volume. An output of $0.5-1$ ml kg^{-1} h^{-1} is considered satisfactory.

Temperature

The continuous monitoring during anaesthesia and surgery may be of therapeutic and prognostic value. The usual method is the monitoring of rectal temperature using a thermistor probe.

Nowadays multiple sensors are used for determinations of skin temperature of various parts of the body. Thermal pads, warm blankets and blood-warming systems are accessories for the maintenance of constant temperature. Major surgical intervention of long duration is accompanied by a decrease in body temperature. A compensatory reaction is an arteriolar vasoconstriction with a redistribution of circulating blood volume and metabolic changes resulting in a decrease of pO_2 and tissue acidosis. Reperfusion with the reopening of small arteries can break this vicious circle and restore the homeostasis.

Blood loss

The anaesthesiologist should make accurate determinations of blood loss and its replacement. An underestimation aggravated by an unnoticed accumulation of blood in sterile drapes results in a rapidly diminished circulating blood volume and the initial stage of shock.

Particularly in children, conscientious estimations of blood loss and monitoring of pulse and blood pressure are mandatory. Sudden tachycardia under balanced anaesthesia and adequate analgesia should lead to suspicion of diminution of the circulating blood volume. Fluid balance should be calculated hourly during surgery and 24-hourly postoperatively, considering the restriction of fluid intake during the hours preoperatively and loss per 'perspiration insensibilis'. Two veins, cephalic and saphenous, are cannulated for separate fluid and drug administration.

DELIBERATE HYPOTENSION

The aim of the anaesthesiologist is to provide good operating conditions for the surgeon (Clement 1978). The introduction of modern anaesthetic techniques and the application of invasive monitoring of vascular parameters have extended the indications for controlled hypotension (Beare 1985). Hypotension may not reduce operative bleeding sufficiently if it is not accompanied by correct posture of the patient on the operating table and suitable changes in haemodynamics (e.g. reduction of venous tone, decrease of cardiac preload or blocking of sympathetic activity).

Controlled hypotension should not be used after a massive haemorrhage, but rather initially with the aim of reducing the blood loss and to facilitate the surgical dissection. A low rate of complications is only attainable if a high degree of proficiency using the hypotensive technique is available. It is important to stress that some hypotensive drugs, such as sodium nitroprusside, may interact with the flow : pressure ratio in the brain and an increase in intracranial pressure may follow!

Deliberate hypotension can be used if the following general conditions are fulfilled:

1. Invasive monitoring of arterial and central venous pressures is available.
2. There is no previous hypovolaemia, anaemia, respiratory or cardiac diseases.
3. Agreement exists between the surgeon and the anaesthesiologist about the indication and both have understood the implications of the technique.
4. The anaesthesiologist is well versed in the method and the pharmacological action of hypotensive drugs used.

In our clinics the drug of choice is sodium nitroprusside, owing to easy titration for circulatory control in the older patient. In children the risks of delibrate hypotension probably outweigh the benefits and therefore this is not practised routinely.

POSTOPERATIVE TREATMENT

The type and extent of surgical intervention may necessitate further management in a suitably equipped intensive care unit. If necessary, respiratory support can be provided for the first 24 hours after operation. This is required in the case of regional oedema, wound bleeding, $2\times$ exchange transfusion and hypothermia (despite all efforts).

In the case of difficult intubation or intermaxillary fixation the patient is allowed to breathe spontaneously through the tube if possible and left intubated for 48 hours or longer. In those cases extubation should be performed in the theatre with the always present tracheotomy tray and a surgeon at hand.

With this course of treatment, tracheostomy following early extubation and sudden upper airway obstruction is avoided. Controlled ventilation with adequate alveolar gas exchange plays a role in the prevention of cerebral oedema and avoids also respiratory depression due to the use of high doses of analgesics in the early postoperative period. In our clinic we attempt to extubate the patient after surgery is completed, in the presence of spontaneous breathing and full consciousness, where the blood gas values are normal and where there are no alterations in neurological score and haemodynamics. A gastric tube, often inserted before operation, controlled for the correct position, guards against aspiration through continuous suction. It serves also for gastric nutrition. High carbohydrate and high protein diets should be given as soon as gastrointestinal function resumes. No problems in nutrition are to be expected when the postoperative course is uneventful.

Prevention and therapy of cerebral oedema

The correction of craniocerebral malformations is combined with a neurosurgical intervention — open craniotomy — and some aspects relating to neuroanaesthesia should be mentioned: (1) adequate fluid, electrolytes and blood volume substitution during surgery; (2) use of osmotic agents and corticosteroids; and (3) controlled intermittent positive pressure ventilation (IPPV).

The development of cerebral oedema and an increase in intracranial pressure are serious complications, which should be prevented and therapy started as soon as possible (Jones et al 1981, Jupa-Marcinkowski 1980, 1981). Signs occurring postoperatively, such as diminished consciousness, headache and vomiting, suggest increased intracranial pressure. Prevention begins before the craniotomy has been started, with modest head-up tilt, hyperventilation (Pa $CO_2 \pm 25$–30 mm Hg) and with the use of osmotic and oncotic agents (mannitol and human albumin). Mannitol is initially given as a 20% solution of 200–1000 mg kg^{-1} over a period of 30 min. It may be repeated three times within a period of 24 hours. The osmotic effect may be increased by an administration of oncotics: salt-poor human albumin (125 ml in 20% solution). After its use the cerebral perfusion should be adequate and haemoconcentration avoided. The value of corticosteroids in reducing cerebral oedema is well known and their actions include a potentiation of osmotic agents,

decrease in vascular permeability and stimulating reabsorbtion of cerebrospinal fluid. If necessary, corticosteroids are given parenterally as dexamethasone in doses of 0.25 mg kg^{-1} per 24 hours. Controlled ventilation producing a decrease in CO_2 tension and cerebral vasoconstriction may lead to a diminution of cerebrovascular volume and intracranial pressure.

Prevention of infections

After surgery and anaesthesia, especially after neurosurgical procedures, a period of reduced immunological defence is counteracted by administration of immunoglobulin (i.m. and i.v.) (Jupa-Marcinkowski 1981) and antibiotics.

Fluid electrolytes and acid–base therapy

The basis for the appropriate management of all disturbances is a 24-hour analysis of the deficit and a replacement of fluids and electrolytes (Weil & Hennin 1978). An examination of the skin, mucous membranes and continuous monitoring of vascular parameters help in the assessment of the state of hydration.

Postoperative hypotension

This may be a symptom of a serious disorder after surgery: cardiac arrhythmia, controlled ventilation with positive-endexpiratory pressure (PEEP) and sepsis, should both be suspected as causes of observed hypotension. Hypovolaemia is the most frequent cause of hypotension. This may be due to a loss of: (1) extracellular fluid; (2) whole blood or plasma; or (3) extracellular fluid and blood.

It is well known that hypoalbuminaemia occurs after major surgical operations (Skillman & Weintraub 1975).

Table 19.1 Serious anaesthetic and operative complications

Respiratory	Difficult intubation
	Airway obstruction (blockage, kinking of tube, disconnection, misplacement, overinflation, herniation of cuff, intraoral oedema, oropharyngeal oedema)
Vascular	Massive blood loss (sagittal sinus bleeding)
Neurological	Brain oedema + increase of intracranial pressure
	Haematoma
	Sinus thrombosis
	Seizures
	Liquor leakage
Fluid, electrolytes, blood component disturbances	
Infections and sepsis	
Coagulopathy	

The decrease in total circulating albumin content can reach 30% of the total amount. Infusion of albumin solution preoperatively and in the early period after operation may preserve the stability of the intravascular volume and serum oncotic pressure and prevent the risk of pulmonary and cerebral oedema and cardiac disturbances during this period.

Table 19.1 gives a summary of serious anaesthetic and operative complications. It is beyond the scope of this chapter to give detailed information about every aspect of the anaesthesiologist's work. Without an optimally functioning intensive care unit, and without the teamwork of medical and nursing staff, there can be no excellent operative results.

REFERENCES

Artru A A 1987 New concepts concerning anesthetic effects on intracranial dynamics: cerebrospinal fluid volume and cerebral blood volume. ASA 38th Annual Refresher Course lectures, Atlanta, No. 133

Beare R 1985 Indications for hypotensive anaesthesia. In: Enderby G E H (ed) Hypotensive anaesthesia. Churchill Livingstone, Edinburgh. pp 99–108

Berry F A 1986 Anesthetic management of difficult and routine pediatric patients. New York. Churchill Livingstone, Edinburgh. p 119

Betts E K, Nicholson S C, Downes J J 1985 Monitoring the pediatric patient. In: Blitt C D (ed) Monitoring in anesthesia and critical care medicine. New York. Churchill Livingstone, Edinburgh. p 603

Bourke D L, Katz M D, Tonneson A 1985 Nebulized anesthesia for awake endotracheal intubation. Anesthesiology 63: 690

Broennle A M 1985 Preanesthetic considerations in pediatric anesthesia. International Anesthesiology Clinics 23: 1

Christianson L 1985 Anesthesia for major craniofacial operations. International Anesthesiology Clinics 23: 117

Clement A J 1978 Hypotension in anaesthesia. In: Churchill-Davidson H C (ed) A practice of anaesthesia. Lloyd-Luke, London. p 594

Cote C J 1986 Blood replacement and blood product management. In: Ryan J F, Todres I D, Cote C J, Goudsouzian N G (eds) A practice of anesthesia for infants and children. Grune & Stratton, Orlando. pp 123–132

Davies W, Munro I R 1975 The anesthetic management and intraoperative care of patients undergoing major facial osteotomies. Plastic and Reconstructive Surgery 55: 50

Deléque L, Guilbert M 1985 Management of airway problems during the repair of craniofacial anomalies in children. In: Caronni P (ed) Craniofacial surgery. Little Brown, Boston. pp 141–148

Diaz J K, Henling C E 1982 Pneumoperitoneum and cardiac arrest during craniofacial reconstruction. Anesthesia and Analgesia 61: 146

Ferguson D J M, Barker J, Jackson I T 1983 Anesthesia for craniofacial osteotomies. Annals of Plastic Surgery 10: 333

Fromme G A, MacKenzie D O, Gould A B Jr, Lund B A 1984 Does controlled hypotension really improve quality of the surgical field? Anesthesiology 61: A42

Furman E B, Roman D G, Lemmer L A S et al 1975 Specific therapy in water, electrolyte, and blood volume replacement during pediatric surgery. Anesthesiology 42: 187

Handler S D et al 1978 Airway management in the repair of craniofacial defects. Cleft Palate Journal 16: 16–23

Handler S D 1985 Upper airway obstruction in craniofacial anomalies: diagnosis and management. Birth Defects 21: 15

Handler S D, Beaugard M E, Whitaker L A et al 1979 Airway management in craniofacial repair. Cleft Palate Journal 16: 16

Handler S D, Keon T P 1983 Difficult laryngoscopy/intubation. The child with mandibular hypoplasia. Annals of Otology, Rhinology and Laryngology 92: 401

Holliday M A, Segar W E 1957 The maintenance need for water in parental fluid therapy. Pediatrics 19: 823

Jones R F C, Dorsch N W C, Silverberg G D et al 1981 Pathophysiology and management of raised intracranial pressure. Anaesthesia and Intensive Care 9: 336–351

Jupa-Marcinkowski V 1980 Use of human albumin in neurosurgery. In: Hennesen W (ed) Developments in biological standardization, vol 48. Karger, Basel. p 62

Jupa-Marcinkowski V, Lachitjaran E G, Reusen E 1981 The prophylactic use of immunoglobulins in prevention of infections in neurosurgical patients. In: Brükner J B (ed) Proceedings Zentral European Anaesthesie Kongress, Berlin

Jupa-Marcinkowski V 1981 Osmotic and oncotic therapy in neurosurgical practice. In: De Vlieger M, de Lange S A, Beks J W F (eds) Brain oedema. Wiley, New York. 155

Pagar D M, Kupperman A W, Stern M S 1978 Cutting of nasoendotracheal tube. An unusual complication of maxillary osteotomies. Journal of Oral Surgery 36: 314

Patel C, Cotten S, Turndorf H 1980 Partial severance of an oronasotracheal tube during a Le Fort I procedure. Anesthesiology 53: 357

Scholtes J L, Thauvoy C, Moulin D et al 1985 Craniofacial synostosis: anesthetic management and perioperative management. Acta Anaesthesiologica Belgica 3: 176

Skillman J J, Weintraub R M 1975 Hypotension. In: Skillmann J J (ed) Intensive care. Little, Brown, Boston. p 495

Sklar G S, King B D: Endotracheal intubation and Treacher Collins syndrome. Anesthesiology 44: 247

Stark D C (ed) 1974 Practical points in anaesthesiology, 1st edn. Huber, Bern

Vries J K, Bechler D P, Young H F 1973 A subarachnoid screw for monitoring intracranial pressure. Technical note. Journal of Neurosurgery 39: 416

Waters D J 1963 Guided blind endotracheal intubation. Anaesthesia 18: 158

Weil M H, Hennin G R J (ed) 1978 Handbook of critical care medicine, 1st edn. Symposia Specialists, Miami

Winn H R, Jane J A 1987 Chronic measurement of intracranial pressure. Review of 142 cases. Submitted for publication

Whitaker L A, Broennle A M, Kerr L P et al 1980 Improvements in craniofacial reconstruction. Methods evolved in 235 consecutive patients. Plastic and Reconstructive Surgery 65: 561

Whitaker L A, Munro I R, Salyer K E et al 1979 Combined report of problems and complications in 793 craniofacial operations. Plastic and Reconstructive Surgery 48: 533

Wilton T N P, Cochrane D F 1980 Anaesthesia for plastic and facio-maxillary surgery. In: Gray T C, Nunn J F, Utting J E (eds) General anaesthesia. Butterworth, London. p 1267

20. Surgery

M. Stricker, J. Van der Meulen, B. Raphael, R. Mazzola

PRINCIPLES

The correction of craniofacial malformations is defined by the following characteristics:

it is a surgical discipline;
it has the craniofacial area as its domain;
it is devoted to the treatment of congenital anomalies.

Surgical discipline

The techniques employed in craniofacial surgery must follow the essentials common to all surgical disciplines: asepsis, haemostasis and gentle tissue manipulation. In addition the surgeon must be extremely painstaking and vigilant during long periods in the operating theatre.

Craniofacial topography

General surgical principles are adapted to the specific requirements of the craniofacial territory. The surgery should be conducted:

extradurally in the cranial cavity;
extraperiosteally in the orbital and facial areas;
extramucosally in the nasal fossae and accessory air sinuses;
extraolfactory.

The close confines in which the surgeons are working therefore calls for a team whose thoughts and actions are well integrated. The proximity of the cranial and facial zones and the resultant continuity of the surgical fields is a matter of concern to the neurosurgeon who is anxious to safeguard the contents of the cranium against contamination.

Malformative aetiology

The nature of this type of surgery also presents the surgeon with a number of specific problems.

THE COMPLEXITY OF THE MALFORMATION

This aspect requires a thorough knowledge of the anatomy, a precise analysis of the condition and systematic surgical planning. The goal is to achieve harmony by reconstruction of elements that are defective or even completely absent and by mobilization of dystopic parts.

THE PLURALITY OF TISSUE INVOLVEMENT

Only rarely is the skeleton alone deficient; most frequently the soft parts are affected as well, whether these be the muscles, the skin, the nerves, the mucosa, or even the periosteum, which forms the bond between the bone and its environment. This tissue plurality varies with the topography and differentiation between centrofacial and laterofacial involvement is therefore necessary. In everyday life it is the central facial area which is exposed to view and which is thus the most important.

THE SUSCEPTIBILITY OF THE RECONSTRUCTED PARTS FOR ADVERSELY ACTING FACTORS

Morphological correction of the malformation is indeed rarely definitive. The area involved remains subject to the quirks of individual growth and the contracting qualities of scar tissue. The time element plays an important role and craniofacial surgery is in fact four-dimensional surgery.

THE TEAM

Craniofacial surgery is by definition teamwork. It is more than mere collaboration for it presupposes a common line of thought and action which links the two disciplines of neurosurgery and facial surgery.

This concept of teamwork is not confined to the operative treatment itself but should begin immediately after birth as a dialogue with the paediatrician, continuing throughout the phase of special examination carried out by facial specialists, and reaching its climax during the treatment, which is itself the result of collaboration between the anaesthetist, the neurosurgeon, the facial surgeon and the orthodontist.

The assistance of diverse medical specialists is obviously beneficial but one must not forget that each tends to be an individualist by nature. Moreover, their medical backgrounds may lead them to place different emphasis on each problem and finally cooperation between specialists is logistically difficult without combined meetings of those involved. This does not imply that decisions must be collective, since the final responsibility should ideally rest with one surgeon only.

Centres for craniofacial surgery

Craniofacial surgery should only be undertaken at a limited number of special centres where a considerable number of patients are seen. The surgeons who perform this kind of surgery should be well versed in both skeletal surgery and the surgery of soft tissues. This means that training facilities should also be available. In craniofacial surgery, just as in any other type of surgery, two years of general surgery is a minimum requirement, and this should preferably include some orthopaedic experience. This basic surgical exposure must be complemented by apprenticeships in neurosurgery and facial surgery. The latter should incorporate stages in both maxillofacial surgery, with its systematic and analytical approach to the many occlusal problems, and in plastic surgery, where accent is put upon the repair and reconstruction of soft tissues. Such a training should remove the current distinction between those craniofacial surgeons who are 'soft-tissue technicians', ill at ease when dealing with the skeleton and with virtually no knowledge of occlusal problems, and those who are maxillofacial specialists skilled in the correction of malocclusion and maxillary surgery but unused to dealing with the soft tissues.

Preparation

The preparation of the operating field involves three elements:

the skin, a considerable area of which is hair-bearing;
the external orifices, which are easily accessible;
the internal cavities, in particular the nasopharynx.

The Skin

The bitemporal route for the approach to the upper areas is situated within the hair-bearing zone and this calls for special care. Some surgeons do not shave the scalp but are content to rely on a preoperative shampoo with disinfection of the scalp.

The hair is then tied up in very tight plaits before the operation is begun. However, most surgeons prefer to have the scalp shaved on the morning of the operation in the hope that the re-emergence of bacteria contained in the depths of the hair follicles will be prevented. The residual portion of the craniofacial skin must also be subjected to scrupulous disinfection.

The external orifices

These include the nasal vestibules, external auditory meati and buccal vestibule, all of which are cleaned at the same time. It goes without saying that good dental hygiene is a prerequisite and carious deciduous teeth should also be properly treated before surgery.

The internal cavities

These are not readily accessible for direct aseptic preparation and an attempt should be made to sterilize them with antibiotics.

Waldeyer's ring constitutes an additional source of bacterial infection in the nasopharynx. Lavage of the nasal cavities is useful. Adenoidectomy or tonsillectomy may sometimes be indicated.

Currently prophylactic antibiotics are administered in one single loading dose whilst the choice of antibiotic is influenced by the operative site and on occasions an antibiogram. There is in effect a bacteriological 'map' of the nose and nasopharynx which assists in the forecasting of the risks of infection (Fig. 20.1). Prophylaxis is mainly aimed against anaerobic organisms and the antibiogram usually gives information on the sources of infection one can expect in the postoperative phase.

Basic techniques

Craniofacial surgery had its origins in the critical reflection of surgeons confronted with the correction of facial trauma in wartime. In these traumas parts of the facial skeleton were frequently displaced in a posterior direction. It appeared therefore possible to bring these bony units forward by a surgical procedure. Not surprisingly Gillies & Harrison (1950) were the first to attempt an osteotomy of the middle third of the face.

The surgical correction of the soft tissues and the skeleton differs to some extent. The bony corrections are precise and the fragments readily manipulated so that the end result is predictable. Soft tissue surgery on the other hand is less precise and plans must be frequently modified and adapted to suit each individual case.

ROUTES OF APPROACH

There are of two types of approach; the cutaneous and the mucosal (Fig. 20.2).

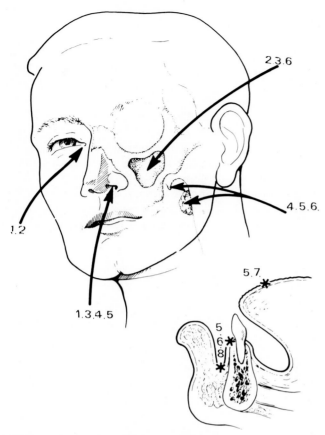

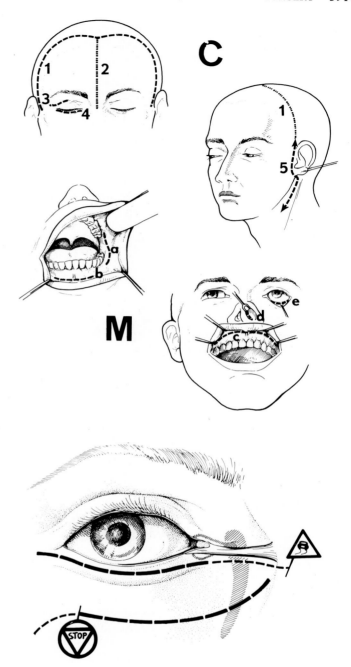

Fig. 20.1 The bacteriological map. (1) Staphylococci, (2) *Haemophilus*, (3) *Streptococcus pneumoniae*, (4) *Neisseria* (meningococcus, etc.), (5) streptococci, (6) anaerobes, (7) veillonellae, (8) *Actinomyces*.

Cutaneous approaches

THE CORONAL ROUTE

The Cairns–Unterberger bitemporal coronal approach, has been described by Unterberger to give access to the frontal sinus. This technique has long been known to neurosurgeons and the bilateral frontal variation is used by them for access to the anterior cranial fossa.

The incision runs across the scalp posterior to the anterior hair margin (Fig. 20.2); as a rule it begins just above the ears but can be extended inferiorly, in the preauricular and retromandibular areas for extensive lateral approaches to the face. Sometimes the incision is made more posteriorly when access to the region of the lambda is required. It is prudent to preserve the superficial temporal artery in order to keep one's options open.

As a preliminary, xylocaine combined with a vasoconstrictor is injected and some minutes later the skin incision is made and carried down to the epicranium.

Following haemostasis, towels are clipped to the wound margins, and the frontal flap is reflected forward, keeping the plane of dissection superficial to the epicranium. The dissection is carried out with a scalpel as far as the supraor-

Fig. 20.2 Routes of approach. C = cutaneous: (1) coronal (Cairns–Unterberger), (2) mediofrontal extension, (3) superior palpebral, (4) inferior palpebral, (5) lateral extension. M = mucosal: (a) inferior lateral, (b) inferior anterior, (c) superior vestibular, (d) unilateral interseptocolumellar, (e) conjunctival.

bital ridge. Once this level is reached, the epicranium is incised and the flap is raised in the subperiosteal plane.

At this stage, it is possible to continue the dissection further in three directions: the cranial, the midfacial and the lateral facial area.

In the cranial area, the frontal flap is designed either as a whole or pedicled on one of the temporal arteries.

In the midfacial area, the orbital periosteum is freed from the orbital rim: resistance is met at three points of attachment: along the frontomalar suture, at the emergence of the supraorbital nerve and at the pulley of the superior oblique muscle. Occasionally it is necessary to perform an osteotomy of the supraorbital margin in order to free the nerve and keep its attachment to the flap intact. Once these three points of attachment have been freed the orbit can be easily cleared in its upper half and the dissection can be continued towards the middle zone, where there is also firm attachment of the periosteum along the frontonasal suture. The skin of the nose and periosteum is dissected free as far as the upper margin of the pyriform aperture and the medial canthal region exposed by detaching the medial canthal ligament. The lacrimal fossa is exposed, and the lacrimal sac is displaced downwards and forwards so as to bypass it and reach the orbital floor.

It may be necessary at this stage to control bleeding from the anterior ethmoidal artery. Periosteal elevation is carried out simultaneously behind and in front of the lacrimal ducts so that by freeing them circumferentially they are better protected. The upper part of the canine fossa is thus easily reached.

In the lateral facial area the temporal muscle is detached from the semicircular line. Following periosteal incision on the lateral orbital wall and elevation of the periosteum from the lateral orbital wall, the muscle is freed from the temporal fossa, the ascending ramus of the malar bone and the orbit as far as the sphenomaxillary fissure and then turned downwards. Thus the edge of the malar bone is reached and the lateral plane of dissection 'linked up' with the area dissected in front of the inferior orbital margin. The upper edge of the zygomatic arch is also cleared of periosteum as a prelude to freeing the temporalis muscle. The muscle is thus largely separated from the soft parts and one is able to transpose it at will. It is useful to divide the anterior aponeurotic reflection extensively.

It will be noted that this approach in itself affords extremely wide access, both to the cranium and facial skeleton and that the other incisions are indicated only as supplementary measures.

The periosteal dissection is carried as low down on the face as possible and the periosteal layer is widely released by means of multiple vertical incisions. These incisions are situated at the midline on the dorsum nasi, and laterally over each ascending ramus of the malar bone. The periorbital ring is interrupted by complementary parallel incisions. Closure of the scalp incision is best performed by a continuous suture, leaving a drain in the temporal fossa. No suction is required if the cranium has not been opened. An extradural suction drain is, however, indicated after a subfrontal approach. Postoperatively there is considerable oedema which may persist for a week and extend to the lower part of the face. In particular, the eyelids become very swollen.

THE LATERAL ROUTE

This approach, which may or may not be used in conjunction with an extension of the previous technique, corresponds essentially to the classical curved preauricular bayonet incision described by Redon and extends beyond the mandible along the upper cervical crease (Fig. 20.2).

The technique requires preliminary exposure of the facial nerve trunk with dissection of its branches. It is therefore necessary to reflect the skin flap and carry out a preliminary parotidectomy so that wide access to the temporomandibular region can be gained.

Following this approach closure is by suture in two layers, with suction drainage. Conservation of the superficial preparotid fascia is sufficient to maintain the natural contour.

THE PALPEBRAL ROUTE

This provides an alternative to the transconjunctival route for access to the orbital floor. The localization of the incision in the lower lid may be superior, intermediate and inferior.

The superior incision is made in the subciliary line (Fig. 20.2). The skin is separated from the underlying muscle in order to reach the orbital margin via the muscular periphery. It is also possible to carry out a dissection that is primarily retromuscular, similar to that used for blepharoplasty.

The intermediate incision is made in the palpebral plane and continued directly between the two parts of the muscle.

The inferior incision is made at the transition of the eyelid and the cheek (Fig. 20.2).

Each incision has its disadvantages: lateral extension of the inferior incision may result in the formation of an ugly scar. Medial extension of the superior incision puts the integrity of the lacrimal system at risk (Fig. 20.2).

Whatever the cutaneous incision, the muscle dissection leads to the orbital margin. The orbital periosteum is incised, and then elevated along the orbital floor above and towards the infraorbital nerve below. The periphery of the orbit is thus completely freed.

THE MEDIO-FRONTONASAL ROUTE

This incision, developed by Cairns, is made vertically along the midline to the tip of the nose, permitting access to the nasal pyramid as a complement to the coronal approach, while also facilitating interorbital cutaneous resection during the preparation of a mediofrontal flap in nasal reconstruction (Fig. 20.2).

If this technique is employed, inferior palpebral access is unnecessary.

Closure is classically in two layers; some recommend a

Z-plasty at the root of the nose in order to achieve a better frontonasal angle.

Mucosal approaches

THE CONJUNCTIVAL ROUTE

Initially devised by Bourguet (1936), this technique has been given prominence by Tessier (1972); the incision is in the lower fornix, following which two alternative techniques are available, either pre- or postseptal (Fig. 20.2). By far the best route is the preseptal, which prevents the loss of fat.

Dissection of the septum leads to the orbital margin, which is stripped of periosteum in the usual way. Instrumental manipulation is more restricted if this approach is used and there is always the risk that the eyelid will be torn.

Repair must be meticulous and in particular vertical telescoping of the septum must be avoided, as this displaces the eyelid downwards. The conjunctiva is closed with a continuous absorbable suture.

THE NASAL ROUTE

This is essentially a unilateral interseptocolumellar incision in conformity with the principles of extramucous rhinoplasty (Fig. 20.3). It frees the internal lining of the nose, thereby reducing the risks of mucosal defect which carries with it the possibility of infection of the bone.

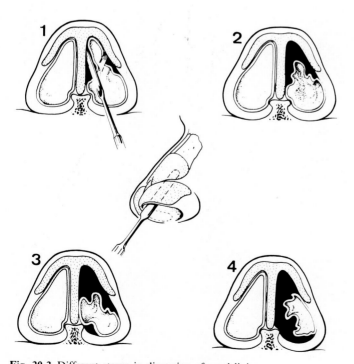

Fig. 20.3 Different stages in dissection of nasal lining.

THE BUCCAL ROUTE

Dependent on the skeletal part to be approached, the maxilla, the mandible or the pterygomaxillary junction, three incisions may be distinguished: the superior vestibular, the inferior vestibular and the palatine incisions.

The superior vestibular incision

The superior vestibular incision (Fig. 20.2) is made above the mucosal reflection straight down to the bone. It can extend from one molar region to the other with a midline deviation at the level of the upper labial frenulum. The exposure of the facial skeleton is carried upwards as far as the orbital margin, laterally as far as the anterior attachment of the masseter, and medially along the periphery of the pyriform aperture. Laterally the dissection is frequently extended as close to the bone as possible in the direction of the pterygomaxillary area. Medially it may expose the floors of the nasal fossae to allow division of the septum with a guided chisel.

The inferior vestibular incision

The inferior vestibular incision consists of one anterior and two lateral parts (Fig. 20.2). The anterior incision should only be made with full appreciation of the risk involved. The mucosa in this area is extremely fragile, threatening the impermeability of the suture line and thus the protection of the bony structures. The danger of disruption is even further increased by the formation of oedema and the pull of gravity. As an intact mucosa is the only guarantee of impermeability, precautions must be taken to ensure its integrity. Thus a mandibular border that is sufficiently wide and thick to permit suture in two layers without tension should be preserved and one should not make a continuous incision from one side to the other. The three usual sites of incision for the performance of a sagittal osteotomy and a genioplasty are the right and left lateral incisions and the medial incision (Fig. 20.2).

The lateral incisions are made as a shallow elongated S, curving inwards, over the medial aspect of the ascending ramus, skirting the last molar and curving outwards in the posterior part of the sulcus. Bone is reached at the lower part of the molar area immediately under the mucosa. Periosteal elevation is carried out from below upwards on the outer aspect of the ascending ramus, following which the anterior border and the inner aspect above the lingula are freed. Some recommend extensive liberation of the muscular attachments of the masseter, and even those of the internal pterygoid, but these manoeuvres do not seem justified.

The medial incision is made on the labial aspect of the inferior sulcus. It extends laterally as far as the second premolar, and ends by curving upwards, thus circumventing the emergent mental nerve. In certain cases it may prove useful either to open the mandibular canal in order to transpose the nerve or to lengthen the extraosseous portion of the nerve by freeing the periosteum and by neurolysis in the lip. If by misfortune the nerve should be divided, it should be repaired by immediate nerve suture. Because of the problems created by gravity and the permanent presence of saliva, the greatest care must be taken in repair of the operation wound. Support of the soft parts must be ensured in the postoperative period by means of an elastic chin-guard.

The palatine incision

This is made over the tuberosity of the maxilla. It affords direct access to the pterygomaxillary region, provided the head can be turned to one side.

SKELETON

Osteotomies

Osteotomies represent deliberate osseous sections with a therapeutic goal. They permit the displacement of a bone or part of it. The bones may be cut with oscillating and reciprocating saws, chisels and osteotomes. The sections are made according to lines corresponding to those of craniofacial fractures.

An osteotomy may serve a dual purpose. It can be used to open a cavity, such as the cranium, the orbit or the maxillary sinus; these access-providing osteotomies are of a temporary nature. It may also be used to correct an anomaly of the craniofacial skeleton by changing its contour. The effect of these contour-correcting osteotomies is then of a permanent nature.

Direct or indirect fixation is important for stabilization of the mobilized portions so that bony union will take place. Direct fixation is the procedure of choice and it is obtained by means of osteosynthesis with or without bone-grafting. Indirect fixation may be indicated in some cases and is then achieved through intermaxillary immobilization or external traction.

ACCESS-PROVIDING OSTEOTOMIES (TEMPORARY)

Craniotomy

Trepanation of a skull by the most direct route, the cranial vault, is an ancient practice, whether for ritual purposes or for the treatment of fractures, etc. Nowadays trepanation is the overture for a more extensive access-providing osteotomy, such as the temporary removal of a bony plate. This plate, usually rectangular, may be pedicled on the homolateral temporalis muscle in order to preserve its blood supply via the pericranium, while remaining an

integral part of the outer table. The risk of bone resorption and sequestration can thus be avoided. More frequently the plate is used as a bone graft with its pericranium attached.

Burr holes are first made to allow the passage of a Gigli saw or an oscillating motor-driven saw. The bone is then removed by the neurosurgeon, who is always confronted by two opposing considerations: the need to limit the number of burr holes, which may impair the frontal contours, and the desire to maintain the integrity of the dural sac. The dura mater is strongly adherent to bone in certain areas, such as at the sutures, in the midline where the superior sagittal sinus is at risk, and over and between bony irregularities of the inner table.

It is essential to avoid any breach of the dura. Should one occur it must be sutured, sometimes with the reinforcement of a pericranial patch. Every dural breach should be covered with a non-interrupted bony surface,

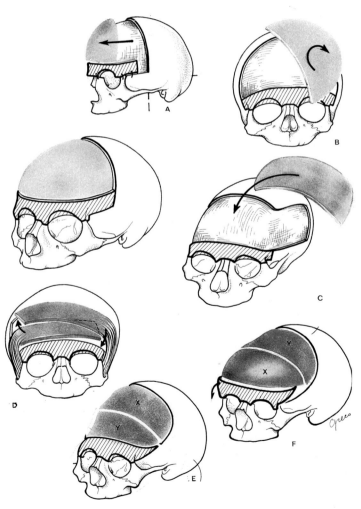

Fig. 20.4 Global forehead remodelling by means of various techniques: (a) advancement of frontal plate; (b) rotation of frontoparietal plate; (c) transposition of parietal plate; (d) transposition of frontal plates (pedicled); (e, f) transposition of frontal plates (free).

otherwise the repair may be inadequate, as may occur in the growing skull fracture in childhood.

Detachment of the dura mater commences at the surface exposed by the craniotomy and is carried on progressively. This is easy over the orbital eminences, difficult in the region of the crista galli, the foramen caecum and the margins of the cribriform plate of the ethmoid, and occasionally awkward over the lesser wing of the sphenoid. Exposure of the anterior fossa is thus completed. In the middle fossa, where the temporal lobe is at risk, some limitation of dural stripping is usually necessary.

In some malformations the middle fossa may almost overlap the orbitomeatal plane in front because of the sagittal shortness of the temporal fossa and the obliquity of the wings of the sphenoid.

Certain mishaps may occur: a dural breach or tear; injury to the emissary veins or superior sagittal sinus (a most unfortunate eventuality) or contusion of the cerebral cortex. An intradural approach is rarely indicated.

Closure of the craniotomy is effected by direct fixation.

Suction drainage is usually applied to prevent the accumulation of fluid and thus enhance healing.

Orbitomaxillotomy

Temporary displacement of part of the maxilla or orbit is a very old practice (Jules Boeckel of Strasbourg). The technique is used to provide access to the deep craniofacial region in case of tumours or traumas and sometimes in cases of meningoencephalocele, when displacement of the superior orbital rim — orbitotomy — may be needed.

CONTOUR-CORRECTING OSTEOTOMIES (PERMANENT)

These osteotomies are made along lines initially defined by the topography of the malformation and the pattern of craniofacial sutures or advocated by different surgeons (e.g. Tessier 1967, 1971, 1972, Converse 1970, 1974). The cuts can be modified as regards site and number in accord-

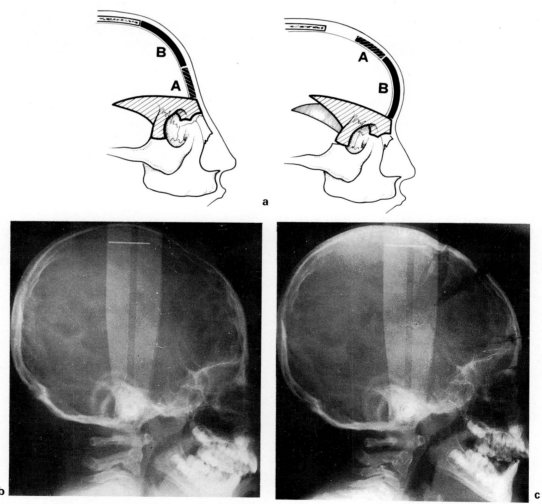

Fig. 20.5 Global forehead remodelling by transposition of frontal plates in combination with Marchac procedure.

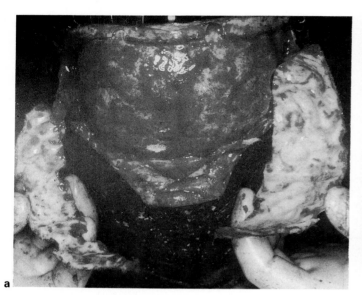
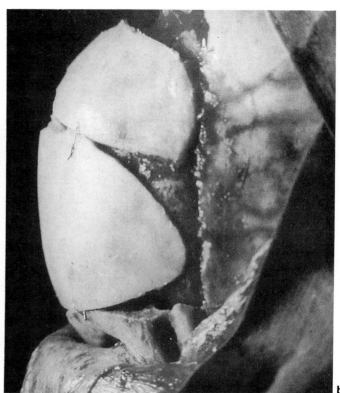

Fig. 20.6 Global forehead remodelling. Peroperative view of: (a) transposition of frontal plates (pedicled); (b) transposition of frontal plates (free).

ance with the type of malformation to constitute a 'free-style' osteotomy.

The cranial vault

Bone segments may be raised in every part of the cranial vault: unilateral frontal, bilateral frontal, temporal, parietal or parietotemporal. Every kind of mobilization in every spacial direction is thus permitted, including transposition, rotation, turning and reversal (Figs. 20.4–20.8). These techniques make it possible to replace a deformed portion of the vault with one of normal curvature.

The pedicled flap technique, readily performed to provide access, is not practicable for contour correction, with the sole exception of the frontal transposition procedure of Montaut & Stricker (1977). Correction of vault anomalies is completed by the use of split skull grafts for closure of remaining defects or by the more delicate technique of remodelling the inner table to restore contour deficiencies in a particular segment. This remodelling procedure by means of a saw must involve the whole length of the concavity in order to prevent a fracture of the outer table.

The orbito-nasofrontal band

The osteotomy requires two preliminary steps: the exposure of the skeleton through a coronal incision; and the mobilization of a bony segment in the cranial vault. After removal of the segment, the osteotomy begins outside the frontomalar junction. The original technique splits the lateral orbital wall vertically, but this line of section, whether inside or behind the pterion, has now been abandoned in favour of an osteotomy around the pterion in the form of a tongue in groove, a spur or a Z-plasty through the frontosphenoidal region (Fig. 20.9). These variations provide more stability and make the interposition of a bone graft unnecessary.

After traversing the smaller wing of the sphenoid, the cut continues across the orbital roof, in its posterior third. It then curves forward in order to avoid the olfactory groove and passes the midline at the level of the foramen caecum. The osteotomy is completed by a horizontal nasofrontal section which is extended in the medial orbital walls to join the cut in the orbital roof.

During mobilization of the band one meets with two difficulties (Fig. 20.10): laterally, in the orbital pillar, which is freed with a chisel while protecting the temporal lobe; and medially, in the thick nasion, where the chisel must avoid the olfactory tracts and respect the integrity of the nasal lining.

After mobilization of the band, it is frequently necessary to remove the lesser wing of the sphenoid and the base of the pterion with a gouge because of the acute inclination

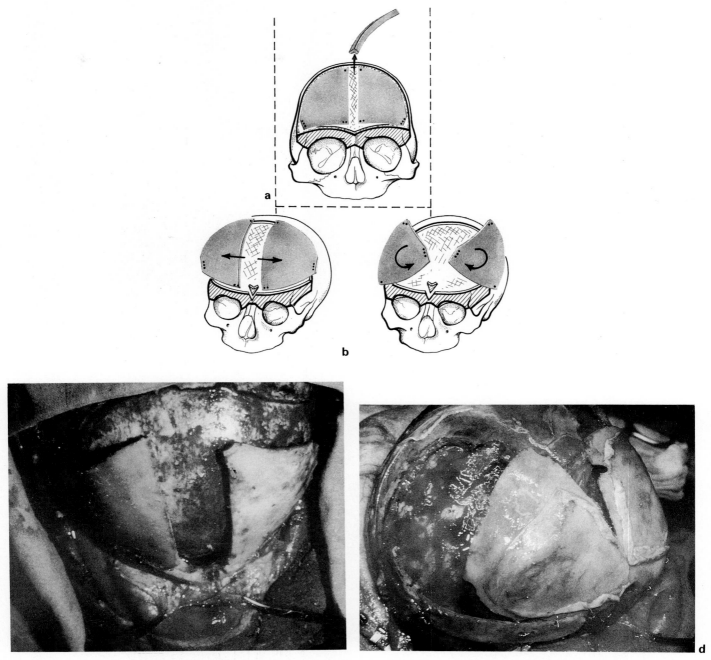

Fig. 20.7 Segmental forehead remodelling (bilateral) by: (a) lateral displacement of frontal plates; (b) rotation of frontal plates; (c, d) peroperative views.

of the orbital roof and the shallowness of the temporal fossae (Fig. 20.11).

The orbito-nasofrontal osteotomy permits much freedom in the design of the band. It may be symmetrical or asymmetrical. The superior rim of the orbit may be removed and substituted by a graft and the same may be done with the inferior part of the frontal plate. The band is moved forward and also rotated downwards. It may be necessary to split and remodel it. A median split will serve to place its lateral part forwards and downwards, whilst multiple cuts allow correction of curvatures (Fig. 20.12).

Orbital osteotomies

In order to obtain complete exposure of the orbit, several routes are required. The coronal route gives access to almost all of the orbital contours but the safety and precision of the procedure as to the mobilization of the

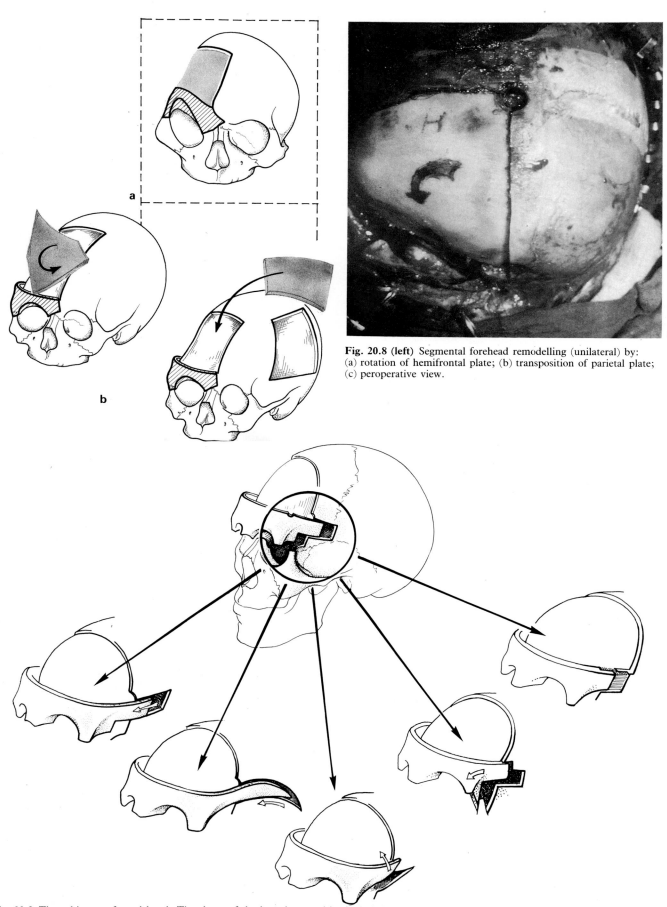

Fig. 20.8 (left) Segmental forehead remodelling (unilateral) by: (a) rotation of hemifrontal plate; (b) transposition of parietal plate; (c) peroperative view.

Fig. 20.9 The orbito-nasofrontal band. The shape of the lateral extremities is designed in accordance with the direction into which the band is to be moved.

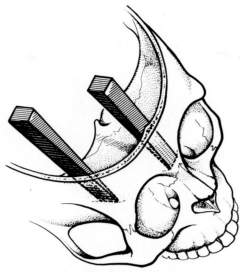

Fig. 20.10 The two areas of resistance in the mobilization of the orbito-nasofrontal band: (a) laterally in the pterion; (b) medially in the nasion.

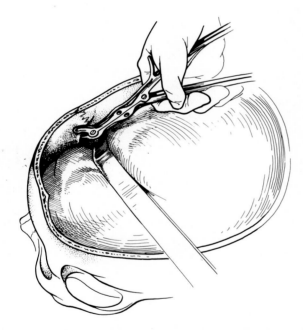

Fig. 20.11 Removal of the external part of the lesser wing of the sphenoid by means of a gouge.

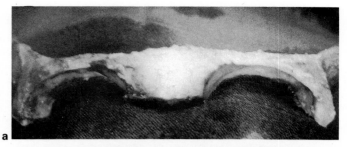
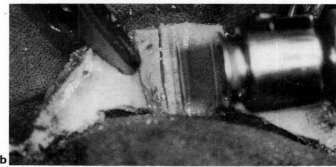
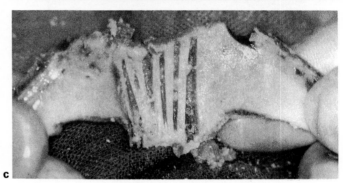

Fig. 20.12 Remodelling of orbito-nasofrontal band by multiple corticotomies of its interior aspect.

inferior part are not guaranteed. A direct route through the lower eyelid is ordinarily used in conjunction, except when the procedure involves a medial cutaneous interorbital approach. Exposure of the orbit is facilitated by detachment of the medial canthal tendon. An osteotomy of the orbit involves its anterior ring (the movable orbit or 'orbite utile of Tessier'). This ring can be divided into several segments, which can be moved separately or in combination with each other.

Total osteotomy (Fig. 20.13). The orbits are mobilized by osteotomies which are made at two different levels: one anteriorly around the orbital rim and one more posteriorly inside the orbital cavity.

At the anterior level, a horizontal osteotomy is made in the supraorbital region. The cut runs parallel to the inferior edge of the frontal defect and extends somewhat more laterally. A bar is thus preserved which later serves as line of reference and can also be used in fixation for the transposed orbit. A vertical cut is made down the malar bone to a point slightly below the level of the infraorbital foramen. From this point a horizontal incision is continued in the maxillary body towards and into the pyriform aperture, below the inferior concha. The infraorbital nerve may have to be liberated when the incision is made at a more superior level, to avoid dental buds. A second vertical cut through the nasal roof and through the frontal sinus completes the osteotomy at the anterior level.

At the posterior level the movable orbit is mobilized by

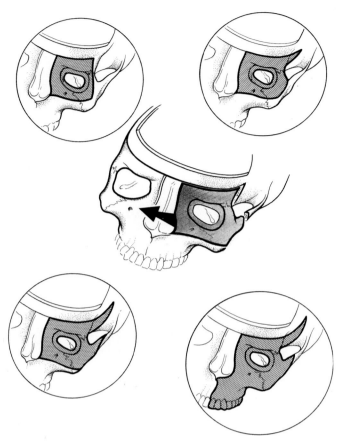

Fig. 20.13 Total orbital osteotomy and variants.

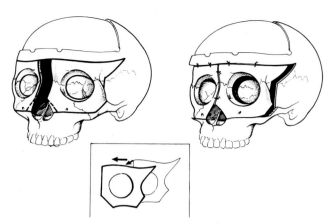

Fig. 20.14 Medialization of the two orbits using the original Tessier procedure.

a circular osteotomy, which starts in the inferior orbital fissure and is carried up and into the anterior cranial fossa. At the pterion a bifurcation is formed into an external cut which joins with the lateral extension of the supraorbital osteotomy and an internal cut which runs across the orbital roof and continues downwards in the medial wall. This part of the osteotomy is completed by a cut which traverses the orbital floor behind the lacrimal fossa and below the infraorbital nerve to join the inferior infraorbital fissure.

To avoid pitfalls special attention should be paid to the mobilization and translation of the orbit.

Mobilization — The orbital osteotomy may meet some resistance in two areas: laterally in the zygoma, where the cut is completed by chiselling obliquely in the direction of the temporal fossa, and medially in the maxillocanine pillar.

Translation — Once freed, the orbital framework may be moved in the required direction. In the majority of cases this is medially (Fig. 20.14). The integrity of the facial skeleton, however, shows three dimensions and it should thus be realized that medial dislocation and correction of the position of the orbital aperture is not so much obtained by a linear as by a rotatory movement along a curved line defined by the cranial contour. The nature of

this movement depends on the degree to which the medial walls of the orbit can be displaced medially. If these walls can be moved over the same distance, the orbital transposition will consist of a single rotatory movement around an imaginary craniocaudal axis, which corresponds to the line of osteotomy through these walls. The movement will inevitably result in an anterior projection of the lateral wall. The orbit is thus enlarged, predisposing to enophthalmus, and the temporal fossa is deepened, creating a depression (hourglass deformity).

Orbital transposition becomes more complex when the anteroposterior divergence of the orbits is associated with caudocranial divergence. In these patients, the superior interorbital distance is greater than the inferior interorbital distance, and orbital approximation will be associated with a second rotatory movement around an anteroposterior axis through the medial wall of the maxillary sinus. The latter movement will obviously be followed by a cranial displacement of the lateral wall of the orbit and Tessier (1971, 1972) therefore has very wisely suggested the preservation of a frontal crown as a safeguard against the projection of the orbital frames.

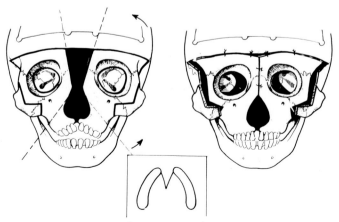

Fig. 20.15 Medialization of the two orbits using the 'medial faciotomy' procedure (Van der Meulen).

Variants. Several modifications have been described for the osteotomy of the lateral wall (Fig. 20.13).

It may split the orbital rim over its whole length in an interior and exterior section, thus limiting displacement of the movable orbit.

It may split the lateral wall partially in its inferior part, thus facilitating the procedure and improving stability, but also introducing a discrepancy between the superior and inferior relief.

It may include a large sphenofrontal spur, making translation of the orbital block more accurate while increasing its stability.

The orbits can also be moved in combination with the maxilla. Pterygomaxillary disjunction and a midpalatal osteotomy are then required for mobilization (Figs. 20.13, 20.15).

Partial osteotomy (Fig. 20.16). The orbit can be divided into four segments: mediofrontal, laterofrontal, maxillary and malar. The term 'one-quadrant' osteotomy is applied when one of these fragments is mobilized. A U-osteotomy or two-quadrant osteotomy may be used when two adjacent quadrants are moved as one unit. Four different U-osteotomies may thus be distinguished: cranial or

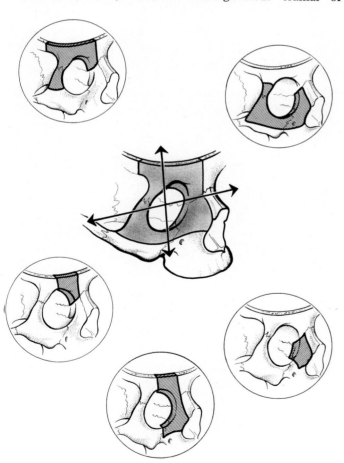

Fig. 20.16 The four segments of the orbit and the different types of partial orbital osteotomies.

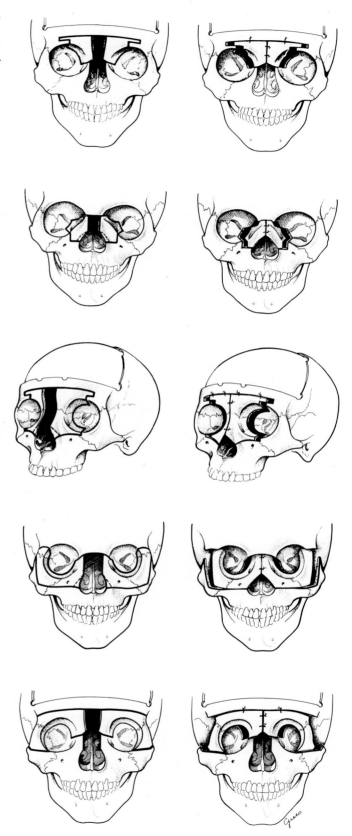

Fig. 20.17 Reduction of the interorbital distance using various types of partial orbital osteotomies.

superior, subcranial or inferior, nasal or medial and temporal or lateral.

Subtotal osteotomies may also be designed as C-osteotomies and in fact in every conceivable way, provided of course that the principles of craniofacial surgery are respected and the envisaged correction achieved (Fig. 20.17).

Interorbital osteotomy (Fig. 20.18)

Movement of the orbits towards the midline requires the resection of a rectangular segment of bone in the fronto-nasal area. The size of this segment is first measured and then delineated by two horizontal and vertical cuts.

The superior horizontal cut is made in continuity with the supraorbital osteotomy. An inferior horizontal dissection is carried out between the border of the nasal bones and the triangular cartilages. It serves to separate the mucosa from the nasal roof, taking care to preserve the olfactory nerves.

The vertical osteotomies pass through the frontal sinus in their upper part to enter the anterior cranial fossa (Fig. 20.19). In their lower part they cut through the nasal roof and the ethmoidal sinus.

The nasal roof is removed, exposing and preserving the mucous domes. The central bony block can then be mobilized by an incision through the nasal septum and through the floor of the anterior cranial fossa at the site of the frontoethmoidal junction.

The exenteration of the interorbital region is completed by the resection of the deformed part of the septum and of the ethmoidal sinus. The integrity of the olfactory nerves is preserved.

Orbito-nasomaxillary osteotomy (Le Fort III)

The osteotomy (Fig. 20.20) separates the facial bones from the cranium and has therefore been named after the Le Fort III fracture. The coronal incision is the principal route of access. Additional routes are provided by bilateral inferior palpebral and interseptocolumellar incisions. Submucous dissection in the nose via the interseptocolumellar incision is necessary to protect against septic contamination. The dissections expose the malar bones, the orbits and the nasal roof. Detachment of the medial canthal tendon may therefore be required. Access to the pterygomaxillary junction may be obtained via vestibular or palatine incisions. The lateral wall of the orbit is divided transversely at the frontomalar suture line. Posteriorly the line of osteotomy is carried downwards into the infraorbital fissure.

Sectioning is then continued in two directions: medially, the osteotomy traverses the orbital floor and the medial wall of the orbit behind the lacrimal fossae to reach the frontonasal suture; laterally and downwards, it runs across

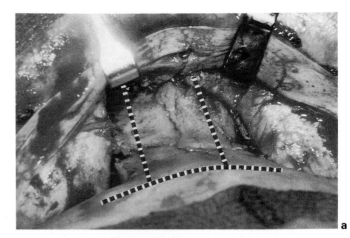

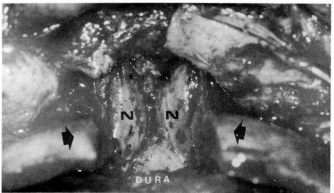

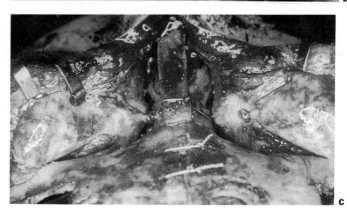

Fig. 20.18 Interorbital resection: (a) exposure of the interorbital region and line of osteotomy; (b) exposure of the mucous nasal domes; (c) nasal reconstruction by means of a bone graft following medialization of the orbit.

the posterolateral wall of the maxilla into the pterygoid groove area, where disjunction may be performed in a variety of ways.

Position and direction of the cut in the malar area are indicated by the specific requirements of the case. Tessier (1967) originally described a sagittal cut through the lateral orbital rim in combination with a medially directed step-osteotomy of the malar bone.

In the sagittal plane the perpendicular plate of the

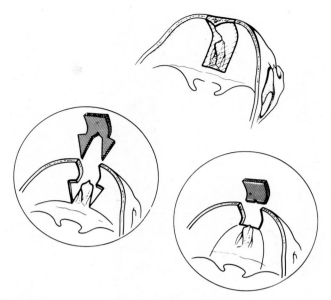

Fig. 20.19 Interorbital resection. The lines of osteotomy pass through the anterior cranial fossa. The integrity of the cribriform plate is to be respected.

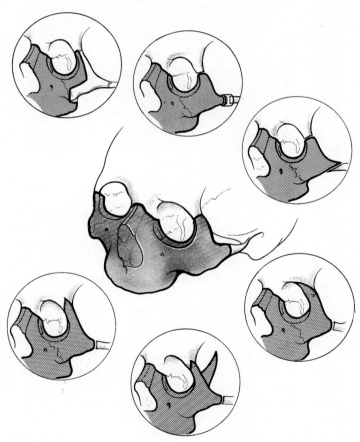

Fig. 20.20 Le Fort III osteotomy and its variants: (I) Tessier I procedure; (II) Tessier II procedure (types a and b); (III) Tessier III procedure; (IV) Tessier IV procedure; (V) Tessier V procedure.

ethmoid and the vomer are severed with the osteotome through the transverse cut at the nasofrontal junction. While performing these steps, it is extremely important to keep clear of the cribriform plates, the position of which should be carefully checked on the preoperative X-rays.

If there is doubt about the condition of the mucosa, exenteration of the ethmoidal sinuses is advised. Coagulation of the anterior ethmoidal artery is usually indicated.

The mobilization manoeuvres are performed with Rowe and Killey or Freidel disimpaction forceps. Sometimes it is also necessary to use additional traction posterior to the tuberosity with the instrument designed by Tessier or with a wide, blunt hook.

Variants (Fig. 20.20). Since Tessier (1967) first reported his revolutionary procedure, several alternatives and modifications have been described. They serve to obtain better stabilization or to advance part of the frontal bone in conjunction with the orbito-nasomaxillary block. These variations mainly involve the lateral wall of the orbit.

In the Tessier I procedure a sagittal cut is made in the inferior part of the lateral wall, which is continued with a step osteotomy in the malar bone. The latter cut can also be made in the zygomatic arch, either vertically or obliquely (Tessier II). Tessier later extended the osteotomy into the upper part of the lateral wall. Three modifications of this technique have been described.

The medial frontal spur procedure (Tessier III) — this alternative makes it possible to advance the lateral part of the orbital rim. Control of the osteotomy is through a burr hole in the anterior cranial fossa.

The lateral sphenofrontal spur procedure (Tessier IV 1970). This technique offers excellent stability but one must pay the price of a craniotomy.

The vertical frontal spur procedure (Tessier V) — The osteotomy was designed as a Z to improve stabilization. Direct control is provided in these cases by a burr hole in the medial cranial fossa.

The first of these variations can be performed without neurosurgical control, but in the other osteotomies, which pass through the wall of the anterior or middle cranial fossae, direct control by means of a burr hole (craniotomy 'à crâne fermé' (Tessier)) or a craniotomy is required.

The frontofacial monobloc procedure (Le Fort IV) (Fig. 20.21a)

Used but rejected by Converse (Firmin et al 1974) this procedure was first advocated by Ortiz-Monasterio et al in 1978. The technique makes it possible to advance the maxillomalar complex and the orbito-nasofrontal band as a whole.

To avoid communication of the cranial with the nasal cavities and adjacent sinuses and prevent injection by maintaining the integrity of the anterior cranial fossa and

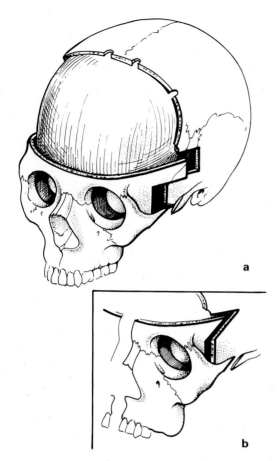

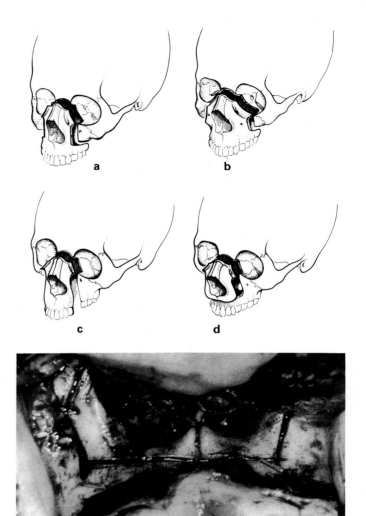

Fig. 20.21 Frontofacial osteotomies: (a) the monobloc procedure (Ortiz-Monasterio); (b) the hemifacial monobloc procedure (Van der Meulen).

Fig. 20.22 Le Fort II osteotomy and its variants.

supraorbital bar, Anderl et al (1983) have advocated differential advancement of the forehead and maxilla.

The hemifacial monobloc procedure (Fig. 20.21b)

This 'medial faciotomy', 'facial bipartition' or 'split face, produce was first described by Van der Meulen (1974, 1976, 1979). A complementary midpalatal osteotomy enables the surgeon to advance and rotate one or both facial halves and thus correct orbital hypertelorism at the same time.

Nasomaxillary osteotomy (Le Fort II)

Access to the skeleton is obtained via the vestibular mucosa and via the skin, either indirectly through the coronal route or directly through the internal canthus bilaterally. The transnasal incision is to be condemned because it tends to produce a conspicuous scar. The nasal lining is dissected via an interseptocolumellar incision. The midfacial 'degloving' procedure of Casson et al (1974) incorporates the risk of a nasal cavity stenosis, which is generated by the circumferential incision of the nasal lining.

The osteotomy (Fig. 20.22a) mobilizes the central facial pyramid with the nose as in the Le Fort II fracture, but in this case the osteotomy line differs from that of the classical fracture at two sites: it runs medial to the intraorbital canal and it interrupts the nasal prominence at its junction with the forehead.

In its superior part the osteotomy is similar to that used for the Le Fort III procedure. In the inferior part it is identical to that to be described for the Le Fort I technique. The osteotomy is characterized by its transmaxillary course, which runs below the malar bone and infraorbital nerve and then cuts through the orbital rim lateral to the lacrimal apparatus.

Disjunction, should be performed with care because of the fragility of the ethmoidonasal portion. Additional traction posterior to the tuberosity may be of use.

Variants. Tessier (1977) describes a line of osteotomy which runs lateral to the infraorbital nerve and includes a part of the malar bone (Fig. 20.22b). Alternative intermediate lines of osteotomy have been described by Converse et al (1970) (Fig. 20.22c) and by Psillakis et al (1973) (Fig. 20.22d). The nasomaxillary osteotomy of Converse cuts across the alveolar process between the canine and the first premolar and traverses the maxillary sinus up and into the orbital floor. The perinasal osteotomy of Psillakis also frees the nasal pyramid, but does not involve the palatodental plateau. The osteotomy line runs a dangerous course between the dental apices and the nasal spine and then joins the classical route of the Le Fort II trajectory. The mobilization of the osseous perinasal block is quite delicate. The ambiguous term 'intermediate' does not correspond to reality and these procedures are in fact very different and rarely indicated.

Maxillary osteotomy (Le Fort I)

A vestibular incision is made above the mucosal reflection and the exposure of the maxilla then proceeds cranially towards the rim of the orbital floor. The nasal lining is elevated within the nasal apertures in continuity with the vestibular dissection. Elevation of the fibromucosa in the direction of the teeth is to be condemned.

The osteotomy (Fig. 20.23) frees the palatoalveolar complex in accordance with the upper apical fracture line of Guerin. Cutting with a saw or Lindemann burr starts anteriorly in the pyriform aperture and continues horizontally through the maxillary sinus, 4 mm above the canine tooth, to end at the maxillary tuberosity at the level of the lower third of the pterygoid process. Separation of the pterygoid and maxilla is performed with a curved chisel, either via the vestibular incision with the back of the chisel pressing against the pterygoid, which often breaks, or via a counter-incision in the palate just posterior to the tuberosity. This latter approach is more anatomical.

The osteotomy line courses between the dangers of the canine apex below, and the lower concha of the nose and the infraorbital nerve above. A so-called high variant can be used to bring the lower part of the nose anteriorly. The mobilization of the bony block requires complementary incisions in a sagittal plane: in the midline, where the vomer is cut after elevation of the mucosal lining on both sides and then laterally on the inside of each maxillary sinus, taking care not to damage the descending palatine arteries which pass through the mucoperiosteum and assure the vascularization of the osseous block. In this way the vitality of the teeth is preserved, although the sensitivity of the teeth may disappear for a period of several months.

The obligatory transection of the maxillary sinus poses no problems when its lining is normal. When the mucous

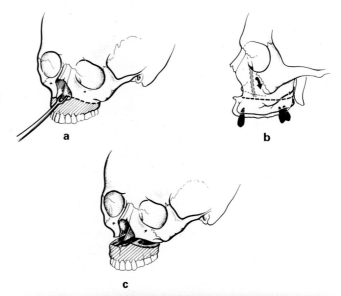

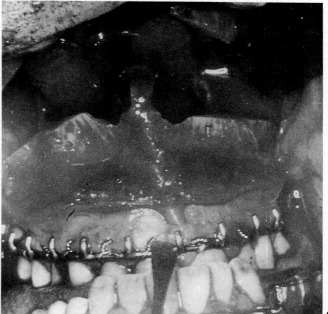

Fig. 20.23 Le Fort I osteotomy: (a) line of osteotomy; (b) the dangers; (c) mobilization of the maxilla in the midline; (d) peroperative view.

membrane is diseased, drainage of the sinus by an inferior nasal incision is indicated.

The osteotomized portion contains two strong areas in the canine (tooth) pillars and two somewhat weaker ones in the tuberosity region, all of which can be used for fixation. The dental fixation is an obligatory safety measure which is performed by means of a plate that is fastened to the inferior orbital rim.

Variants. In the intermediate osteotomy described by Popescu (1974) and advocated by Souyris et al (1973), the incision is carried into the lateral orbital wall, which is split sagitally in its inferior part. This procedure seems rarely indicated since its purpose is to accentuate the zygoma. We believe, however, that the form of the zygoma largely depends on the soft tissues covering it.

Partial osteotomies (Fig. 20.24) The idea of dividing the alveolodental arches in groups — although very old — (Wassmund 1935, Schuchardt 1959), has been successfully rejuvenated by the works of Bell, (1973), Epker (1964) and Schendel (1970). These authors have shown that vascularization of the segment remains adequate when the integrity of the fibromucous gingiva and the lining of the hard palate is preserved. The vertical segmentary cuts through an adherent mucoperiosteum have their origin in the Le Fort I osteotomy line, the course of which is changed in the sense that it ends in the lower part of the tuberosity. The need for a pterygomaxillary disjunction is thus eliminated. All combinations of segments may be considered but these procedures require excellent prosthetic preparations, permitting immediate stabilization of the segment in a thin intercuspidation plate fixed to the inferior orbital rim.

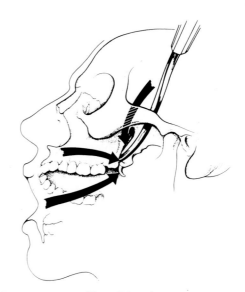

Fig. 20.25 The pterygomaxillary disjunction.

The pterygomaxillary disjunction

The pterygoid groove serves as a fixed reference for the osteotomy routes that traverse the face, and the separation of the pterygomaxillary junction is mandatory. The danger of haemorrhage is grave, either from the internal maxillary artery of from a venous origin, because of the presence of the pterygoid plexus.

The approach to the groove varies (Fig. 20.25). It may be: inferiorly, by an incision close to the tuberosity with the chisel in the line of separation, far from the vessels; anteriorly, via an vestibular incision; or superiorly, through the temporal fossa. The latter approach is more elegant but involves a greater risk of bleeding.

The question may be raised whether a bone graft is necessary once the disconnection has been achieved. Lachard et al (1973) have shown in an experiment that the pterygoid is usually fractured. Therefore stabilization will be illusory when this occurs.

The mandible

The mandible is frequently the site of osteotomies (Fig. 20.26) The following points should be noted:

1. The conditions for healing are adversely influenced by the mobility of the mandible, the thickness of its cortex and the fact that the sites of osteotomy are subjected to the forces generated by masticatory muscles, and by occlusion.
2. Exposure of the bone is primarily through a mucosal incision, S-shaped in its posterolateral part, where it crosses the anterior ridge of the ramus, and linear in its anterior part.
3. A complementary cutaneous incision below the mandibular angle is indispensable for surgery on the ramus.
4. The sites of the osteotomies are dependent on the presence of the dental nerve, which passes through the bone.

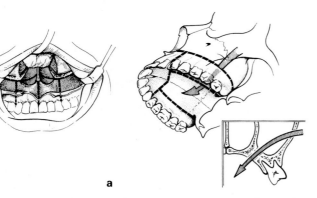
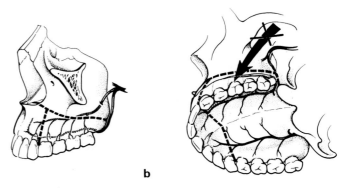

a   b

Fig. 20.24 Partial osteotomies: (a) techniques described by Bell, Epker and Schendl; (b) vascular distribution in relation to the techniques.

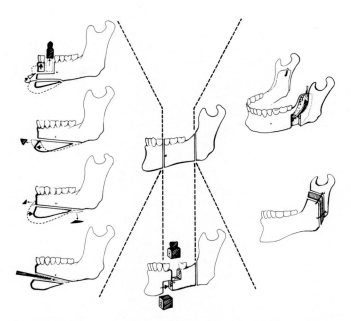

Fig. 20.26 The three sectors of the mandible and their respective sites of osteotomy.

The following three segments may be distinguished (Fig. 20.26): an anterior segment in front of the mental foramen; a middle segment between the lingula and the mental foramen; and a posterior segment formed by the ramus.

Anterior segment. Deformities of the chin are corrected by a genioplasty, a complementary procedure which is as common as it is useful. The dissection of the anterior surface of the mandible is carried in a lateral direction until the mental neurovascular bundle is identified and exposed. Of the basilar rim only its anterior part is freed, respecting the muscular insertions and their vascular supply. The rim is detached by cutting below the apices and below the level of the mental foramen. The mobilized block may then be moved in several directions: occasionally backward; more commonly upward, forward or laterally. It is moved upwards following the resection of an intermedial segment of bone to reduce the vertical dimension of the chin, forwards in conjunction with a bone-grafting procedure to fill the resulting defect or lateral when asymmetry is to be corrected. The osteotomy may be used to detach the alveolodental segment in some patients with abnormal occlusion (Köle 1959). Immobilization is obtained by bilateral osteosynthesis using wires or screws.

Middle segment. The presence of the inferior dental nerve is the main reason that osteotomies and ostectomies in this part of the mandibular body are rarely considered. A step osteotomy passing through a toothless area may, however, be used for shortening in selected cases and will require the identification, mobilization and rerouting of the nerve. The procedure has also been used for lengthening.

Posterior segment. The ascending ramus is the part favoured by most surgeons when shortening or lengthening of the mandible is considered. The following techniques have earned prominence in this respect.

1. Sagittal split procedure. This technique, already conceived by Schuchardt (1955), was introduced and perfected by Trauner & Obwegeser (1957) and modified by Dal Pont (1961). The osteotomy divides the ascending ramus in two halves: an external portion that carries the temperomandibular joint and the coronoid process, and an internal portion that contains the vascular, nervous and dental elements. To achieve this objective the lateral and medial aspects of the ramus are first exposed. The insertion of the temporal muscle is identified and the dissection restricted to an area which is sufficient for the osteotomy. Starting above the lingula the line of osteotomy runs horizontally at first. It is then continued downwards along the internal oblique line. Outside, its course is carried somewhat more obliquely, either backwards for repositioning of the mandible or forwards across the flat retromolar part to obtain a longer external portion and thus bring the mandible forward.

2. Inverted L-procedure (Trauner). The osteotomy, this time bicortical, was devised by Trauner (1955). The cut transects the anterior half of the ramus horizontally above the lingula and is then carried orthogonally towards the inferior rim of the mandibular angle. This procedure depends on the following requirements: a cutaneous incision below and behind the mandibular angle (Sebileau–Risdon) this approach passes through the platysma, avoiding the facial vessels and nerves and reaches the bone to free the elevator sling; a bone graft is used for lengthening the ramus, its dimensions being dictated by occlusion and by the projection of the mandibular angle. The procedure of Mehnert (1976) allows one to avoid bone grafts in some cases. The mandibular osteotomies that have been described are generally associated with a maxillary osteotomy when used to re-establish skeletal and occlusal balance. Their combination permits correction in all directions: vertically, anteroposteriorly and horizontally (Fig. 20.27).

3. Temporomandibular joint and ramus. The congenital temporomandibular bony ankylosis does not exist. The articular structures are altered, often severely in the lateral malformations, but mobility is rarely compromised. The condylar process and the glenoid fossa with the adjacent musculature, more particularly the lateral pterygoid, may be deficient or even absent. The ramus may be short, malformed and retruded, distorting the hemimandible. The zygomatic arch, malar bone and hemimaxilla participate so that the occlusal plane is elevated and retracted on the affected side. Sometimes the masseter muscle is hypoplastic, or one discovers fused temporal and masseter muscles. It is important to re-establish the equilibrium of the face with reference to the sagittal, median and

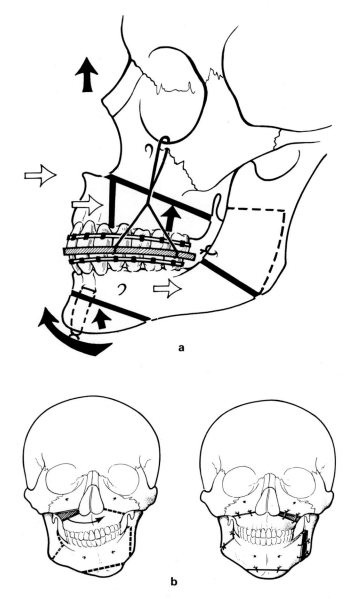

Fig. 20.27 Combinations of maxillary and mandibular osteotomies allowing movement in vertical and anteroposterior and horizontal direction: (a) lateral view; (b) frontal view.

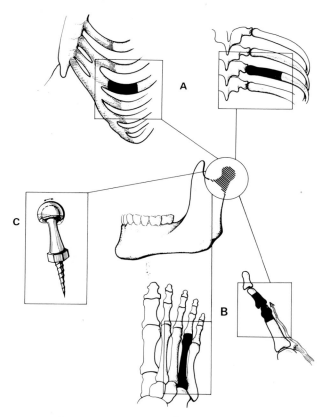

Fig. 20.28 Procedures used for reconstruction of the temporomandibular joint: (a) a chondrocostal or costovertebral (a2) graft; (b) the fourth metatarsus as a graft or revascularized according to Sheng-Chang; (c) a prosthesis according to Stricker and Flot.

horizontal plane. In order to do this one had to: lengthen the affected ramus and bring the mandibular angle downwards and forwards; level the occlusal plane by a bilateral maxillary rotation; rotate the mandible using a short sagittal osteotomy on the normal side if necessary; and reconstruct the defective or absent articulation (Fig. 20.28), either with the cartilaginous portion of a chondrocostal or metatarsal graft, or by insertion of an articulated prosthesis (SF prosthesis) on top of a free vascularized bone graft. In this case the posterior part of the iliac crest is used with its muscular layer pedicled on the circumflex branch of the posterior iliac artery.

Fixation

The new position of bony parts may be maintained directly or indirectly.

DIRECT FIXATION

This goal may be achieved in various ways: by osteosynthesis, by bone-grafting or by bone carpentry.

The osteosynthesis (Fig. 20.29) is performed according to the rules which are set by the particular architectural condition of the craniofacial skeleton, such as the very fragile cortex and the predominant role of the periosteum in consolidation. Wire sutures and most frequently miniature screws or plates are used for fixation.

A bone graft (Fig. 20.30) stabilizes the site of the osteotomy and promotes consolidation. Its importance is directly proportional to the range of displacement and its nature may be cortical, corticospongious or spongious, depending on the forces to which it is submitted.

Bone carpentry (Fig. 20.30) by tenon in mortise or tongue-in-groove designs permits secure fixation per se in many cases.

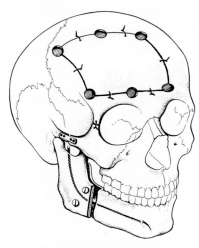

Fig. 20.29 Direct fixation by means of wire sutures, screws and plates.

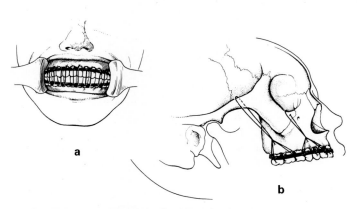

Fig. 20.31 Indirect fixation by means of: (a) arch bar and intermaxillary fixation; (b) subcranial suspension.

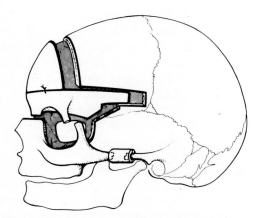

Fig. 20.30 Direct fixation by means of bone grafting or bone carpentry.

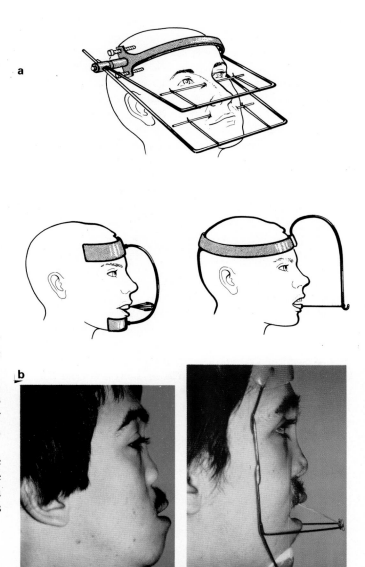

Fig. 20.32 Fixation to the cranium: (a) various methods; (b) application following Le Fort II osteotomy and nasal reconstruction.

INDIRECT FIXATION

The purpose of indirect fixation is to reposition the structures and connect them to the cranium. The teeth serve as anchors and as reference point for correct occlusion. The dental anchors consist of archbars (Fig. 20.31), bonded brackets, splints and intercuspidation plates. This material is fixed to an underlying structure by cranial or subcranial suspension. Subcranially the infraorbital rim, the zygoma or the lateral orbital wall may be used.

Fixation to the cranium (Fig. 20.32) may also be achieved by means of a pericranial crown such as those developed by Tessier & Delbet (1971), Georgiade & Nash (1966) and many others or by the use of headgears described in the section on orthopaedics (Ch. 18).

Bone supply

BONE GRAFTS

Continuity of bone after an osteotomy must be restored by

bone grafts. Restoration of contour is effected or completed by onlay grafting, which was formerly the only technique available for correction of dysmorphism. When the decision to use a graft is made, several important aspects have to be considered.

The first is the survival potential of a graft. The transplantation of a graft is followed by necrosis of most of the cellular elements. Autografts are, however, better than any other graft because of the uncertainty surrounding the antigenic behaviour of homografts (allografts) or heterografts (xenografts). Banked bone (allografts) may be useful in the reconstruction of a large defect, provided one achieves stringent asepsis and watertight wound closure, but heterografts (xenografts) are not recommended.

The second consideration is the donor site. Membranous grafts are revascularized earlier then endochondral grafts and will contain a greater percentage of living bone (Zins & Whitaker 1983). Grafts including periosteum are superior to those without, for the same reason (Knize 1974).

The third consideration is the size of the graft. Since reabsorption is directly proportional to the thickness of the grafts there is little to be gained by overcorrection in order to compensate for resorption.

The fourth consideration is the stability of the skeletal assembly. Immobility of the graft is a prerequisite for good revascularization and perfect fixation is therefore needed.

The fifth consideration is the vascularity of the recipient area. The better it is the more bone will survive. A final factor to be considered is the morbidity of the donor site.

Donor sites (Fig. 20.33)

The cranium is the donor site now favoured by many craniofacial surgeons. In the newborn, the capacity for re-ossification of the vault from the dura mater permits extensive bone removal in the parietal regions, obviating the need for grafts from remote sites; however, a drawback to this type of graft is its rigidity. In the older child and even in the adult a rich source of bony material can be obtained by splitting the thickness of a bone flap and using the inner table as a graft or simply removing the outer table and using this. Ribs may be preferred in both children and adults because rib grafts are pliable once split and because of the negligible associated morbidity.

The iliac crest offers the advantage that it can provide larger pieces of bone which are principally cancellous. This bone can be used for both support or for reshaping. However, the risk of resorption is higher and the morbidity greater. The scar is more prominent and lateral femoral cutaneous nerve paresthesiae can be troublesome. In the child one should take care to preserve the cartilaginous iliac crest. It is a vain hope to expect retention of the growth potential in the transplant by removing the bone, cartilage and junctional zone in one piece.

The tibia, finally, provides an excellent source of cancellous bone.

Complications

Care should be exercised in avoiding technical mistakes such as pleural tears or injury to the lateral femoral cutaneous nerve. Infection may cause the loss of the graft and this itself is linked either to a collection of blood or serous fluid, or to a failure to secure watertight closure of the skin or mucosal layers.

BONE FLAPS

The reconstruction of a skeletal part or the restoration of contour with a bone flap instead of a graft may have distinct advantages.

The first of these concerns the survival of bone when transferred as part of an osteomuscular flap. Comparing the fate of pedicled and free bone grafts by histology, autoradiography, fluorescein microscopy and injection of vessels, Baadsgaard & Medgyesi (1965) were able to show that pedicled bone grafts survive while free bone grafts resorb. Rhinelander et al (1968) explained the survival of these flaps by a reversal of the normally centrifugal blood supply into a centripetal flow that will maintain the viability of the bone. This view is consistent with the observations made by McGregor & Morgan (1973), who demonstrated that dynamic vascular territories in flaps do not parallel anatomical territories delineated by injection studies. The boundaries of dynamic vascular territories are dependent on pressure differentials. Brookes (1971) added the provision that revascularization of the periosteum from capillaries at the receptor site occurs, which is in agreement with the fact that grafts with periosteum undergo less resorption than grafts deprived of periosteum.

The second advantage relates to the osteogenic potential of the cambium layer of the periosteum, which is at its maximum in young animals. Early transfer of a viable osteomuscular flap will take full advantage of this potential. It will definitely result in better healing and perhaps help to increase the volume of the transferred bone. In addition, spontaneous closure of some donor defects can also be expected. The younger the child, therefore, the better the conditions for optimal repair.

The third advantage is that the cambium layer of the periosteum is a 'going concern'. It maintains growth and reacts to stimuli. There is evidence now that periosteum responds to surface tension and that detachment or transposition of some muscles is followed by changes in the craniofacial morphology. Whether the transposition of a hypoplastic muscle has the same effect remains questionable but the possibility should not be overlooked. At the time of writing, evidence continues to increase that

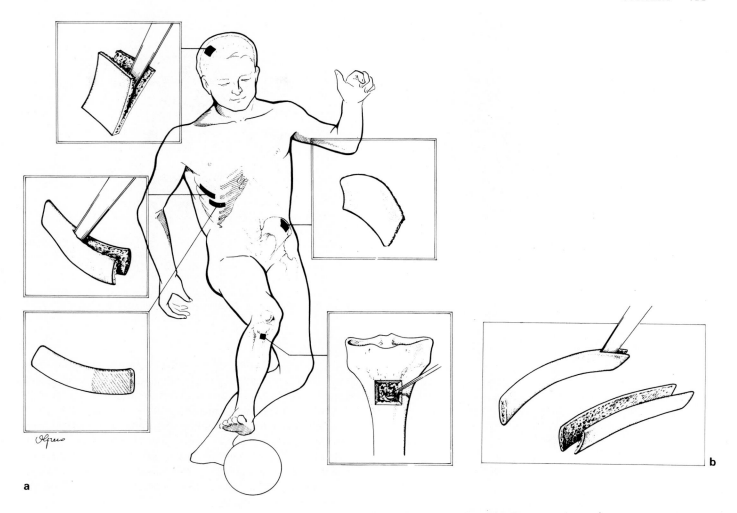

a

b

Fig. 20.33 Bone grafts: (a) different donor sites; (b) split-rib graft for nasal reconstruction; (c) peroperative view.

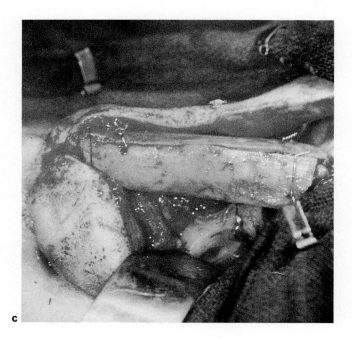

c

compound flaps will prove to be of great value for the treatment of patients with craniofacial dysplasias.

Donor sites

Compound flaps may be designed as an osteocutaneous, osteofascial, osteomuscular or osteo-musculocutaneous flap. Medgyesi (1973) compared osteocutaneous and osteomuscular flaps in goats by ink perfusion of the vascular connection between soft tissues and bone and observed poor filling in the osteocutaneous flap. In spite of this, viability of these flaps could be demonstrated by sequential tetracycline labelling.

Osteocutaneous flaps have been transferred incorporating the frontal bone, the clavicle and the rib, but their role in craniofacial surgery is distinctly less important than that of the osteofascial flaps incorporating a part of the vault (McCarthy et al 1984). Osteomuscular flaps (Fig.

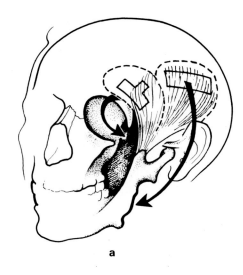

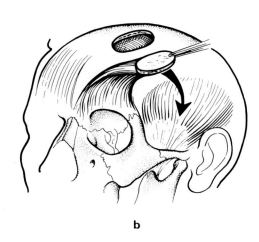

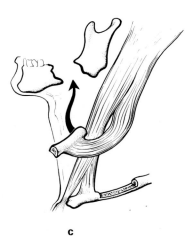

Fig. 20.34 Pedicled osteomuscular flaps: (a) on the temporal muscle; (b) on the galea; (c) on the sterno-cleidomastoideal muscle.

(McKee 1978, Ariyan & Finseth 1978), by the intercostal artery (Serafin et al 1977), by the latissimus dorsi (Schmidt & Robson 1982), or by the serratus anterior (Takayanagi & Tsukie 1982). A scapular flap (Dos Santos 1980, 1984) or its extension, a parascapular flap (Nassif et al 1982), are also possibilities.

In addition it is possible to harvest bone in more distant donor sites (Fig. 20.35) such as the iliac crest (Daniel 1978, Taylor 1978), the radius (Soutar et al 1983) and the ulna (Lovie et al 1984).

Cartilage supply

Restoration of contour is the main objective of cartilage grafts. They may be used for reconstruction of the nasal cartilages, the tarsal plates, the malar prominence and the framework of the ear. Since the avascular cartilage graft is nourished by imbibition and therefore provokes very little antigenic response, it can also be used as a stored homograft (Fig. 20.36a). This requires stringent standards for removal, together with strict standards of storage in an organized bank. Naturally aseptic and atraumatic conditions must apply during surgery. The use of blocks has been discontinued by some in favour of diced cartilage.

Donor areas

The costal cartilages as donor areas provide the maximum quantity of material. For reconstruction of the helix it is only here that sufficient material is found. The external ear, the septum and the triangular cartilages provide only limited amounts of fibrocartilage (Fig. 20.36b) These sites may, however, serve as a source for composite grafts.

20.34) have rapidly become another valuable part of the surgeon's armamentarium. They may be designed as a temporal flap pedicled on the temporalis muscle (Conley 1972, Van der Meulen et al 1984), a clavicular flap pedicled on the sterno-cleidomastoid (Blair 1918, Siemssen et al 1978), a sternal flap pedicled on the sterno-cleidomastoideus (Esser 1918) or on the pectoralis major (Green et al 1981), a costal flap pedicled on the pectoralis major (Cuono & Ariyan 1980), on the latissimus dorsi (Maruyama et al 1985) or on the serratus (Richards et al 1982); a scapular flap pedicled on the trapezius has also been described (Panje & Cutting 1980).

The indications for each of these osteomuscular flaps are determined by the vascularity of the supporting pedicle, its arc of rotation and the possible morbidity of the donor site.

The introduction of microvascular techniques in craniofacial surgery has made it possible to transfer some of the flaps mentioned above; examples of this development are a costal flap vascularized by the internal mammary artery

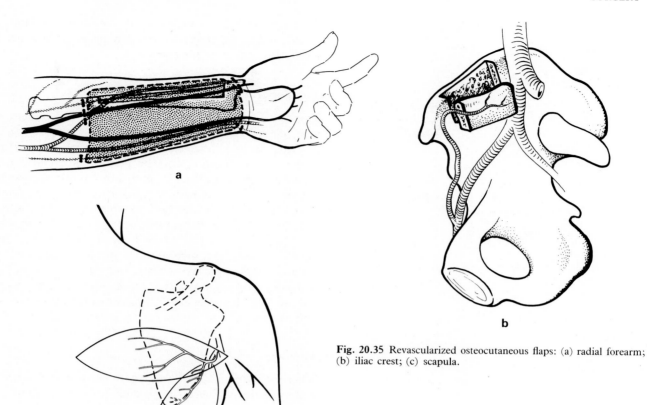

a

c

Fig. 20.35 Revascularized osteocutaneous flaps: (a) radial forearm; (b) iliac crest; (c) scapula.

Complications

The drawbacks are scars at the donor site and the risk of infection, as in bone-grafting. There is no unanimity as regards the degree of resorption.

Implants

The use of implants seems justified only as a last resort and in very strictly defined circumstances, given the risks of infection and occasionally of skin necrosis. Methyl methacrylate or a metal mesh can be used for repair of the cranial vault, provided the implant can be immobilized and the overlying tissues are of good quality. The implant must not be in communication with septic cavities, the facial sinuses and zones of friction. Flexible silicones may, in exceptional cases, be used to correct a contour deficiency.

PERIOSTEUM

This structure forms the boundary and the bond between the skeleton and the soft parts. As an envelope of the bony

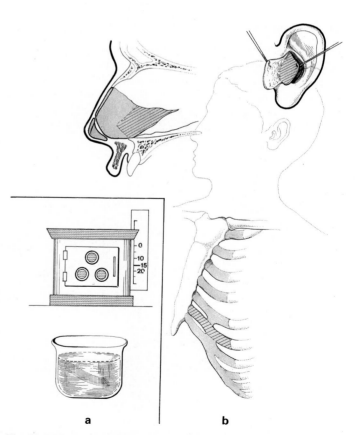

a   b

Fig. 20.36 Cartilage grafts: (a) storage of homografts in freezer (1) or in cialit (2); (b) donor sites of autologous grafts.

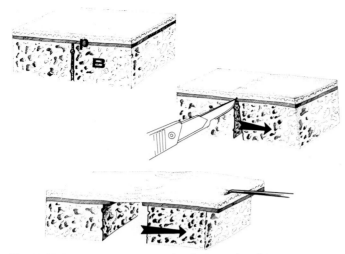

Fig. 20.37 Periosteotomy to allow for displacement of bony parts.

element, it reproduces the latter shape in such a way that the soft parts can be mobilized only if the periosteal sheath is interrupted. This technique of freeing the periosteal envelope, called periosteotomy (Fig. 20.37) is a ritual in the surgery of malformations and particularly important at certain sites.

The cranial vault

The characteristics of the periosteum and the dura mater might suggest that the former could be used to extend the dural sac in the child, but this practice is both dangerous and useless. It is useless because the elasticity of the dura mater is such that the dead space caused by the expansion of the bone normally disappears after a few weeks. It is dangerous because continuity of the dural envelope is indispensable for bony consolidation, as evidenced by serial observation of fractures.

The periorbital sac

This layer faithfully reproduces the form and dimensions of its cavity. Once the orbit has been modified as regards its situation and dimensions, the adaptation of container to contents is possible only by periorbital expansion, an expansion brought about by means of circular section and closure of the defect with an epicranial graft (Fig. 20.38). This concept is valid for both exorbitism and telorbitism.

In addition, the periorbital sac must also be detached from the inner canthus at the level of the palpebral ligament. Indeed, the repositioning of a canthus en bloc without periosteotomy carries the risk of incomplete correction or of recurrence of canthal dystopia, the correction of which necessitates extensive dissection of the canthus and an elective procedure on the ligament.

The face

Whenever bone is mobilized, even minimally for a limited synostosis as may occur in plagiocephaly, it is essential to open the contracted periosteal sheath in order to enable the soft parts to accompany the skeleton. This act is facilitated by the expansion of the periosteum by multiple interrupting incisions, thus forming a net (Fig. 20.39). Particular attention must be paid to the temporal muscle: The latter, freed from its bony insertion and detached from the zygoma, is transferred with the mobilized bony block. The fixation of the muscle to the lateral rim of the orbit will determine its new position.

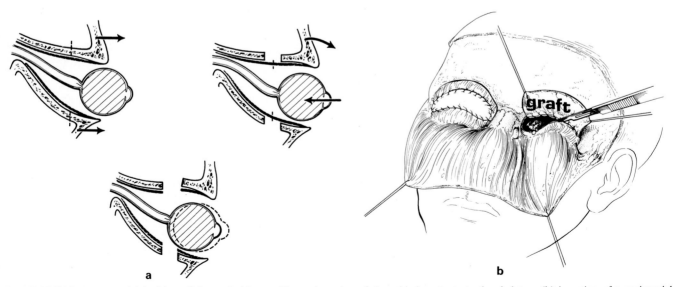

a   b

Fig. 20.38 Periosteotomy: (a) incision of the periorbit to achieve adaptation of the orbital contents to the skeleton; (b) insertion of a pericranial graft into the periorbital defect.

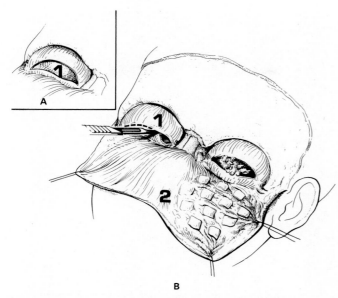

Fig. 20.39 Periosteotomy: (a) incision of the external part of the palpebral ring without grafting (1); (b) multiple incisions used for periosteal expansion (2).

As it reflects the alterations of a bony structure, the periosteum itself is sometimes part of the malformation, together with the bone. In such a case it is difficult to conclude which is primarily responsible, the periosteal deficiency provoking the osseous abnormality, or vice versa. The periosteum is the intermediary between the skeleton and the soft tissues, in particular the muscles, which promote periosteal ossification by their action. In this capacity the periosteum is not only the victim and witness of a skeletal abnormality, but it is also useful as a producer or a transporter of bone.

The osteoformative role of the periosteum in children lies at the origin of periosteal grafting, the technique used to produce bone in skeletal defects. The transport of bony segments is possible because of a generous blood supply, particularly in the cranial vault. The vascularization of bone usually passes through the periosteum, except in the presence of a nutritional or dominant artery. Numerous composite bone flaps therefore depend on the periosteum for adequate nourishment.

SOFT TISSUES

The interest of the soft tissues is of a static and of a dynamic nature. They serve to protect the bony reconstruction, to restore facial contours, both in surface and in volume, and to re-establish an equilibrium within the craniofacial regions.

Intimately attached to the skeleton by various means of fixation, the soft tissues are frequently involved in the malformation. Their ability to grow is dependent on the restoration of balance in morphology and function and this balance may be achieved occasionally by the mobilization or transposition of cutaneous and muscular tissues. The role of the mucosa is in this respect of limited importance.

In the craniofacial complex four different layers may be distinguished: the fascia, the muscle, the mucosa and the skin.

Fascia

The musculoaponeurotic system in skull and face forms a continuous covering, interrupted by the orifices and the various salients. Its structure is very different in the skull and the face. The galea aponeurotica, separated from the pericranium by an easily dissectable plane of areolar tissue, is a thick layer, attached to the occipital muscles posteriorly and the frontal and temporal muscles anteriorly. In the temporal region it forms a connection with the superficial fascia of the face, originally named after Charpy but rebaptized SMAS by Tessier and his collaborators (Mitz & Peyronie 1976). This layer incorporates the layer of mimic muscles.

As a carrier of blood vessels with a wide arch of motion the galea is the material of choice in restoring contours, because its vascular reliability is protective to bone grafts while also conferring safety and viability and thus good contour in the long term. Flaps may be designed with an anterior or lateral pedicle, allowing for tissue transfer to the face or to the cranial base (Fig. 20.40).

The importance of the galea has recently been recognized by various authors, especially in ear and socket reconstruction. In contrast with the galea, the superficial fascia of the face is not of much practical use, except in the cervical region, where it becomes the platysma.

Muscle

The muscular layer serves many purposes: the stimulation of growth, the establishment and maintenance of form, the animation of the face, the opening and closing of orifices, the mastication of food. Muscles may be interrupted, hypoplastic or absent.

The palpebral sling of orbicular muscles is most often interrupted.

The masticatory muscles are affected differently: the pterygoids, of which especially the lateral pterygoid is responsible for lateral movements, may be hypoplastic or absent, whereas the temporalis and masseter sometimes fuse into a single muscle in certain lateral dysostoses.

In the correction of craniofacial anomalies muscles occupy a prominent position as: a passive element for the restoration of contour; an active element for the restoration of function and the transfer of bone (see section on compound bone flaps).

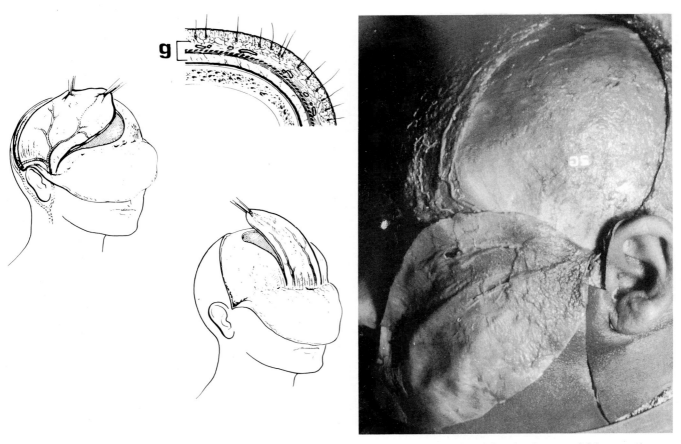

Fig. 20.40 The galea (g): (a) laterally and anteriorly based galeal flaps; (b) dissection of laterally based flap showing superficial temporal artery.

The temporal muscle contributes to laterofacial morphogenesis and dystopia of its cranial insertion will therefore affect the position of the mandible. Because of its strategic position at the transition of cranium and face it is of great value to the surgeon (Fig. 20.41).

Transposition is effected on an inferior pedicle, thus preserving its innervation and vascular supply. Total and partial transposition are possible (Fig. 20.42). Total transposition serves to restore its normal axis of action. Most frequently the muscle is advanced to accompany craniofacial propulsion. Sometimes it is used to fill a cavity, such as the orbit. Partial transposition concerns the anterior part of the muscle and is used with three objectives: to correct a contour deficiency; to transfer an osseous segment of the vault; and to reanimate a paralysed face. The resulting frontotemporal contour deficiency is closed by forward transposition of the posterior part of the muscle. Severe facial abnormalities may be corrected by the transposition of calvarial segments with a pedicle based either on the galea (superficial temporal a., McCarthy et al 1984), or on the temporal muscle (deep temporal a., Van der Meulen et al 1984).

The first of these techniques allows for a wide range of motion and may therefore be used for mandibular recon-struction. A pedicle based directly on the temporal muscle has a smaller range of motion and its use is therefore restricted to malar reconstruction.

The platysma muscle was originally described as a carrier of an island of supraclavicular skin (Fig. 20.43). It is now also used as a muscle flap to correct contour deficiencies of the lower third of the face by upward rotation. The latissimus dorsi represents an excellent alternative when transposition of substantial amount of tissue is required (Fig. 20.44). Partial transfer of a revascularized latissimus dorsi using the portion around the neurovascular pedicle permits restoration of the palpebral sphincter. Total transfer of a muscle may finally be performed with the purpose of contour restoration.

Mucosa

Mucosal layers prevent desiccation of the cornea, moisten the air on its way through the nose and lubricate the oral cavity. These layers are interrupted in some clefts and they may be hypoplastic or absent in other malformations. The correction of mucosal deficiencies is usually obtained by approximation of adjacent tissue, by the transplantation of a graft or the transposition of a flap.

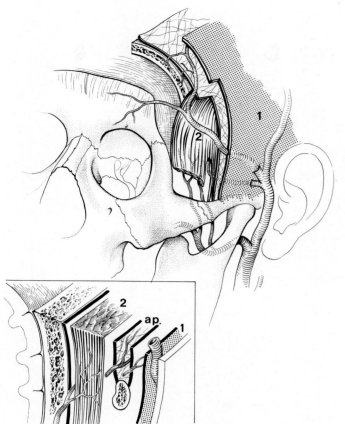

Fig. 20.41 The temporal muscle and its aponeurotic and vascular relationships.

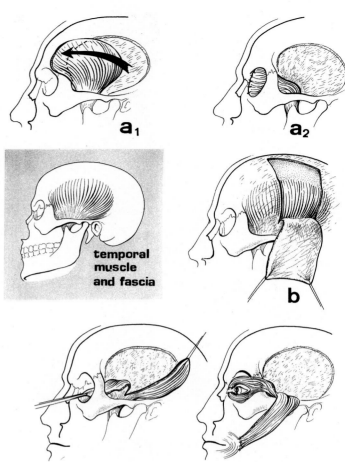

Fig. 20.42 Different modalities of temporal muscle and fascia transfer: (a, b) total muscular transposition; (c) fascial transposition; (d, e) partial muscular transposition.

Skin

The cutaneous layer provides protection to the underlying structures and preserves facial contour by its fixation to skeleton and muscle at strategic points. Malformations resemble those observed in the mucosal layer. Skin malformations call for special treatment because of the difficulties of mobilization and provision in the infant and the inevitable scarring following surgery.

Minor anomalies can be repaired using the classical procedures of approximation, rotation or transposition. In more severe malformations, however, a flap must be tailored with a blood supply adequate to ensure regional growth. Preference should then be given to an axial pattern flap or to a free flap, incorporating skin, fat, muscle or even bone.

Skin expansion to correct craniofacial malformations appears to have great potential; its merits are to be explored for future cases. The indications vary with the site but also with the type of abnormality, keeping in mind that the vault is the site of election for atrophy of the skin and the face for dimensional insufficiencies, especially in the lateral areas. A dynamic equilibrium in the malformed area is the only real guarantee of a subsequent capacity for growth, provided it does not result in constrictive scarring.

Conclusions

Form and function are the yin and yang of craniofacial surgery. The integrity of the face with all its qualities is based on that of the skeleton, the fascia, the muscle, the mucosa and the skin. Re-establishment of this integrity in facial malformations may therefore require:

1. The reconstruction of a supporting skeleton, using orthopaedic or surgical methods.
2. The reanimation of movable parts by reinsertion, transposition or transfer of muscles.
3. The reproduction of mass and contour by the reinsertion of a muscle, transposition of galea, muscle (temporalis, platysma) or skin with fat; the transfer of skin, fat, muscle or omentum (Fig. 20.45) by revascularization procedures.

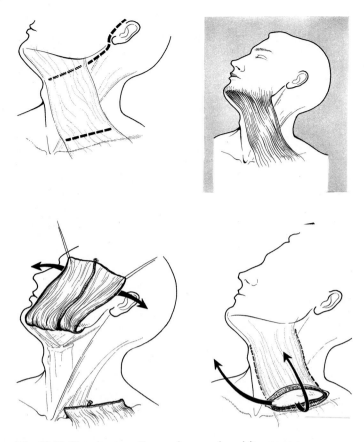

Fig. 20.43 The platysma. Route of approach and its use as a musculocutaneous or muscular flap.

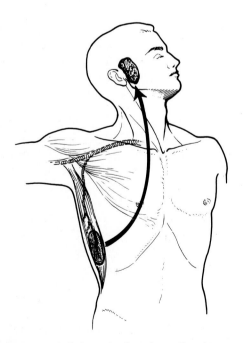

Fig. 20.44 The m. latissimus dorsi used as a flap; its range of motion.

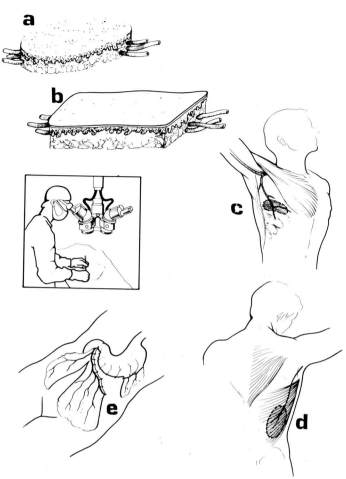

Fig. 20.45 The restoration of facial contour using microsurgical techniques for the transfer of: (a) dermis and fat; (b) skin and fat; (c) muscle; (d) muscle and skin; (e) omentum.

4. The restoration of a mucosal or cutaneous surface in harmony with the skeleton and muscles.

All these objectives must be achieved with a minimum of scarring, particularly when it concerns the skin. Scarring, it cannot be stressed sufficiently, is frequently the culprit when the result falls short of expectation. Many faces can be and have been ruined where a more judicious approach would have worked wonders. Application of the following rules may help to avoid a disappointing outcome.

The first rule concerns *postponement*. This is in fact a variation of the old Gillies rule and means 'do not do today what can honourably be put off until tomorrow'. In terms of craniofacial surgery it means that scarring should be avoided if there is any chance that the condition will improve spontaneously or can be improved by skeletal restoration.

The second rule concerns *planning*. Scarring cannot always be avoided but if incisions are to be made they should: (1) not cross the midline of conspicuous areas such as the nasal dorsum or the philtrum; (2) be hidden in creases or folds whenever this is possible; (3) run parallel to the lines of minimal tension.

The third rule concerns *performance*. When incisions are to be sutured it is not always sufficient to do this in a flawless fashion. Even when situated parallel to the lines of minimal tension the resulting scar may be subject to tangential or shearing forces. The effect of these forces is particularly harmful in the early postoperative period when scar tissue is still young and this may jeopardize its final appearance. Anchoring the skin to the skeleton, for instance in the medial and lateral canthal area, and careful repositioning of muscles whenever this is required, will help to promote good scar formation.

REGIONAL PROBLEMS OF SOFT TISSUES

Dural sac

The dura mater forms a continuous envelope which is closely related to the internal surface of the cranium. It is tightly attached at the central part of the skull base in the area of the adherent dura mater, but easily detached from the bone at the vault and over the orbital roofs where the dura is free.

Two layers can be distinguished: an external layer, periosteal and osteogenic, which forms an osteodural unit with the bone, and an internal meningeal layer, associated with the leptomeninges and related to the CSF. Because of these facts, surgery of the dura mater also has two aspects.

The first aspect concerns its osteogenic potential. The external layer is involved in the premature fusion of sutures, where it is thickened and adherent. Reduction of the osteogenic potential of the dura mater is therefore one of the objectives of the treatment in synostoses. However, chemical destruction is dangerous for the cortex and splitting, as advocated by Van der Werf (1966, 1971) may cause fissures and leaks of CSF. The current dural procedure combines mild electric cauterization with bipolar forceps at the convexity and splitting with extirpation of the external layer at the lower part of the coronal suture in a zone of extreme reinforcement and thickening.

The second aspect is related to the continuity of the dural sac, which is essential not only to ensure impermeability but also to allow osseous consolidation. Dural tears must be sutured and if necessary reinforced with a piece of pericranium fixed with biological glue.

CSF AND INTRACRANIAL PRESSURE

Obstruction to the free circulation of CSF leads to ventricular dilatation, increased intracranial pressure and eventually central atrophy in extreme cases. Hydrocephalus may be communicating or due to obstruction when the aqueduct is stenosed: a quite rare eventuality (5 cases out of 161 in the series of Nancy). The physiopathology of this type of hydrocephalus is very debatable. Compression of the arteries of the base and of the aqueduct by the basal deformation (Gross 1957), venous compression (Hoffman & Hendrick 1979) and meningeal fibrosis (Esbough 1948) are some of the causative mechanisms suggested in the literature.

Hydrocephalus calls for rerouting of the CSF into the peritoneum by means of a valve with a variable flow. Extensive excisions of the dura mater at the sutural site with replacement by a pericranial are unacceptable because they cause postoperative hydrocephalus. The increase in intracranial pressure, as indicated clinically and radiologically, initially almost asymptomatic, is measured directly by inserting a transducer on the dura mater; these measurements are made over a period of 24 hours (Renier & Marchac 1987).

The conjunctival sac

ANOPHTHALMIA

When the eye is absent, expansion of the conjunctival sac may be obtained by orthopaedic means or by surgery.

ORTHOPAEDIC DILATATION

Expansion of the conjunctiva and indirectly also of the eyelids should start as early as possible, preferably in the first weeks following birth when growth potential of the tissues is still present. For this purpose conformers have been made of different design and material. Initially such a conformer should be replaced every two weeks by one of a somewhat larger size and this strategy should be continued at gradually increasing intervals until completion of orbital growth. Additional pressure on the conjunctival sac may be obtained by fixation of the prosthesis. For this treatment to be succesful (Fig. 20.46) it is crucial that the prosthesis fits accurately and is worn comfortably. Failures may occur when the palpebral fissure does not permit the placement of a larger prosthesis.

SURGICAL DILATATION

Expansion of the conjunctival sac by surgical means is performed by first making a transverse incision to open the floor of the sac and lenghten the palpebral fissure. The conjunctival defect is then expanded by a second complementary incision in the lateral part of the sac. This incision runs at right angles to the first. The resulting anchor-shaped defect may be closed with a mucosal graft, which should always be of full thickness to limit subsequent contraction. The dimensions of the newly formed cavity

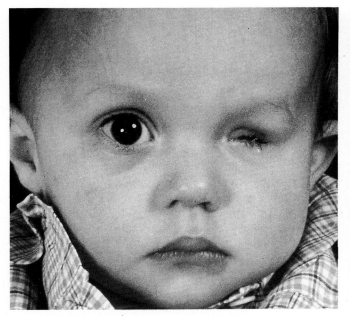
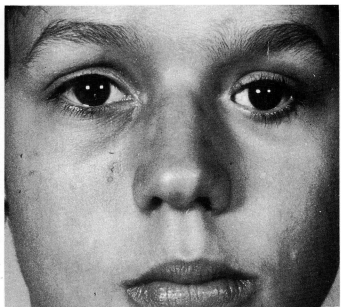

Fig. 20.46 Patient with anophthalmia: (a) before correction; (b) after correction.

are maintained by a conformer which may be held in position by means of a blepharorrhaphy and by a lateral canthopexy.

Normally contraction of a full-thickness graft is not as severe as that observed following application of a split-thickness graft. Extrusion of the conformer may occur with graft contracture. This phenomenon is probably related to the particular qualities of the receptor site, which consists of inadequately vascularized and extremely mobile fatty tissue, and to the excessive contractile potential exhibited by young children.

SKIN FLAPS

The development of new techniques has made it possible to reconstruct the conjunctival sac with skin from the retroauricular region. The skin flap originally described by Washio (1969) is nourished by the posterior branch of the superficial temporal artery and it may be transferred to the socket either by a two-stage procedure in which the pedicle must be severed at a second stage (Van der Meulen 1985) or as an island flap in a one-stage procedure (Fig. 20.47) (Guyuron 1985, Van der Meulen 1985).

The presence of an eye, however small, offers the advantage that it induces orbital growth. Enucleation is therefore never indicated. Expansion of the palpebroconjunctival sac can be accomplished with a scleral conformer that leaves the cornea free. If this is not succesful the fornices may be deepened with a mucosal graft. The orbital volume is rarely too small, but if it is surgical expansion of the orbital aperture will be indicated.

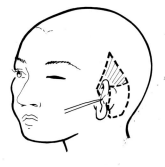
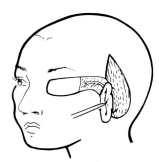

Fig. 20.47 Retroauricular island flap.

Eyelids and adnexa

THE EYELIDS

Craniofacial malformations may be associated with eyelid abnormalities such as ptosis or blepharophimosis. Their treatment has been described in many oculoplastic textbooks and is therefore beyond the scope of this work.

In this section we will restrict ourselves to the correction of colobomata of the upper and lower eyelid. Following birth immediate protection of the eye may be required and this can be obtained by ocular ointment, an hourglas bandage or a tarsorrhaphy. The procedure to be used is first of all determined by the nature of the coloboma. It may involve only the skin or both skin and conjunctiva. The defect can be found in the medial, central or lateral part of one eyelid or in both eyelids.

The skin

In theory closure of a skin defect may be obtained either by apposition of the edges of the coloboma or by transposition or transplantation of tissues. In practice, however, closure by simple apposition is never indicated because of the almost inevitable contracture that may follow.

Transposition of skin may be performed in many ways (Fig. 20.48), but the donor skin must match that of the receptor area if possible (Fig. 20.49). Transplantation of skin is indicated when transposition is not possible or when additional scarring is to be avoided for some reason. Several donor areas are available but here again the first choice should always be the upper eyelid, because of the perfect match. Retroauricular and preauricular skin are the second choice. A full-thickness graft taken from the inside of the upper arm or another hairless body area that is comparable is the next choice. The last choice, only to be used in emergency or as a temporary measure, is the split-thickness graft. There is too much contraction of these grafts and the hyperpigmentation which inevitably occurs makes them undesirable from a cosmetic point of view.

Mucosa and skin

In congenital anomalies of the eyelids mucosal defects are always observed in combination with a skin defect. Repair of the mucosal lining should always precede that of the skin, but the range of possibilities for closure of a conjunctival defect is small compared to that for the skin.

Closure of a conjunctival defect by approximation of its edges is virtually always possible if less than one-third of the eyelid rim is to be reconstructed. Once this objective has been attained it is only the skin defect that remains to be closed and this can be done by apposition, transposition or transplantation of skin. The procedures that are most useful for this purpose are shown in Fig. 20.48.

Closure of a conjunctival defect larger than one-third of the eyelid rim can no longer be achieved by approximation of its edges and since transposition of conjunctival flaps is inadvisable, particularly in children who have a limited amount of tissue available, it is only by transplantation of mucosa that repair can be effected.

Transplantation of mucosa is without question the most useful technique for the closure of defects involving more than one-third of the eyelid rim. The graft takes in the majority of cases and there are several donor areas in the

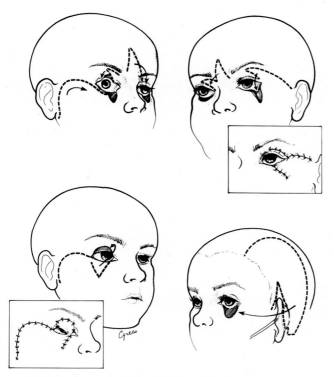

Fig. 20.48 Different techniques for upper and lower eyelid reconstruction.

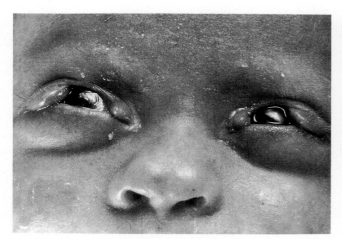
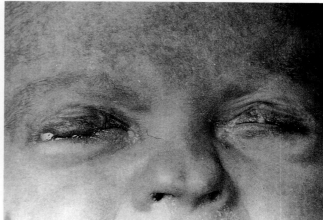

Fig. 20.49 Patient with upper eyelid colobomas corrected by local rearrangement of mucosa and skin.

immediate vicinity. A conjunctival graft with or without tarsus from the upper eyelid is ideal in terms of quality. Unfortunately only a small amount can be taken. A nasal graft with cartilage from the septal or upper cartilage areas is a good alternative if one prefers to include cartilage. An oral graft provides excellent replacement material if one feels that the inclusion of cartilage is not essential.

The use of a mucosal graft for the closure of an eyelid defect (Van der Meulen 1982) has important advantages over other techniques. It is in general a one-stage procedure. The conjunctival lining of the upper eyelid can be left intact and inspection of the eye remains possible. The graft can be covered with a wide variety of flaps raised in the temporal area as well as in the upper or lower eyelid. The transfer of this flap may leave a substantial defect in the donor area but this defect in its turn can always be closed with a skin graft.

ADNEXA

Lacrimal tract

In cranial dysplasias, anomalies of the lacrimal tract usually appear within the bony rather than within the palpebral part. Various manifestations may be observed, such as lacrimal fistulas due to a deficiency of skin, or canalicular dystopia or ectopia, caused by clefting in naso-maxillary or in maxillary dysplasia. Aplasia or hypoplasia of the excretory system, resulting in atresia and stenosis, is particularly common in severe forms of nasal dysplasia.

Inadequate drainage is a possible cause of infection. Relief of an obstruction in the upper part of the lacrimal tract can sometimes be achieved by probing and irrigation. Topical application of antibiotics and massage of the infected area is also helpful.

Relief of an obstruction in the lower part by reconstruction of an absent lacrimal duct is very difficult, if not useless.

Reconstruction of an ectopic canal can be attempted by closure of the skin over a buried strip of mucosa and congenital fistulas can be closed in a similar manner. A dacryocystorhinostomy will usually solve the problem of epiphora when other methods have failed. Fortunately nasal drainage involves only a part of the lacrimal secretion. The majority of tear volume is by evaporation and few patients therefore complain of epiphora.

The medial canthal area

Abnormalities in the medial region may have their origin in the skeleton, the canthal tendon or the skin. The skeleton is involved in cases of fronto-nasoethmoidal dysplasia (orbital or interorbital hypertelorism), the canthal tendon in canthal dystopia and the skin in patients with epicanthus.

The skeletal changes in the position and configuration of the lateral wall of the fronto-nasoethmoidal complex must be normalized before surgery of the canthal tendon or skin is to be performed. Dislocations of skeletal parts may be corrected by an osteotomy and relocation of the displaced segment or by its removal and replacement with a graft in the correct position and with a normal contour. Bony defects and other contour deficiencies may be repaired by the reduction of prominent parts or by the closure of defects with a bone graft.

The canthal tendon. Canthal dystopia due to a deficiency of the tendon or to its faulty position is frequently observed. Most commonly there is lateral or caudal dystopia. If an osteotomy is indicated in the case of skeletal abnormalities one may consider leaving the insertion of the tendon intact and correcting its dislocation in combination with that of the skeleton. Usually, however, a canthopexy is indicated (Fig. 20.50). The reinsertion of the medial canthal tendon in its proper position, i.e. deep behind the line connecting the corneas, is not an easy task. The insertion site should be placed far back in the lacrimal fossa. Accuracy is most important here and failure to achieve a good result is mainly due to technical problems. The position of the canthal insertion makes it awkward to burr a transnasal tract from one side of the nose to the other and pressure on the eye may be difficult to avoid with the apparatus normally used. Many surgeons therefore perforate the nasal bone and septum with an awl — a less elegant procedure.

Procedure. A hole is burred at the site of insertion of the canthal tendon or more posteriorly with a diameter sufficiently wide to allow the tendon to be inserted as deeply as possible. After identification of the tendon, it is secured with an Ethilon monofilament 3–0 suture, leaving both ends long. Then, parallel to and just below the bridge of the nose, two holes are burred on the contralateral side. The direction of the canals is such that the tip of the burr becomes visible in the hole that was previously made. Through these canals two hollow needles are passed, and these serve as guides for the ends of the sutures. The needles are then withdrawn and the procedure is concluded with the tying of a firm knot. It is most important that medial movement of the canthal tendon is not prevented by tethering adhesions of the structures. Extensive freeing of the orbital rim and occasionally incision of the periorbit are indicated.

The skin. Contour deficiencies of the skin in the medial canthal region are characterized by a lack of adherence between the skin and the skeleton and by a shortage of skin in the medial canthal region. This may be diffuse or localized. The lack of adherence and the inherent mobility are the reasons why displacement of skin by lateral or caudal forces may be produced. The shortage of skin may result in a variety of phenomena, such as: (1) flattening of the nasal root sulcus and an obtuse angle between the

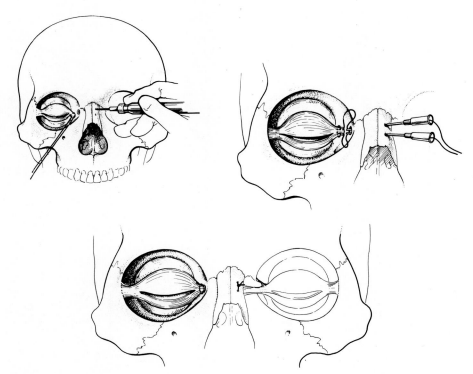

Fig. 20.50 Medial canthopexy.

medial canthal region and the upper eyelid; (2) an epican-thal fold with a relative surplus of skin on the medial site of the demarcation line and a relative shortage on the lateral site. Correction of these deformities is based on the following principles: reattachment of the dermis to the periosteum by carefully placed sutures — this step is facilitated by the resection of fatty and other tissues between the skin and the skeleton; redistribution of skin by a variety of methods, which are demonstrated in Figure 20.51.

Complications. Canthal drift is a common complication following the correction of interorbital deformities. This phenomenon may consist of the following anomalies: tele-canthus, flattening of the nasal root sulcus and epicanthus. Telecanthus is due to detachment of the canthal insertion. This phenomenon probably has its origin in the continuous traction of the orbicularis muscle. Its pull will have little effect when the canthopexy is performed according to the principles outlined above but faults in technique will in-evitably result in telecanthus. Flattening of the nasal root sulcus may follow separation of skin and periosteum or periosteum and bone by sharp dissection. Once healing is in progress the traction of the orbicularis muscle in the upper eyelid and the contraction of newly formed scar tissue in the orbital region may result in remodelling of scar tissue and flattening of the nasal root sulcus. An epicanthal fold is formed when the lateral pull of the orbicularis muscle in both eyelids joins forces with the downward pull of gravity. A line separating the loose, mobile, relatively redundant skin over the nasal dorsum from the more adherent skin over the origin of the canthal tendon and over the eyelids will then appear. Canthal drift may finally be enhanced by the production of fibrous tissue between skin and periosteum and by the production of new bone in children between the cambium layer of the periosteum and the bone.

The lateral canthal area

As in the medial canthal area abnormalities in the lateral canthal area may have their origin in the skeleton, the canthal tendon or the skin. The skeleton plays a role in fronto-nasoethmoidal dysplasia and malar dysplasia, the canthal tendon in canthal dystopia and the skin in canthal obliquity or diastasis.

The skeleton. The manner in which correction of the skeletal malformations in the lateral canthal area must be achieved is dictated by the position and configuration of the lateral orbital wall. Lateralization, retrusion and caudalization should be corrected by osteotomies and re-location of the displaced parts. Skeletal defects must be repaired with a bone graft or a compound flap.

The canthal tendon. An abnormal insertion of the canthal tendon may be due to a deficiency of the tendon itself or to a faulty position of an otherwise normal tendon. In both cases reconstruction is based on a canthopexy (Fig. 20.52).

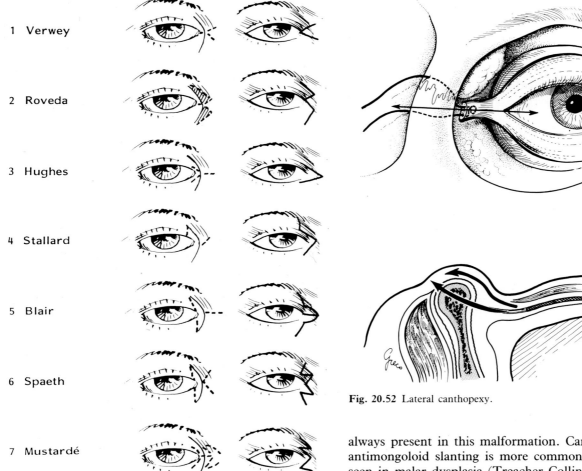

1 Verwey

2 Roveda

3 Hughes

4 Stallard

5 Blair

6 Spaeth

7 Mustardé

Fig. 20.51 Different methods for correction of epicanthal folds.

The procedure is as follows: two small holes are burred in the lateral wall of the orbit, directly behind the rim. The lateral canthal tendon is secured with an ethylon monofilament 3–0 suture and both ends are left long. Hollow needles passed through the holes serve as a guide for the ends of the tendon suture. The needles are withdrawn as soon as the suture ends become visible at the other end of the needle. A firm knot is then tied. The restoration of contour in the lateral canthal area demands the close approximation of skin to the underlying skeleton. This may be achieved by fixation of the dermis to the periosteum of the lateral orbital rim using one or two sutures.

The skin. It is almost inevitable that abnormalities of the skeleton and the canthal tendon may also be associated with skin anomalies. Canthal diastasis is sometimes seen in this area. This palpebropalpebral cleft and the epibulbar dermoid with which it is accompanied can be corrected by simple resection of the interfering tissue and linear closure of the resulting defect (Fig. 20.53). A skeletal defect is not

Fig. 20.52 Lateral canthopexy.

always present in this malformation. Canthal obliquity or antimongoloid slanting is more commonly observed. It is seen in malar dysplasia (Treacher Collins' syndrome) and can be corrected by repositioning of the lateral canthus, following its release from all tethering structures and the closure of the lower lid defect with a V-shaped advancement rotation flap from the upper eyelid and temporal area.

Eyebrows

The eyebrow marks the superior orbital margin. Distortion, interruption or deficiency of one or both eyebrows is sometimes seen and correction, frequently difficult, may be obtained by the application of one of the following principles:

1. By reorientation of the distorted parts. This requires transposition of one of the ends, in general the external end, by means of a Z-plasty (Fig. 20.54).
2. By restoration of the continuity. Certain colobomas traverse the eyebrow, leaving a bare area. An H-plasty is useful in such a case (Fig. 20.54).
3. By reconstruction of defects. This goal can be achieved with hair from the other eyebrow or of the hairy scalp and with a graft.

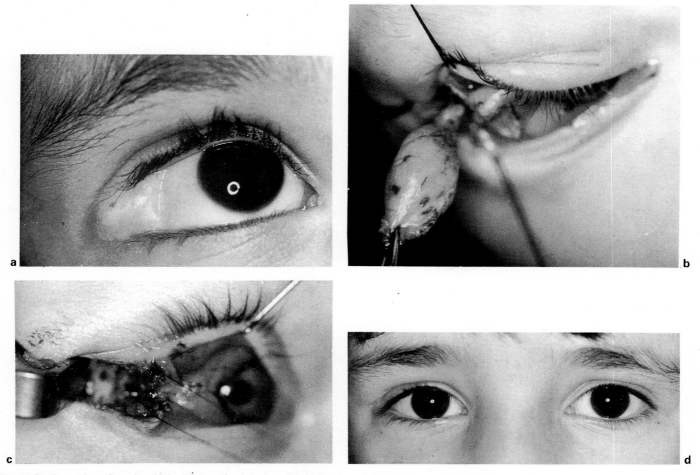

Fig. 20.53 Correction of canthoschizis: (a) preoperative view; (b) extirpation of lipoma; (c) canthopexy; (d) postoperative view.

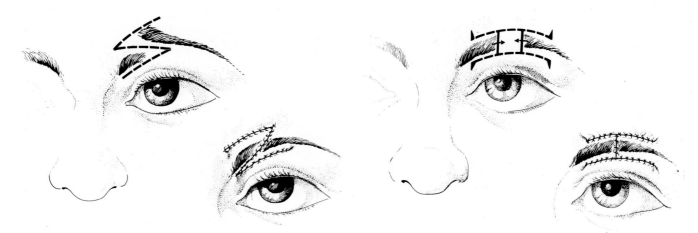

Fig. 20.54 Eyebrow reconstruction by local rearrangement of tissue: (a) Z-plasty; (b) H-plasty.

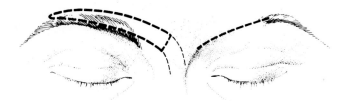

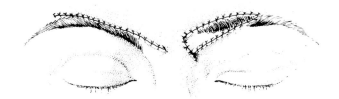

Fig. 20.55 Eyebrow reconstruction by use of its contralateral partner.

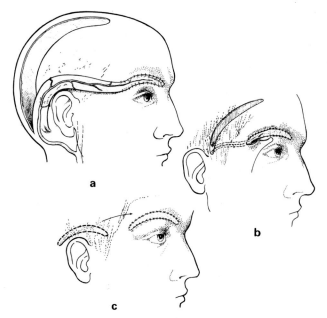

Fig. 20.56 Eyebrow reconstruction by use of the scalp: (a) as a free graft; (b) as an island flap based on the superficial temporal artery; (c) as a flap based on the occipital artery.

The first of these two alternatives provides the best aesthetic result, but the technique demands a thick, hairy eyebrow and a very short interophryal distance, if the splitting procedure described by Morax is to be used (Fig. 20.55).

The scalp (Fig. 20.56) has a very different quality of hair as regards density, orientation and colour and should only be used as a second choice, even when transferred as an island flap. Adequate make-up is frequently the best solution for a woman.

The nose

Optimal correction of nasal malformations, the final step in centrofacial rehabilitation, requires (1) the restoration of a skeleton that is sufficiently slender and solid to maintain function and form (projection and symmetry); (2) a mucosal lining of adequate dimensions; and (3) a skin cover with a perfect colour match and no conspicuous scars.

THE SKELETON

The restoration of the nasal skeleton consists of the following consecutive steps:

1. Dissection of the mucosal lining.
2. Resection of the malformed portion of the cartilaginous skeleton.
3. Reconstruction of the nasal profile with a bone graft.

This graft, which is taken from the iliac crest or the cranial vault, can be used in various ways (Fig. 20.57). It may be modelled as a triangular segment. It may be T- or L-shaped or it may be composed of two parts: one to reconstruct the nasal dorsum, and the other to be used as a columellar strut. Such a strut helps to provide adequate forward projection of the tip of the graft, but this objective can also be achieved by tight fixation of the graft to the nasal bones in a correct position using one or two circumferential wires or by pegging it into the bone at the nasofrontal angle. The graft should always be made sufficiently long to give adequate projection.

Discontinuity between the nasal graft and the surrounding pyriform aperture may be restored with the help of a split rib or split calvarial graft, fixed to the main body. The domes of the lower cartilages are finally draped over and in front of the tip of the bone graft in the midline and fixed with a few absorbable sutures. If this is not possible, the placement of a septal or conchal graft over the tip of the graft will help to prevent perforation of the skin and give a better contour.

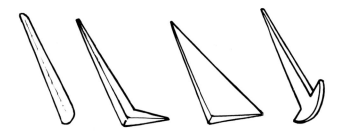

Fig. 20.57 Various designs of bone grafts for nasal reconstruction.

THE SOFT PARTS

Deficiencies in the mucosal lining can be corrected by:

1. The mobilization and rearrangement of the available mucosa, a method which is usually sufficient.
2. The transplantation of grafts, which may be either mucosal, cutaneous or composite.
3. The transposition of flaps from adjacent skin.

Reconstruction of the nasal lining by infolding of flaps carries the risk that the nostrils become too thick, obliterating the nasal aperture. This tendency can usually be overcome by the application of stents or moulds which are to be worn for a period of several months or by secondary thinning procedures.

The use of turnover flaps raised in the nasolabial or frontal area (Fig. 20.58) is associated with the formation of conspicuous scars and should therefore be avoided in children.

Correction of skin deficiencies can be obtained in several way, depending on the nature and severity of the condition.

The first method is by wide undermining and stretching of the local skin cover; this situation can be maintained by the insertion of a bone graft. Xenografts such as chondroplast and alloplastic implants (silicon) are not recommended. The application of a Radovan skin expander may offer the best solution.

The second method is by the transposition of nasal or paranasal skin (Figs. 20.59, 20.60). This technique offers the advantage of a perfect skin match but the resulting scars may be conspicuous when they cross the midline.

The following donor areas are to be considered for rotation or V-Y advancement of skin.

1. The midfrontal area.
2. The nasofrontal area, the rotation flap originally described by Rieger (1967) and modified by Marchac & Toth (1985) is particularly useful.
3. The nasal area.
4. The midlabial area.

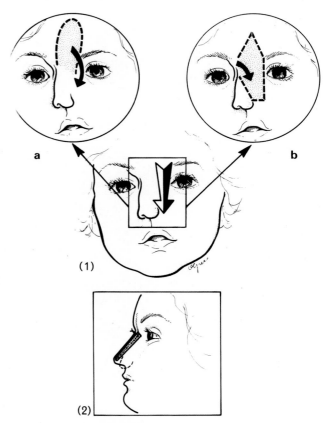

Fig. 20.59 Nasal and paranasal donor sites used for local (1) rearrangement of skin: (a) mediofrontal; (b) nasofrontal (Rieger flap modified by Marchac); (2) bone graft for nasal projection.

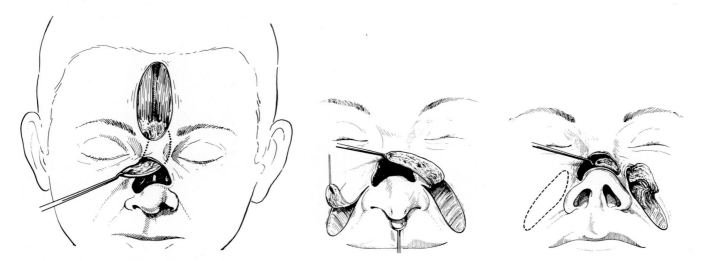

Fig. 20.58 Turnover flaps for reconstruction of the nasal lining.

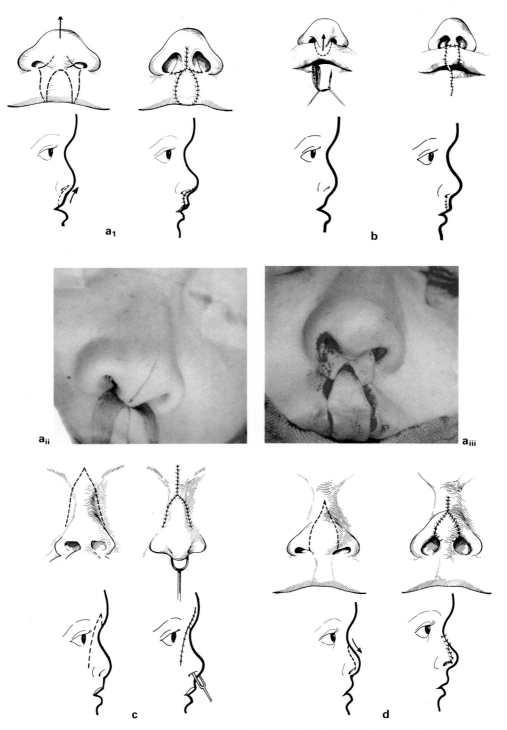

Fig. 20.60 Lengthening of the nasal dorsum. Lengthening of the nasolabial area: (a) columellar release associated with forked flap procedure of Millard; (b) columellar release associated with heterolateral flap transposition procedure of Sabattini-Abbe (Brown procedure). Lengthening of dorsonasal areas: (c) nasofrontal V-Y procedure; (d) dorsonasal V-Y procedure.

The third method is by the transfer of skin from a more distant donor area (Fig. 20.61). A considerable amount of skin with an acceptable colour match may thus be obtained. There may, however, be some donor-site morbidity and the resulting nasal scars will tend to be of inferior quality when the principles outlined in the introduction of this chapter are not respected.

Ears*

Despite considerable improvements in techniques and results over the last ten years, reconstruction of the auricle remains one of the most difficult problems with which the plastic surgeon is confronted. This is not surprising when one considers the anatomical complexity of the ear.

At one time, before the results of reconstruction were really presentable, the use of artificial ears constructed of acrylic or rubber was popular. Patients with these prostheses have often found them unsatisfactory and in the long run prefer surgical reconstruction of the ear. The major controversy for many years has centred round the method of reconstruction.

Although the use of pedicles may occasionally be required in cases of trauma, this technique has given way to the subcutaneous implantation of a skeletal framework

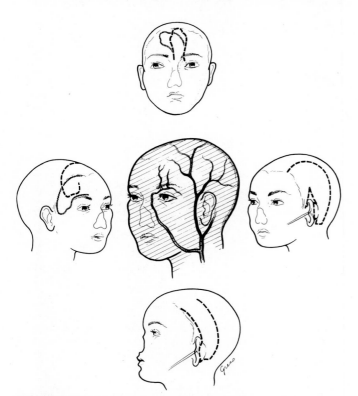

Fig. 20.61 Distant donor sites used for nasal reconstruction.

*The author of this section is L. Barinka

in the region of the auricle. Of the various prefabricated artificial frameworks, silicone has given the best results, but its disadvantages are well known. Following trauma, skin necrosis or the development of a seroma with infection, removal of the silastic implant may be necessitated. Despite modifications such as covering the silastic with dacron or temporal fascia, it is nowadays the opinion of many that the autogenous cartilage is the most suitable material for construction of the framework.

Cartilage has several advantages over other materials, the chief of which being its ability to withstand trauma and the maintenance of elasticity, shape and volume. Following small skin defects it is possible to obtain healing over exposed cartilage, whereas exposed silastics usually require removal or radical salvage measures. The chief drawbacks to the use of cartilage are that it maybe difficult to obtain enough material, and the carving and modelling of the cartilage makes great demands on the surgeon's skill.

To those who argue that reconstruction is unnecessary if the missing ear is covered with long hair one can reply that at some stage in their lives the patients may need to wear glasses, in which case an ear becomes important.

The descriptions and remarks which follow are based on research and clinical experience extending over 23 years and 148 cases.

PRINCIPLES OF RECONSTRUCTION

The method we use was first described in 1958 and is really a modification of the technique practised by Tanzer (1959, 1971) and Converse (1950, 1958). It was our aim to overcome some of the technical problems associated with their procedures and to improve the end result.

The following are the important principles of the reconstruction:

1. The cartilaginous framework is preferably modelled from one block of cartilage, but if necessary several blocks can be pieced together with catgut sutures.
2. The framework is thinned out to a thickness of 2–3 mm, so that the normal elasticity of the ear is reproduced, and also to keep the weight of the ear to a minimum.
3. Several holes are drilled through the cartilage, which allow connective tissue to grow through.
4. The upper two-thirds of the ear is supported by the cartilage graft, which is itself fixed to the ventral surface of the mastoid area following sharp dissection.
5. A conchal hollow, blind meatus and tragus are reconstructed, where necessary, as a second-stage procedure.
6. When the lobule is absent or atrophic, it is constructed from a long neck flap which is folded on itself. This is raised at the same time that the cartilaginous skeleton is separated from the temporal bone.

Since the adoption of these principles our end results have been far more satisfying. Because the skin used comes mainly from the position where one finds a normal ear, the colour and sensitivity of the skin are virtually normal.

The entire reconstruction, although making great demands on the surgeon's skill, can be completed within six months, which means that the patient is relieved of considerable stress and inconvenience as compared with the effect of procedures involving the transfer of tubed pedicles.

TOTAL AURICULAR RECONSTRUCTION

Preparation (Fig. 20.62)

A linen pattern of the normal ear is made and the normal ear is painted with a solution of methylene blue in alcohol.

The pattern is then moistened with alcohol and an imprint of the major features is obtained by pressing the pattern against the ear. These lines are now reproduced at the site of the future ear by simply reversing the pattern, which gives a mirror image.

It is important to determine the exact position of the upper pole of the new ear by comparing it with the normal side and also the correct vertical axis of the ear. This is done by measuring the distances between the external palpebral angle and the otobasion and the superior and inferior extremities of the ear, and by reproducing these distances on the side to be reconstructed.

Operative procedure

First stage (Fig. 20.63). An incision of approximately 3 cm is made 2 cm behind the posterior edge of the new

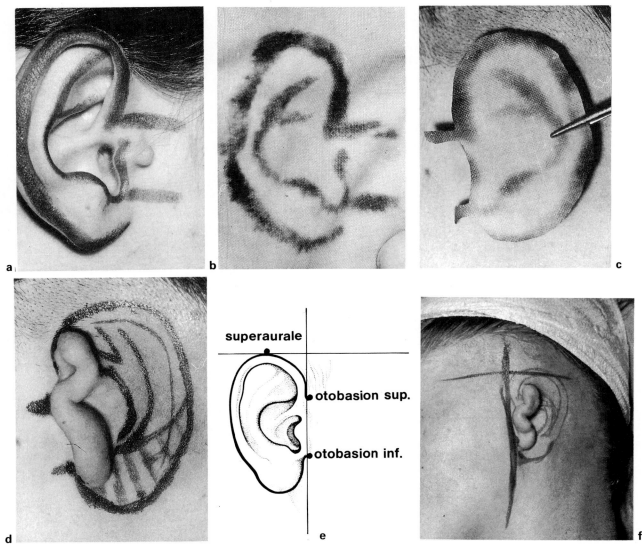

Fig. 20.62 Auricular reconstruction (Barinka). Preparation: (a) the normal ear is painted with a solution of methylene blue in alcohol; (b) a linen pattern is moistened in alcohol and pressed against the ear; (c) the linen pattern is reversed; (d) the lines of the normal ear are reproduced at the site of the malformed ear; (e) the site of the new ear is determined by comparing on the normal side the distances between the otobasion and the external palpebral angle, and; (f) by reproducing them on the affected side.

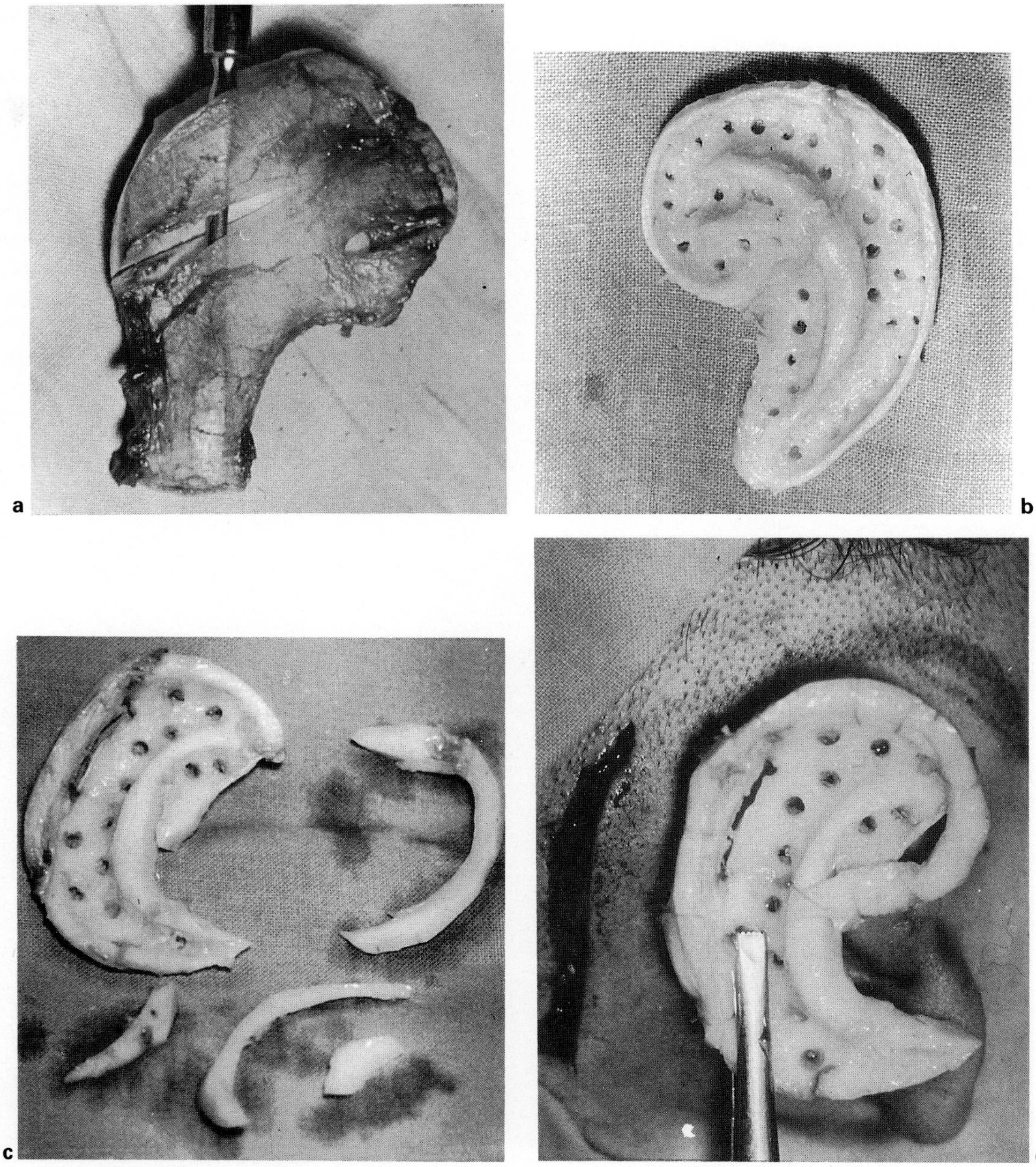

Fig. 20.63 Auricular reconstruction (Barinka). First stage: (a) removal of the perichondrium from the cartilage graft; (c) the auricle is created as a single piece; (d, e) using different pieces of cartilage.

ear and the skin over the whole area of the new ear is undermined. The plane of dissection is between the dermis and the subcutaneous fat, so that the thickness of the skin is almost that of a 'full-thickness' graft. If necessary, hair-bearing skin is also elevated as this can be replaced by a graft at the second stage.

A full-thickness cartilage graft is now removed from the junction of the 6th and 7th costal cartilages via a curved incision about 10 cm in length just above the margin of the cartilage. The right side is preferred, so that the risk of damage to the pericardium is excluded. In a 10-year-old it is always possible to obtain enough cartilage from this site. The exact amount of cartilage is gauged from the sterile linen copy of the original ear pattern and it may be necessary to excise two or more pieces of cartilage in continuity, which must be reinforced with sutures before carving begins. The junction between the two main pieces of cartilage should if possible be orientated in the longitudinal axis of the scapha, and the perichondrium is included with the cartilage. The wound is closed in layers, with drainage, and special care is taken to approximate the muscle and fascia.

Modelling of the cartilage graft — the perichondrium is first removed from the cartilage and the shape and contours are then carefully made with scalpels and chisels. Then follows the completion of the modelling with drills, which are rotated slowly in order to prevent overheating of the cartilage. Perforations approximately 3 mm apart are now made in the cartilage and final reinforcing catgut sutures placed where needed. The through growth of connective tissue has been found to strengthen the cartilaginous skeleton. Sharp edges and points are carefully smoothed off and the graft is now inserted in the subcutaneous pocket, care being taken to orientate it according to the preoperative measurement.

The skin incision is now closed and modelling sutures inserted through the skin and cartilage behind the anti-

helix, the helix and in the fossa triangularis. These sutures are tied over acriflavine wool to accentuate the ridges and hollows of the ear. The ear is then covered with a bulky dressing which is removed after 24 hours to check that there are no pressure areas jeopardizing the vitality of the skin.

Second stage (Fig. 20.64). Two to three weeks later the second stage is carried out, in which any useful rudiments are transposed to improve the shape of the ear. The lobe is switched inferiorly and cartilage from the upper part of the rudimentary ear used to create a tragus. The advantage of this method of approach is that the rudiment can be put to better use and the implantation of cartilage is not vitiated by scars.

Third stage (Fig. 20.65). Six months following the

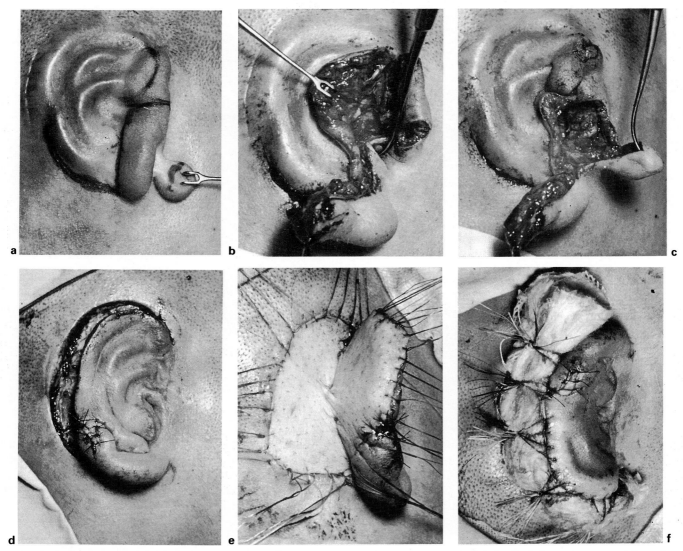

Fig. 20.64 Auricular reconstruction (Barinka). Second stage: (a–c) use of the rudiments to create the lobule; (d–f) the ear is separated from the head and the raw surface covered with a split thickness skin graft.

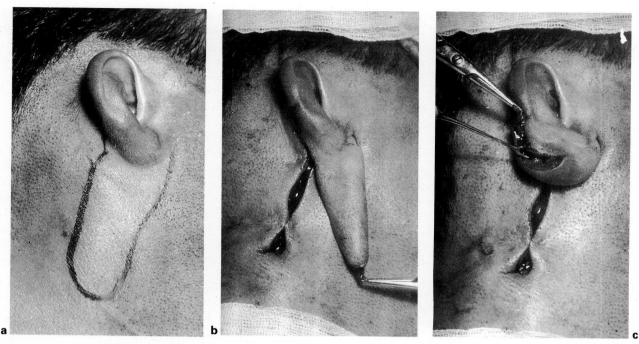

Fig. 20.65 Auricular reconstruction (Barinka). Third stage: construction of a lobule using an upper-based neck flap. This procedure is carried out only in case of an atrophic lobule.

second operation the ear, including the lobule, is separated from the head and the raw surfaces covered with a medium-thickness split-skin graft. Care is taken not to expose the cartilage and the plane of cleavage is just superficial to the temporal fascia.

PARTIAL RECONSTRUCTION OF THE EAR

Only 12 out of 60 cases required partial reconstruction. Many different types of deformities, ranging from simple absence of the lobule to microtia, are encountered and as a rule reconstruction tends to be more complicated, requiring more operations.

It is often necessary to expand the deformed ear to its normal size and then proceed with reconstruction of the missing portion. However, cartilage grafting follows the same principles as outlined in the section on total reconstruction. Later, with the implanted cartilage being fixed to existing cartilage the ear is raised and skin-grafted.

The buccal orifice (lips, vestibule and tongue)

A strong interdependence is observed between the composing structures of the buccal orifice. On the one hand there exists an intimate relationship between the upper and lower lip, resulting in a permanent equilibrium. On the other hand there is the constant balance between the pressure of lip and tongue, producing a neutral zone

which is secured by the vestibules. This zone determines the position of the dentoalveolar arches and thus occlusion.

THE LIPS

Labial competence supposes the integrity of each lip and a correct bilabial relation in every plane. Correction of an imbalanced lip may be achieved by means of a homolabial procedure. A disturbed relationship between two lips requires the use of a heterolabial procedure such as that of Sabattini (1838) and Abbe (1898).

THE VESTIBULE

Adequate depth of the vestibule is a prerequisite for independent mobility of the lips, and an adherent fibromucosa is indispensable to secure dental eruption in a proper direction. The purpose of a vestibuloplasty may therefore be twofold. It may serve to restore the depth of a vestibule by fixation of the detached mucosa to the periosteum in a correct position or resurface a fibromucosal defect with a cutaneous or palatal graft. The adherence of these grafts is superior to that of a mucosal graft.

THE TONGUE

The position, size and range of action are important qualities of this organ. Their restoration or preservation may require the release of adherent bands or a short frenulum. Tongue reduction and correction of a bifid tongue may also be indicated to improve function.

Airway

The concept of the 'respiratory tract', which is fundamental in the context of morphogenesis and growth, involves a group of anatomic components:

the nasopharynx, determined by the position of the sphenoid, the opening of the sphenoclival angle and the divergence of the petrous pyramids. Its actual dimensions are defined by the pterygoids;
the palate, arranged in two parts — the anterior bony palate, maxillopalatine, designed as a closed partition, and the posterior musculomucosal palate, designed for mobility.

Position and dimensions of the palate and depth of the nasal fossae and the choanae are determined by the site and size of the maxillae.

Centrofacial malformations intrinsically affect the dimensions of the respiratory tract and disturb ventilation. The nasopharynx is not accessible to surgical remodelling, except in the case of choanal atresia, but skeletal mobilization may affect the palate and nasal fossae, changing their position, modifying their dimension and possibly deranging their functions.

SURGICAL TREATMENT OF CRANIOFACIAL MALFORMATIONS (INDICATIONS)

INTRODUCTION

Having made the exact diagnosis, the decision to operate and the selection of an appropriate technique require a full understanding of the relation between treatment and growth in the affected region. The surgery of malformations, especially of craniofacial malformations, is a surgery of interception, designed to restore the balance between structures so that they may find their proper place in the programme of growth.

The course of growth, which determines the quality of the final result, depends on: (1) the type of malformation; (2) the outcome of the surgical intervention; and (3) the effect of complementary, especially orthopaedic, measures. An analysis of these three factors allows the planning of a treatment programme over a period of time. It is legitimate to attempt to codify the prognosis for growth on the basis of the above-mentioned factors:

The growth potential inherent in the type of malformation = G.

The morphological repercussions determined by the severity of the malformation and the effects of surgery = M.
The effectiveness of extrinsic orthopaedics or intrinsic surgical stimulation = D.

G

The growth potential of tissue, a non-quantifiable characteristic, approaches zero when there is involvement of the brain and the placodes (cerebrofacial dysplasia). It is impaired when the bone is altered (dysostosis), either in quality or in quantity, but it is fortunately adequate when there is only a single obstacle to development, as in synostosis. The intrinsic situation, specific for each malformed patient, is influenced both by surgical intervention and postoperative stimulation.

M

The morphological consequences stem from the severity of the malformation, i.e. from the amount of residual useful tissue, as well as from the surgical intervention. The surgical procedure modifies the form, may ameliorate the potential for local development and removes the obstacles to normal dynamics, but at the inevitable cost of a scar. The effect of this scar is felt at all tissue levels, but varies in relation to the procedure required: a section of bone, a subperiosteal dissection, or a reunion of soft parts.

The essential question is whether the surgical operation is detrimental to a structure while in the course of its development or capable of development. If the answer is in the affirmative, we have the classical, even antiquated, admonition of 'no surgery before the end of growth'. To deny surgery is to assume total responsibility of the consequences. 'No, but . . .' seems to be the correct reply. The harm is not inherent in the surgery but in the manner in which it is performed, in relation to the age of the patient and the region treated.

The morphological outlook must be a dynamic one, in keeping with growth. This evolutionary potential will vary with the topography, and if the face is devoid of intrinsic stimulation additional measures must be used.

D

The skull and the face form two systems which are fundamentally opposed as regards postoperative outcome. The skull has its own dynamics, brain growth being superior to any orthopaedic force. As the face has no such stimulus, it is essential to rely on the extrinsic force provided by dentofacial orthopaedics, although its efficiency is undeniably limited. Sometimes muscle surgery, by transferring an attachment or transposing one or more muscles, may provide the necessary stimulus favourable to growth. Such an objective analysis of the gamut of indications calls for greater modesty in the surgeon. It would be foolhardy to pretend that the difficulties can be resolved in every case.

Three groups of malformations stand out in the realm of therapy and prognosis.

First are those with a poor prognosis, in which it seems logical to abstain except in special cases; the cerebrocraniofacial malformations.

Second are those with a good prognosis, in which early operation is justified, in order to allow growth to catch up, but where the result will vary with the region; the cranial synostoses. The procedure gives long-term improvement when the vault of the skull is concerned and short-term improvement at the base of the skull and the face, thus requiring a further operation in adolescence; the craniofacial dysostoses and synostoses and the facial synostoses. Orthodontic treatment is an indispensable aid in improving the initial result and enabling the patient to traverse the crucial stages of growth, which are characterized by the

eruption of the permanent teeth and the prepubertal growth spurt of the mandible.

Third are those craniofacial malformations which, although similar in morphology, arise from different causes and therefore require a different therapeutic approach; the craniofacial dysostoses.

CEREBRO-CRANIOFACIAL MALFORMATIONS

In malformations where brain and placodes are affected, any surgical procedure serves merely a morphological purpose. It may be beneficial from a psychological point of view but a positive effect on growth is not to be expected.

Hypotelorism

Early treatment is indicated in spite of the severity of the

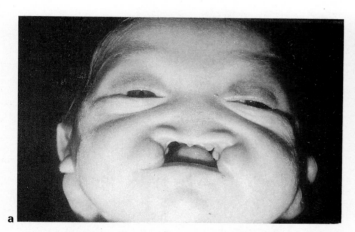
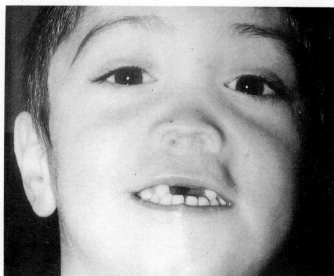
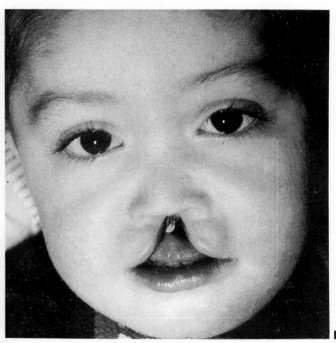

Fig. 20.66 (a) Holoprosencephaly without premaxilla and with median cleft of the lip. (b) Correction of the palatal cleft by tibial periosteal graft. (c) Repair of the cleft lip with a Sabatini–Abbé flap. Note the morphological change following the palatal repair.

condition, which frequently causes these children to die within a year.

Surgery concerns the palatal cleft and the hypoplastic derivatives of the median nasal process (prolabium, premaxilla and vomer). The palatal cleft is closed, respecting the principles of reconstruction of the velophar-

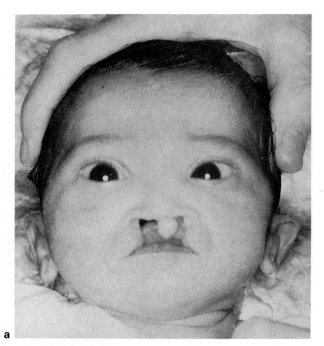

yngeal sphincter mechanism. The defect in the alveolus and the anterior palate is bridged with a periosteal graft from the tibia. Repair of the median defect in the upper lip may require the transposition of a heterolabial flap (Sabattini & Abbe) (Fig. 20.66).

Correction of the hyporhinia must be envisaged at a later stage in view of the fact that the creation of a nasal pyramid with growth potential is illusory (Fig. 20.67). Hypotelorism, a pathognomonic sign, may theoretically be corrected by separation of the two orbits (Converse et al 1975) but this procedure should not be considered, in our opinion, as a simple detachment of the medial canthi is probably just as effective.

Hyporbitism

Development of the eye is rapid: with a diameter of 17 mm and a volume of 2.5 ml at birth the eye will already have completed its growth at the age of 3 years. Its diameter will then be 24 mm and its volume 6.5 ml. The height, width and depth of the orbit will measure 35, 40 and 45 mm, respectively, and the volume of the orbital contents will be approximately 30 ml.

Fig. 20.67 Holoprosencephaly with hypoplastic premaxilla and median cleft lip: (a) as a newborn; (b, c) as an adult.

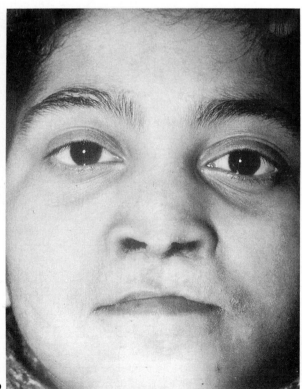

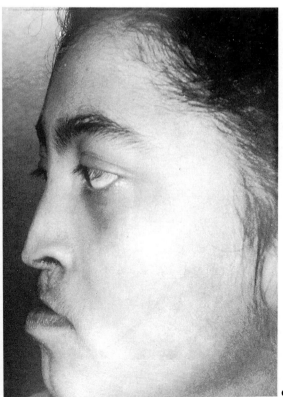

The orbit will fail to expand in patients with anophthalmia, and correction of this hyporbitism will consist of the following three steps:

1. Expansion of an orbit which is too small.
2. Formation of a socket of adequate dimension.
3. Insertion of a prosthesis to achieve symmetry.

ORBITAL EXPANSION

Dilatation of an anophthalmic orbit by insertion of conformers with progressively increasing dimensions or by an expander is an efficient procedure, although time-consuming and fastidious for the patient, the family and the surgeon. The use of an intraorbital expander may, however, provide an excellent alternative. A prosthesis with a diameter of 20–24 mm has a volume of not more than 2–3 ml. In order to contain a prosthesis of this size it is usually sufficient to dilate the orbital aperture by an expansion osteotomy, the site of which varies with the type of malformation, while direction and amplitude of the necessary movements are being defined by computerized scanning. Depending on the information so obtained, several procedures have been described, such as:

1. The resection of part of the orbital rim.
2. The translation of parts of the orbital rim
   a. in all directions (Converse et al 1974);
   b. in a lateral direction (Tessier 1977);
   c. in a lateral and superior direction (Marchac 1977);
   d. in a medial direction (Van der Meulen 1983);
   e. in an anterior, lateral and superior direction (Stricker) (Fig. 20.68).

Rarely also in patients with severe frontal retrusion it may be necessary to reconstruct an orbit by the apposition of bone. Dilatation of an anophthalmic orbit must be accompanied by expansion of the conjunctival sac.

SOCKET FORMATION

Reconstruction of a mucosal cavity of adequate dimensions is feasible but extremely difficult to realize. Failures may be due to excessive scar contraction in childhood, occasionally aggravated by complications of an inflammatory nature.

Orthopaedic dilatation by conformers of progressively increasing dimensions or by an expander should start as early as possible. The conformer must be changed every two weeks and this requires an optimal cooperation between the surgeon, the ocularist, the patient and parents if treatment is to be completed before the child goes to school. If one of these parties cannot muster the patience and perseverance that are needed the result is doomed to failure.

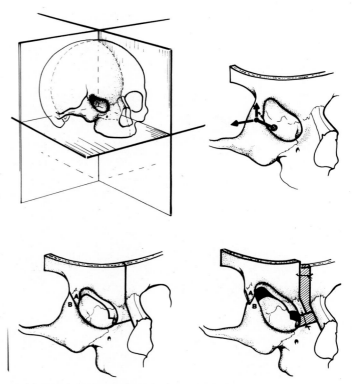

Fig. 20.68 Orbital expansion, according to Stricker.

Surgical expansion by incision of the sac and resurfacing of the resulting defect with a split skin graft is generally associated with severe contraction in spite of adequate splinting by conformers.

To prevent extrusion of the conformer several possibilities are available. A tarsorrhaphy is probably the most reliable, but fixation of the conformer to the orbital rim has also been recommended. In spite of these measures failures are known to occur. Rupture of the tarsorrhaphy and retraction of the eyelids into the orbit or perforation of the eyelids can occur. Results of socket reconstruction using full-thickness mucosa or skin grafts are better but they also contract, although to a much lesser degree.

Reconstruction of the socket with regional skin flaps may provide a solution to this problem but experience with this approach is still limited (Fig. 20.69).

Quality and dimensions of the eyelids vary considerably and the restoration of these structures deserves much attention. Orthopaedic expansion may increase the transverse diameter of the eyelids and make it necessary to anchor the extremities of the palpebral fissure with a canthopexy. Reconstruction of the upper eyelid by transposition of the lower eyelid is an alternative that may be considered (Esser 1918, Mustardé 1966).

Retention of a prosthesis requires the presence of a socket of adequate dimensions. The fornices must be sufficiently deep and to obtain this goal some authors

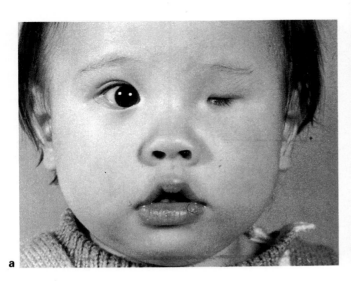
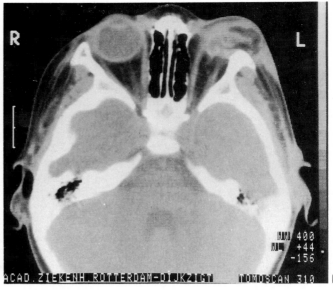
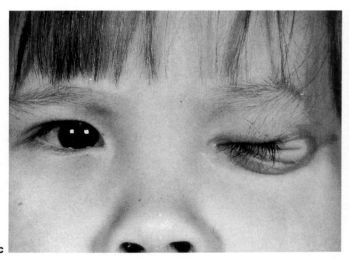
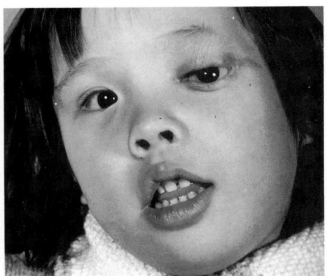

Fig. 20.69 Microorbitism: (a) preoperative appearance; (b) scan shows transverse dimensions of abnormal orbit; (c) reconstruction of the socket with a Washio flap and expansion of the orbit by an osteotomy; (d) postoperative appearance.

prefer to use composite chondromucosal or chondrocutaneous grafts.

The role of the ocularist is important by virtue of his or her ability to choose the correct colour of the iris and to adapt the shape of the prosthesis to that of the conjunctival sac. In microphthalmia, correction may be obtained by the application of a precorneal lens.

Surgical protocol is dictated by the following considerations: (1) ocular growth is completed at 3 years of age; (2) orbital size is almost definite at 8 years of age. Orthopaedic expansion of the mucous sac, when indicated, should be carried out as soon as possible to allow the prosthesis to be held in place before school age. Surgical expansion in successive bony, mucosal and prosthetic steps

should begin by 7–8 years of age. The classical difference between anophthalmia and microphthalmia is the subject of an old dispute. The orbit is small in both conditions but a microphthalmic eyeball should always be preserved. Cryptophthalmia constitutes a very special case, and the only indication for extirpation of the ocular rudiment (Fig. 20.70).

CRANIAL SYNOSTOSIS

Premature closure of a suture produces a cranial malformation and forms an obstacle to further expansion of the

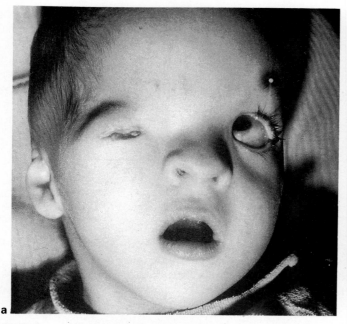
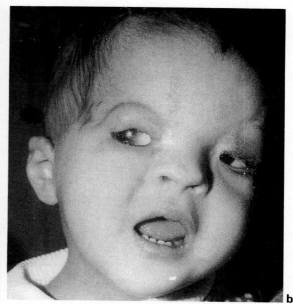

Fig. 20.70 Cryptophthalmia associated with cryptotia, coloboma of the contralateral upper eyelid and malformation of the urogenital apparatus. Treatment involved excision of the rudiment of the eyeball, reconstruction of the eye socket by two island flaps and application of a prosthesis: (a) before treatment; (b) after treatment.

brain. Surgical correction is based on the following three objectives:

the resection of the fused suture to decompress the brain and allow its expansion;

the prevention of premature reossification by alteration, destruction or reduction of the osteogenic potential of the external dural layer (Fig. 20.71);

the restoration of a normal morphology by cranial and facial remodelling.

Instant correction may be achieved by the mobilization and transposition of bony segments, free or pedicled. Long-term improvement may be obtained by the dynamic forces of unrestricted cerebral growth, which guarantees the normal development. We therefore distinguish between:

synostosis of the cranial vault, under the direct influence of the encephalic thrust, which has an excellent prognosis;

synostosis of the face and even more so the dysostosis combined with synostosis, which are devoid of stimulation following surgery and have a worse prognosis.

Surgery may be performed from the age of 3 months onwards. It must be early to free the brain in patients at great functional risk (brachy- and oxycephaly) and to draw maximal benefit from the cerebral expansion which will have increased to 75% of its adult volume at the end of the first year.

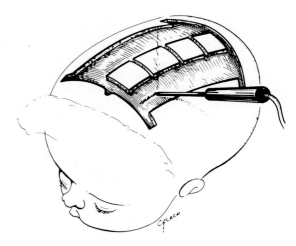

Fig. 20.71 Bipolar destruction of the dura mater.

The effectiveness of this remodelling thrust diminishes with time and becomes less efficient in the anterolateral part of the cranial vault in areas deformed by plagiocephaly. Early intervention is therefore advocated in all cases and appropriate measures must be taken to prevent rapid reossification of the bony defect, such as wide resection of the fused sutures, or destruction of the external layer of the dura mater. Linear destruction with the bipolar thermocauter advocated by the school of Lille is the procedure of choice (Dhellemmes) (Fig. 20.71). Fulfilling a crucial role in the treatment of scaphocephalies, this technique is systematically used in all forms of synostoses, but in the lower part of the coronal suture, where the dura is thick, dedoubling is mandatory. Cauterization excluded, the integrity of the dura must be respected.

Expansion plasties are useless because the dural sac will fill the postoperative dead space quite rapidly (Montaut & Stricker 1977). Resection of the dura is dangerous.

A fracture of the cranial vault will not ossify in the presence of a dural defect and attempts to prevent ossification by dural resection at the sutural site have resulted in reactive hydrocephaly. Measurement of intracranial pressure pre- and postoperatively is advisable.

Pachycephaly

Correction of this rare malformation is quite simple and involves the removal of bone on both sides of the synostosis to avoid bleeding from underlying veins and the linear destruction of the external dural layer with the thermocauter.

Scaphocephaly

Treatment of the classic form with a normal forehead requires freeing of the synostosis by formation of a parasagittal trench on each side (Fig. 20.72). Extirpation of the fused suture with possible damage to the longitudinal sinus can thus be avoided.

Fragmentation of the sagittal crest is, however, indicated. Anteriorly the craniectomy is continued transversely along the coronal suture and posteriorly along the lambdoid suture. The external dural layer is destroyed by linear application of the thermocauter. Mobilization and separation of two large parietal segments is indicated exceptionally in older children. Anteroposterior remodelling of the cranial vault, advocated by Marchac & Renier (1979) is not necessary in newborns but may have a place in children.

Additional procedures are required when forehead malformations are present. Correction of these anomalies may be obtained by lateral fronto-orbital advancement, by the transposition of bony segments restoring contour, and by reduction of the height of the cranial vault in leptocephaly. Spontaneous and progressive remodelling in babies who have been operated on (Fig. 20.73) will reproduce an almost normal morphology in the years following surgery (Fig. 20.74).

CRANIAL SYNOSTOSIS WITH FACIAL INVOLVEMENT

Trigonocephaly

Synostosis of the metopic suture produces a triangular forehead and alters the configuration of the orbits. The orbital malformations are characterized by retrusion of the superior orbital rim and by verticalization and elongation of the median wall.

Extirpation of the suture is first indicated. This step is

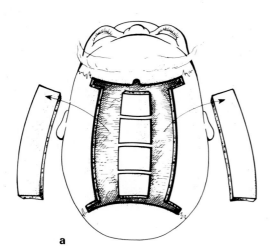

a

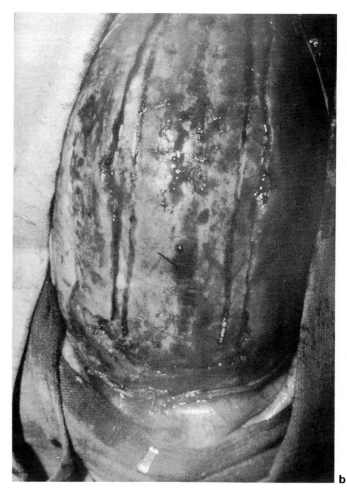

b

Fig. 20.72 Correction of scaphocephaly: (a) technique; (b) peroperative view.

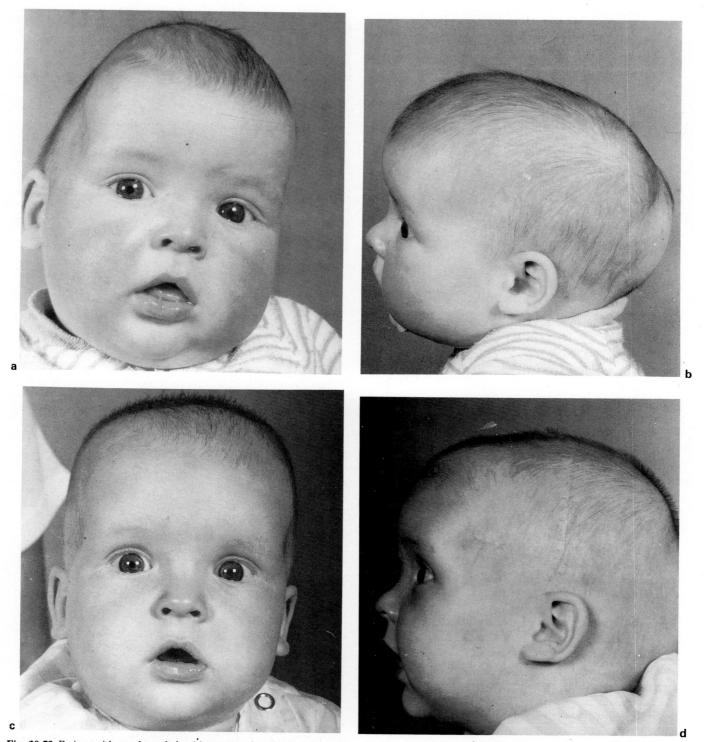

Fig. 20.73 Patient with scaphocephaly: (a) preoperative views; (b) postoperative views (several weeks later).

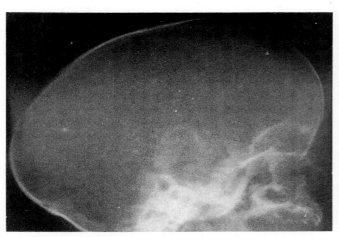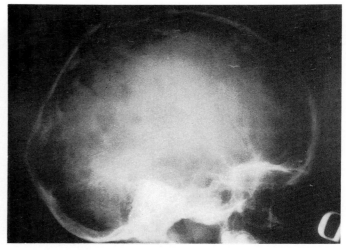

Fig. 20.74 Remodelling of scaphocephalic skull following correction: (a) preoperative view; (b) postoperative view.

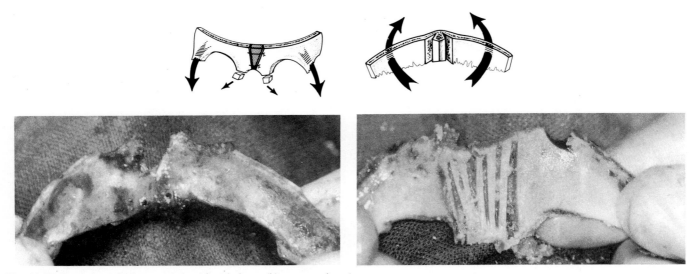

Fig. 20.75 Correction of trigonocephaly: (a) technique; (b) peroperative views.

facilitated by the fact that damage to the sagittal sinus in its anterior part is relatively easy to avoid. Resection of the metopic suture is carried towards and up to the frontonasal suture.

Frontal remodelling may be obtained in several ways: by lateral translation of the two frontal halves, by rotation of these halves, or by transposition of a parietal segment (Marchac 1978) with a curvature somewhat different from that of the forehead. The choice between these options is dictated by the prominence of the metopic crest and its cranial extension. Tessier (1986) has advocated correction of trigonocephaly by differential straightening of horizontal segments taken from the frontal part of the cranial vault.

Remodelling of the frontonasal segment is more complex (Fig. 20.75). Mobilization in several directions is required to achieve the transformation of the anterior angulation into a harmonious curvature and restoration of the orbital contour. Correction of the V-shaped angulation is obtained by differential propulsion of the fronto-orbitonasal band. Splitting of the internal cortex by one median or multiple cuts along its length permits forward displacement of the lateral extremities of the band.

Downward displacement of these parts is made possible by the formation of a greenstick fracture in the upper part of the midline. The median defect thus formed must be closed with a triangular bone graft. Downward displacement may produce a discrepancy between the vertical dimensions of the lateral and medial orbital wall as the latter remains too high. This inadequacy may be corrected by the removal of a small part of the medial wall and by lowering of the fronto-orbitonasal band as a whole.

The morphological result is generally good (Figs. 20.76,

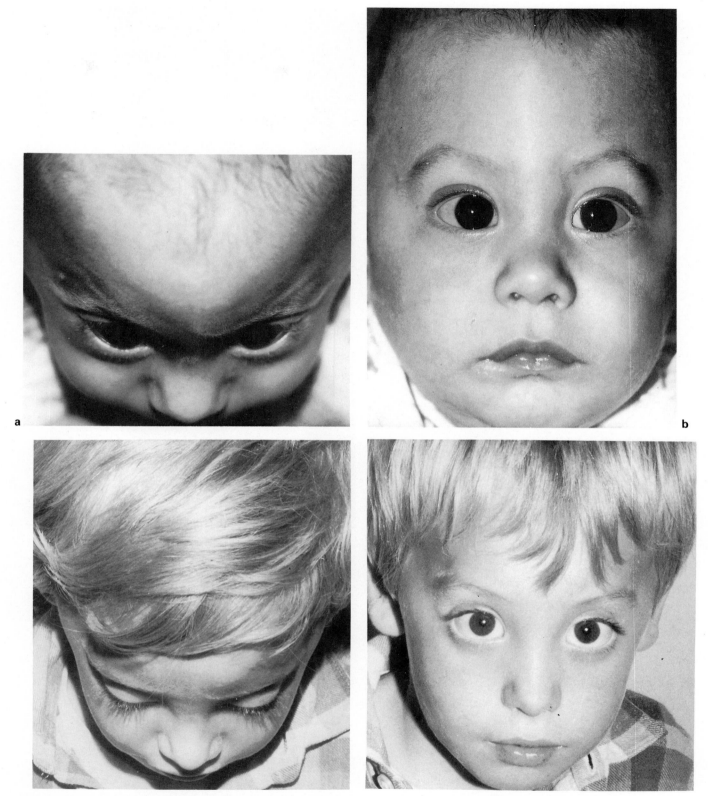

Fig. 20.76 Patient with trigonocephaly: (a) preoperative views at 1 month of age; (b) postoperative views at 4 years of age.

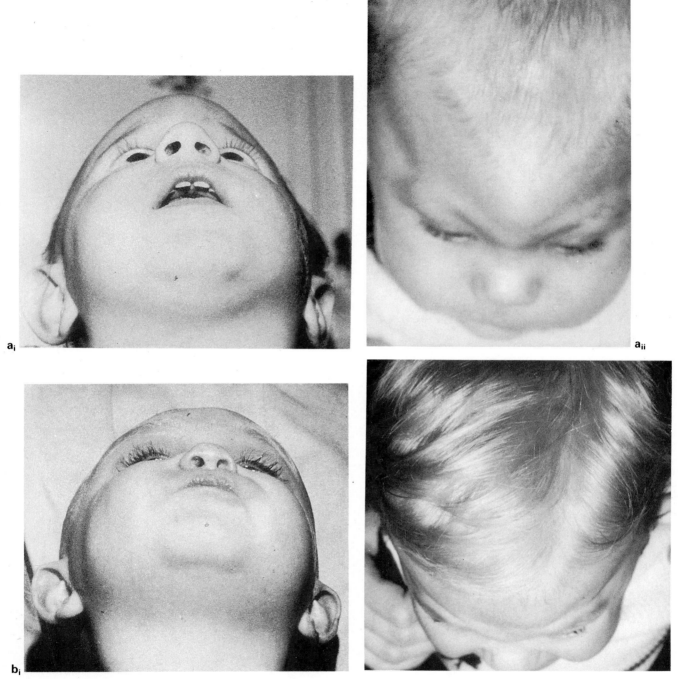

Fig. 20.77 Patient with trigonocephaly: (a) preoperative views; (b) postoperative views.

20.77), although it sometimes falls short of expectations owing to the residual transverse shortness of the forehead, which is accentuated by the flat lateral parts and the presence of hypotelorism. In patients with cerebral abnormalities the result is always poor.

Plagiocephaly

Correction of these anomalies is difficult. The malformation may affect the face and the lateral aspects of the cranial vault from the front to the back of the head, in all degrees of severity. The prognosis of surgical correction is variable because of the reduced effect of the cerebral thrust on skeletal remodelling in the lateral areas. Early intervention is therefore strongly advocated. Three fields of surgical action may be distinguished: the cranial vault; the fronto-orbitonasal junction; and the face.

THE CRANIAL VAULT

Correction of the cranial malformation involves the formation of a hemifrontal plate that includes the coronal suture. The contour of the vault is then restored by rotation of the plate or by transposition of a parietal segment from the other side. Some authors prefer to correct the entire frontal area.

THE FRONTO-ORBITONASAL JUNCTION

Correction by advancement of the retruded area on a median axis may be obtained in two different ways.

The first method is by the formation of a bilateral band with a tenon-shaped extension on the affected side (Fig. 20.78). Part of the rotation takes place on the normal side.

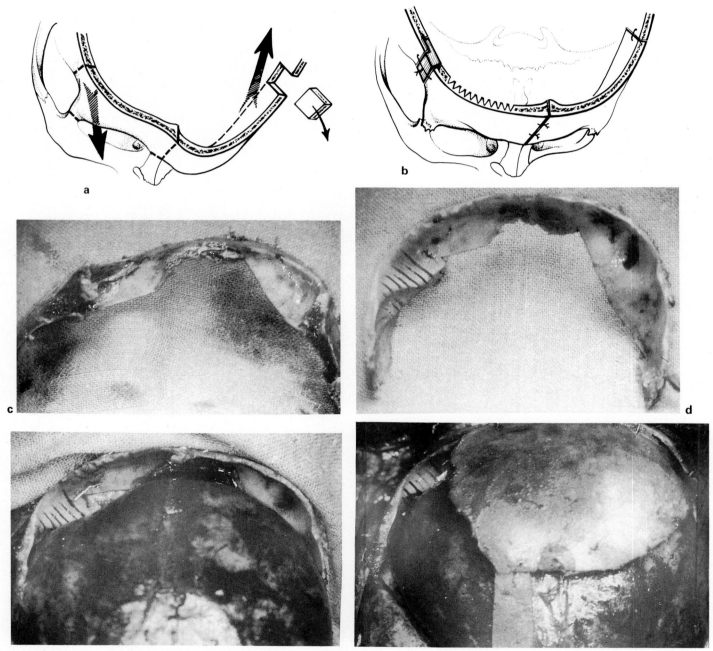

Fig. 20.78 Correction of plagiocephaly by bilateral remodelling: (a, b) technique; (c–f) operative views.

This procedure is indicated when the normal half of the forehead has become very prominent and restoration of symmetry may be obtained by retropulsion of the protruding part and propulsion of the affected side.

The second method is by the formation of a monolateral band with a tenon-shaped extension on the affected side and a tongue-in-groove connection with the non-affected side, permitting differential propulsion of its lateral extremity (Fig. 20.79). This technique is useful when the non-affected part of the forehead has a normal contour.

The orbital anomaly is characterized by the ovalization of the superolateral quadrant. Correction involves mobilization of the orbital roof by partial resection of the pterion. The deformity of the orbital rim persists, however, and remodelling of the hemiband by corticotomies or replacement of the superior arch with a calvarial graft may therefore be required.

An extended periosteotomy is indicated to open the periosteal envelope widely. An incision of the anterior layer of the periorbit is also useful, because the periorbital sac is laterally retracted, reflecting the malformation of the orbital skeleton. The results of correction are generally satisfactory (Figs. 20.80–20.85) but exceptions are seen occasionally (Fig. 20.86).

FACIAL CORRECTION

To correct facial deformities some authors advocate osteotomies of the roof of the nose and the maxillomalar

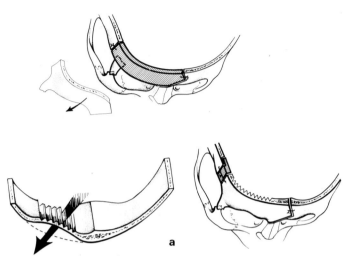
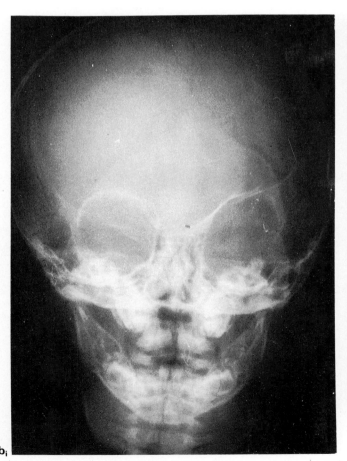
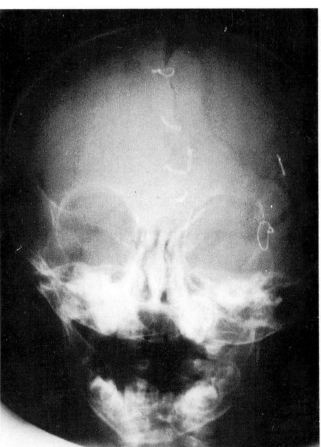

Fig. 20.79 Correction of plagiocephaly by unilateral remodelling: (a) technique; (b) X-rays, pre- and postoperative.

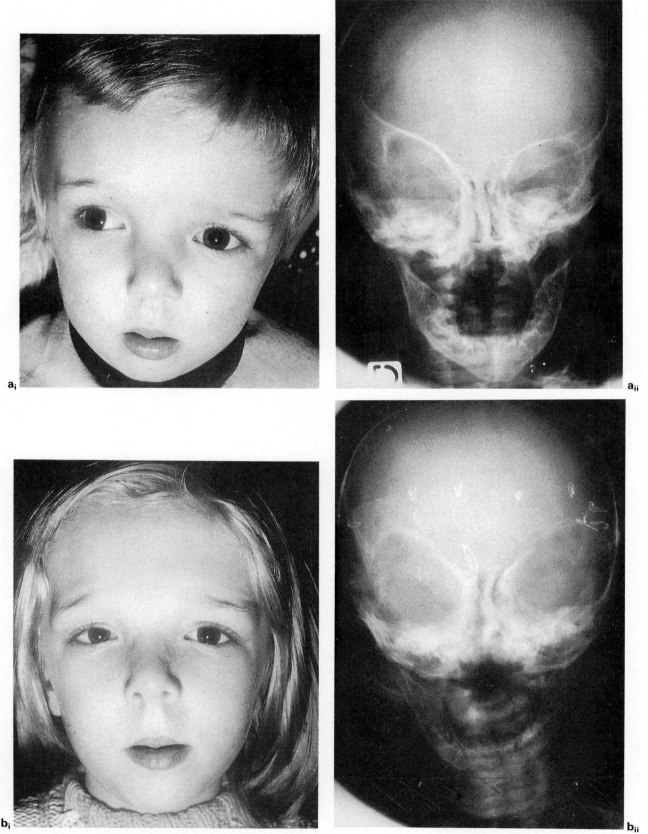

Fig. 20.80 Patient with right-sided plagiocephaly. Correction by bilateral remodelling:(a) preoperative views; (b) postoperative views.

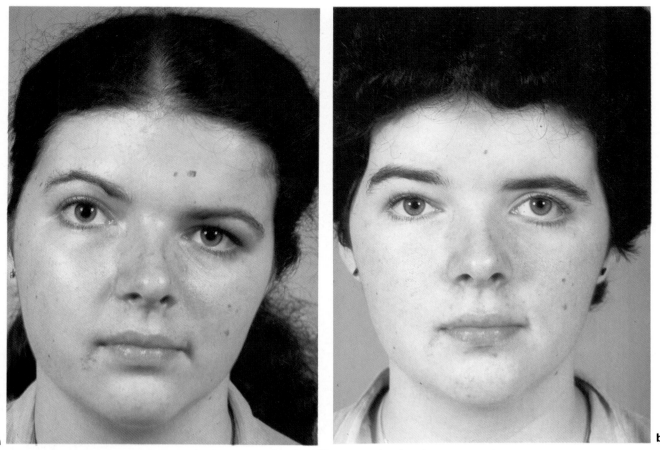

Fig. 20.81 Patient with right-sided plagiocephaly: (a) preoperative view; (b) postoperative view.

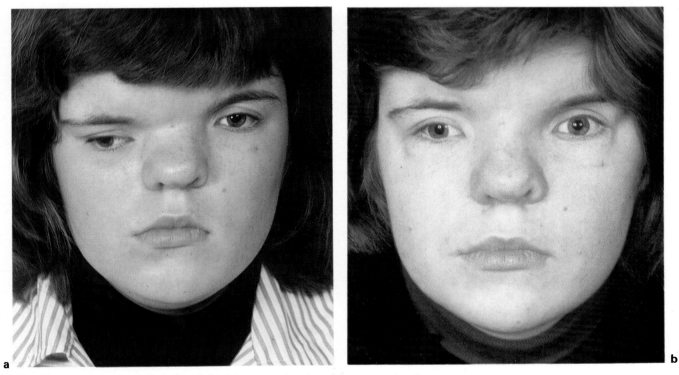

Fig. 20.82 Patient with left-sided plagiocephaly: (a) preoperative view; (b) postoperative view.

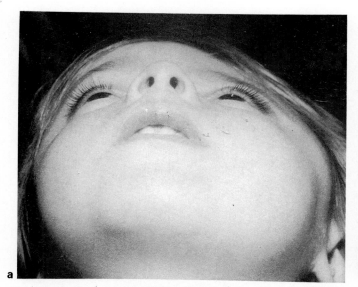
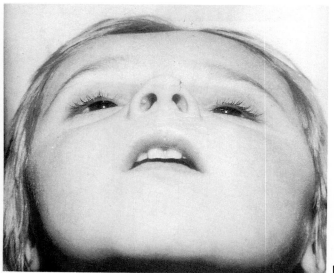

Fig. 20.83 Patient with left-sided plagiocephaly: (a) preoperative view; (b) postoperative view.

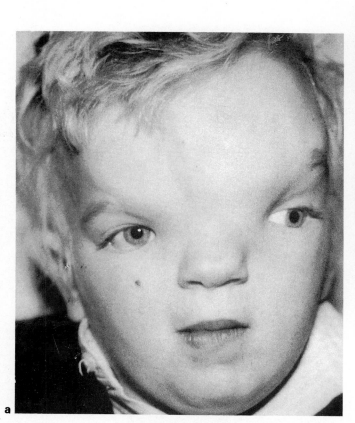
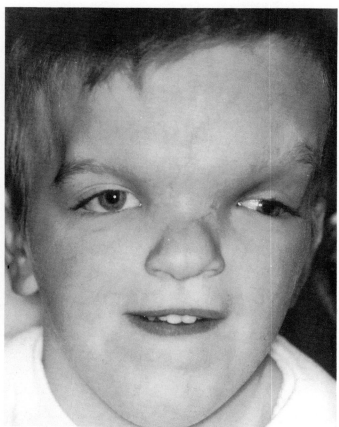

Fig. 20.84 Patient with left-sided plagiocephaly and teleorbitism. Correction by bilateral remodelling and reduction of interorbital distance: (a) preoperative view; (b) postoperative view.

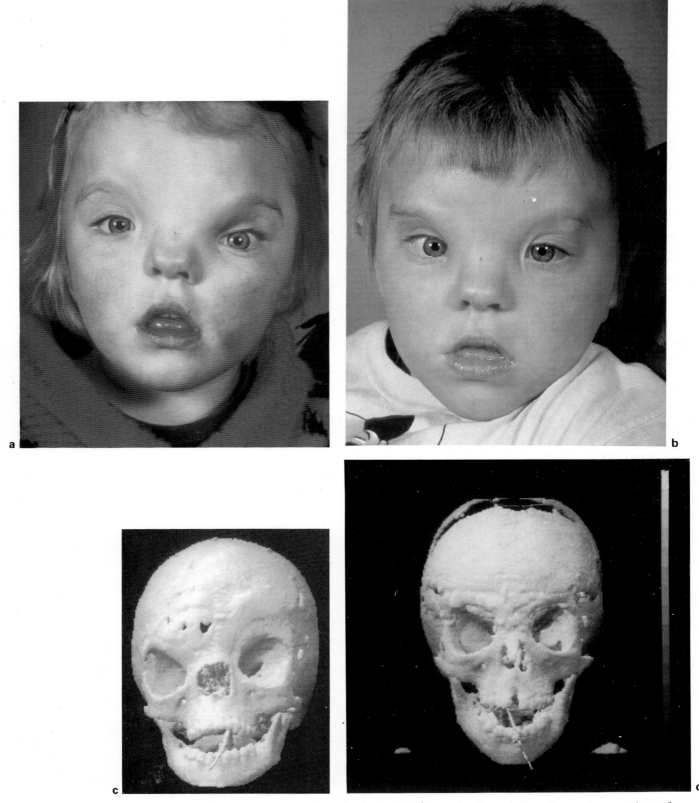

Fig. 20.85 Patient with right-sided plagiocephaly and teleorbitism. Correction by 'medial faciotomy' and remodelling of upper inner quadrant of right orbit: (a) preoperative view; (b) postoperative view; (c) 3-D CT reconstruction (preoperative); (d) 3-D CT reconstruction (postoperative). Note: residual epicanthal folds require secondary correction.

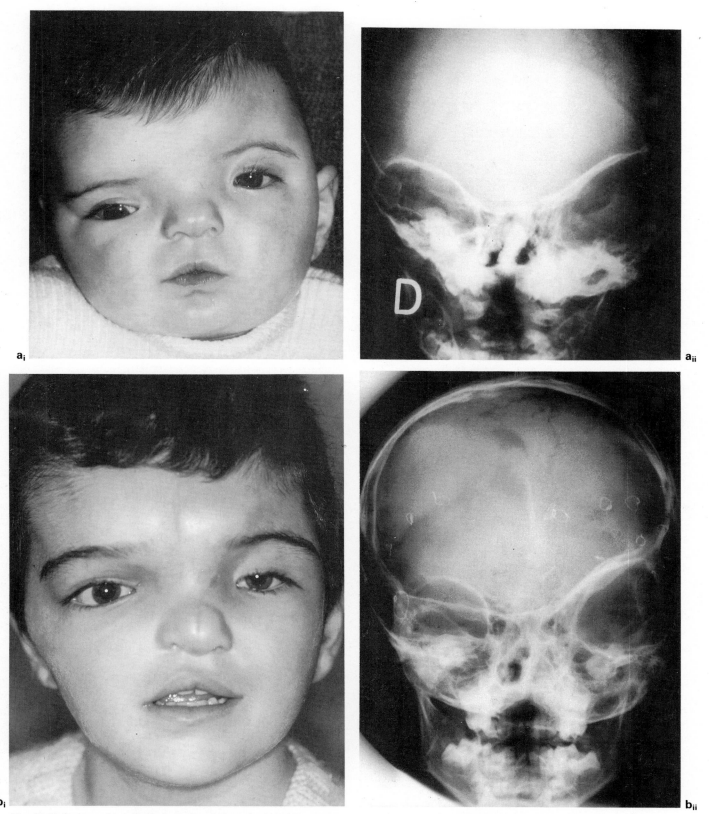

Fig. 20.86 Patient with left-sided plagiocephaly and teleorbitism. Correction by unilateral medialization of orbit. The result is unsatisfactory: (a) preoperative views; (b) postoperative views.

complex. Justified as this approach may be in adolescents or adults we consider it dangerous with a poor prognosis in childhood. On the other hand, transposition of the temporal muscle is extremely important. Its sphenoidal insertion lies too far backward, and forward transposition will serve to maintain the anteroposterior enlargement of the temporal fossa and to promote mandibular symmetry.

Brachycephaly

Anteroposterior shortness of the cranial vault and of the part anterior to the coronal suture in particular frequently occurs and also affects the face. In the past, attempts at correction solely concerned the frontal bone. Nowadays the principles are always the same and include:

1. Frontal remodelling by transposition of an adequately shaped segment from the cranial vault.
2. Fronto-orbitonasal propulsion with forward rotation to restore the frontonasal angle.
3. Temporal correction if necessary.

Reduction of the height of the cranial vault is indicated in patients with acrocephaly and may be achieved by more extensive remodelling involving the parietal bones.

FRONTAL REMODELLING

The transposition of frontal segments, initially pedicled, later free, was described in 1977 by Montaut & Stricker. The idea was to replace the dysplastic segment by one of normal contour, while also preserving its vascular supply by means of the temporal muscle and periosteum. Marchac (1978) advocated and popularized this concept, coining the imaginative term 'floating forehead' for this procedure. In fact, the forehead does not float but remains anchored to the anterior part of the cranial base.

Frontal transposition by lowering of a superiorly situated bipedicled visor-like segment is the procedure of choice, but the transposition of a free segment is of similar usefulness in all cases in which vascularization of the segment is difficult to preserve.

FRONTO-ORBITONASAL PROPULSION

The type of osteotomy is dictated by the specific demands posed by the malformation in question. A tenon-shaped extension is used for horizontal advancement, and a Z-shaped transposition (Marchac 1978) for all other cases.

TEMPORAL CORRECTION

The temporal fossa is usually short and depressed. The malformation may be corrected by various methods: by extirpation or inversion of the anomalies segment, by

replacing it with a graft or by exchanging it with that of the opposite side.

Results obtained with the use of these techniques are generally good in uncomplicated cases (Figs. 20.87–20.91) but somewhat less when facial involvement exists (Fig. 20.92).

Oxycephaly

Correction of this special form of brachycephaly associated with scaphocephaly is subject to the same surgical objectives. The bregma may have to be removed, especially if it is responsible for a 'clown's cap' malformation.

The results are generally of good quality (Fig. 20.93) but there are cases in which a discrepancy occurs between a normal forehead and facial retrusion over the years. This situation is seen in some patients operated on for brachycephaly and is probably due to minor degrees of facial dysostosis or synostosis previously unnoticed. Facial stenosis in the newborn with Crouzon's deformity (Fig. 20.94), except when spectacular exorbitism exists (Fig. 20.95), is not always obvious. Facial correction may therefore seem of less importance.

Three types of brachycephaly can in fact be distinguished:

1. True brachycephaly, which is a brachycrany, without facial retrusion.
2. Brachyorbitism, in which the retrusion affects the orbital and fronto-orbital level.
3. Brachyprosopy, in which facial retrusion only becomes obvious at a later stage.

In the majority of patients with scaphocephaly there is no indication for forward advancement of the frontonasal band. Postoperatively however, some of these cases develop brachycephaly with or without a rise of the intracranial pressure (ICP). In other cases visual problems may be observed after many years. Regular, clinical control and measurement of ICP, when in doubt, is therefore imperative.

FACIAL SYNOSTOSIS

Synostosis of one or more facial sutures, whether isolated or in association with synostosis of the cranial vault, introduces a negative element in the prognosis of growth. The effect of cerebral growth on the face is only felt indirectly and remains restricted to its upper part.

The morphological results of surgical correction show no improvement apart from that produced by normal growth. This pessimistic but realistic notion influences the age at which surgery can best be performed. In spite of this it is useful to distinguish between craniofacial

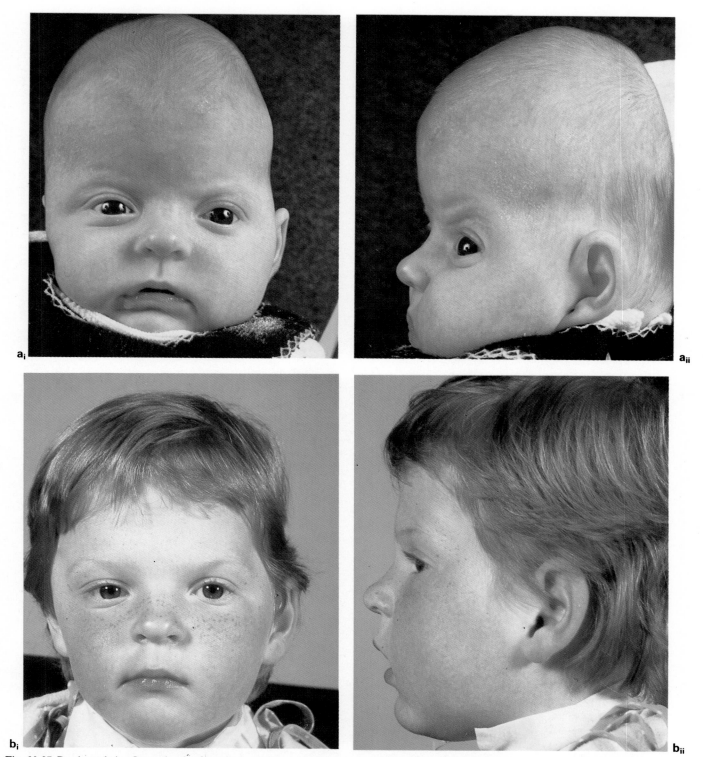

Fig. 20.87 Brachycephaly. Correction by frontal advancement: (a) preoperative views; (b) postoperative views.

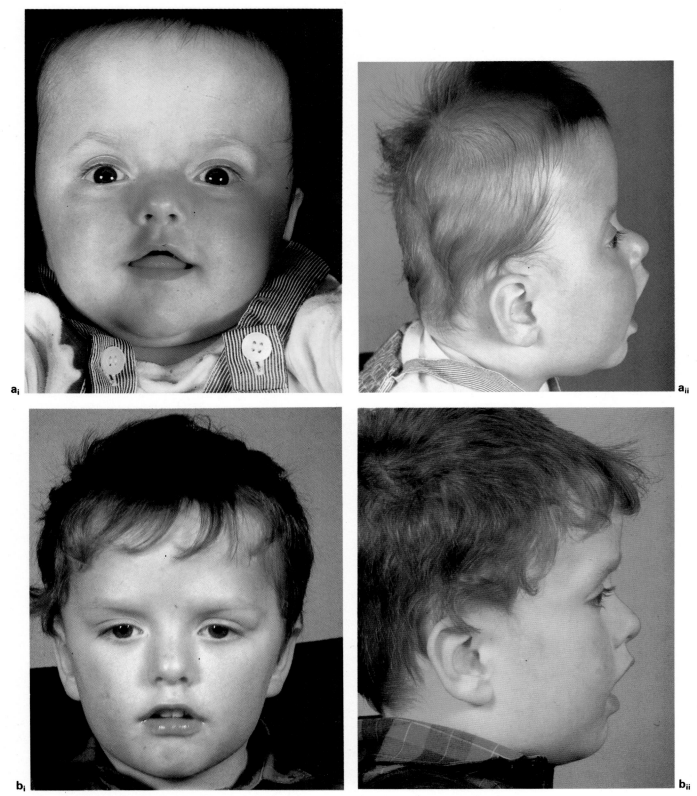

Fig. 20.88 Brachycephaly. Correction by frontal advancement: (a) preoperative views; (b) postoperative views.

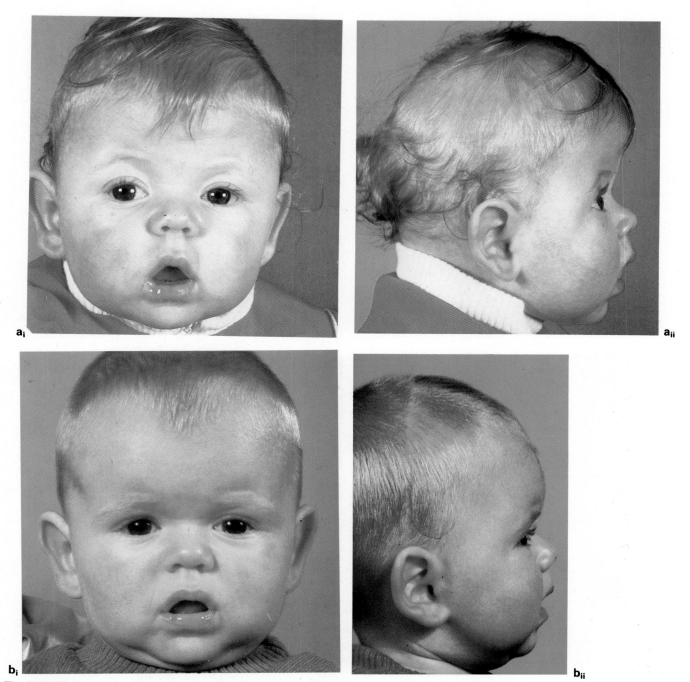

Fig. 20.89 Brachycephaly — note retrusion of orbital roof: (a) preoperative views; (b) postoperative views.

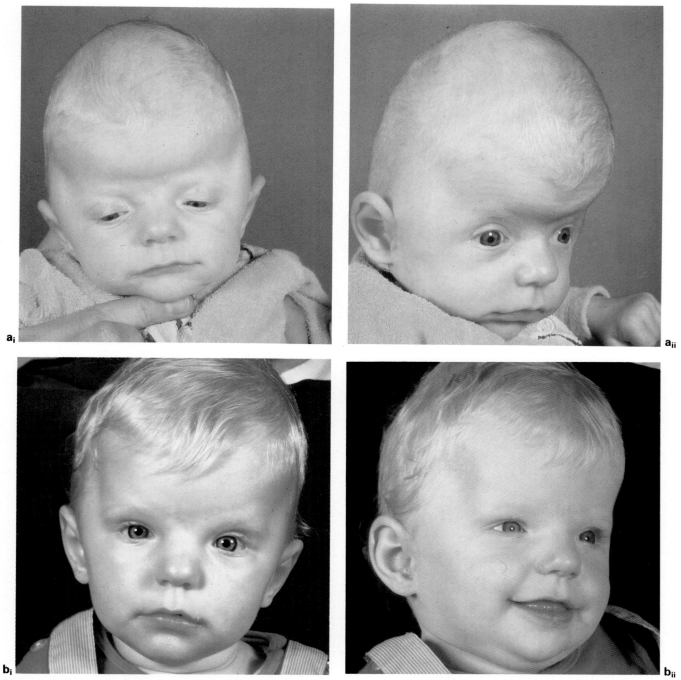

Fig. 20.90 Brachycephaly — note frontal bossing. Correction by frontal advancement and remodelling: (a) preoperative views; (b) postoperative views.

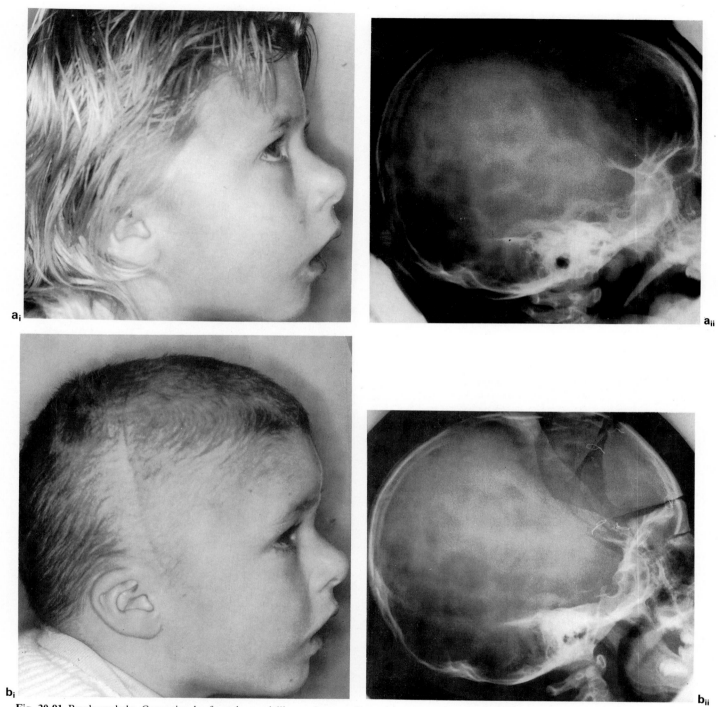

Fig. 20.91 Brachycephaly. Correction by frontal remodelling at 3 years of age: (a) preoperative views; (b) postoperative views.

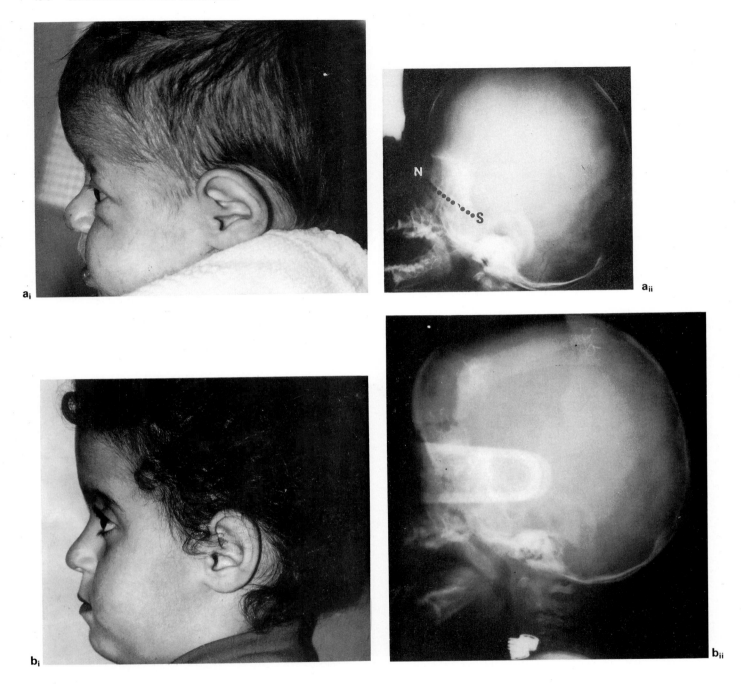

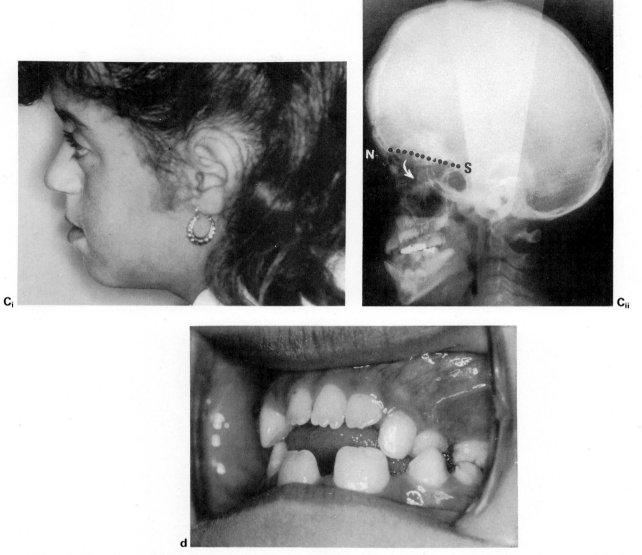

Fig. 20.92 Transitional form between brachycephaly and Crouzon. Early diagnosis is difficult. (a, b, c) Evolution shows the presence of facial retrusion at different stages of development, and X-rays confirm this. (d) Occlusion.

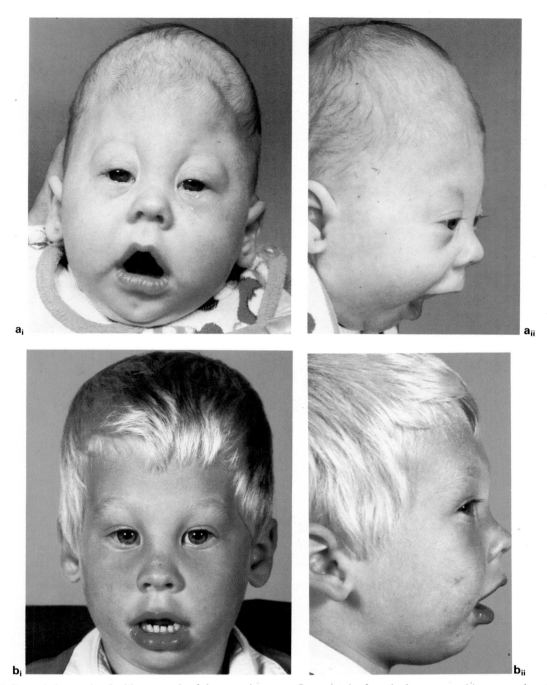

Fig. 20.93 Oxycephaly associated with synostosis of the metopic suture. Correction by frontal advancement: (a) preoperative views; (b) postoperative views.

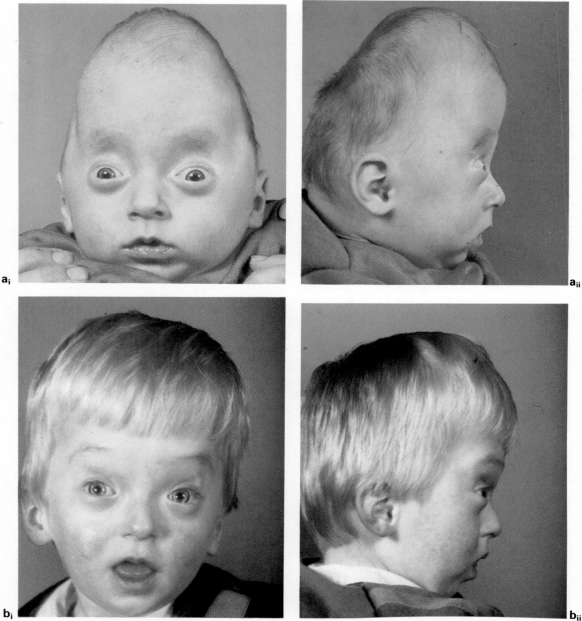

Fig. 20.94 Oxycephaly associated with orbital retrusion (Crouzon's syndrome). Correction by frontal advancement: (a) preoperative views; (b) postoperative views.

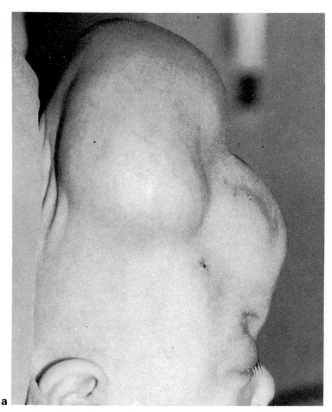
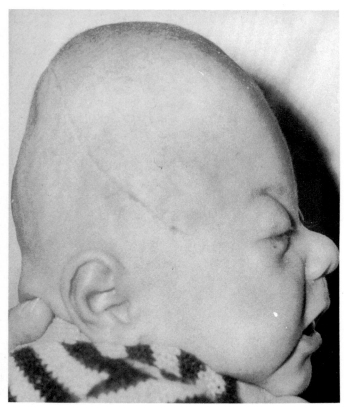

Fig. 20.95 Triphyllocephaly. Correction by cranial remodelling: (a) preoperative view; (b) postoperative view.

synostosis and isolated facial synostosis, since it is in the first group that the cranial intervention, which is necessary to free the brain, will be associated with a release of the facial skeleton — without hope, however, as to a better long-term result.

Three typical forms may be distinguished: orbitosynostosis, retromaxillism (Fig. 20.96) and Binder's syndrome (Figs. 20.97–20.99).

The lack of an intrinsic dynamic mechanism in the postoperative period and the absence of any risks of functional deterioration are reasons to postpone surgical treatment until

1. orbital development is completed at the age of 8 years in patients with orbitosynostosis;
2. the canine tooth has erupted at the age of 11 years in cases with retromaxilly; and
3. adolescence where Binder's syndrome is concerned.

Here it must be stressed that the use of orthopaedic appliances has no effect on the stenotic structures.

Secondary correction

Correction postponed until adulthood combines orthodontics and surgery in different protocols.

In Binder's syndrome there are two options:

1. Orthodontic treatment to harmonize the alveolodental arches in occlusion and bone-grafting in the deficient area or a supra-alveolar perinasal osteotomy according to Psillakis et al (1973).
2. A naso-maxillary monobloc osteotomy (Converse 1970), which brings the retruded area forward.

Transverse reduction of the upper lip, a genioplasty and projection of the nasal bridge by means of a graft are complementary procedures. In retromaxillism orthodontic treatment is limited to harmonization of the alveolodental arches, facial correction being obtained by Le Fort I or II osteotomies.

CRANIOFACIAL DYSOSTOSIS AND SYNOSTOSIS

In the past correction of craniofacial dysostosis and synostosis, such as Crouzon's and Apert's syndromes, was

Fig. 20.96 (right) Faciostenosis. Retromaxillism with promandibulism. Correction by Le Fort I osteotomy and sagittal splitting of the ramus: (a) preoperative views; (b) postoperative views.

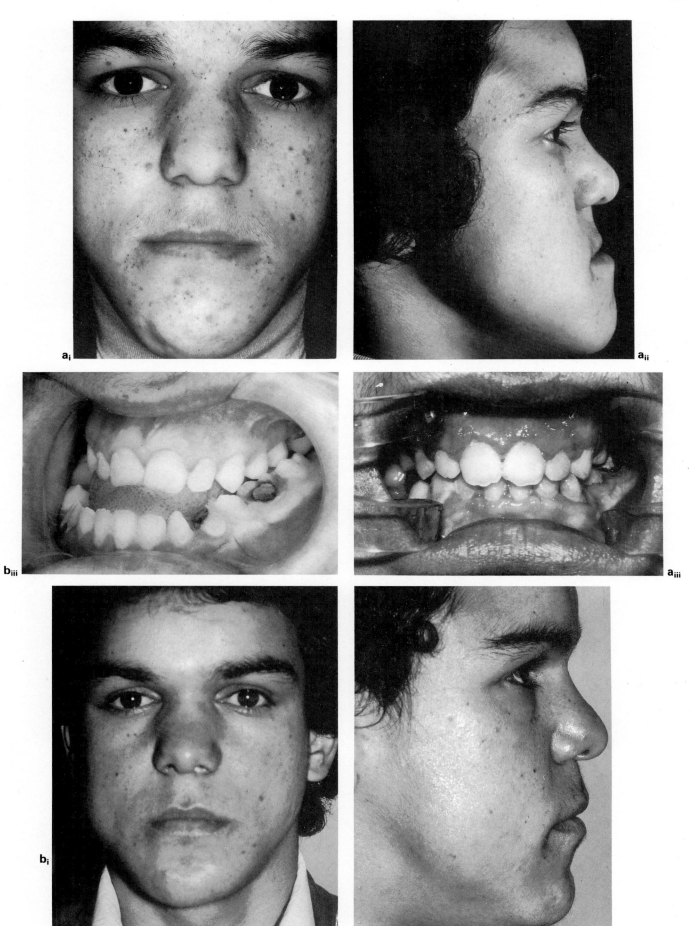

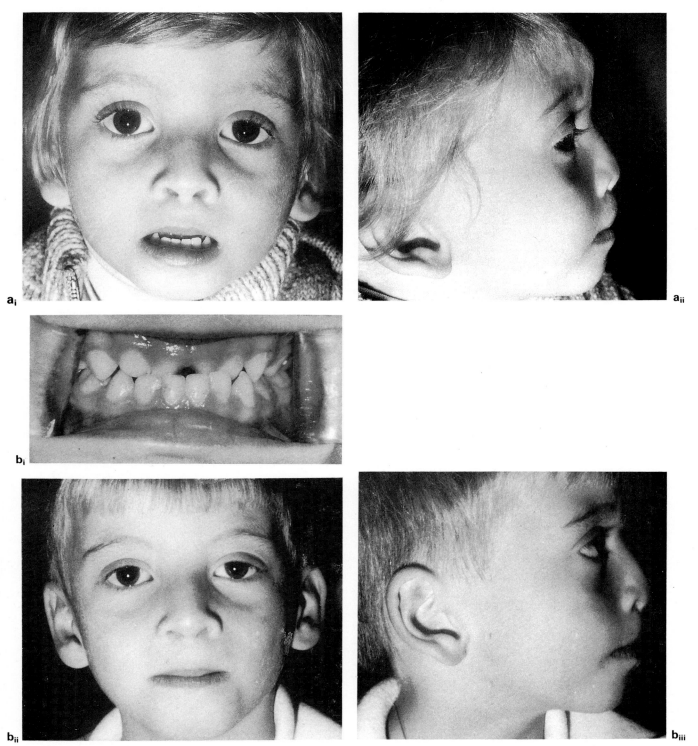

Fig. 20.97 Binder's syndrome. Unfavourable result following osteotomy of the vomers–premaxillary complex and orthopaedic treatment: (a) preoperative views; (b) postoperative views.

Fig. 20.98 (right) Binder's syndrome. Mild degree of occlusion disturbance. Correction of facial balance by bone grafting to the dorsum of the nose, onlay genioplasty and medial approximation of the orbicularis oris.

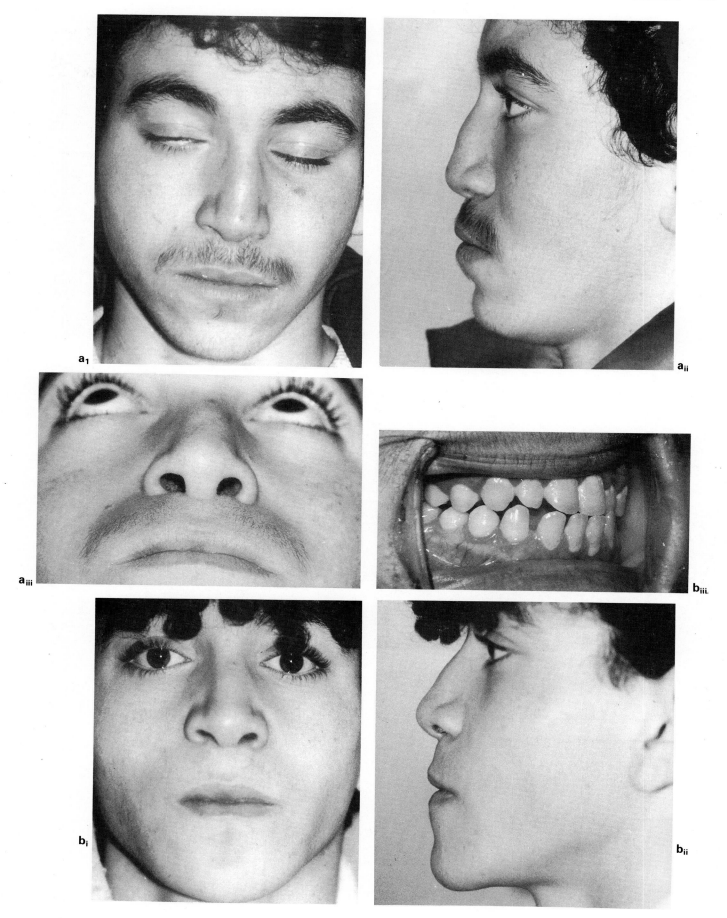

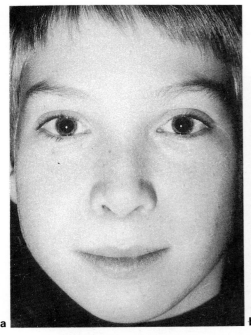

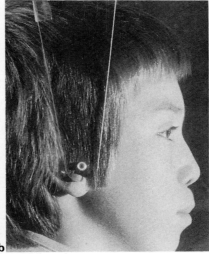

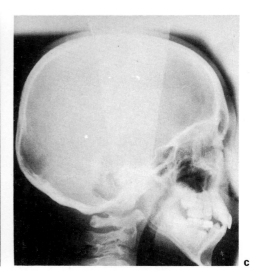

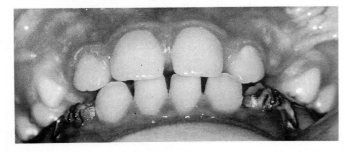

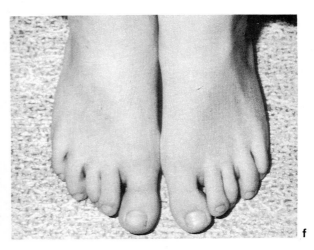

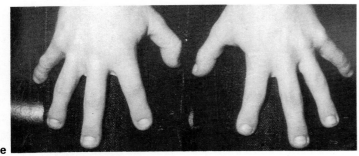

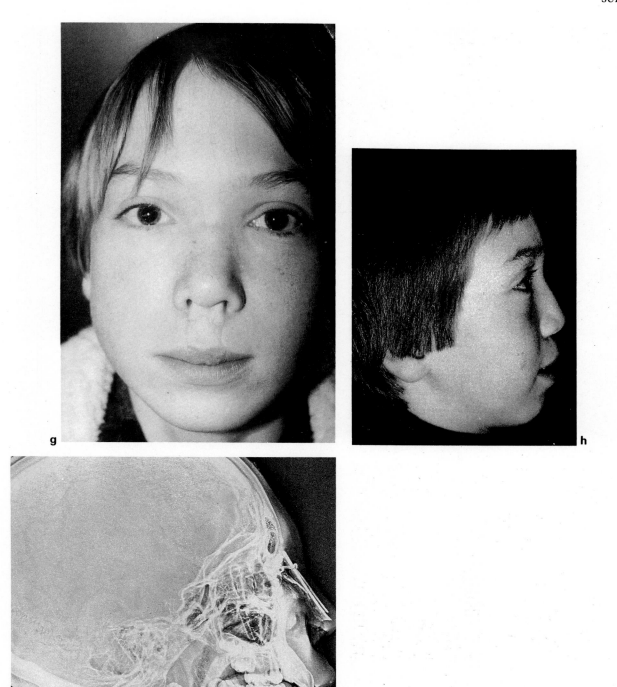

Fig. 20.99 Binder's syndrome: (a–f) clinical aspect suggests a Binder's syndrome. However, occlusion is normal and hands and feet are abnormal. Histological examination of the septum revealed cartilaginous pathology. Treatment consisted of columellar lengthening (g) and restoration of the nasal projection (h) with bone graft (i).

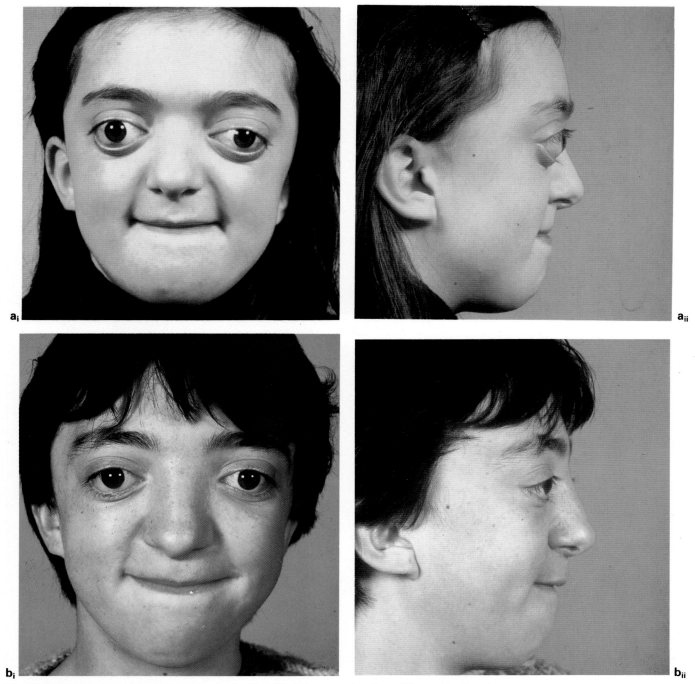

Fig. 20.100 Crouzon's syndrome. Correction by Le Fort III: (a) preoperative views; (b) postoperative views.

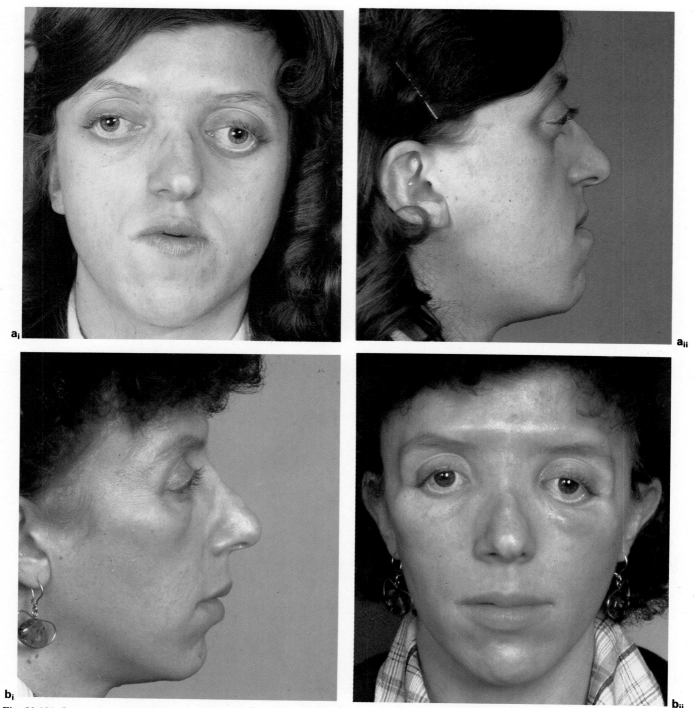

a_i

a_ii

b_i

b_ii

Fig. 20.101 Crouzon's syndrome. Correction by Le Fort III: (a) preoperative views; (b) postoperative views.

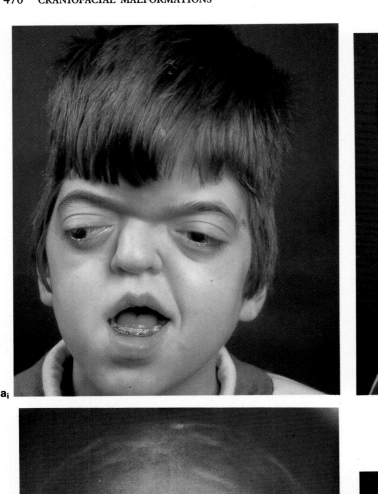

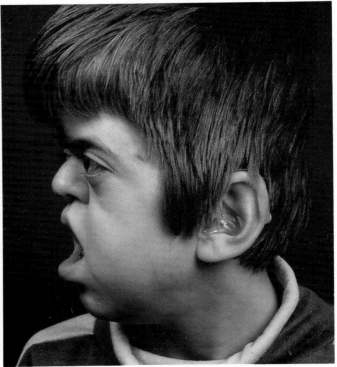

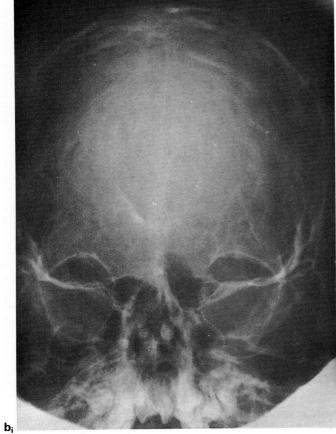

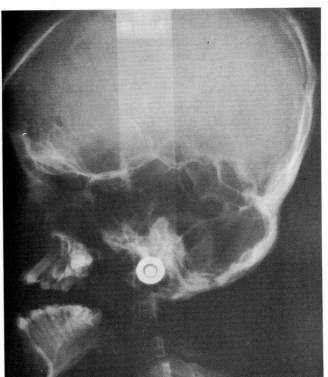

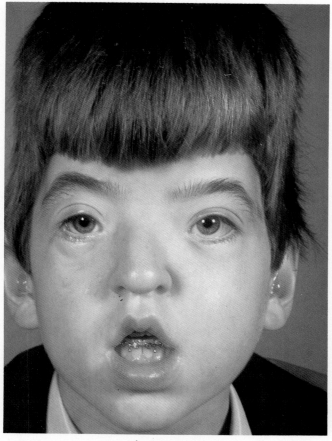
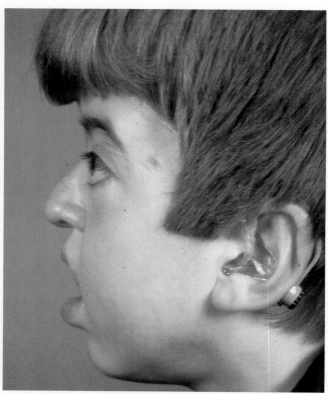

c_i   c_ii

Fig. 20.102 Apert's syndrome associated with loss of vision. Correction by Le Fort III: (a) preoperative views; (b) X-rays show teleorbitism and and maxillary retrusion; (c) postoperative views.

mainly performed in adolescents and adults. A Le Fort III or rarely a Le Fort II osteotomy was the treatment of choice. If necessary it was combined with frontal remodelling. In general results were satisfactory (Figs. 20.100–20.104). Onlay grafting to correct orbital retrusion provided an alternative when disimpaction was impossible or inadvisable for some reason (Fig. 20.105).

Nowadays treatment of these patients is started at a much earlier age. The correction of cranial and facial synostosis may, however, pose many technical difficulties in the newborn. Surgery of the cranial vault is similar to that used for the correction of brachycephaly, with the restriction that a frontofacial monobloc or Le Fort IV osteotomy is indicated in most of the symmetrical cases. The forehead is advanced or replaced by transposition of a frontal segment of the vault.

Timing of treatment

Early operation is indicated in view of the risks of functional deterioration, but the time of surgery should be delayed in view of the extended operating time and the additional hazards associated with total facial disimpaction. Severe exorbitism in Crouzon's disease (Fig. 21.106) and an obstructed airway in acrocephalosyndactyly are the two functional indications.

Type of procedure

Technical difficulties vary in accordance with morphological types. Disimpaction of the face is always perilous. It can be achieved by a Le Fort III osteotomy following fronto-orbital remodelling at an early age (Figs. 20.107, 20.108) or by a Le Fort IV (frontofacial monobloc) procedure (Figs. 20.109, 20.110).

In cases of Apert's syndrome, frontofacial asymmetry due to plagiocephaly and teleorbitism are commonly seen. Initially masked by the facial retrusion, the interdacryal distance (IDD) is accentuated in some cases as a result of the forward movement of the face (Fig. 20.111). Correction requires the formation of a fronto-orbitonasal band and reduction of the interorbital distance by medialization of the two halves of the band occasionally by a subethmoidal osteotomy at a second stage. The nasal corridor is,

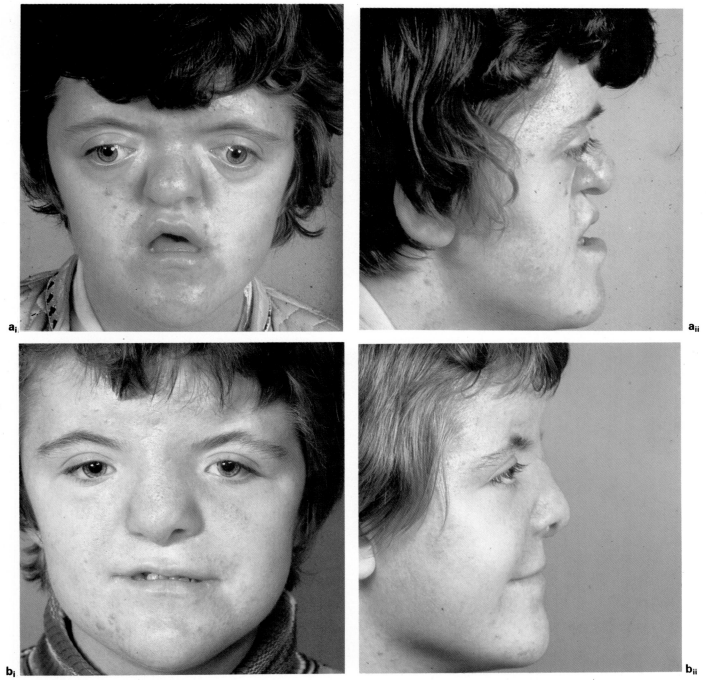

Fig. 20.103 Apert's syndrome. Correction by Le Fort III: (a) preoperative view; (b) postoperative view (with permission of the editor of *Annales de Chirurgie Plastique*, vol 19, 131, 1974).

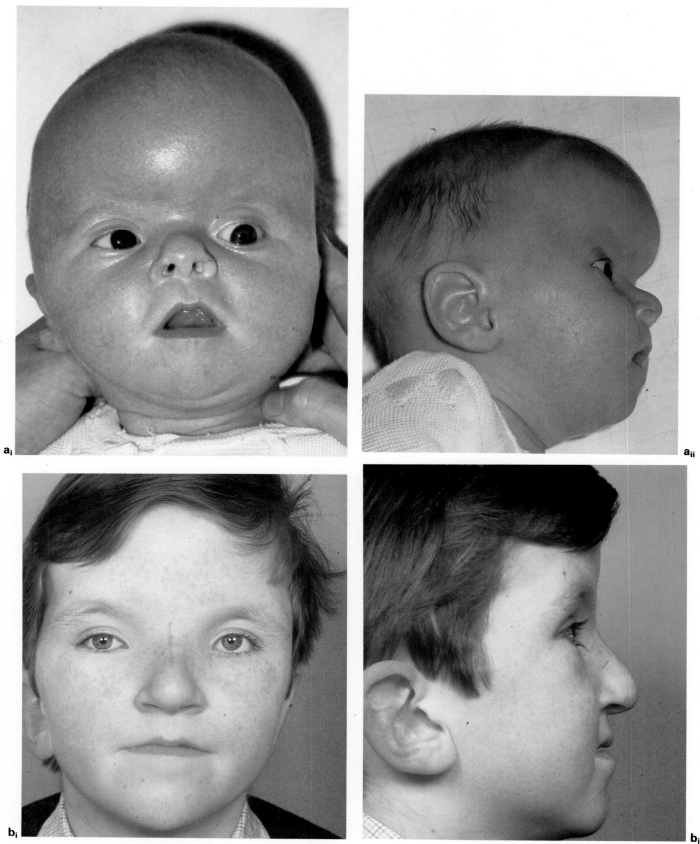

Fig. 20.104 Apert's syndrome. Correction by Le Fort II: (a) preoperative views; (b) postoperative views.

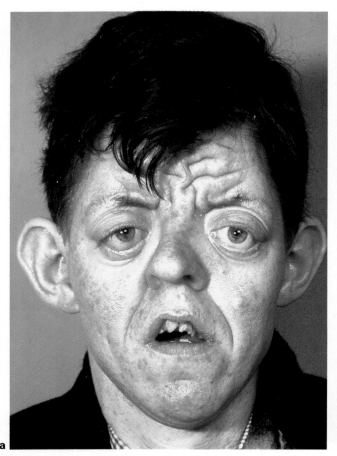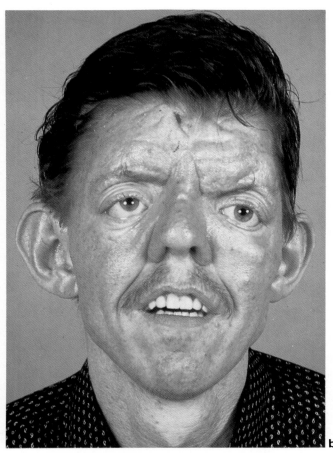

Fig. 20.105 Apert's syndrome. Correction by frontal advancement and onlay rib grafts in the infraorbital region: (a) preoperative view; (b) postoperative view.

however, narrow and the pharyngeal cavity small and filled by adenoid tissue. Bipartition of the frontofacial monobloc (Van der Meulen 1979) combining a triangular-shaped interorbital resection and an intermaxillary disjunction may be needed in some of these cases.

These surgical protocols are adapted to the specific requirements of each case. A periosteoplasty is always required to allow its expansion and a periorbitoplasty is indispensable in patients with exorbitism.

Prognosis of growth

The facial Le Fort III or frontofacial monobloc, Le Fort IV freed from above, is advanced, but instead of being fixed in this position orthopaedic stimulation is applied on the disimpacted skeleton by exerting forward traction 'en bloc' through a palatal plate, itself fixed by perizygomatic wires (Fig. 20.112).

Deprived of intrinsic stimulation the facial complex is, however, unable to pursue a normal growth. What then is the effect of orthopaedic treatment? The procedure is

technically difficult and long-term appliance probably illusory. We now attempt to prevent the relapse of stenosis and to stimulate facial advancement by partial transposition of the temporalis muscle (Stricker) (Fig. 20.113). The anterior half of this muscle, pedicled on the coronoid process and retaining its neurovascular bundle, is passed behind the face through the pterygomaxillary fossa and fixed to the pharyngeal sling in front of the pterygoid.

CRANIOFACIAL DYSOSTOSIS

The topographical order in which the indication for correction of dysplasias with dysostosis will be discussed follows that of the craniofacial helix. To prevent overlap and repetition it seems, however, logical to regroup the indications in accordance with their respective region. Each of which corresponds to specific surgical objectives and therefore demands different techniques. Five regions may thus be distinguished within the craniofacial skeleton (Fig. 20.114):

the cranio-orbitonasal region
the nasomaxillary region
the lateral craniofacial region
the oromandibular region
the dentoalveolar region.

The aetiology of the malformation is a decisive factor in the timing of surgery. The prognosis is determined by the presence of the intrinsic growth potential.

Cranio-orbitonasal region

The cranial cavity and more particularly its frontal part is the common denominator in this region. Most of the osteotomies pass through the anterior fossa and through one or both orbits. The objectives of surgery are therefore dictated by the need to preserve olfaction and oculopalpebral function. They concern:

1. The restoration of the continuity of the floor of the anterior cranial fossa and the contour of the cranial vault.
2. The mobilization of the orbits and their reconstruction.
3. The reconstruction of a nose. This is an important step which must not be underestimated because, as Tessier has said, in its final meaning the correction of teleorbitism is surgery of the nasal pyramid.

One is justified in operating early because the growth of the malformed region is seriously compromised. Surgical correction improves the morphology and consequently the 'body image' and mentality of the patient. In addition it diminishes the residual deformities, minimizing the importance of the secondary correction.

SPHENOFRONTAL DYSPLASIA

The appearance of the patient resembles that of a plagiocephaly but the skeletal anomaly is usually more severe and associated with a coloboma of the upper eyelid and a variety of soft tissue anomalies (widow's peak, etc.).

Protection of the eye has priority and it can be obtained by means of ocular unguents or an hourglass bandage. A temporary tarsorrhaphy carries the risk of an amblyopia. This strategy means that future craniofacial surgery is not compromised by scarring.

The skeleton

The dural deficiency in this area is marked by a band which may be released by a Z-plasty. The anomalies of the orbital roof and lateral orbital wall can be corrected by rotation of the upper half of the orbital rim, including a segment of frontal bone, around a craniocaudal axis at or near the midline. The resulting defects are closed with

bone grafts, and these, together with the displaced orbital rim, are stabilized in their new position. It should, however, be emphasized that the effect of cerebral thrust may be disappointing and that secondary corrections may have to be performed.

The soft tissues

The coloboma of the upper eyelid is usually repaired by transposition and advancement of conjunctiva and skin following mobilization of these structures and by release of retaining bands in the immediate vicinity of the defect (Fig. 20.115). A widow's peak should be resected and the defect closed by transfer of adjacent skin.

Ptosis of the upper eyelid should be anticipated and the repair of the coloboma provides an excellent opportunity to explore the orbit for the levator muscle. If this structure or remnants of it are found, tarsal reinsertion should be performed. In the absence of a levator, frontalis suspension may still be considered, provided of course this muscle is functional. Associated deficiency of tissue in the medial part of the eyelid and in the medial canthus may finally have to be corrected in an appropriate manner.

FRONTAL AND FRONTOFRONTAL DYSPLASIA

The skeleton

Malformations of the forehead (Fig. 20.116) are mainly characterized by skeletal defects and anomalies of the hairline, the eyebrow and the skin, which may be covered with dystopic patches of hair.

From a clinical point of view two different skeletal anomalies may be distinguished. The first relates to the presence of a malformation which is associated with a bony defect and as a whole will correspond to a cerebromeningeal anomaly (meningoencephalocele).

The second concerns the interruption of the superior orbital margin and eyebrow (coup de sabre) between the medial and lateral part of the frontal bone.

Correction of minor irregularities of the frontal bone is usually straightforward. They can be repaired by flattening of the more prominent parts and levelling of remaining depressions with bone grafts.

Closure of skeletal defects (Figs. 20.117, 20.118), however, requires a more cautious approach. The edges of the defect are meticulously dissected, taking care not to perforate the dura. Once they are free any protruding mass of brain tissue is either repositioned or removed and the defect is then bridged with bone grafts made of split skull or rib.

The soft tissues

Depending on the severity of the malformation,

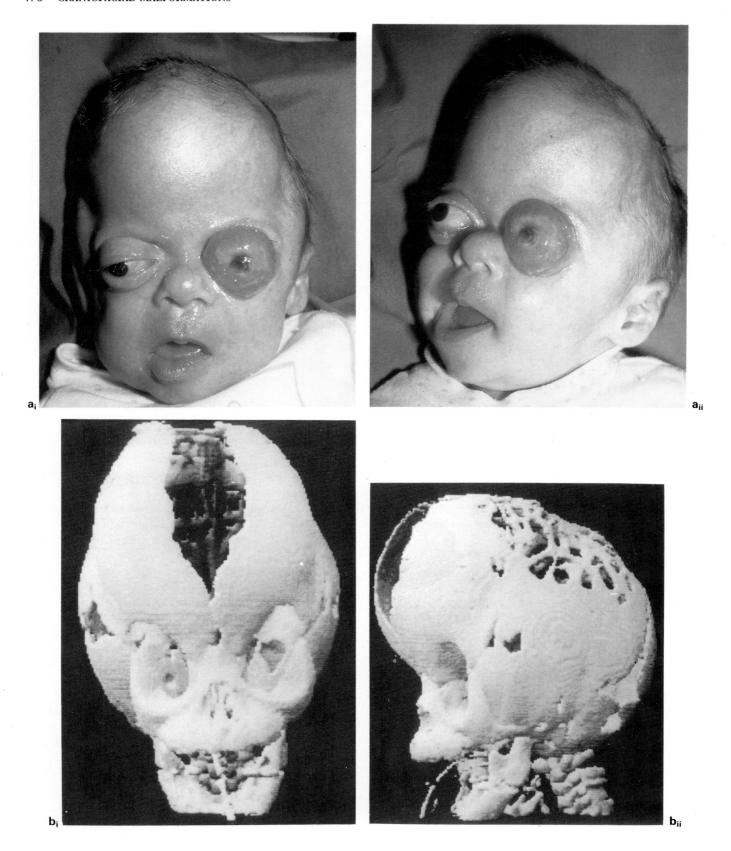

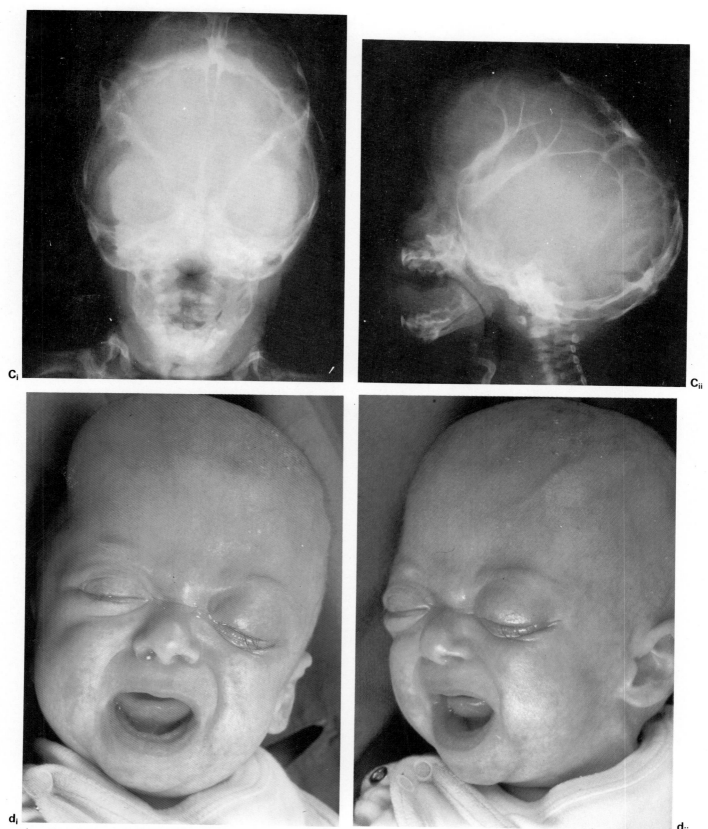

Fig. 20.106 Crouzon's syndrome associated with triphyllocephaly and extreme exorbitism. Failure of tarsorrhaphy necessitated early correction by frontofacial advancement (Le Fort IV): (a) preoperative views; (b) 3-D CT reconstruction; (c) X-rays shows trilobar configuration; (d) postoperative views.

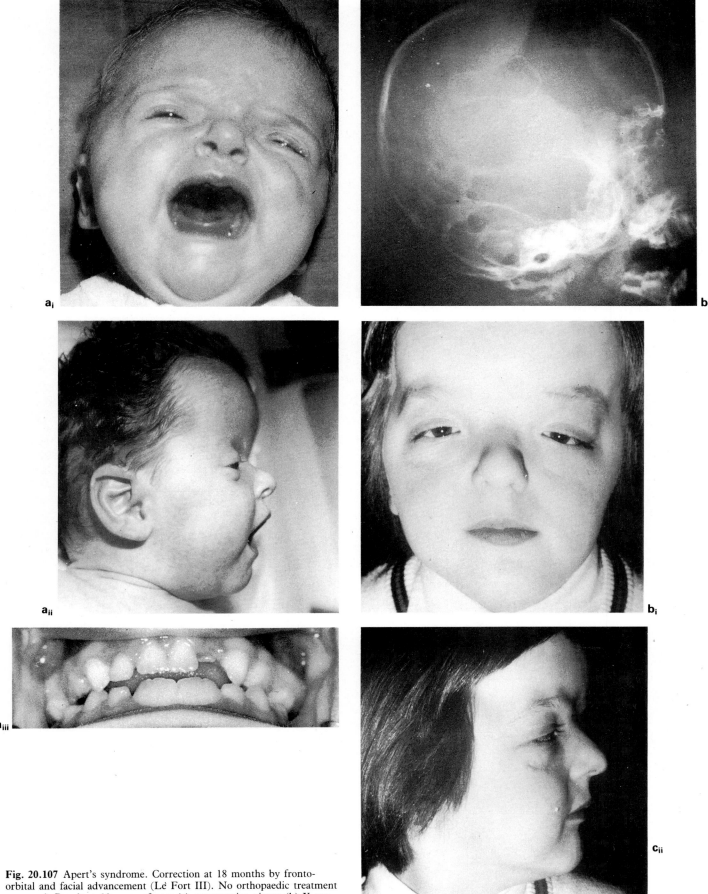

Fig. 20.107 Apert's syndrome. Correction at 18 months by fronto-orbital and facial advancement (Lè Fort III). No orthopaedic treatment was used. Result at 10 years of age: (a) preoperative views; (b) X-ray shows frontal advancement; (c) postoperative views.

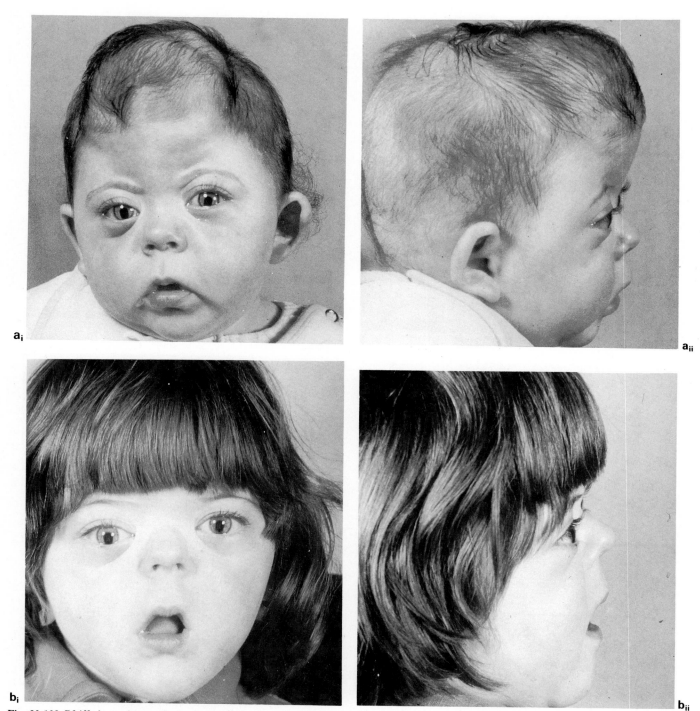

Fig. 20.108 Pfeiffer's syndrome. Correction by frontal remodelling: (a) preoperative views; (b) postoperative views. Facial advancement remains to be done.

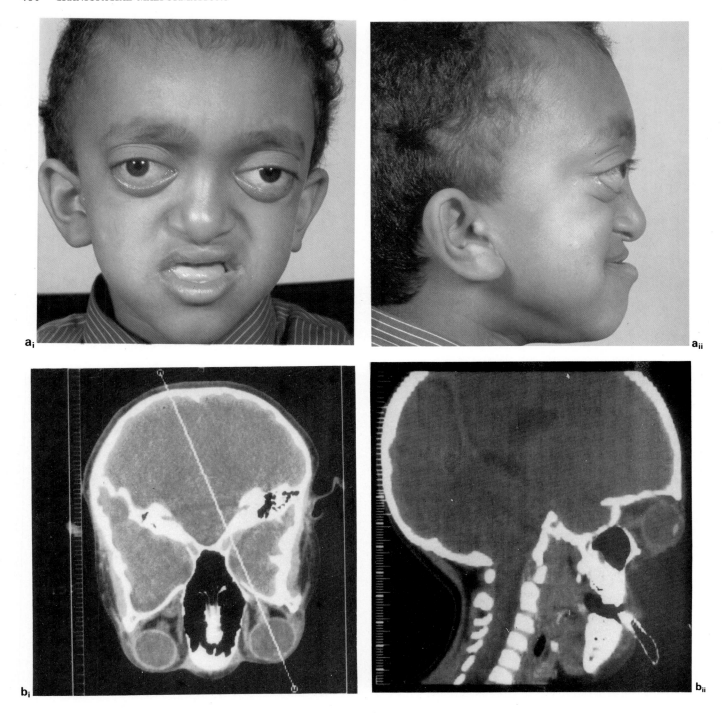

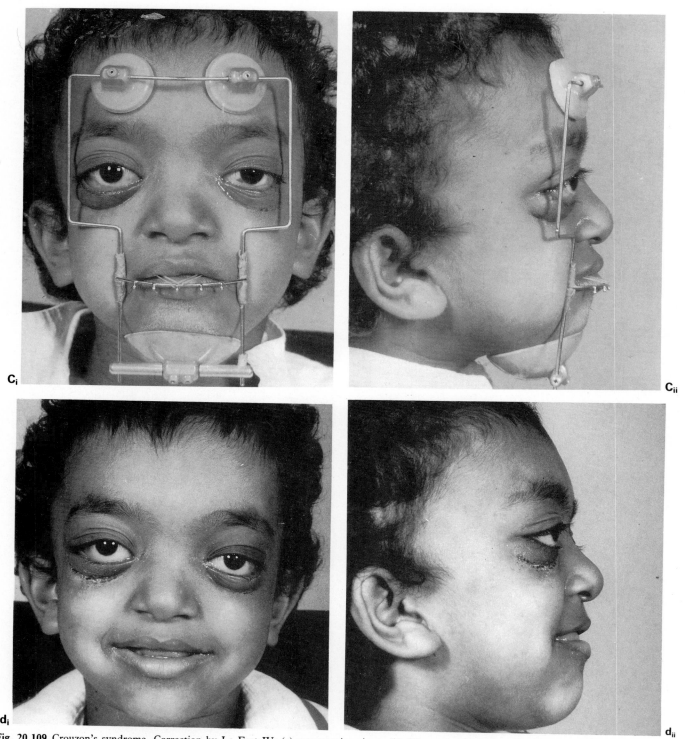

Fig. 20.109 Crouzon's syndrome. Correction by Le Fort IV: (a) preoperative views; (b) CT scans; (c) orthopaedic treatment; (d) postoperative views show early result.

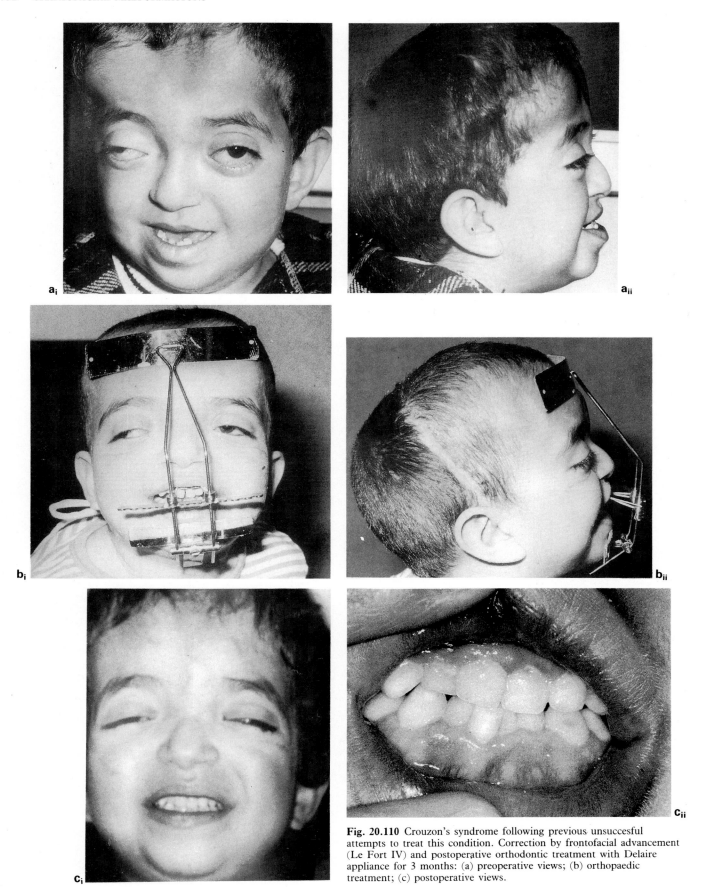

Fig. 20.110 Crouzon's syndrome following previous unsuccesful attempts to treat this condition. Correction by frontofacial advancement (Le Fort IV) and postoperative orthodontic treatment with Delaire appliance for 3 months: (a) preoperative views; (b) orthopaedic treatment; (c) postoperative views.

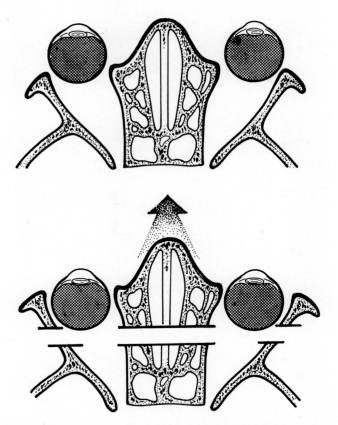

Fig. 20.111 Accentuation of teleorbitism following facial disimpaction.

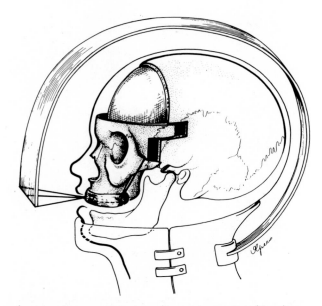

Fig. 20.112 Forward traction 'en bloc' following facial disimpaction.

irregularities of the hairline and of the eyebrow can be treated in one or several stages by excision or revision of a widow's peak, an ectopic streak of hair or a coloboma of the eyebrow. Resulting defects should be closed by advancement or transposition of normal skin. The use of a skin graft or skin flap or a galea flap covered with a skin graft may be indicated in exceptional cases.

FRONTO-NASOETHMOIDAL DYSPLASIA

Interorbital anomalies

The interorbital space may be compared to a two-floor building, each with two compartments. The frontal sinus and anterior cranial fossa constitute the upper floor and the nasal cavity with the ethmoidal sinus, the lower. The space filled by these compartments is always subject to changes in an absolute sense and in relation to each other. Normally these alterations are minor and of little significance.

Important changes may, however, be produced by the displacement of the cribriform plate and medial wall of the orbit in craniosynostoses, by protrusion of an encephalocele through a defect in the floor of the anterior cranial fossa, by enlargement of the frontal sinus, by expansion of the ethmoidal sinus and by other space-occupying processes (fibrous dysplasia, craniotubular dysplasia) in this particular region. As a result, abnormalities in composition, dimension and configuration of the interorbital space will be observed.

Orbital anomalies

Contrary to the interorbital space, the orbit is only a one-compartment structure. Its formation responds to a dynamic process of adjustment designed to accommodate the growing brain and eye.

This process may be altered by developmental disturbances affecting the eye itself (cerebro-craniofacial dysplasias) or the surrounding skeletal structures (craniofacial dysplasias). As a result abnormalities in dimension (retrusion and constriction), configuration (vertical or oblique ovalization) and position (lateralization, verticalization and rotation) may be observed. In combination the interorbital and orbital anomalies may produce an almost infinite spectrum of malformations, some symmetrical, some asymmetrical with one abnormal orbit. Analysis by CT scanning is always required for accurate planning of the osteotomies and the precise direction in which the orbital segment will have to be moved.

Correction of interorbital or orbital hypertelorism is based on the following steps:

1. Removal of interorbital obstacles.
2. Preservation of the cribriform plates.

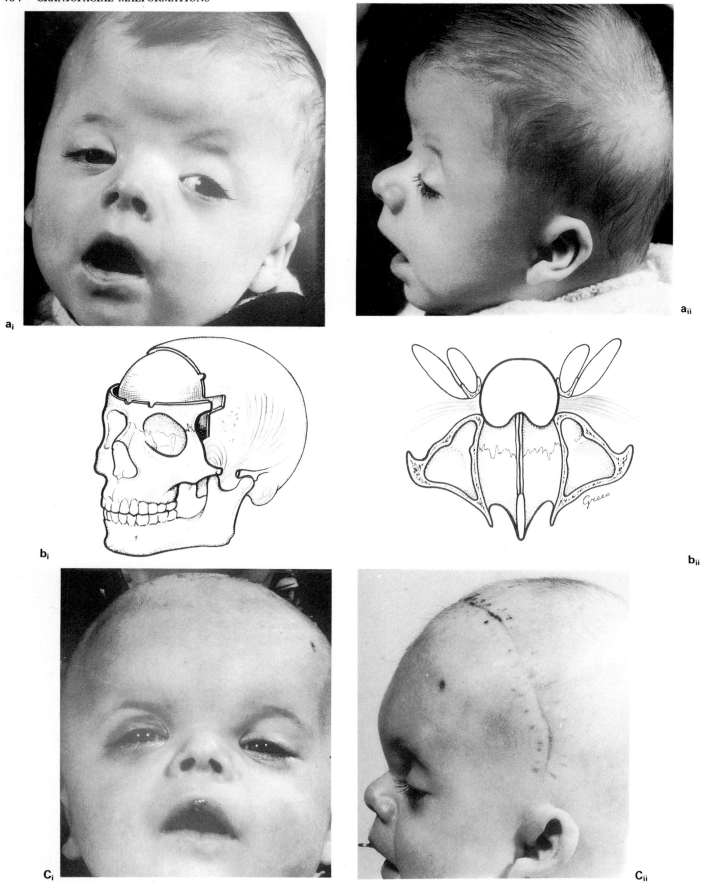

Fig. 20.113 (left) Crouzon's syndrome. Correction by frontofacial advancement (Le Fort IV) supported by retromaxillary transposition of the anterior half of the temporal muscle. Postoperative orthopaedic treatment by traction on palatal plate fixed by zygomatic suspension: (a) preoperative views; (b) operative technique; (c) postoperative views show early result.

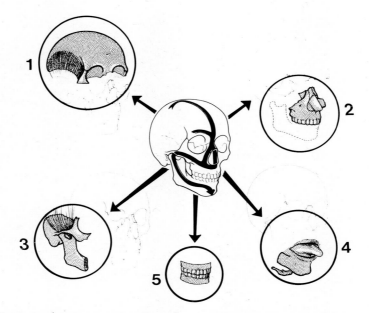

Fig. 20.114 Surgical sectors:(1) Cranio-frontonasal, (2) nasomaxillary, (3) temporomandibular, (4) dentoalveolar, (5) oromandibular.

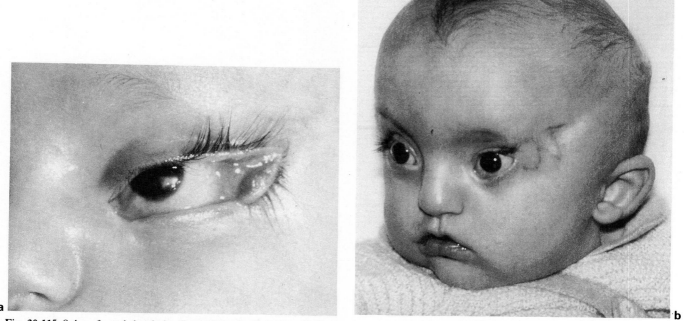

Fig. 20.115 Sphenofrontal dysplasia. Correction of palpebral malformations by local rearrangement of flaps:(a) preoperative view;
(b) postoperative view.

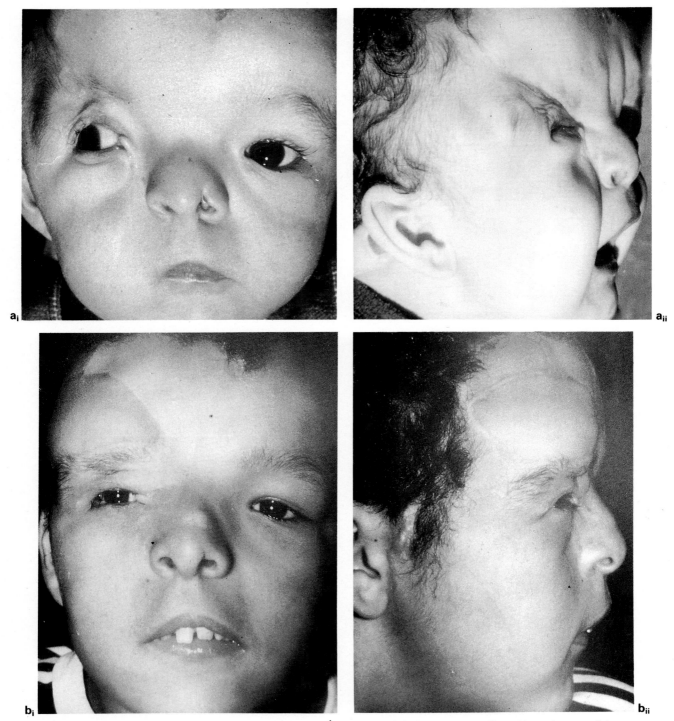

Fig. 20.116 Frontal dysplasia with ophryal distorsion, plagiocephalic deformation of forehead corresponding with contracture of dura mater, upper eyelid coloboma, telecanthus and notch in left nostril. Correction by Z-plasty of dura, fronto-orbital advancement, free flaps in frontal region and local rearrangement of skin: (a) preoperative views; (b) postoperative views.

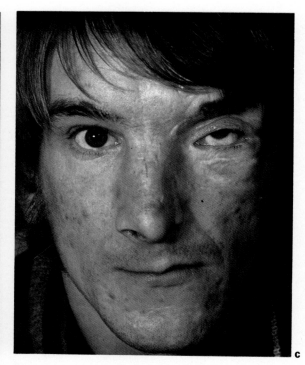

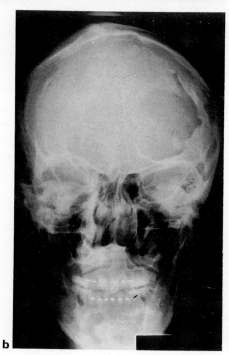

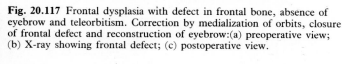

Fig. 20.117 Frontal dysplasia with defect in frontal bone, absence of eyebrow and teleorbitism. Correction by medialization of orbits, closure of frontal defect and reconstruction of eyebrow:(a) preoperative view; (b) X-ray showing frontal defect; (c) postoperative view.

6. Relaxation of the periosteum and reattachment of a mobilized temporalis muscle.
7. Fixation of the skin by means of a canthopexy.
8. Adaptation of the soft tissues to the skeleton by resection and rearrangement.

Removal of the interorbital obstacles may be achieved by the resection of brain tissue, ethmoidal cells, the perpendicular plate of the ethmoidal bone, the septum and the turbinates. The integrity of the cribriform plate and the nasal mucosa is to be respected. In some patients with a good profile it may be advisable to preserve the midline of the nasal dorsum and restrict the resection to the removal of parasagittal blocks.

Reduction of the interorbital distance requires approximation of the interface between the interorbital space and the orbit. The manner in which the orbit is moved, in part or in toto, by single-quadrant osteotomies (mediofrontal or maxillary), by two-quadrant osteotomies (nasal or medial, subcranial or inferior, cranial or superior, U-shaped or C-shaped) or by movement of the entire orbital aperture alone or in combination with the maxilla, depends on a number of factors.

The dimension of the orbit. This is usually normal in interorbital hypertelorism. It may, however, be abnormal

3. Reduction of the interorbital distance by medial displacement of the orbit in part or in toto, sometimes by movement of the orbitomaxillary complex as a whole.
4. Restoration of the continuity of the cranial base.
5. Reconstruction of the nasal pyramid.

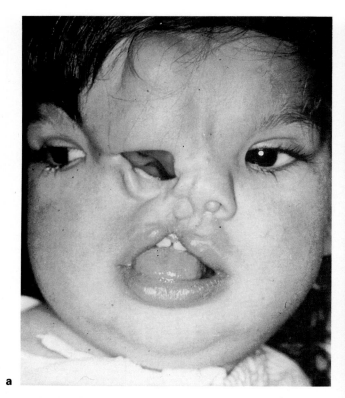

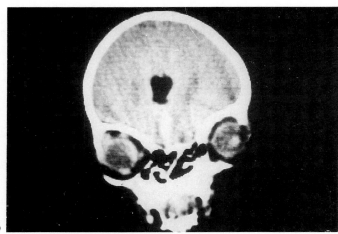

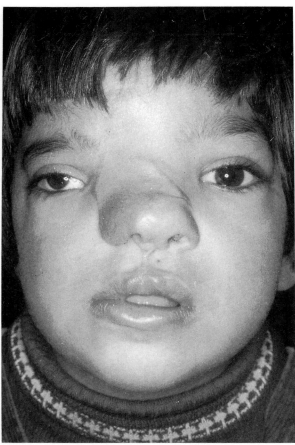

Fig. 20.118 Frontofrontal dysplasia associated by with severe teleorbitism and nasoschizis. Correction by closure of midfrontal defect, medialization of orbits and nasal reconstruction using regional skin surplus: (a) preoperative view; (b) CT scan; (c) postoperative view (with permission of the editor of the *Annals of Plastic Surgery*).

in some patients with teleorbitism (symmetrical or asymmetrical). Exorbitism in Apert's syndrome and microorbitism are typical examples. In the first example, correction of the retruded orbit and of teleorbitism is achieved by propulsion, translation and rotation of the entire orbital aperture. In the second example, correction of the restricted orbit and of teleorbitism may be obtained by nasal U-osteotomy and by medialization of the mobilized segment.

The configuration of the orbit. Abnormal configuration may be observed in both interorbital and orbital hypertelorism. The type of treatment, always by partial osteotomies, is determined by the site(s) of the abnormality and

the level of the cribriform plate. Interorbital hypertelorism (caused by encephaloceles, pneumatoceles, synostoses, etc.) is usually corrected by mobilization and medialization of a superior skeletal quadrant. Remodelling of the medial orbital wall and closure of the defect in the anterior cranial fossa with a bone graft can, however, be sufficient in some patients with frontonasal or frontoethmoidal encephaloceles. The surgical protocol should always be adapted to the specific requirement posed by each case (Figs. 20.119–20.123). Inferior quadrant osteotomies are rarely indicated. The correction of orbital disfiguration and teleorbitism seen in some synostoses, such as Cohen's syndrome and plagiocephaly, requires more extensive partial osteotomies incorporating the lateral wall. Superior two-quadrant U-osteotomies or even better C-osteotomies are used for this purpose, but additional remodelling of the orbital roof to correct the inward bulging of the medial wall and the outward bulging of the lateral wall may be required.

The position of the orbit. This is normal in interorbital

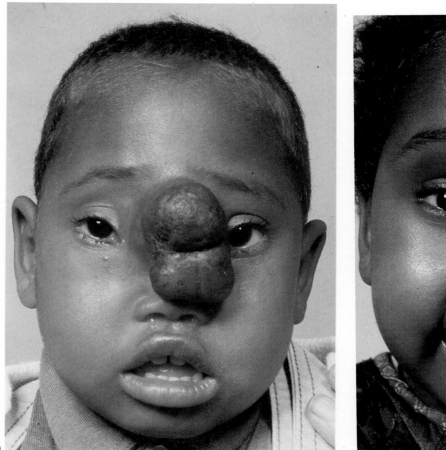
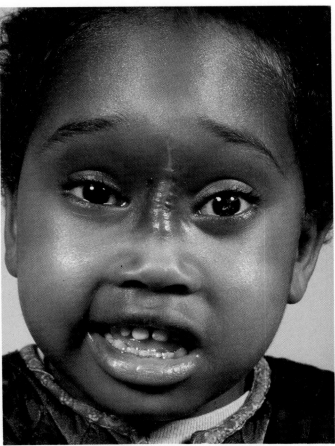

Fig. 20.119 Frontonasal meningoencephalocele. Correction by medialization of the superomedial quadrants of the orbit, and closure of the remaining osseous defects with a graft and canthopexies. Reconstruction of the nasal dorsum is indicated: (a) preoperative view; (b) postoperative view (early) (with permission of the editor of *Plastic and Reconstructive Surgery*).

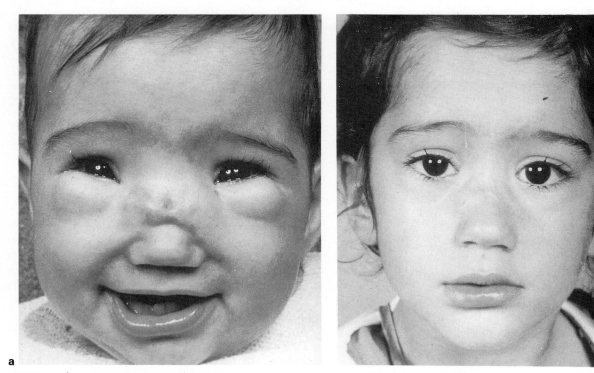

Fig. 20.120 Frontonasal meningoencephalocele. Correction by closure of osseous defect: (a) preoperative view; (b) postoperative view.

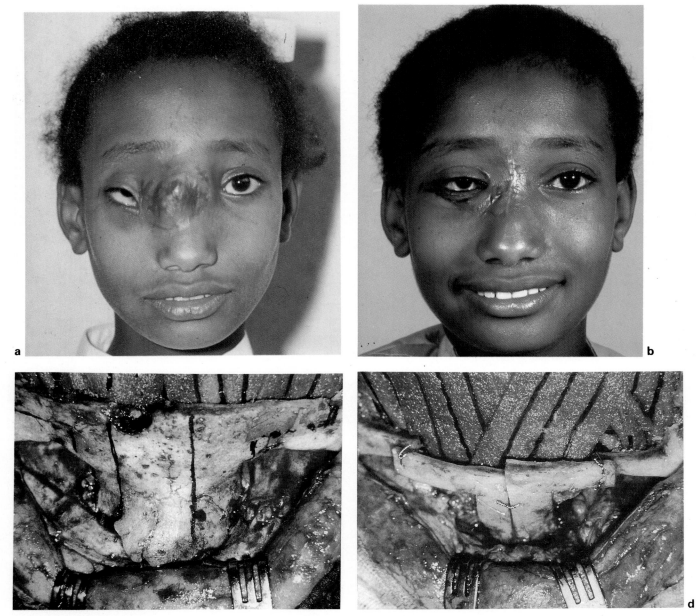

Fig. 20.121 Frontoethmoidal meningoencephalocele (lateral). Correction by medialization of the superomedial quadrants of the orbit, palpebral relocation and canthopexies: (a) preoperative view; (b) postoperative view (early); (c, d) operative technique.

hypertelorism and abnormal in orbital hypertelorism or teleorbitism. Correction can best be obtained by translation and rotation of the orbit as a whole (Fig. 20.124).

The position of the maxilla. The combination of teleorbitism and positional abnormalities of the maxilla is quite common in patients with craniofacial dysplasias with dysostosis (internasal, nasal and nasomaxillary dysplasia) and with synostosis (Cohen's syndrome, Apert's syndrome). In these patients, correction of teleorbitism by a medial faciotomy or by facial bipartition may be indicated.

The age of the patient. This factor may finally play a role when the type of orbital osteotomy is chosen. A four-quadrant osteotomy cuts across the maxilla and may inhibit growth when used at an early age (Mulliken et al 1986). The disadvantages of a medial faciotomy in terms of growth are not known but the magnitude of this procedure at an early age is such that it should only be used in selected cases after full consideration of the risks involved.

Restoration of the continuity of the cranial base over an intact nasal mucosa is of the utmost importance. It should

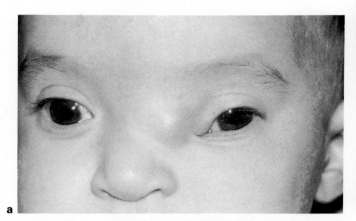
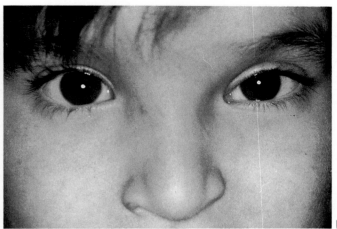
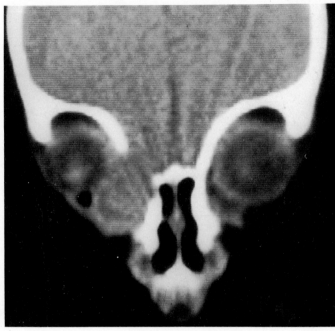

Fig. 20.122 Frontoethmoidal meningoencephalocele (lateral):
(a) preoperative view; (b) postoperative view; (c) scan shows defect in medial orbital wall.

this new position. Fixation of the canthi to the naso-orbital skeleton is extremely important.

Adequately performed canthopexies will anchor the soft tissues to the bone and help in preventing the formation of secondary deformities due to the presence of lateral forces generated by the orbicularis muscle and the contraction of newly formed scar tissue in the orbital region (Fig. 20.126). Telecanthus, epicanthus, canthal dystopia and flattening of the nasal roof sulcus may thus be produced.

To overcome these problems and adequately correct the different anomalies one should resect as much of the redundant skin as possible and thin the remaining tissues in order to enhance solid reattachment, since firm fixation is only achieved over a period of time. In some less severe cases one should even consider waiting for the correction of teleorbitism until adulthood is reached (Fig. 20.127). Adaptation of the soft tissues by resection of the redundant skin and rearrangement of the residual tissues in harmony with the orbital and nasal skeleton will complete the operation.

INTERNASAL DYSPLASIA

Internasal dysplasia is usually associated with hypertelorism. The wider the cleft and the greater the interorbital distance, the shorter the nose and the more arched the maxillary vault.

When the maxillary deformity is of little importance, reduction of the interorbital distance by medialization of the orbits alone is obviously the procedure of choice. Medialization of the orbit and maxilla by means of a medial faciotomy may, however, be indicated in cases with a more pronounced maxillary deformation.

The idea of transposing the orbit and the maxillary

be achieved by the medial movement of the skeletal segments. The closure of a small defect with a bone or a pericranial graft or even by the transposition of a galeal or pericranial flap is, however, occasionally indicated.

The reproduction of a nasal skeleton must be seen as the 'grand finale' of each hypertelorism correction and this step may be particularly difficult when the nose itself is abnormal (Fig. 20.125). The quality of this rhinoplasty is to a large extent responsible for the overall result of the performance and the principles of nasal reconstruction should therefore be strictly adhered to. Relaxation of the periosteum by multiple incisions through the periorbital ring and in the immediate vicinity of the orbital aperture will serve to readapt this tissue to the displaced skeletal segments and reattachment of the mobilized temporalis muscle to the lateral wall of the orbit will help in retaining

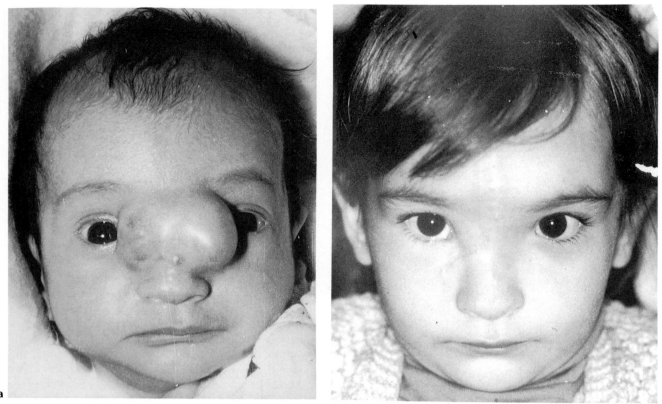

Fig. 20.123 Frontoethmoidal meningoencephalocele (lateral): (a) preoperative view; (b) postoperative view.

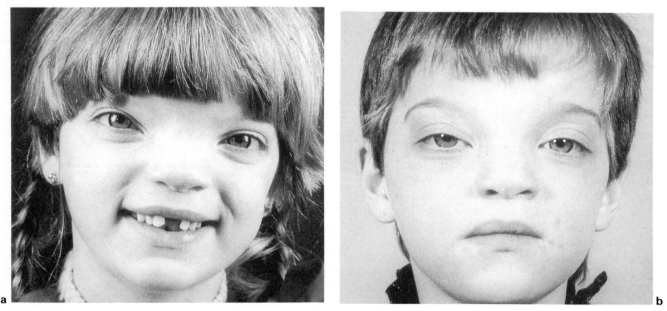

Fig. 20.124 Teleorbitism. Correction by medialization of orbits: (a) preoperative view; (b) postoperative view.

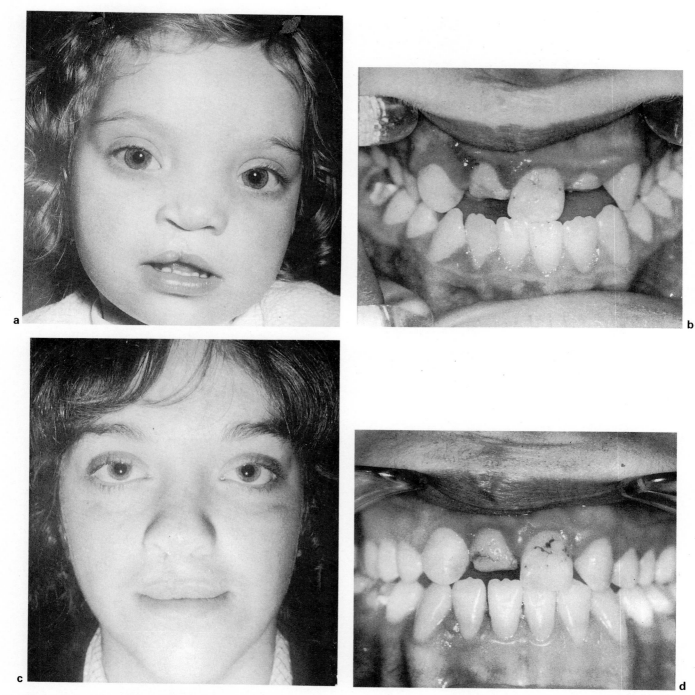

Fig. 20.125 Teleorbitism with cleft lip and palate. Correction by medialization of orbits at an early stage followed by orthopaedic treatment of maxillary retrusion, reconstruction of the nose by split-rib graft and revision of the lip deformity: (a) preoperative view; (b) occlusion before orthopaedic treatment; (c) postoperative view; (d) occlusion after orthopaedic treatment.

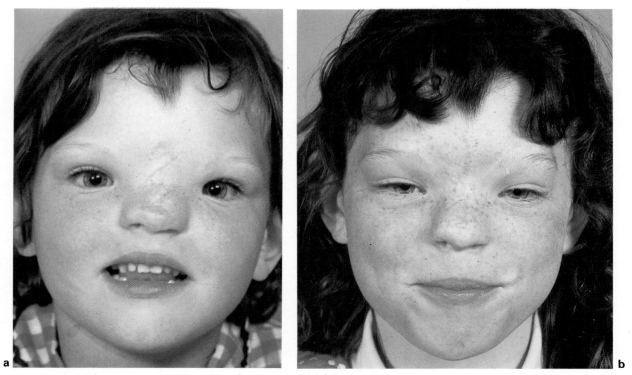

Fig. 20.126 Teleorbitism. Correction by medialization of orbits: (a) preoperative view; (b) postoperative view — residual telecanthus, probably due to canthal relaxation or secondary bone formation.

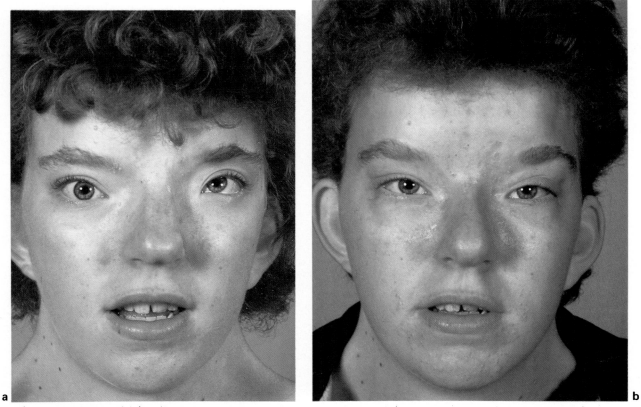

Fig. 20.127 Teleorbitism. Correction by medialization of orbits: (a) preoperative view; (b) postoperative view shows stability of result when correction is performed in adulthood.

segment as one unit was conceived when the association of hypertelorism and maxillary malformations was observed and the possibility of correcting these skeletal anomalies in one procedure was considered (Van der Meulen 1974, 1976, 1979, 1983). It was, however, first put into practice in patients with severe hypertelorism and median nasal clefting. The technique permitted a rotatory movement in each facial half, reducing the interorbital distance and lowering the height of the palate (Figs. 20.128, 20.129). Its potential for the correction of patients with craniofacial synostosis and hypertelorism (Apert's syndrome and Cohen's syndrome) was then also fully realized (Van der Meulen 1979). Correction of the nasal anomaly usually involves the cartilaginous skeleton as well as the skin.

The skeleton

In minor degrees correction may be achieved by extensive mobilization of the paramedian structures and repositioning of the alar cartilages (Fig. 20.130). Further augmentation of the nasal tip by cartilage grafts may be needed in some cases. In the more severe anomalies, reconstruction of the skeleton will require the following measures: removal of the anomalous cartilaginous tissue; restoration of a nasal framework; and medialization and fixation of the alar cartilages and redraping of skin over the new skeleton (Fig. 20.131).

The soft tissues

Correction of the skin deficiency in the nasal tip may be achieved in several ways, depending on the degree of severity. Linear closure of the dorsal defect following redistribution of skin over the depressed area and resection of redundant tissues is usually successful. Advancement of the contracted skin towards the tip of the nose in a V–Y manner and the transposition of flaps over the dorsum carry the risk of conspicuous scarring and these procedures should therefore be performed with utmost attention to detail (Figs. 20.132, 20.133). Rotation of a forehead flap has always been an excellent alternative when the anomaly cannot be corrected by local rearrangements of skin, but the results obtained by skin expansion may well make this technique the procedure of choice in the future.

NASOSCHIZIS

The severity of the anomaly ranges from a small coloboma of the ala to complete absence of one nasal half, providing direct access to the pyriform aperture. Choanal atresia has been reported, demanding immediate attention and early correction. Hypertelorism is always present in the more severe cases, while clefting of the alveolar arch may be observed. Reduction of the interorbital distance is obtained

by movement of the orbit in toto or by rotation of a hemifacial monobloc to correct both hypertelorism and the maxillary anomaly in one stage (Van der Meulen 1974, 1976).

The skeleton

Restoration of a nasal framework is required in the more severe cases. A costal or calvarial graft is preferably used, bearing in mind that this framework never grows and that the risk of some degree of resorption is real. It is for this reason that the cover of the graft should consist of well-vascularized tissue.

The soft tissues

Minor degrees of nazoschizis are usually corrected by simple rearrangement of skin. In the more severe cases reconstruction proceeds as follows.

The dislocated cartilages are first identified and dissected. The nasal lining is then restored by mobilization and apposition of the mucosal edges. This procedure is usually sufficient to create a passage of adequate dimensions. The final step concerns the nasal coverage, introducing the familiar problems related to scar formation and different colour match.

Unfortunately one cannot predict the behaviour of scars running across the bridge of the nose, since they may be scarcely visible or quite conspicuous. Nor is it possible to guarantee that texture and colour of the normal ala will match with that of the remaining part of the dorsum (Fig. 20.134).

To solve these problems it is in the first place better to provide coverage by rotation of the available surplus of skin in the nasal dorsum and glabella, a procedure which is facilitated by a back-cut in the medio-frontonasal region (Fig. 20.135). Secondly, one can remove the skin of the ala on the affected side up to its rim and close the resulting defects by judicious and economic use of the rotation flap. This approach provides a new cover with the final scars on the lateral aspect of the nose and in the alar rim, where they are least visible. It avoids scarring of the nasal dorsum (Fig. 20.136).

The nasomaxillary region

The centrofacial block, which predominantly is formed by the maxilla, benefits only little from cerebral expansion. Its main purpose is to protect the inferior respiratory part of the nose (Zuckerkandl 1882) and to support the orofacial muscular sling over its entire surface. Its sagittal growth is determined by the chondrocranium, more in particular by its nasal projection, the septum.

The surgical objectives specific for this region concern preservation of nasal permeability, reconstruction of the

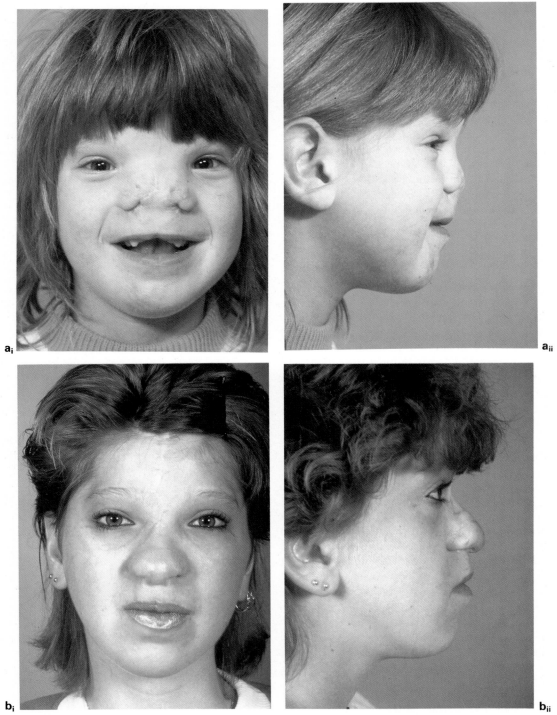

Fig. 20.128 Internasal dysplasia associated with severe teleorbitism. Correction by medial faciotomy (facial bipartition) and reconstruction of nose using forehead flap: (a) preoperative view; (b) postoperative view (with permission of the editor of the *British Journal of Plastic Surgery*.

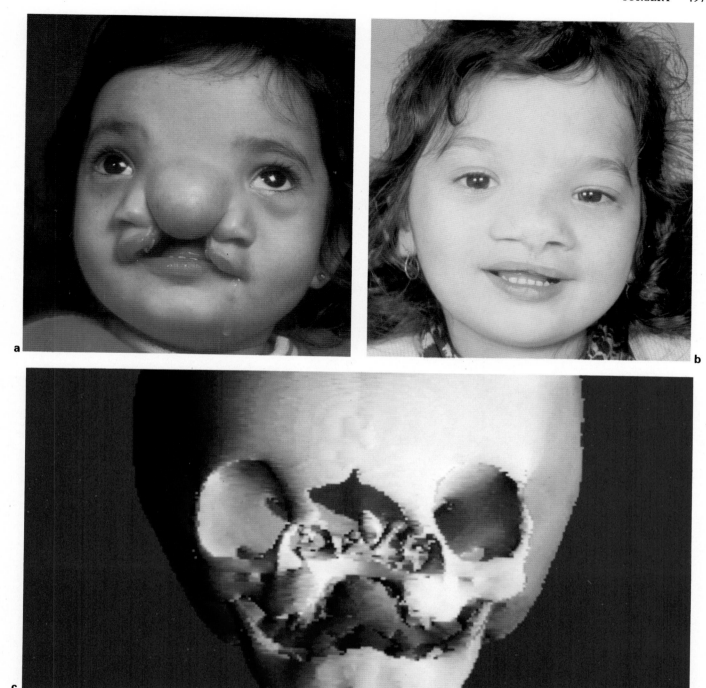

Fig. 20.129 Internasal dysplasia associated with extreme teleorbitism. Correction by medial faciotomy (facial bipartition) and resurfacing of the nasal dorsum using local surplus of skin: (a) preoperative view; (b) postoperative view; (c) 3-D CT reconstruction, frontal view (preoperative); (d) 3-D CT reconstruction, frontal view (postoperative); (e) 3-D CT reconstruction, cranial view (preoperative); (f) 3-D CT reconstruction, cranial view (postoperative); (g) 3-D CT reconstruction, sagittal view (preoperative); (h) 3-D CT reconstruction, sagittal view (postoperative).

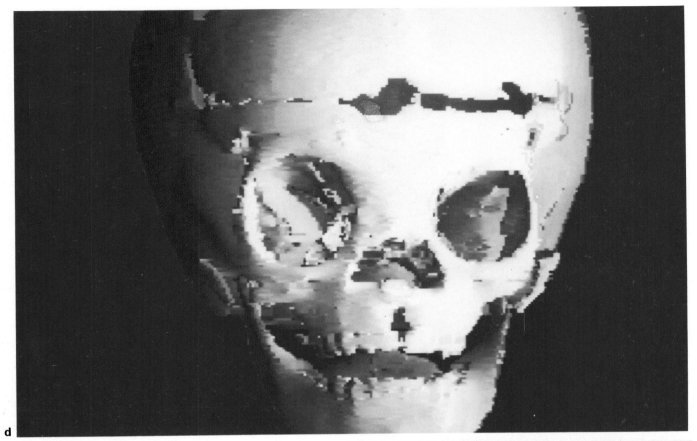

d

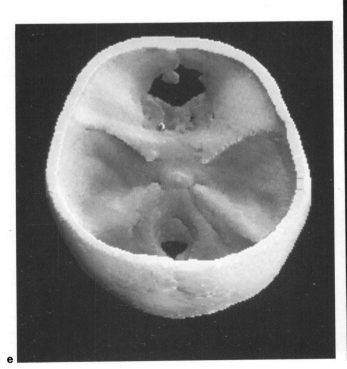

e

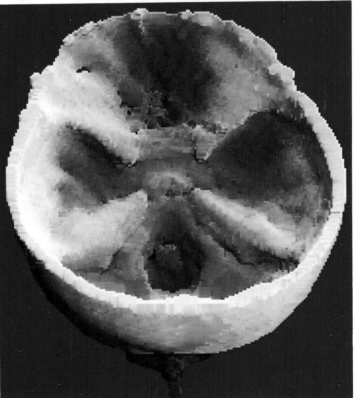

f

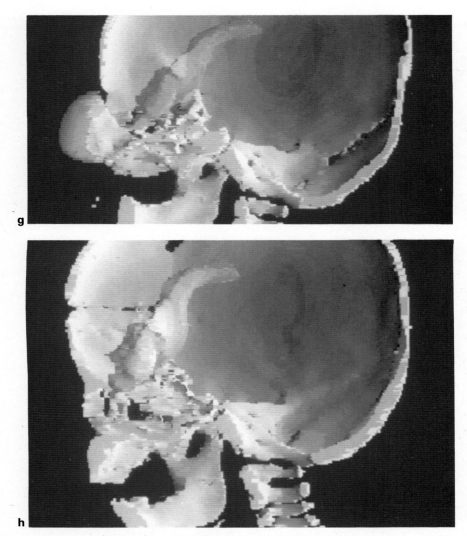

Fig. 20.129 Internasal dysplasia associated with extreme teleorbitism. Correction by medial faciotomy (facial bipartition) and resurfacing of the nasal dorsum using local surplus of skin: (a) preoperative view; (b) postoperative view; (c) 3-D CT reconstruction, frontal view (preoperative); (d) 3-D CT reconstruction, frontal view (postoperative); (e) 3-D CT reconstruction, cranial view (preoperative); (f) 3-D CT reconstruction, cranial view (postoperative); (g) 3-D CT reconstruction, sagittal view (preoperative); (h) 3-D CT reconstruction, sagittal view (postoperative).

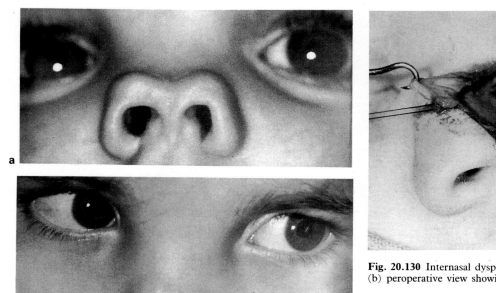

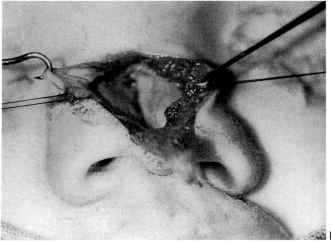

Fig. 20.130 Internasal dysplasias: (a) preoperative view; (b) peroperative view showing bifid septum; (c) postoperative view.

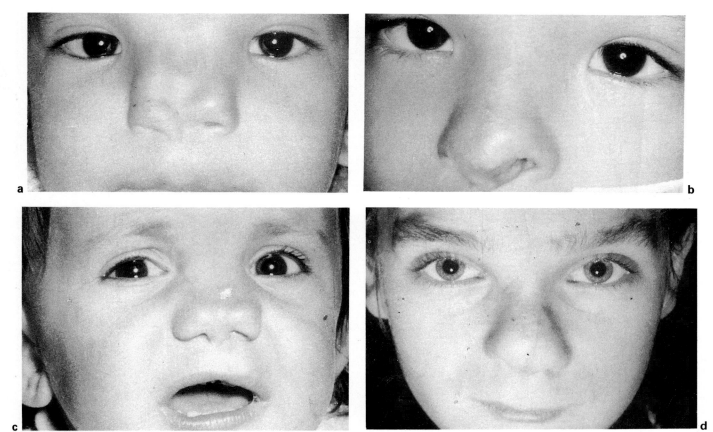

Fig. 20.131 Internasal dysplasia. Correction by approximation of two halves of the septum: (a, b) pre- and postoperative views; (c, d) pre- and postoperative views.

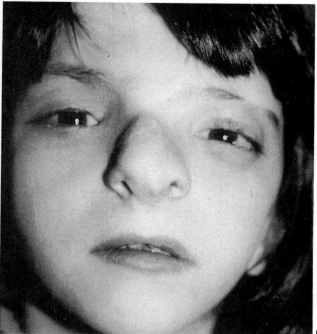

Fig. 20.132 Internasal dysplasia associated with nasal dysplasia. Correction by local rearrangement of skin and reconstruction of nasal framework: (a) preoperative view; (b) postoperative view.

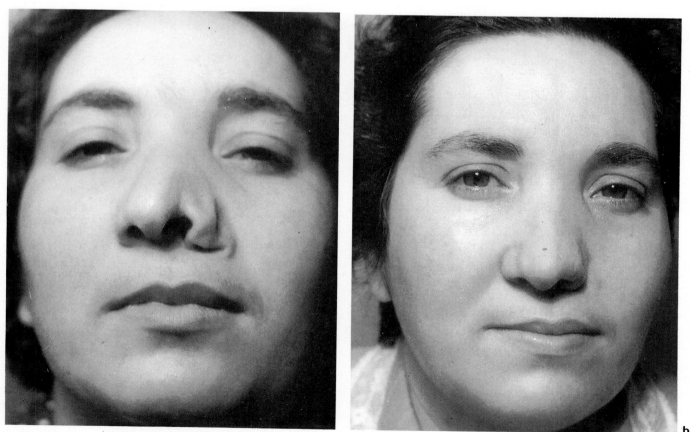

Fig. 20.133 Nasal duplication. Correction of internasal dysplasia by resection of redundant tissue in the middle and approximation of nasal halves. A cartilage graft was inserted in the new columella to improve tip projection: (a) preoperative view; (b) postoperative view.

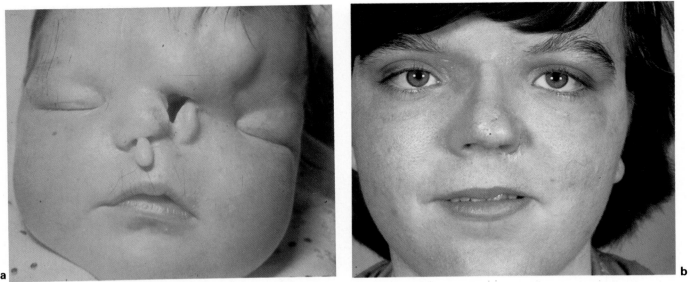

Fig. 20.134 Nasoschizis (unilateral), with teleorbitism. Correction by medialization of orbits and reconstruction of nostril with bilobar flap. (a) preoperative view (shortly after birth); (b) postoperative view (with permission of the editor of the *British Journal of Plastic Surgery*).

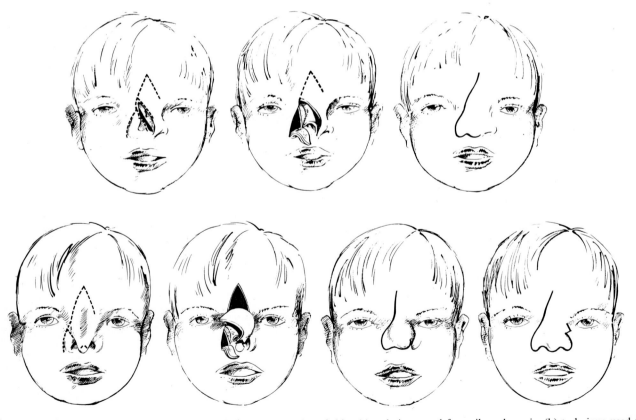

Fig. 20.135 Nasoschizis. Correction by transposition of regional surplus of skin: (a) technique used for unilateral repair; (b) technique used for bilateral repair.

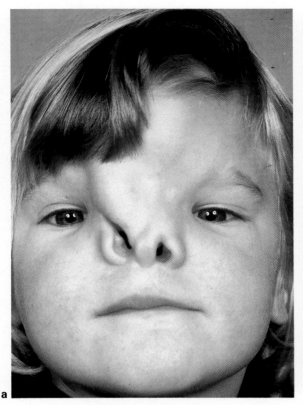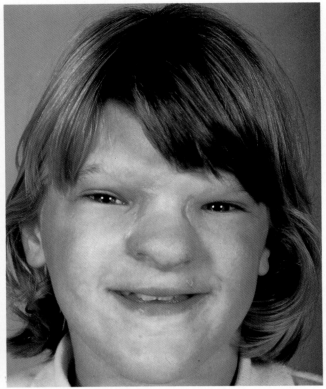

Fig. 20.136 Nasoschizis (bilateral) with teleorbitism. Correction by medialization of orbits and reconstruction of nostrils. (a) preoperative view; (b) postoperative view (with permission of the editor of *Plastic and Reconstructive Surgery*).

nasal pyramid, harmonization of the maxillary block with the upper arcade used for reference, and restoration of oromuscular continuity.

Malformations to be discussed are:

1. nasal aplasia
2. nasal aplasia with proboscis
3. nasal dyschondrosis
4. choanal atresia
5. premaxillomaxillary and intermaxillopalatine clefting (cleft lip and palate)
6. nasomaxillary and maxillary dysplasia.

NASAL APLASIA

Nasal aplasia represents the unilateral form of an extremely rare condition called arhinia. Surgery fails to restore a functional nose, in most instances producing only an improved cosmetic result.

The skeleton

The creation of a functional nasal airway is the theoretical goal. In fact, the bone can easily be perforated and the created tunnel lined with mucosa or skin, but whether such a procedure has ever made normal breathing possible is extremely doubtful. It therefore seems wiser to accept defeat and be satisfied with the construction of a nasal pyramid, if only to improve cosmesis.

Skeletal restoration may not be needed in nasal aplasia, when a septum is present. However, in arhinia — the bilateral form of the anomaly — the creation of two nostrils will have to include the construction of a skeletal framework.

The soft tissues

In nasal aplasia the so-called normal side is deviated from the midline towards the affected side. Reconstruction includes formation of the missing nostril and realignment of the normal half of the nasal pyramid. This objective may be achieved with a folded forehead flap (Fig. 20.137). It should, however, be kept in mind that such a procedure may result in conspicuous scarring over the nasal dorsum, a different colour match and possibly stenosis of the new aperture.

There is much to be said for complete nasal reconstruction in which the lining of the new nostril is obtained by the turned-over skin from the normal side, and the nasal pyramid completely resurfaced by means of a forehead

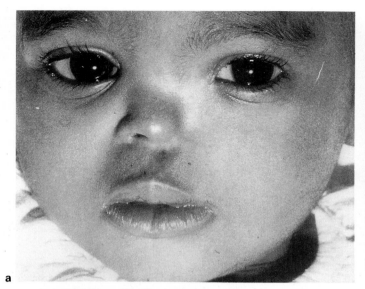

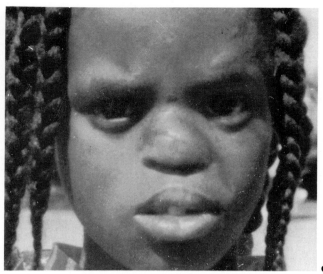

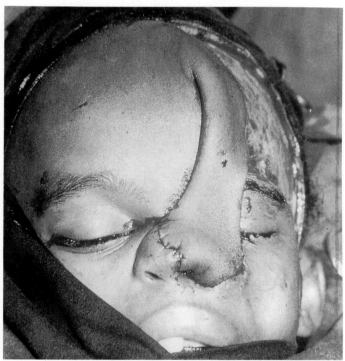

Fig. 20.137 Nasal aplasia. Correction by reconstruction of missing nostril with forehead flap: (a) preoperative view; (b) operative technique; (c) postoperative view.

flap. This procedure does not apply to arhinia. In this exceedingly rare condition the nasal pyramid is reconstructed with a forehead flap.

NASAL APLASIA WITH PROBOSCIS

As in nasal aplasia, attempts to reconstruct a functional nasal airway are futile since it is impossible completely to resurface the tunnel with the deficient lining of the proboscis. All efforts should therefore be directed at the formation of the missing dorsum and nostril. The presence of a proboscis appears to facilitate the fulfilment of these objectives. Its use as a donor site is generally recommended, in spite of the difficulties related to the absence of adequate drainage facilities of the mucous lining. A short proboscis, or one that has its origin in an abnormally high position, should first be moved downwards with a caterpillar procedure.

Classical procedures

Two different approaches have been reported.

Decortication of the proboscis and tunnelling. The skin of the proboscis is removed, with the exception of a small cuff at its distal margin, and the tube is then buried in a tunnel parallel to the normal half. The preservation of an intact nasal lining is a distinct advantage of this procedure, but attempts to reproduce a normal-looking nostril have not always been successful owing to stenosis.

Incision of the proboscis and appositioning. The proboscis is longitudinally opened over its posterior aspect. The floor of the nasal aperture is restored with local skin and the remaining nostril lining with that of the proboscis. The nasal dorsum is reconstructed by rearrangement of skin (Fig. 20.138).

NASAL DYSCHONDROSIS

Achondroplasia or hypochondroplasia produce a craniofacial malformation characterized by a discrepancy between a skull with well-developed mesenchymal components and a deficient nasal capsule with retrusion and shortness of the

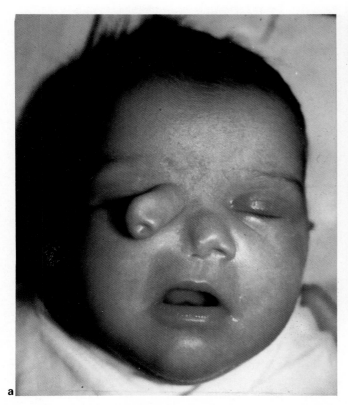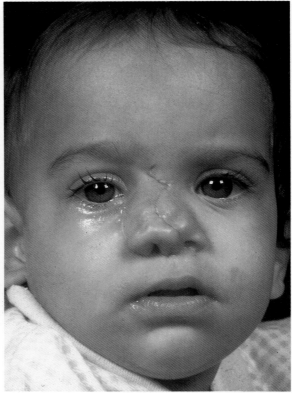

Fig. 20.138 Nasal dysplasia with proboscis. Correction by reconstruction of missing nostril with proboscis: (a) preoperative view; (b) postoperative view. (Van der Meulen, in press)

nose. The maxilla is indirectly affected because of the absence of a sagittal thrust, but the vomer remains normal.

The nose, which is short and wide, seems impacted in the middle third of the face. The interorbital region is flat. Occlusion is slightly modified and the upper incisors are usually retruded, exhibiting mild inversion. The cartilages of the tip are not always involved and may even show a paradoxically hypertrophic appearance. Occasionally, the malformation is characterized by a protrusion of the upper alveolar sector. It is important to remember that the anomaly is fundamentally different from vomeropremaxillary synostosis (Binder's syndrome).

The surgical objective, which is difficult to achieve, involves forward displacement of the nasal skeleton and restoration of a nasal dorsum. Perinasal osteotomy (Psillakis et al 1973) respecting the dentoalveolar process mobilizes an extremely fragile paranasal segment, whose projection is maintained by bone grafts.

Restoration of a nasal profile requires ancillary procedures. Hypertrophic alar cartilages may supply material for backward rotation in a flying-wing fashion, but this alone is not sufficient. An additional bone graft is mandatory and it seems wise to defer this step until after the osteotomy.

A wired iliac graft, anterior to which the alar cartilages are modelled, may be resorbed over the years to a degree that cannot be foreseen. A graft from the cranial vault with the shape of an anchor to project the tip is a challenging technique (Fig. 20.139) and the use of a revascularized bone graft represents an alternative, although this is rarely indicated.

Early surgery is not justified, as the reconstructed nose is not patent. Therefore it is advisable to wait until the postpubertal period to repair the deformity. Attempts to stimulate osteogenesis by the transfer of a tubed periosteal flap, suggested by Tessier (1976), or by the insertion of demineralized bone as proposed by Mulliken & Glowacki (1980), have been performed but without manifest success.

CHOANAL ATRESIA

Obstruction, uni- or bilateral, may be caused by a membrane or by a bony block. Respiratory troubles affect newborns in particular, unable as they are to breathe through their mouths during sucking. Bilateral atresia is thus an emergency.

One has to be aware of the caudalization of the sphenoid, which causes the axis of the nasal fossa to be directed towards the cranial base, a true danger in removal

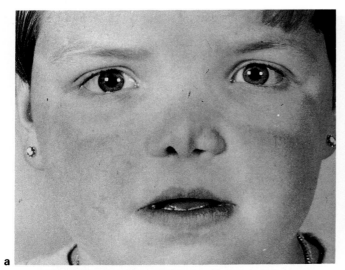

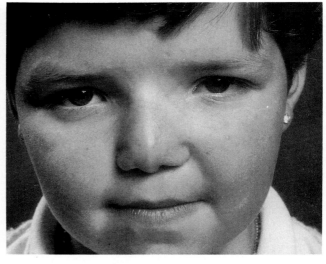

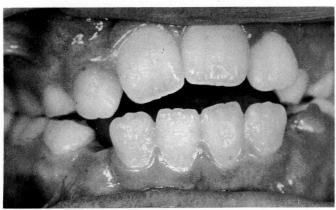

Fig. 20.139 Nasal dyschondrosis. Correction by extensive mobilization of the soft tissues of the nose followed by insertion and fixation of an anchor-shaped calvarial bone graft: (a) preoperative view; (b) postoperative view; (c) maxillary deformity.

conformer must be kept in position for at least six months. Local infection is frequent and the child with unilateral atresia must be trained to use the newly opened airway. Prognosis is, however, doubtful: nasal ventilation may be reduced, owing to residual constriction or improper use; sagittal growth of the maxilla as a result of surgery or dysostosis, or the orientation of the dentoalveolar arches may not be harmonious.

PREMAXILLOMAXILLARY AND INTERMAXILLOPALATINE CLEFTING

Premaxillomaxillary dysostosis (or cleft lip) and intermaxillopalatine dysostosis (or cleft palate) have three main characteristics:

they create a disequilibrium of forces within the orofacial muscular sling, which is interrupted at both extremities (Fig. 20.140);

they cause a maxillary, alveolar and palatal gap, a sort of congenital pseudoarthrosis;

they disturb the so-called orality, the ensemble of sensory and motor functions formed by sucking, tongue proprioceptivity and phonation (Fig. 20.141).

Morphologically there are two clinical types: incomplete or complete and uni- or bilateral. The centrofacial region is severely affected in complete forms (Fig. 20.142). A description of the many aspects would, however, go far beyond the scope of this book.

The principles of primary repair can be summarized as follows:

of the bony block. The malformation not only affects the sphenoid but also the palatine bone and the vomer, which converge to form an osseous funnel, which is narrow or obliterated (Fig. 9.32).

Radiological examination by lipiodol injection and tomography or CT scan demonstrates the choanal condition, and treatment varies with the type of malformation present.

When there is a membranous obstacle, nasal perforation is carried out. When the obstruction is bony, removal is performed by a palatine approach. In both cases a stent is inserted. The palatine approach describes a continuous retroalveolar arch incision close to the gingival rim, extending from one tuberosity to the other. The palatal mucoperiosteum is elevated up to its vascular pedicles. The vault is trephined and the bony block removed. The correct orientation of the instruments is constantly controlled since the danger of intracranial penetration is real.

Prognosis is dependent on the quality of the new airway lining. The nasal mucosa is therefore carefully dissected and distributed along the passage as far as possible. The

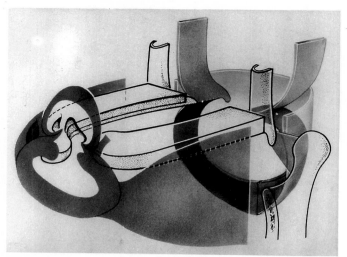

Fig. 20.140 Muscular imbalance due to interruption of the facial slings.

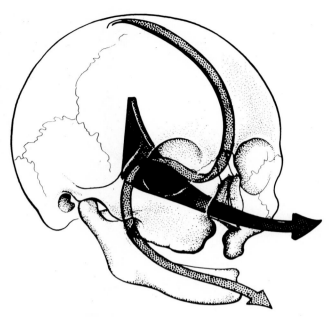

Fig. 20.142 Disturbance of the sagittal thrust in unilateral clefting.

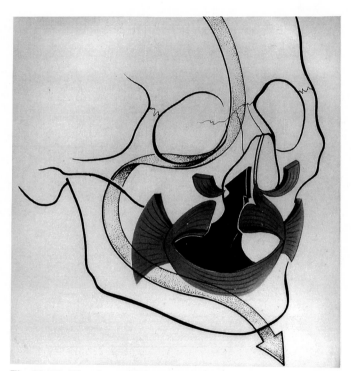

Fig. 20.141 Disturbance of the orofacial function.

reconstruction of the anterior nasolabial muscular sling;
restoration of a watertight palatal partition;
closure of the posterior velopharyngeal muscular sling to obtain velopharyngeal competence.

The surgeon should avoid concentrating on a specific structure at the expense of another and the procedure should respect the growth capacity of the affected region which is present in the majority of cases.

Timing of surgery

The therapeutical protocol (Fig. 20.143) consisting of various important surgical orthopaedic and orthodontic steps, which follow each other in a logical order, is inspired by the normal evolution of craniofacial growth represented by the temporospatial helix described in Chapter 4. It is adapted to the abnormal circumstances seen in each individual patient.

Primary repair is carried out from anterior to posterior, the anterior step being performed once sagittal growth is accomplished (6 months), while the posterior or velopharyngeal repair is done about the age of 1 year. Malek and Psaume (1983) advocate a posteroanterior correction. Both approaches meet at the alveolar level, where future expansion should not be limited. A free periosteal graft from the tibia is perhaps the best solution in this area.

Use of periosteum in clefts

The treatment of the soft tissues and skeleton of labial, alveolar and palatal clefts has attracted much attention, but periosteum, the fundamental element, has largely been ignored. In Veau's monumental work (1931) it is hardly named, although Ollier's textbook on osteogenesis was published 70 years before (1867).

The periosteal envelope

The periosteum — the interface between the skeleton and its muscular environment — holds a key position in congenital malformations. It contributes first to the

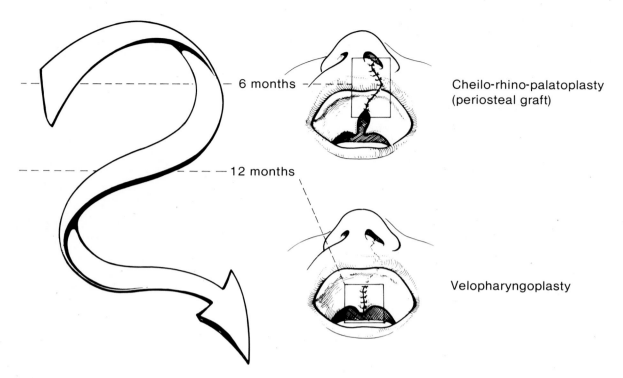

— 6 months

— 12 months

Cheilo-rhino-palatoplasty
(periosteal graft)

Velopharyngoplasty

Fig. 20.143 Protocol of cleft lip and palate repair — basic steps.

formation of the skeleton and then to its organization. It is in fact the privileged layer between the bony scaffold and adjacent soft tissues, particularly in the midface or maxillary region.

Two opposing features of the periosteum demand attention: the first is negative, owing to lack of its extensibility. It keeps the soft tissues in a position dictated by that of the skeleton (Fig. 20.144); the second is positive, owing to its osteogenic capacity (Fig 20.145) within the cleft. This quality, induced by the contact between nasal and buccal periosteum, is well recognized.

Trauner (1948) shifted a small flap of local periosteum across the cleft, and Ross & Johnston (1972) found bony nuclei in the repaired cleft (Fig. 20.146). Tord Skoog (1965, 1967) can undoubtedly be considered the father of the use of periosteum as a bone inducer.

Periosteum surgery fulfils two goals: the first one, common to any sort of surgical procedure, aims to release the periosteal envelope shortened by malformation or retracted by trauma and to allow its expansion. This periosteotomy permits full mobilization of the soft tissues and on occasion of the body components following osteotomies. Wide release of the periosteum is not only obtained by detaching it from the underlying bone but also by interrupting its surface by variously oriented single or multiple cuts.

The second goal, specific for clefts, uses the normal

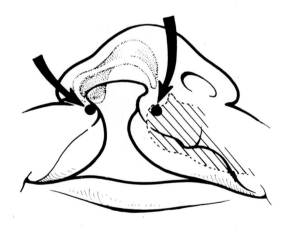

Fig. 20.144 Site of periosteal attachments which unite the soft tissues and the bony edges of the cleft.

periosteum, taken from elsewhere (usually the tibia). The graft is transplanted to the cleft and induces bone formation and epithelialization.

Skoog periosteoplasty

The idea of routine use of maxillary periosteum to form bone in clefts of the primary palate (the boneless bone

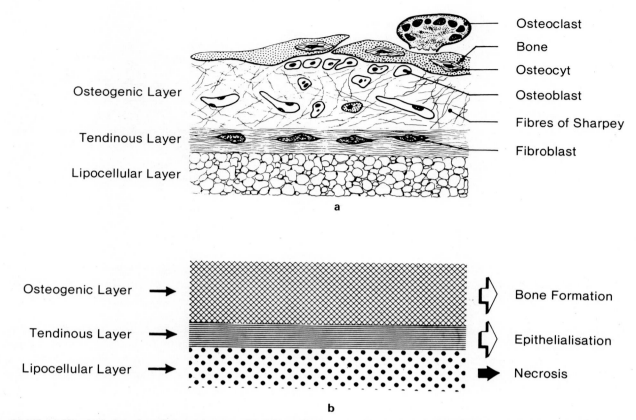

Fig. 20.145 (a) Histological section of the periosteum; (b) Schematic representation of the periosteal graft and the destination of each layer.

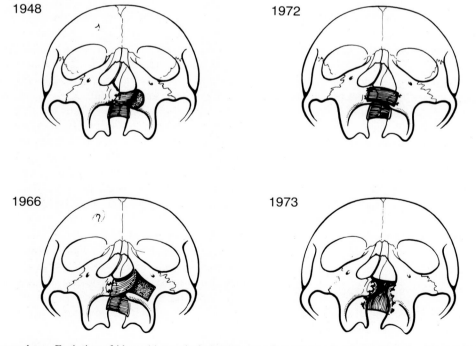

Fig. 20.146 The periosteoplasty. Evolution of ideas: (a) marginal alveolopalatal flap (Trauner); (b) maxillary flap (Skoog); (c) anterior tibial graft (Ritsila); (d) anterioposterior tibial graft (Stricker).

graft) was reported by Skoog in 1965 (Fig. 20.146). In re-establishing the periosteal continuity across the cleft with a wide maxillary mucoperiosteal flap, three main premises were stated:

1. The periosteum covering the maxillary segments possesses normal growth potential.
2. Denuded bone in this area will regenerate normal periosteum.
3. The re-established interaction between growth centres on the medial and lateral sides will determine the growth and development of the united maxilla.

We are in favour of the first two concepts, but we cannot agree with the third one, particularly in the way it is worded.

The periosteoplasty, a pseudo-flap based on a questionable pedicle, should supply a bony complement for mobilized teeth during early orthodontic treatment as carried out by Hellquist (1971), in the deciduous or mixed dentition. To secure a matrix for ossification, Surgicel was used, thus rendering the procedure very complicated. Surgicel, repeatedly used in different operations, would theoretically regulate the volume and shape of the newly formed bone. The periosteal maxillary flap was part of Skoog's philosophy: to respect the medial side; to mobilize the lateral side; to re-establish periosteal continuity; and to prevent malocclusion.

This technique, used by some of us for three years from 1970 to 1973, was disappointing: quantitatively it is difficult to raise a viable flap of periosteum with a wide enough base in the infraorbital region, and to transpose it to fill in the wide cleft; qualitatively there is a lack of good bone production by the resorptive nature of periosteum at this site as demonstrated by Enlow (1968).

Ritsila (1972a,b), aware of these disadvantages, reported on the use of a free graft of periosteum taken from the anterior tibia to obtain an abundant bone formation to close the defect of the alveolar cleft. They placed the transplanted free tibial periosteum graft transversally over the cleft from one alveolar segment to the other (Fig. 21.146).

One of us, dissatisfied with the Skoog periosteoplasty, had the idea in 1973 of using the periosteal tibial free graft in an anterocaudal direction within the cleft, from the floor of the nostril to the posterior border of the bony palate (Fig. 20.146).

The philosophy of free tibial periosteal grafting

Some authors erroneously believe that the sole purpose of this technique consists of bone production within the cleft, but free tibial periosteum grafts fulfil two goals.

The major interest lies in the formation of a buccal plane, i.e. in carrying out a uranoplasty without using the

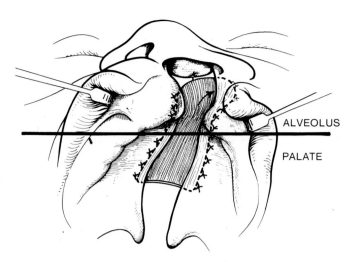

Fig. 20.147 The two areas closed by the periosteal graft — alveolar and palatal.

palatine fibromucosa in a critical area where the release of this fibromucosa may cause a future maxillary collapse. This concept comes directly from Dunn's (1952) and Stenstrom & Thilander's (1974) ideas. These authors, concerned about the palatal mucoperiosteum, covered the oral side with a skin graft. Others, later, used a mucosal graft from the dorsal aspect of the tongue (Chancholle 1980).

The second point is the degree of bone formation within the cleft. The alveolar region, and also at the edge of the piriform aperture under the alar base, must be built up.

The periosteal graft incorporates two different territories (Fig. 20.147). The anterior one (alveolar) is in a favourable situation because it is protected and fed by the repaired orbicularis muscle. The amount of bone produced at this level is detectable (Fig. 20.148).

The posterior one (palatal) is in an unfavourable situation, because of its exposure in a contaminated oral cavity, disturbed by tongue movements. Although the pressure is favourable there is a risk of folding the graft in a forward direction and detaching it from the nasal plane. The amount of bone produced at this level is variable, but the periosteal graft is used as a scaffolding matrix for epithelialization, preventing collapse of the mucoperiosteal edges (Fig. 21.148).

This graft of tibial periosteum is part of our primary repair programme, i.e. a lip–alveolopalatal repair, which is not limited solely to the primary palate but which extends to the posterior border of the palatine bones. With this technique the patient is left with a cleft of the soft palate only, which can be closed at 11 months.

Principles of repair

Free periosteal graft from the tibia. The donor site lies

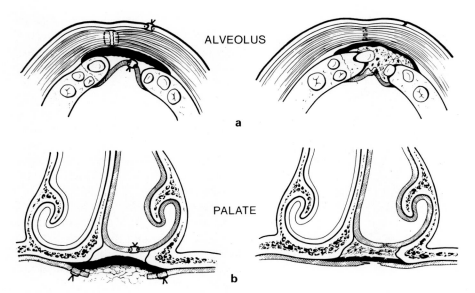

ALVEOLUS

PALATE

Fig. 20.148 The objectives of the tibial graft: (a) the production of bone; (b) the induction of an epithelial lining.

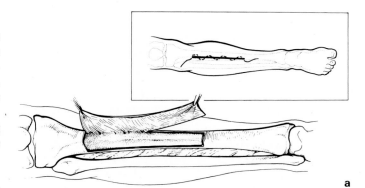

on the anterolateral aspect of the tibia. A skin incision is carried out vertically, lateral to the anterior border of the tibia. The periosteum is bluntly elevated from the underlying bone, thus obtaining a piece measuring 5 × 2 cm. Skin suture should be done with great care and drainage is not necessary (Fig. 20.149).

Cheilorhinoplasty. The cleft edges are incised according to the Skoog procedure, modified over the years in the following ways:

1. By adding a muscle flap from the lateral edge of the cleft to the deficient inner element, to increase the bolstering of the central portion of the vermilion.
2. By freeing the periosteal envelope extensively and by carrying out the periosteotomy on the lateral side of the pyriform aperture. This manoeuvre allows a good advancement of the muscle to the nasal spine with minimal tension (Fig. 20.150).
3. By carrying out a midline columella incision, extending it over the dome. The forward advancement of half the columella on the cleft side shifts it in an upward direction, with a rotational movement identical to that described by Millard (1976–1980) (Fig. 20.151).
4. By rearrangement of the labionasal muscular sphincter: reinserting the external fibres of the orbicularis in front of the nasal spine; shifting the alar base medially by reinserting the common tendon formed by the nasalis muscle and the group of levators.
5. By carrying out, in the case of a bilateral cleft, a primary vestibuloplasty by means of a marginal internal flap, rotated under the prolabium to preserve the sulcus. It should, however, be kept in mind that deepening the sulcus at a later stage is often needed.

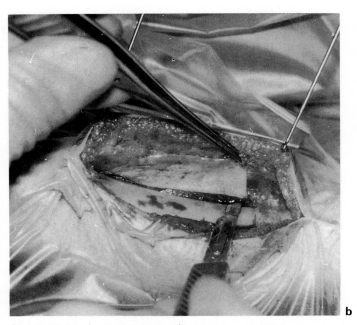

Fig. 20.149 The periosteal tibial graft: (a) donor site; (b) peroperative view.

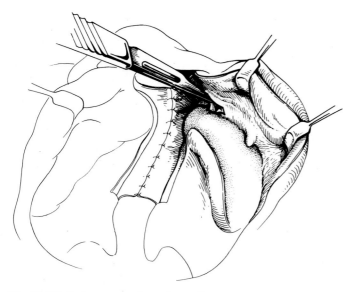

Fig. 20.150 Periosteotomy along the pyriform aperture.

Palatoplasty. This includes two steps. The first step is the restoration of the nasal layer using nasal tissue, by transposing the nasal mucosa laterally and a vomerine mucosal flap from the inner side. This repair of the nasal floor has not changed significantly since Veau (1931). The second step is the closure of the oral layer, which is carried out without using the palatal mucoperiosteum. One should avoid using the nasal or vomerine mucosa for resurfacing the oral layer. In fact, Atherton's (1974) experiments showed that there is a resorptive quality to nasal mucosa, a characteristic which is preserved when it is placed in the

oral cavity. The observation of patients treated by the Schmid–Widmeier procedure (i.e. the turnover of an inferiorly based flap of vomerine mucosa for resurfacing the oral cavity), shows the existence of a depression at the site of the flap.

1. Tailoring the nasal layer — the cleft edges are pared to the posterior margin of the bone. Undermining of the nasal mucosa is done from an anterior to a posterior direction from above downwards, starting from the piriform aperture. The turnover of the nasal mucosa brings in a fibrous marginal crest, which should be excised before starting to suture. The inner edge is incised either along the midline or within the vomerine mucosa in the case of a horizontal vomer. Undermining is easy over the vomer, but is harder behind the alveolus along the premaxilla. The key to correction is by a septal approach. The two detached mucosal flaps are pushed medially, to form the 'nasal chamber'.

2. Preparation of the recipient bed for tibial periosteal graft — the nasovomerine mucosal closure is completed by suturing in the periosteum to form a continuous nasal periosteal bed. The edges are carefully raised with a raspatory to allow acceptance of the graft and to guarantee extra fixation.

3. The application of the periosteal graft — The graft, with the cambial layer applied to the nasal periosteum, is fixed from behind forwards. The posterior border is sutured to the posterior border of the nasal layer, thus avoiding tongue intrusion, which might cause detachment. Suturing starts along the outer edge, which is the most difficult part to join because of the palatine plate lying vertically. The tibial graft is sutured using U-knots to fix

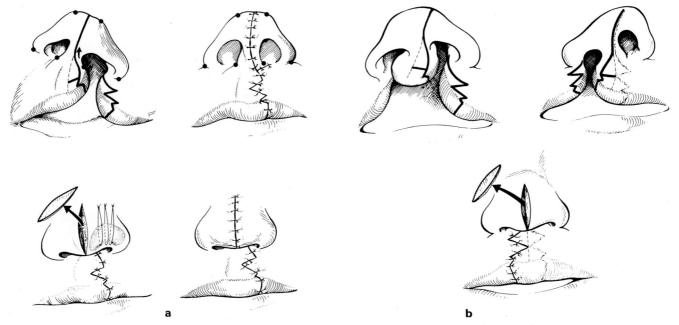

a   b

Fig. 20.151 Modification of Skoog's design according to Stricker and Raphael: (a) unilateral cleft; (b) bilateral cleft.

it under the cleft edges. On the anterior part, the graft avoids the vomeropremaxillary suture and it reaches the lateral periosteum crossing the base of the ala. Bone production should palliate the deficient platform at the level of the ala on the cleft side (Fig. 20.152). The tibial periosteal graft is fixed over the nasal periosteal layer with some stitches. In the postoperative period an appliance is optional, the aim being not to protect the periosteal graft but to prevent alveolar collapse induced by the contracting forces of the reconstructed orbicularis muscle.

4. Evolution — The immediate result is epithelialization. The early aspect is rather disappointing: the graft looks yellowish and suggests necrosis. In fact, tissue loss is only limited to the outer layer while epithelialization progresses. At 15 days postoperatively, little by little the colour improves and a normal mucosal texture is finally visible (Fig. 20.153). Secondary results include three categories:

a. Failures — 1% average. These are due to a technical fault or to a nasopharyngeal infection.

b. Imperfect results — sometimes the graft becomes loose from one of the margins, usually the lateral one. This occurs in approximately 10% of the cases and complicates the secondary velopharyngoplasty. The margins become

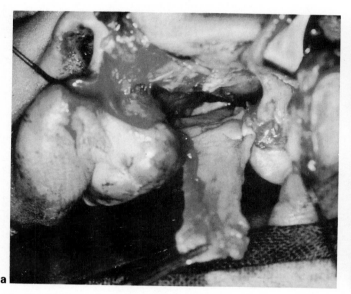
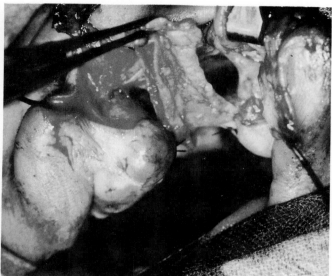

Fig. 20.152 The periosteoplasty: (a) insertion of the graft; (b) fixation of the graft.

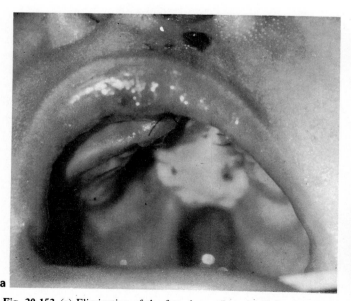
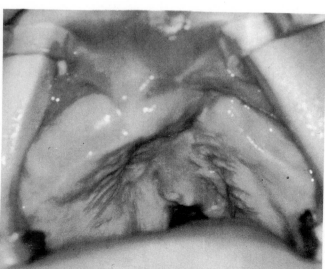

Fig. 20.153 (a) Elimination of the fatty layer; (b) epithelialization of the fibrous layer.

scarred and retracted, and one should use a palatal flap to re-establish a watertight nasal floor.

c. Good results — these include not only the survival of the tibial periosteal graft but also the growth of local alveolar and palatal structures, as manifested by the occlusion and maxillary expansion.

This technique of the tibial periosteal graft developed ten years ago by Stricker et al (1977a) has the advantage of combining a primary palatal repair without the use of local tissues and with a periosteal osteogenesis which fills in the alveolar defect. The procedure used in combination with pre- and postsurgical orthodontic treatment represents one of the most conservative methods of preserving a good dental arch and avoiding transverse collapse (Figs. 20.154–20.156).

Repair of velopharyngeal sphincter. The posterior closure at the site of the velopharyngeal valve is carried out at about 1 year of age, at a prespeech period in order to equip the child with an anatomically functional palate so that speech can develop normally. The technique is mainly based on the Ruding (1964) and Kriens (1969) procedures. A muscular reconstruction with a push back of the sling and limitation of scarring as far as possible are the essentials of this operation (Figs. 20.157, 20.158).

Complementary procedures (Fig. 20.159). Orthopaedic treatment by means of a palatal plate is advocated in all newborns with a complete cleft. This treatment is continued until 3 months, following closure of the palate with a periosteal graft. A vestibuloplasty and an elongation of the columella may be required in bilateral clefts with a lack of tissue in the premaxillary area. A secondary velopharyngeal procedure is occasionally indicated, because competence is not always satisfactory. This may be due to: shortness of the repaired palate, a situation as a rule caused by poor technique; to insufficient mobility of the velum; or to the presence of a congenitally large nasopharynx (Calnan 1954–1971). The indication for a secondary velopharyngeal procedure is based on a careful analysis not only of speech and its imperfections but also of the abnormal sphincter. Either the palate or the lateral or posterior walls of the pharynx may be defective. This examination includes radiography and nasendoscopy. Orthopaedic and orthodontic treatment are recommended when the permanent teeth erupt. Routine assessment of children with clefts must finally include audiological examination, because of the tendency to develop a serous otitis with tympanic membrane deterioration.

NASOMAXILLARY AND MAXILLARY DYSPLASIA

From a surgical point of view the treatment of nasomaxillary and medial maxillary dysplasia show little difference. In both malformations there is shortening of distance between the lower eyelid or medial canthus and the alar base and in both malformations there may be a cleft of the upper lip. Since the severity of these soft tissue defects and of the underlying skeletal abnormalities are intimately related, corrective surgery of skin and mucosa should be preceded by that of the bony structures, and occasionally by orthopaedic measures as well. To avoid unnecessary scarring and loss of time it is essential that the principles of cleft surgery, so well outlined by Tessier (1969), should be strictly adhered to.

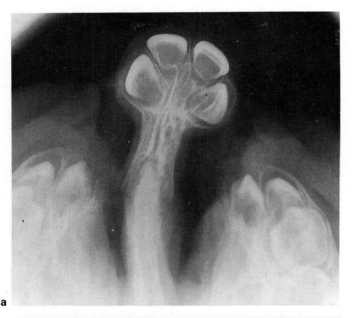

a

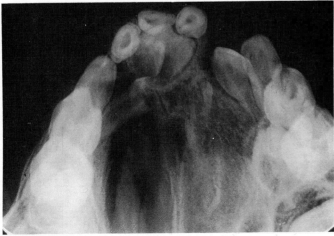

b

Fig. 20.154 (a) Ossification and evolution of the alveolodental arch following (b) insertion of two periosteal grafts in a bilateral cleft.

Fig. 20.155 (right) Result of technique in patient with complete unilateral cleft at 6 years of age: (a) cleft; (b) occlusion; (c) the hard palate; (d) the soft palate; (e) telephotography and teleradiography, frontal view; (f) telephotography and teleradiography, lateral view.

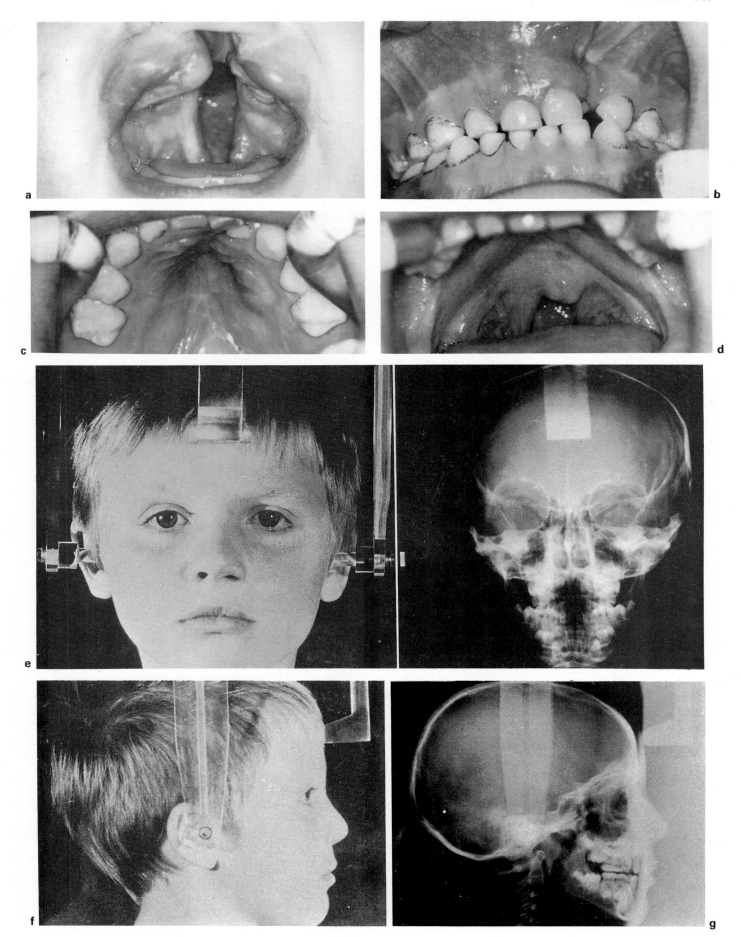

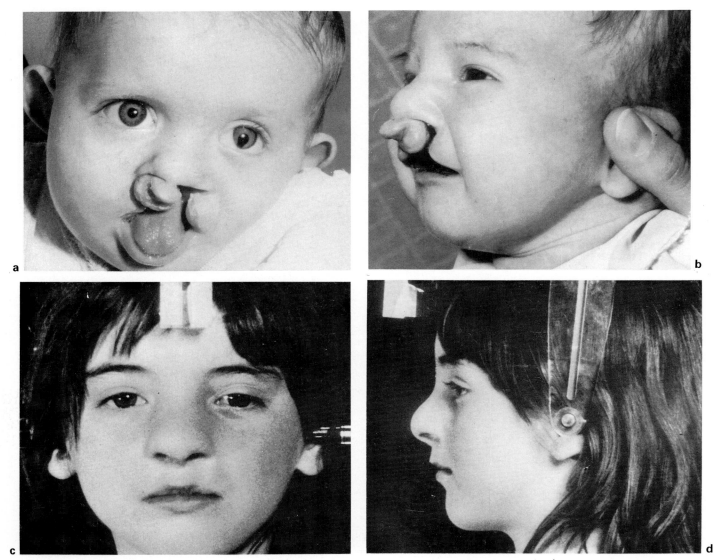

Fig. 20.156 Result of technique in patient with complete bilateral cleft at 10 years of age: (a) clefts, frontal view; (b) clefts, lateral view; (c) telephotography, frontal view; (d) telephotography, lateral view.

The skeleton

Dissection and mobilization of the edges of the cleft are followed by inspection of the maxilla. Here, anomalies are characterized by caudalization of the anterior part of the orbital floor, by lateralization of the medial wall of the future maxillary sinus and by retrusion of the anterior wall of this structure. Correction is obtained by apposition of bone grafts on the orbital floor and on the anterior surface of the sinus.

The bony defect should be left open in order to prevent repositioning of the central structures by the forces that will be generated by closure of the soft tissue defects.

The soft parts

Correction of the soft tissue defect requires repositioning of the medial canthus, of the alar base and of the m. orbicularis oculi and oris. Repair of buccal, nasal and conjunctival lining and finally restoration of the skin are also performed. It is particularly the latter part of these steps which is so difficult.

Reconstruction of the lower eyelid and of the nose requires a significant amount of skin, which can be found on one or more areas: the upper eyelid, the forehead and the cheek. Skin of the upper eyelid may be used for reconstruction of the lower eyelid, but with the disadvantage

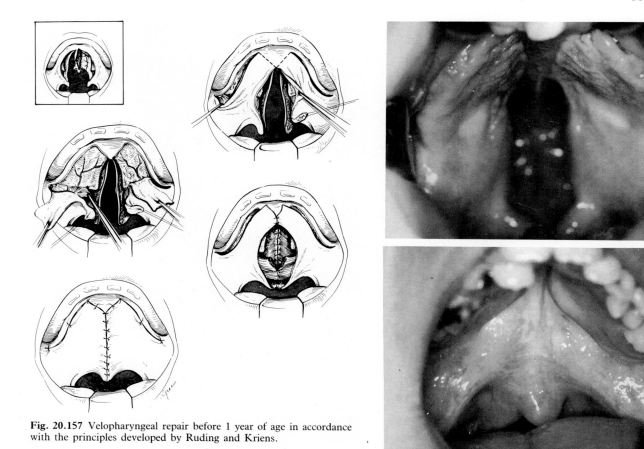

Fig. 20.157 Velopharyngeal repair before 1 year of age in accordance with the principles developed by Ruding and Kriens.

Fig. 20.158 Example of palatoplasty.

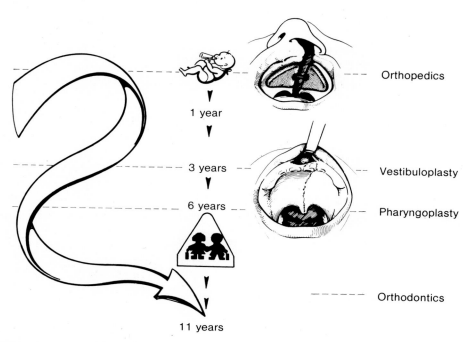

Fig. 20.159 Protocol of cleft lip and palate repair: ancillary steps.

that only small flaps can be transposed. Skin of the forehead is available in sufficient quantity and although its texture and colour leave something to be desired it may be used for reconstruction of the lower eyelid and the medial canthal region.

The surplus of tissue provided by a forehead flap may be of particular value in bilateral forms. In these cases the distal half of the flap serves to close the defect on one side of the face in the first stage, while the contralateral defect and the defect created by the transection of the nasal dorsum may be resurfaced with the pedicles of this flap in a second stage.

Skin of the cheek can be used in a variety of ways and its texture and colour are perfect. The only question is how to take the best advantage of these qualities. Interdigitation of the cutaneous edges of the cleft has been reported by many authors, but the shortage of skin can be so extreme that the result obtained is far from optimal. Rotation and advancement of the cheek (Fig. 20.160), if necessary combined with a forehead flap transfer (Fig. 20.161), has given the best results in our hands. It permits maximal

correction at the expense of minimal scarring and it is therefore advocated as the procedure of choice in the majority of cases. The results obtained with these and other techniques are shown in Figs. 20.162–20.169.

The lateral craniofacial region

The lateral dysostoses are characterized by malformations of the temporal fossa and surrounding structures:

the zygomatic bone or arch, the maxilla and sometimes the orbital region;
the ramus, the temperomandibular joint and its muscular environment;
the external ear and the adjacent soft tissues, the parotid, the facial nerve and the mimic muscles.

The cranial vault and base represented by the insertion sites of the temporal and pterygoidal muscles may be involved, but intracranial correction of these malformations is rarely indicated.

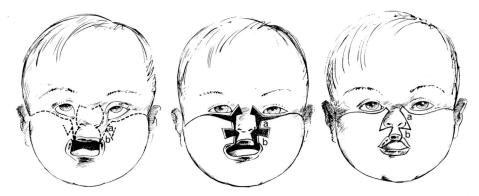

Fig. 20.160 Correction of nasomaxillary and maxillary dysplasia by rotation and advancement of cheek flaps. Note variations in design between left and right side (with permission of the editor of *Plastic and Reconstructive Surgery*).

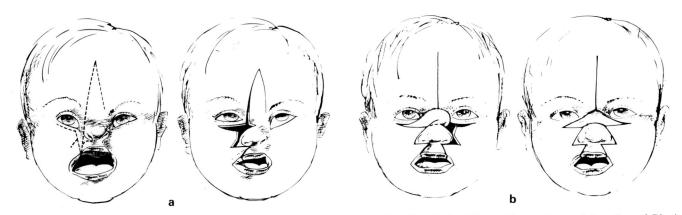

Fig. 20.161 Correction of nasomaxillary and maxillary dysplasia by transposition of median forehead flap (with permission of the editor of *Plastic and Reconstructive Surgery*).

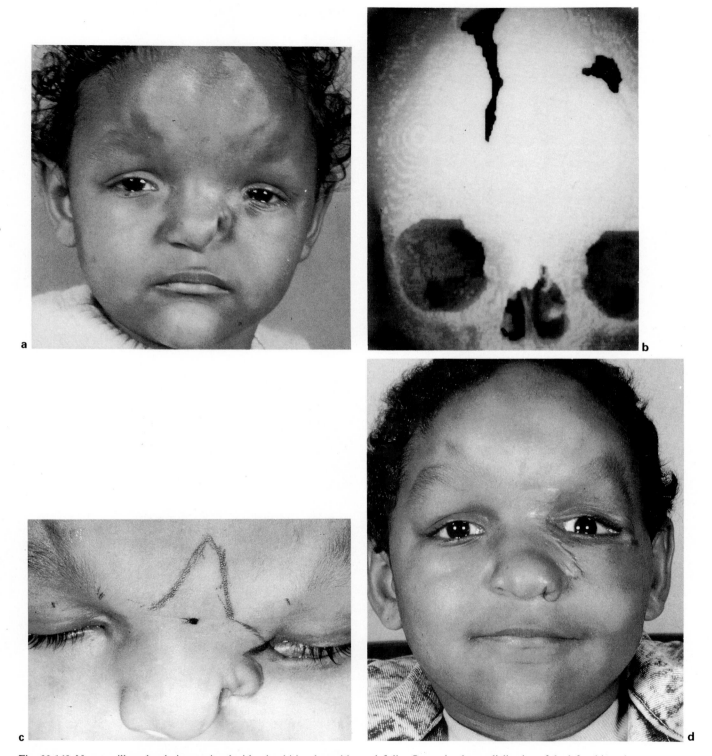

Fig. 20.162 Nasomaxillary dysplasia associated with teleorbitism but without cleft lip. Correction by medialization of the left orbit and transposition of regional surplus of skin: (a) preoperative view; (b) 3-D reconstruction shows teleorbitism and cranial defects; (c) operative technique; (d) postoperative view.

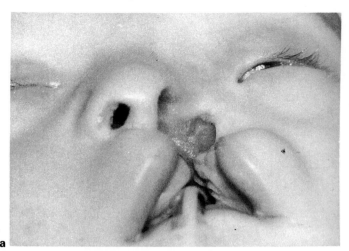

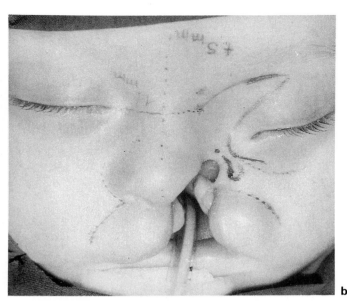

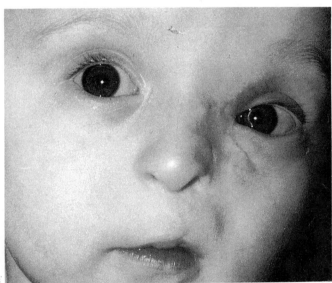

Fig. 20.163 Nasomaxillary dysplasia with cleft lip. Correction by transposition of regional surplus of skin (upper eyelid): (a) preoperative view; (b) operative design; (c) postoperative view.

Three clinical types may be observed:

1. Zygomatic and zygo-auromandibular dysplasia (Treacher Collins' and Francheschetti's syndromes), usually bilateral and mainly affecting the malar bone and zygomatic arch.
2. Temporo-auromandibular dysplasia (or hemifacial microsomia), usually unilateral and mainly affecting the mandible.
3. Temporoaural dysplasia (or microtia), usually unilateral and mainly affecting the auricle.

Establishment of an optimal time for skeletal reconstruction is of crucial importance in this region.

The indication to operate is dependent on the residual growth potential of the dysplastic bone and on the quality of the activating muscles. In this sense the condition of the malar bone and of the mandible appears to be fundamentally different: the zygomatic region is poor in muscle and its growth terminates early. Contrary to this the ramus, rich with muscle, possesses a slow and retarded growth. Abnormalities of the mandible will affect the maxilla through changes in the activity of the facial and masticatory muscles.

Early treatment by bone-grafting in the absence of an intrinsic growth potential will condemn the reconstructed parts to a state of permanent immobility and therefore to the progressive deterioration of the long-term morphological result. The surgeon therefore has only two options: early correction which must be repetitive; or definitive correction which must be delayed.

The transfer of an osteo-musculoperiosteal unit on a pedicle, or revascularized, has recently become possible and it is in this sense that the advantage of early extensive surgery may have to be reconsidered when results obtained with this technique have become known.

PREDOMINANTLY MALAR DYSPLASIA

Malar dysplasia and lower eyelid coloboma are the hallmarks of zygo-temporo-auromandibular dysplasia.

The skeleton

In the past, correction of the malar bone was obtained by using different materials, such as silicone, dermisfat, diced

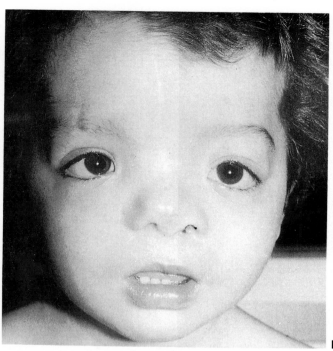

Fig. 20.164 Nasomaxillary dysplasia (unilateral and moderately severe): (a) preoperative view; (b) postoperative view.

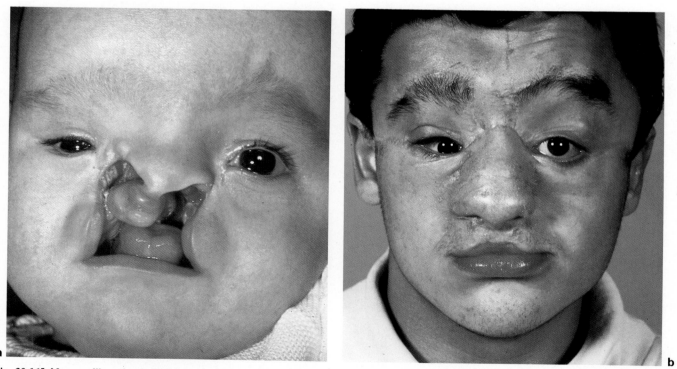

Fig. 20.165 Nasomaxillary dysplasia (bilateral and extremely severe), associated with teleorbitism and microorbitism. Correction by medialization of orbits and transposition of forehead and cheek flaps: (a) preoperative view; (b) postoperative view (with permission of the editor of *Plastic and Reconstructive Surgery*).

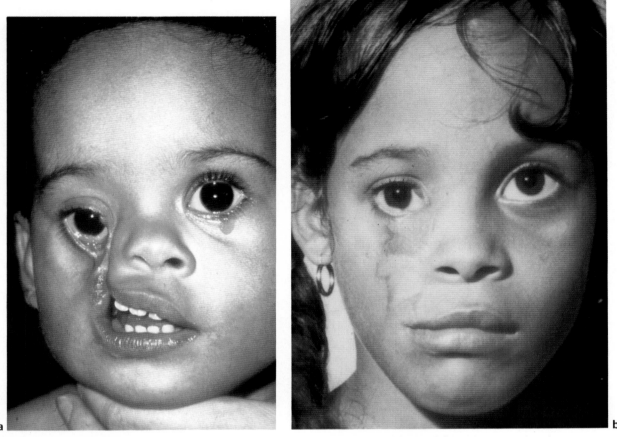

Fig. 20.166 Maxillary dysplasia (unilateral and moderately severe). Correction by transposition of forehead flap: (a) preoperative view; (b) postoperative view (with permission of the editor of *Plastic and Reconstructive Surgery*).

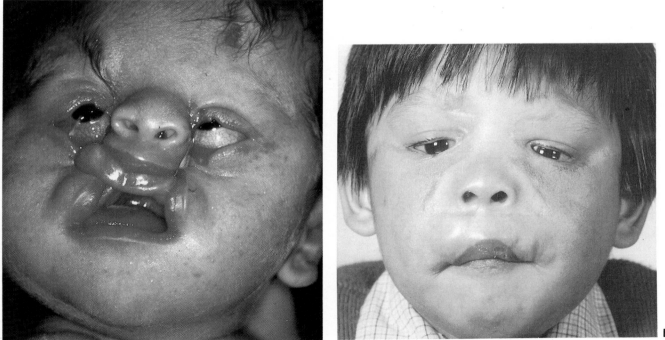

Fig. 20.167 Maxillary dysplasia (bilateral and extremely severe). Correction by transposition of cheek flaps: (a) preoperative view; (b) postoperative view (with permission of the editor of *Plastic and Reconstructive Surgery*).

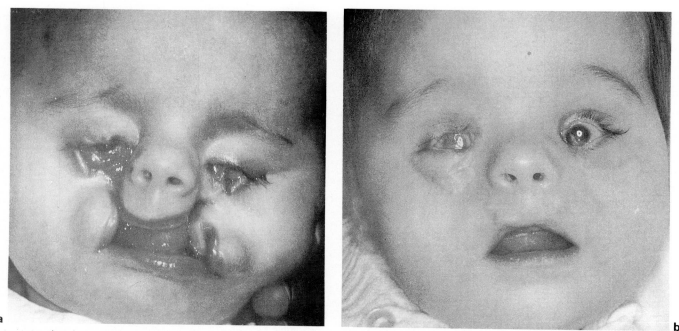

Fig. 20.168 Maxillary dysplasia (bilateral and extremely severe). Correction by transposition of cheek flaps: (a) preoperative view; (b) postoperative view.

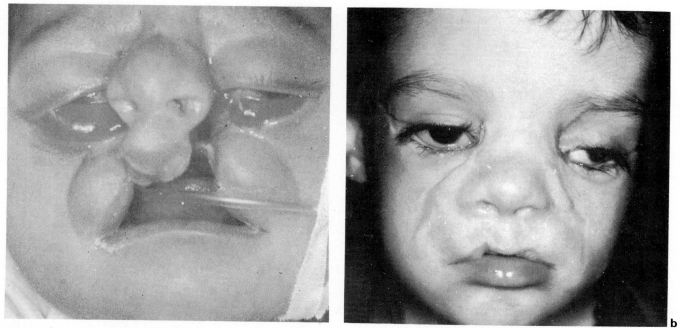

Fig. 20.169 Maxillary dysplasia (bilateral and extremely severe). Correction by transposition of local flaps: (a) preoperative view; (b) postoperative view.

cartilage, split rib and iliac grafts. Recently use of calvarium grafts has been added to this armamentarium.

Autologous costal cartilage is not available in sufficient quantity. Free split-rib and iliac grafts may resorb, necessitating repeated corrections. Calvarial grafts appear to be superior in this respect.

Osteocutaneous, osteomusculocutaneous and osteomuscular flaps have been used successfully for a variety of facial skeletal defects, but until recently not for the reconstruction of the malar bone. Encouraged by these reports and by the results of recent experiments demonstrating the osteogenic capacity of temporoperiosteal flaps transferred from the cranium to the facial skeleton in young animals,

we have used the temporal osteoperiosteal flap for the reconstruction of the malar bone in congenital defects (Van der Meulen et al 1984).

The technique is as follows. A tripod-shaped compound flap is designed in the lower part of the frontotemporal vault, one half covered by the pericranium and one half by the aponeurosis of the temporal muscle. This flap is raised in continuity with the temporal muscle, transposed to the infraorbital area and fixed to the maxilla via a subciliary incision. The vascularization of this flap is provided by terminal branches of the deep temporal artery, contrary to the flap outlined in the upper part of the frontotemporal vault, which is based on the superficial

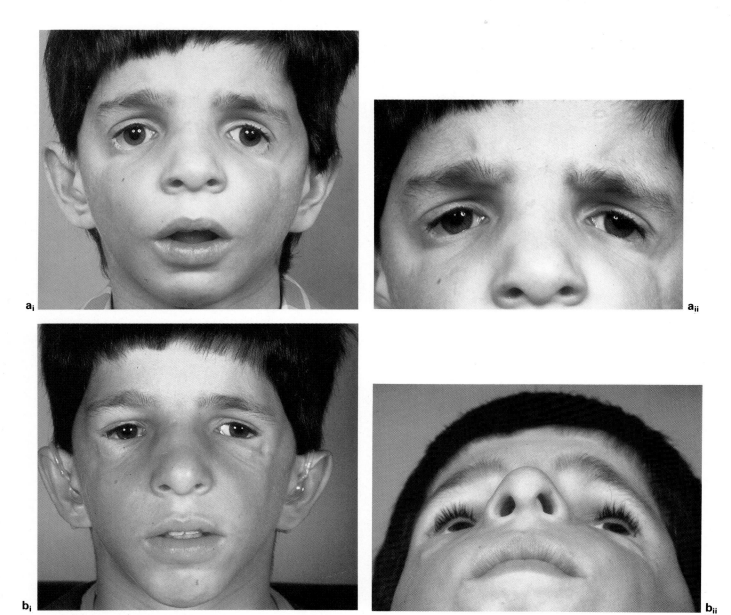

Fig. 20.170 Zygomatic dysplasia associated with marked maxillary protrusion. Correction by transposition of temporal bone flap: (a) preoperative views; (b) postoperative views.

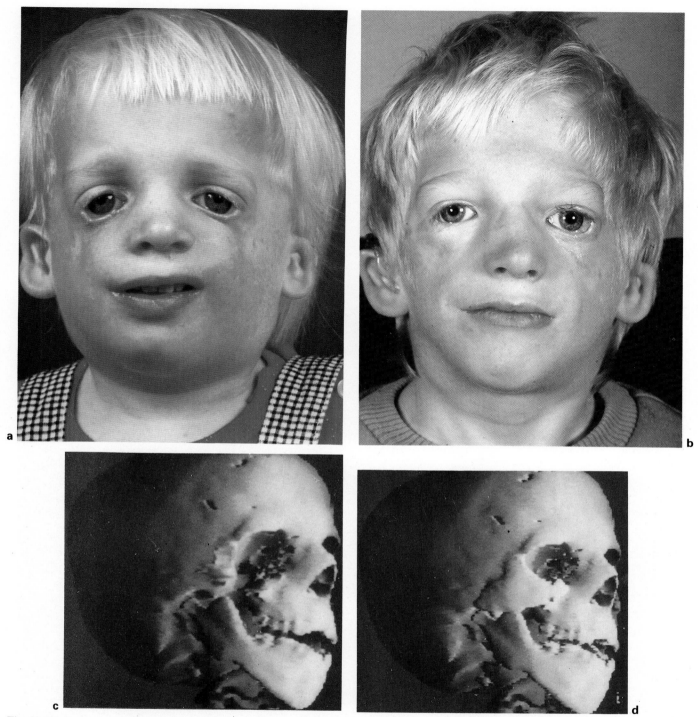

Fig. 20.171 Zygomatic dysplasia. Correction by transposition of temporal bone flap: (a) preoperative view; (b) postoperative view; (c) 3-D CT reconstruction (preoperative); (d) 3-D CT reconstruction (several years postoperative) (courtesy of the editor of *Plastic and Reconstruction Surgery*).

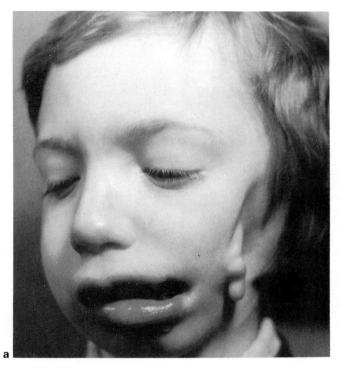

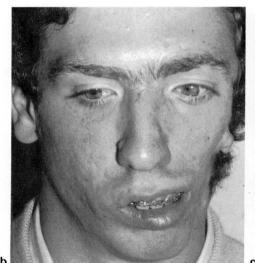

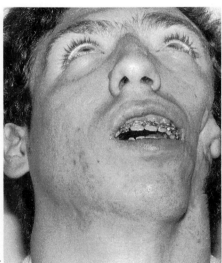

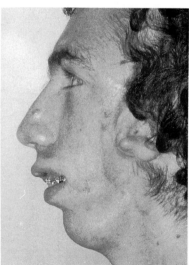

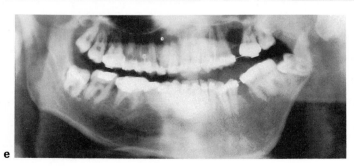

Fig. 20.172 Temporoaural mandibular dysplasia with severe soft tissue deficiency and absence of the ramus, macrostomia: (a) clinical aspect in infancy; (b–e) preoperative views at 20 years of age; (f–h) reconstruction in three steps, by quadruple osteotomy, genioplasty and latissimus dorsi musculocutaneous pedicled flap. Reconstruction of the ramus of a chondrocostal graft and full-thickness skin graft over the de-epithelialized flap to improve colour match.

temporal artery (McCarthy et al 1984) making dissection more difficult. The remaining defect in the orbital floor is closed with a split-thickness graft from the cranium. The full-thickness defect in the frontotemporal area may be left to heal spontaneously in young children. Results obtained with this technique are shown in Figs. 20.170 and 20.171.

Correction of the mandibular abnormalities is usually obtained by an advancement genioplasty. An osteotomy of the mandibular ramus may, however, be required to correct the steep mandibular plane.

Tessier (1987) has recently advocated correction by advancement of midface and mandible using a Le Fort II osteotomy in combination with a reversed V-shaped osteotomy of the ramus.

The soft tissues

In the malar area of patients with zygo-aurotemporal dysplasia, skin is not only deficient but also atrophic. Correction of the coloboma and of the caudal dislocation of the lateral canthus requires the release of skin and periorbit first of all. The resulting defect may be repaired by the transposition of tissue lying in the immediate vicinity of the coloboma, or by transposition of a triangular skin flap from the lateral part of the upper eyelid. A composite flap can be used in cases with deficiency of the conjunctiva (Jackson 1981), but the mucosal shortage in these patients seems to be more apparent than real. We feel that the condition of the soft tissues in this area may benefit when the upper eyelid flap is designed as part of a temporal flap.

The technique is as follows. A palpebrotemporal flap is raised, and the lateral canthus and lower eyelid are released from their tethering structures via a subciliary incision.

The lateral canthus is then fixed in the planned position by a canthopexy and the palpebrotemporal flap transposed into the lower eyelid by rotation and advancement. A surplus of skin is thus produced in the area over the malar bone, where it is most atrophic and deficient. This surplus is trimmed and the wound is closed.

PREDOMINANTLY MANDIBULAR DYSPLASIA (temporo-auromandibular dysplasia)

In this malformation the ramus is affected to varying degrees, ranging from a slightly hypoplastic ramus to complete absence (grades I, II, III of Pruzansky 1969). The impact of the developmental arrest is not limited to the mandible but also involves the maxilla, the muscular masticatory apparatus, the covering tissues and occasionally the zygomatic arch and the orbit.

The skeleton

The philosophy of treatment is determined by the age of the patient, the severity of the anomaly and the growth potential. The literature reveals three attitudes of mind.

Early treatment (about 3 years of age). Early restoration of mandible symmetry by lengthening or reconstruction of the anomalous ramus with a rib graft was advocated by Edgerton & Marsh (1977) in an attempt to limit further deterioration of the malformation. Murray et al (1984, 1985) share their view and now treats his patients at the earliest possible age, consistent with the patients' skeletal classification. According to him, surgery of the mandible may be performed when obliquity of the occlusal place cannot be prevented and as soon as a full complement of deciduous teeth is obtained. The more severe the mandibular

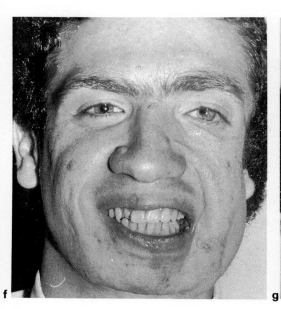
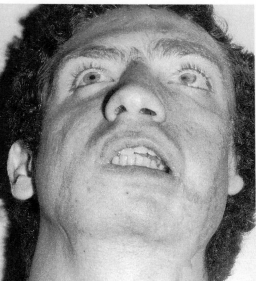
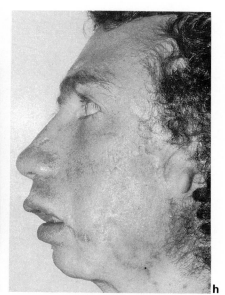

f
g
h

anomaly, the earlier the operation the less interference with maxillary growth. Rowe (1972) and Petrovic & Champy (1982) recommend the use of osteo-chondrocostal grafts, hoping to preserve an intrinsic growth potential. Reconstruction by transplantation and revascularization of the 4th and 5th metatarsus has been suggested by Pruzansky and this procedure is in accordance with our opinion. We agree with Poswillo (1974) on the necessity of a reconstruction by a functional vascularized and dynamic osteomusculoperiosteal unit.

Delayed treatment. Converse et al (1973) combine orthodontic and surgical correction in the following protocol:

1. A first surgical stage at the age of 9 years by a vertical osteotomy of the two rami and by lengthening of the affected ramus with a bone graft. An interocclusal wafer is placed in the created space on the affected side to maintain the horizontal position of the mandible.
2. A second orthodontic stage in which alveolar growth and dental eruption on the affected side is controlled.

3. A third surgical stage in adolescence, in which the remaining deformities are corrected, making use of a wide range of procedures.

Late treatment (in adolescence). Correction of the facial skeleton is performed in accordance with the severity of the malformation. Symmetry is obtained by maxillary and mandibular osteotomies, which also correct the occlusal plane (Fig. 20.172). The mandible and the zygomatic arch are restored by bone-grafting. A deviated chin is realigned by a genioplasty. An abnormal or absent temporomandibular joint is reconstructed and anomalies of the orbit are corrected in the appropriate manner. Temporomandibular joint reconstruction is only justified if it improves mandibular movements (Fig. 20.173). Orbital dystopia or, even more rare, microorbitism calls for primary reposition, expansion or reconstruction of the orbital framework and restoration of the zygomatic contours.

Time for treatment. While agreement between the majority of authors is almost unanimous on the procedures

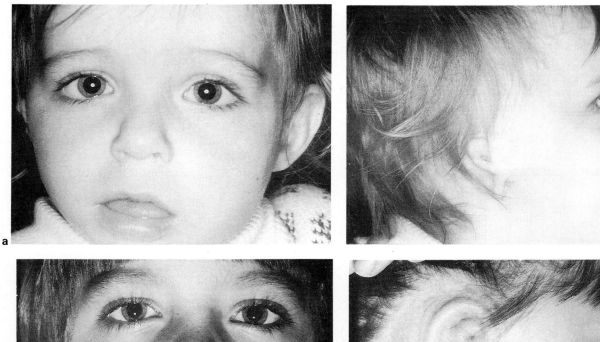

to be used in relation to the different types of malformations, there is no consensus at all on the ideal time for treatment. Munro & Lauritzen (1982–1985) base their classification of the indications for surgery on morphological criteria. While the logic of this attitude cannot be denied when adults are concerned or growth is complete, it may be objected to in children, because it does not consider local dynamic factors. We agree with the principles and conclusions of Harvold (1984), who stresses the role played by the muscles and the importance of investigating them.

In conclusion, an overall morphological repair in childhood is only justified if development of the reconstructed parts is able to progress spontaneously or by orthopaedic stimulation. A surgical procedure, involving the mandible and performed in combination with orthodontic treatment, limits further deterioration of the malformation and presents a constructive approach. In contrast, maxillary osteotomies are to be involved in infancy.

The soft tissues

Deficiencies of the soft tissues may affect the skin, the subcutaneous tissues, including fat, parotid gland, masticatory and mimic muscles, and the facial nerve. Deficiencies of the cutaneous envelope are characterized by a shortened distance between the tragus and the oral commissure, by anterior and inferior dislocation of auricular remnants and by the frequent presence of cysts, fistulas and pretragal tags.

Correction of soft tissue deficiency must accompany the restoration of skeletal balance, particularly in severe forms

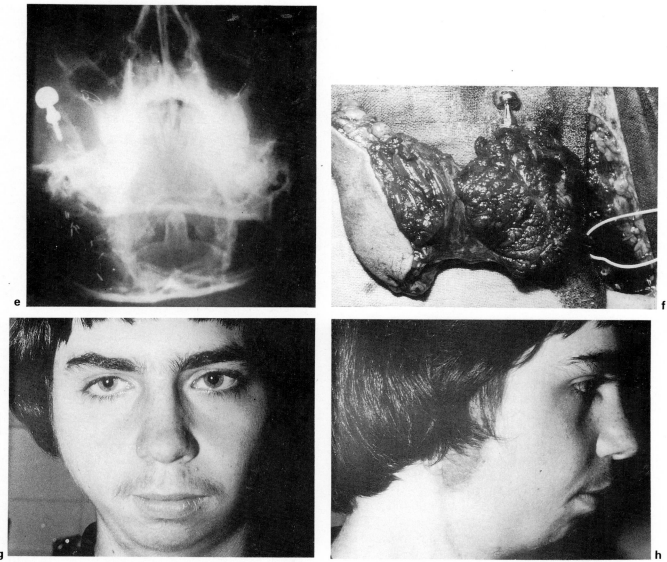

Fig. 20.173 Temporoaural mandibular dysplasia with macrostomia: (a, b) clinical aspect in infancy; (c, d) reconstruction of the auricle. Anterior transposition of the temporalis muscle and orthopaedic treatment; (e–h) reconstruction by free iliac composite flap and temporomandibular joint prosthesis.

when expansion of the skin envelope must precede bony mobilization as a preliminary step. In the past many procedures have been advocated for contour correction, but several of these have been abandoned. The use of a dermal fat graft (Eitner 1920) has become obsolete, because it produces results which are unpredictable owing to volume and contour irregularities, while cyst formation may be observed. The transfer of a de-epithelized tubed flap (Neuman 1953) or a crane flap (Millard 1969) requires many operative stages and is therefore no longer attractive. Silicone as an implant or in the form of multiple small injections (Rees 1973) is a frequent source of complication, because extrusion and migration (Pearl et al 1978) tend to occur.

Today, however, the reconstructive surgeon has better techniques at his disposal. The transfer of muscle and skin, separately or in combination, represents an elegant way to correct both volume deficit and shortage of skin.

1. Deficiency of subcutaneous tissue alone; in such a case correction is possible by the transposition of adjacent flaps and the transfer of distant and revascularized structures.
   a. The platysma can be turned over but this technique (described by Flot et al 1981) has some disadvantages. The vascular supply to the muscle varies and is unpredictable. The use of the flap is subject to the forces of gravity and scar contraction. The muscle itself is often hypoplastic and thus insufficient.
   b. The temporal muscle has been used by some surgeons but the results of this technique are not known.
   c. The galea appears to be the procedure of choice because of its rich vascularization, its wide arch of rotation and its displacement from an upward to a downward position. In addition its viability provides an excellent cover for a bone graft.
   d. Free flaps have long been advocated. The transfer of an inguinal dermal flap was reported by Antia & Buch (1971). The use of omentum was advocated by several authors.
2. Deficiency of subcutaneous tissue and skin. It is advisable to use a single flap to correct both problems. Composite musculocutaneous flaps succeed in achieving this purpose. The latissimus dorsi, preferably used in its musculocutaneous form, makes it possible to solve the most complicated situations. Indeed, its bulkiness is usually sufficient to fill the deepest depressions and its cutaneous surface allows for the correction of skin shortage in the cheek area (Fig. 20.172). The transfer of free revascularized flaps also permits difficult composite tissue reconstructions. The forearm and the back are the donor sites of choice. Use of the latissimus dorsi muscle enables the surgeon to reanimate a paralysed face by correctly orientating the muscle and reinnervating it by the facial nerve.

3. Deficiency of skeleton and soft tissues. Integral correction of temporo-auromandibular dysplasia or hemifacial microsomia may benefit from the development of techniques designed to transport bone and soft tissues 'en bloc' using various donor sites, such as the iliac crest (Fig. 20.173), the transposition of temporal muscle and galea in continuity with a calvarial bone flap (Fig. 20.174), the transfer of revascularized bone segments from the forearm (Fig. 20.175), the scapula and the sternocostal junction.

Facial paralysis

The facial nerve is altered in its passage through the hypoplastic petrous bone owing to alterations in the course and diameter of the aqueduct. The inferior branch of the facial nerve is predominantly affected and spontaneous improvement is sometimes observed. Complete paralysis may, however, be noticed in severe malformations and neurolysis must then be considered.

This procedure is difficult in the newborn. It requires perfect knowledge of dystopic structures and of the anterior and lowered position of the aqueduct. The facial nerve emerges at an abnormal anterior site and is therefore at risk during osteotomies.

AURICULAR MALFORMATIONS*

The question when to operate in children has still not been settled. In adults there is no difficulty as, apart from expecting a co-operative patient, the surgeon should have no difficulty in obtaining an adequate amount of cartilage. Moreover, since growth has ceased it is easy to decide on the size of the auricle to be reconstructed.

In children the difficulties are compounded by the anxiety of the parents and the suggestion of psychologists that early reconstruction is desirable to prevent the development of an inferiority complex, or even worse psychological damage which may persist into adult life.

Our extensive experience and psychological studies have, however, convinced us that postponing initial surgery until the 10th year has produced very little in the way of permanent psychological damage, largely because the adequate amount of available cartilage at this age enables the surgeon to reconstruct a much more presentable ear. We firmly believe that autogenous cartilage is the best material for reconstruction of the ear skeleton in all cases, as demonstrated in Figures 20.63–20.65 and 20.176–20.179. We are also convinced that it is not possible to obtain enough costal cartilage from children for a normal adult-sized ear until the age of 10 years has been reached.

Anthropometric measurements provide information concerning the duration of growth, the size of the ear and its position in relation to other structures. Hajnis et al

*The author of this section is L. Barinka

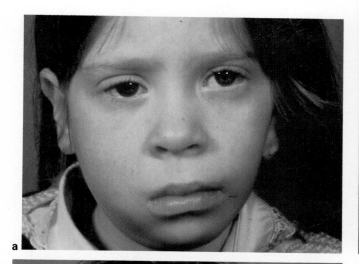

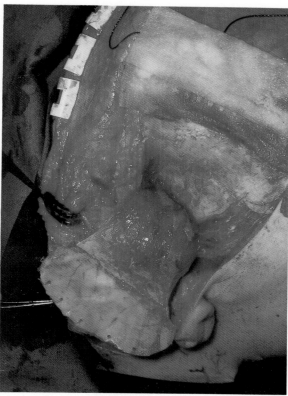

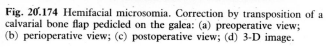

Fig. 20.174 Hemifacial microsomia. Correction by transposition of a calvarial bone flap pedicled on the galea: (a) preoperative view; (b) perioperative view; (c) postoperative view; (d) 3-D image.

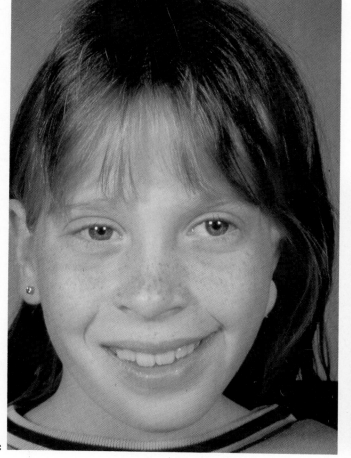

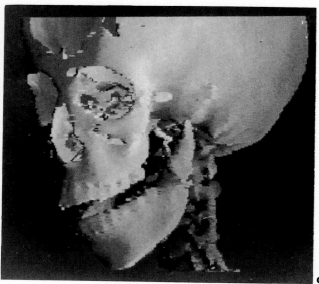

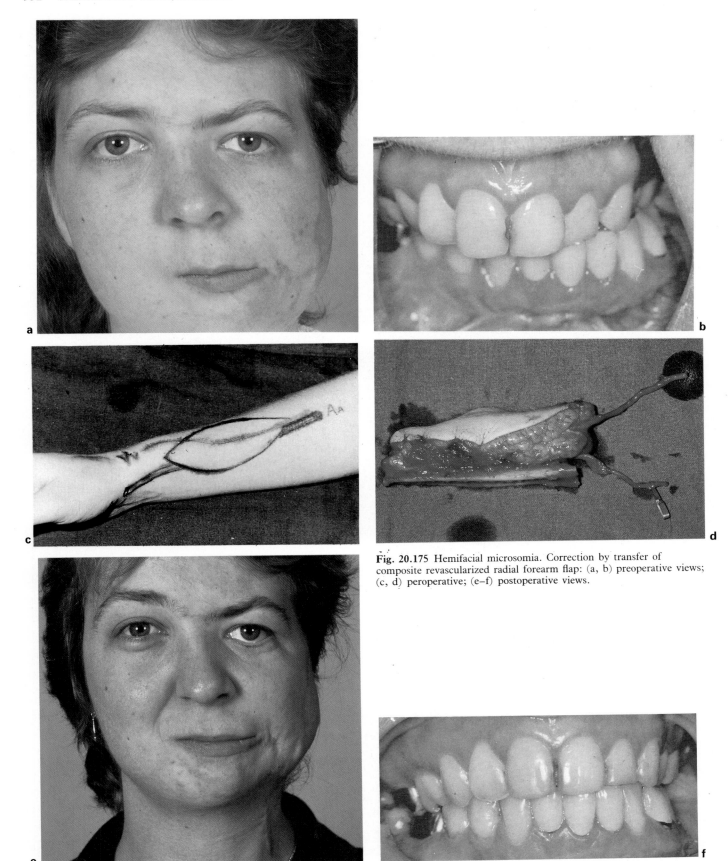

Fig. 20.175 Hemifacial microsomia. Correction by transfer of composite revascularized radial forearm flap: (a, b) preoperative views; (c, d) peroperative; (e–f) postoperative views.

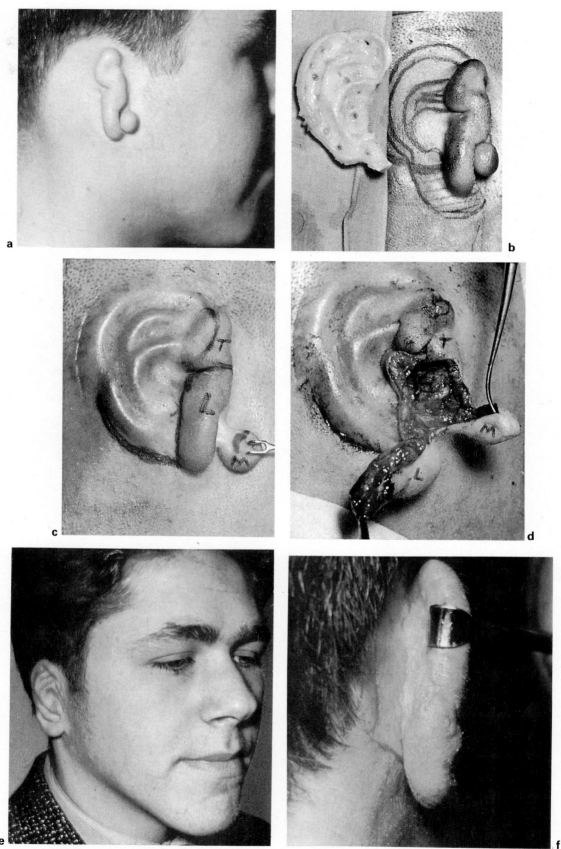

Fig. 20.176 Auricular reconstruction: (a) preoperative view; (b) the cartilaginous implant; (c) postoperative view; (d) formation of lobule and tragus with auricular rudiments; (e) final result.

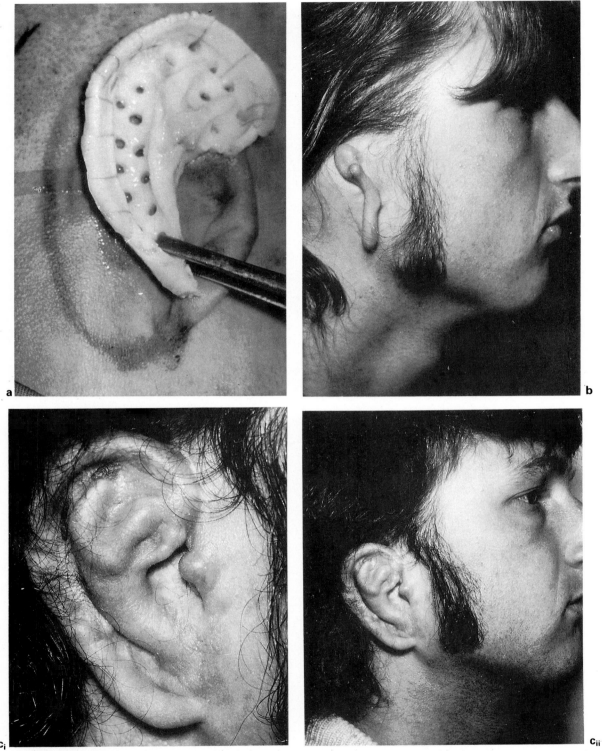

Fig. 20.177 Auricular reconstruction: (a) preoperative view; (b) the cartilaginous implant; (c) postoperative views.

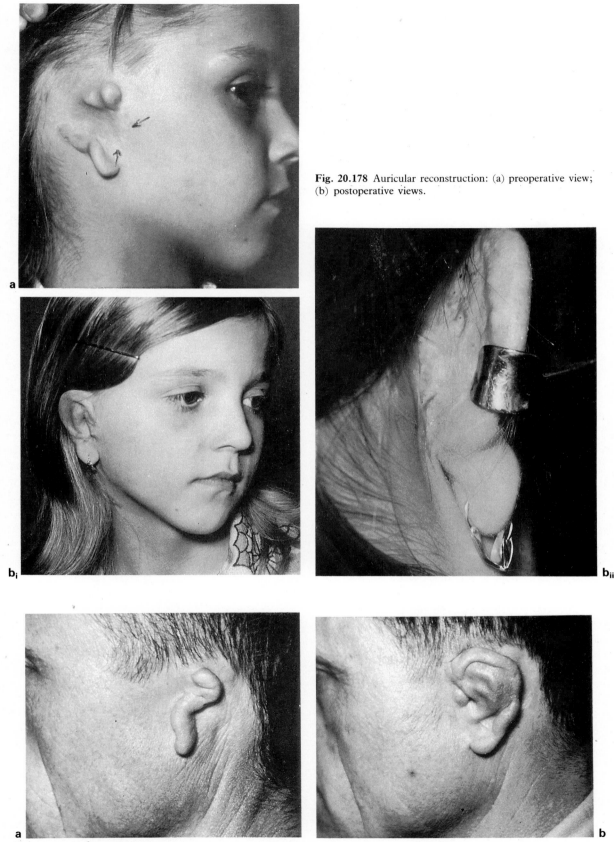

Fig. 20.178 Auricular reconstruction: (a) preoperative view; (b) postoperative views.

Fig. 20.179 Auricular reconstruction: (a) preoperative view; (b) postoperative view.

Table 20.1 Auricle development in vertical dimension (mm)

Age group	Boys		Girls	
	Left	Right	Left	Right
0–9 months	43.9	44.5	40.8	41.3
1 year	49.7	50.2	46.8	46.8
2 years	48.6	50.1	48.5	48.9
3 years	50.2	51.5	49.5	50.8
4 years	51.6	53.0	50.8	51.4
5 years	53.2	54.5	52.0	52.3
6 years	54.8	55.8	53.1	53.9
7–8 years	56.1	56.8	56.5	56.5
9–10 years	57.0	58.3	55.5	58.5
11–12 years	59.7	60.8	57.7	57.9
13–14 years	60.5	60.3	57.0	58.3
15–16 years	62.6	63.4	57.8	58.6
17–18 years	63.4	63.7	58.7	59.3

Table 20.2 Auricle development in horizontal dimension (mm)

Age group	Boys		Girls	
	Left	Right	Left	Right
0–9 months	26.2	27.7	24.8	25.0
1 year	31.0	31.9	28.8	29.4
2 years	31.5	32.4	30.2	31.3
3 years	31.9	32.5	31.1	31.5
4 years	30.8	32.4	31.3	31.5
5 years	33.4	33.2	31.9	32.0
6 years	32.9	33.7	32.4	32.7
7–8 years	33.3	33.8	32.8	32.9
9–10 years	34.8	35.1	32.1	33.0
11–12 years	34.6	35.2	33.1	33.3
13–14 years	34.6	36.3	33.2	34.3
15–16 years	36.7	36.8	32.3	33.9
17–18 years	34.6	36.0	31.7	33.2

(1966) have completed an extensive study on the subject and the vertical and horizontal dimensions of the ear during the period of growth are given in Tables 20.1 and 20.2.

It can be seen that there is virtually no increase in the size of the ear after the age of 10 or 11 years. This confirms the view that reconstruction of the ear should not be undertaken before the age of 10 years.

In cases of unilateral atresia with a normal meatus and normal or good hearing on the opposite side, it is widely agreed that one should not attempt to construct an external auditory canal or explore the middle ear. On the other hand this is indicated in cases of bilateral atresia as the improvement, although small, can have an important effect on the development of speech. Tanzer (1959) reported that an initial improvement by 20 dB later fell to 5 dB in a series of cases.

Oromandibular region

This region concerns the mandible, particularly the body and adjacent structures such as the tongue and the lower lip, including the commissures. Mandibular shortness, rarely a mandibular defect, is the main skeletal characteristic.

The following clinical forms may be distinguished: maxillomandibular clefting (macrostomia); mandibular dysplasia; intermandibular dysplasia (including aglossia).

MAXILLOMANDIBULAR CLEFTING

This malformation is characterized by macrostomia, cutaneocartilaginous rudiments and preauricular fistulas.

Macrostomia (Fig. 20.180)

This cleft extends more or less along a transverse line running from the buccal commissure to the tragus. Its repair is usually undertaken at an early stage for cosmetic purposes and involves reconstitution of the three layers.

Freeing of the mucosal layer is followed by identification of the various muscles situated around the commissure, by reconstruction of the orbicularis sling and by repair of the m. buccinator. The mucosa is then sutured using buried stitches and interdigitation of flaps to avoid a 'dog-ears' excess. Closure of the skin is finally carried out by means of one or more Z-plasties in order to avoid any contracture, which might tend to draw the commissure downwards.

Accurate positioning of the reconstructed commissure is determined in the following manner: in unilateral cases by the position of the normal contralateral commissure, and in bilateral cases by the criteria usually applied for the width of the buccal orifice. These criteria vary with the morphotype of the patient: in a narrow mouth by two vertical lines tangential to the nostrils, and in a wide mouth by two vertical lines passing through the middle of each pupil.

The cutaneocartilaginous rudiments

The cutaneocartilaginous rudiments are situated in front of the tragus or along the groove that separates the maxillary and mandibular process. The superficial tags are easily excised at the time of the first operation.

Preauricular fistulas

One may divide these fistulas into two groups (Arnold 1971).

Type I usually appears in the adult in the form of a painful preauricular cyst, or as a fistula in the parotid region which is often very close to the lower branches of the facial nerve and may extend as far as the temporal fossa.

Type II appears more frequently in childhood. This is a fistula or a superficial cyst situated in the anterior triangle

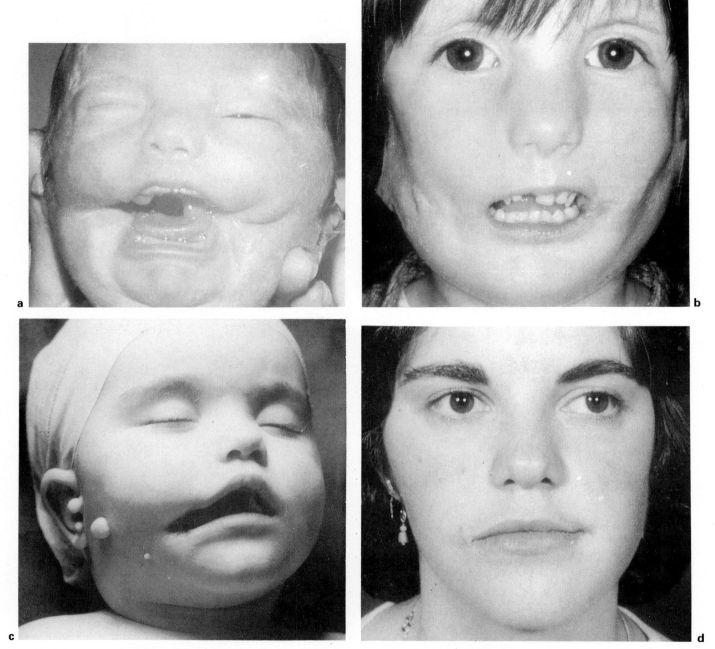

Fig. 20.180 Macrostomia: (a) bilateral, preoperative view; (b) bilateral, postoperative view (Courtesy M. Lincker); (c) unilateral, preoperative view; (d) unilateral, postoperative view.

of the neck; its course extends upwards and backwards to the ear, and is variably related to the facial nerve. The tract ends in the external auditory meatus at the osteocartilaginous junction, or as a blind fistula at the same place.

Surgical excision requires a precise knowledge of the fistulous tract, gained either by fistulography or injection of a dye (Byars & Anderson 1951), in order that removal may be complete. One must not underestimate this procedure. There is frequently a close relationship between the fistula and the facial nerve and one should not hesitate to expose the nerve by means of a superficial parotidectomy (Belenky & Medina 1980).

MANDIBULAR DYSPLASIA (Fig. 20.181)

Micromandibulism may be observed independently from deformities that are associated with temporomandibular ankylosis, caused either by trauma or by infection.

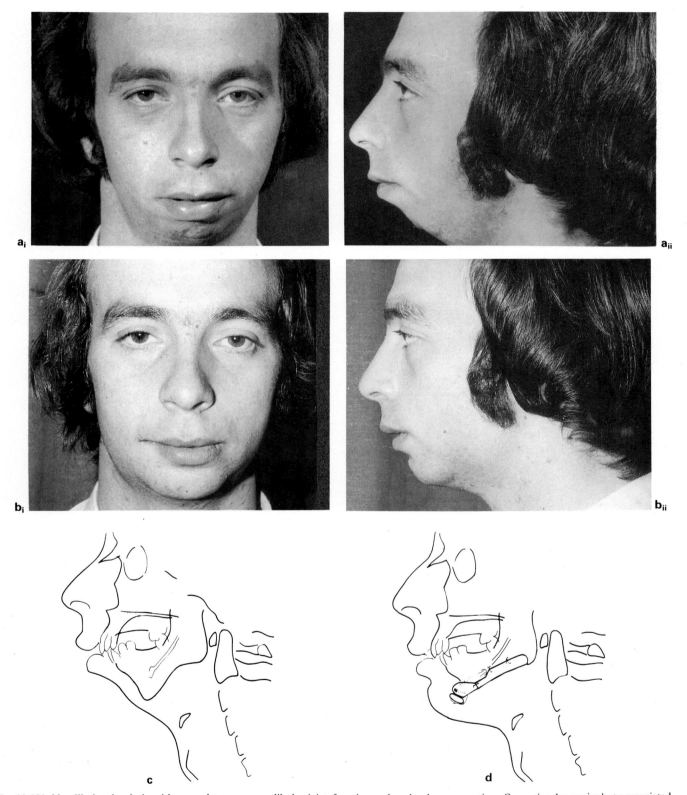

Fig. 20.181 Mandibular dysplasia with normal temporomandibular joint function and occlusal compensation. Correction by genioplasty associated with onlay rib grafts: (a) preoperative views; (b) postoperative views; (c) diagrammatic represention

Sporadic cases are seen in patients with a curiously under-developed lower third of the face, without other associated malformations.

Lengthening of the mandible and forward projection of the chin are the two options that should be considered. Lengthening is carried out in the rami by a combined approach: intraoral, to obtain adequate exposure, and cutaneous for the vertical osteotomy.

In simple cases, the procedure according to Mehnert (1976) is usually sufficient. If not, a bone graft is inserted at the site of the osteotomy, maintaining propulsion. Forward projection of the chin is obtained by a genio-plasty, using an intraoral approach. Harmonization of the arches by preoperative orthodontics is mandatory and calculation of the desired postoperative reference is carried out using a teleradiographic and occlusal simulation study.

The mandibular procedure can be combined with a partial or total maxillary osteotomy and if necessary with additional facial correction in syndromes such as the Hallerman–Streiff malformation.

The Robin Syndrome (pseudomandibular dysplasia)

Some authors have incorrectly considered this syndrome to be a dysostosis, owing to the morphological resemblance to the mandibular anomaly. In fact, the alteration of the structures is essentially functional. The degree of lingual protrusion is a criterion of the evolution of the syndrome.

Surgical treatment is only exceptionally required in the newborn with severe respiratory distress. Fixation of the tongue to the lower lip is a barbaric procedure which should no longer be used. We agree with Moyson (1961) that there is no place for a tracheostomy. Mandibulohyoid fixation is the procedure of choice in emergencies (Sanvenero Rosselli 1960). Forward and upward traction of the mandible by means of a splint is occasionally indicated.

Skilled nursing care with the child in a prone position, maintained by a frame, is the treatment most commonly used (Burston 1969). Application of a palatal plate to hold the tongue in a forward position and lingual rehabilitation by stimulation of suction are complementary methods of treatment.

INTERMANDIBULAR DYSPLASIA

Two forms of very different severity may be observed: the intermandibular cleft not involving the tongue; and the aglossia–adactylia syndrome.

The first form is easily corrected by restoration of the bony continuity using a corticocancellous bone graft and by correction of the soft tissue anomaly in separate mucosal and cutaneous layers. Ultimately closure of the bony defect by means of a free periosteal tibial graft to stimulate bone production may be considered.

The second form is more severe but in patients with microstomia or absence of the tongue correction of the mandible is usually of secondary importance. First of all the oral orifice should be expanded by dilatation of the orbicular muscle using an activator, and the tongue should be freed.

In rare instances of aglossia reconstruction of the tongue by means of a revascularized myocutaneous graft may be considered. The restoration of function, however, requires the presence of adequate innervation.

Dentoalveolar region (occlusion)

Restoration of the occlusion includes: orthodontic alignment as a first step; a meticulous teleradiographic and occlusal study; and a definitive and retentive dentition. For these reasons surgery is to be postponed until the age of 15 years. Surgical–orthodontic rehabilitation is frequently indicated, in particular when dysostosis exists, and it usually concludes the treatment of craniofacial anomalies.

REFERENCES AND BIBLIOGRAPHY

Basic techniques

Abbe R 1898 A new plastic operation for the relief of deformity due to double hare lip. Medical Record 53: 477

Abdul-Hassan H S, Ascher G D, Acland R D 1986 Surgical anatomy of blood supply of the fascial layers of the temporal region. Plastic and Reconstructive Surgery 77: 17

Acland R D 1978 Caution about clinical use of vascularized periosteal grafts. Plastic and Reconstructive Surgery 62: 90

Adekeye E O 1977 Rapid bone regeneration subsequent to subtotal mandibulectomy. Report of an unusual case. Oral Surgery 44: 521

Altonen M, Ylipaavalniemi P, Ranta R 1977 Bone formation with free periosteum around the root of rabbit tooth. Proceedings of the Finnish Dental Society 73: 32

Anderl H, Muhlbauer W, Twerdy K, Marchac D 1983 Frontofacial advancement with bony separation in cranial dysostosis. Plastic and Reconstructive Surgery 71: 303

Angle E H 1907 Treatment of malocclusion of the teeth: Angle's system (7th edn). SS White, Philadelphia

Antonyshyn O, Coleleugh R G, Hurst L N, Anderson C 1986 The temporalis myo-osseous flap: an experimental study. Plastic and Reconstructive Surgery 77: 406

Argenta L C, Vanderkolk C A 1987 Tissue expansion in craniofacial surgery. Clinics in Plastic Surgery 14: 143–153

Argenta L C, Wantanabe J J, Grabb W C 1983 The use of tissue expansion in head and neck reconstruction. Annals of Plastic Surgery 11: 31

Ariyan S 1980 The viability of rib grafts transplanted with the periosteal blood supply. Plastic and Reconstructive Surgery 65: 140

Ariyan S, Finseth F J 1978 The anterior chest approach for obtaining free osteocutaneous rib grafts. Plastic and Reconstructive Surgery 62: 676

Austad E D, Rose G L 1982a A self inflating tissue expander. Plastic and Reconstructive Surgery 70: 107

Austad E D, Pasyk K A, McClatchey K D et al 1982b Histomorphologic evaluation of guinea pig skin and soft tissue after controlled tissue expansion. Plastic and Reconstructive Surgery 70: 704

Avelar J M, Psillakis J M 1981 The use of galea flaps in craniofacial deformities. Annals of Plastic Surgery 6: 464

Baadsgaard K, Medgyesi S 1965 Muscle–pedicle bone grafts. Acta Orthopaedica Scandinavica 35: 279

Barinka L 1966 Congenital malformations of auricle and their reconstruction by a new method. Acta Chirurgiae Plasticae 8: 3

Bell W H 1973 Biologic basis for maxillary osteotomies. American Journal of Physical Anthropology 38: 279–290

Bell W H 1978 Subapical osteotomy to increase mandibular arch length. American Journal of Orthodontics 74: 276–285

Bell W H, Schendel S A 1977 Biologic basis for modification of the sagittal split ramus osteotomy. Journal of Oral Surgery 35: 362

Bell W H, Proffit W R, White R P 1980 Surgical correction of dentofacial deformities. Saunders, Philadelphia

Berggren A, Weiland A J, Dorfman H 1982 Free vascularized bone grafts: factors affecting their survival and ability to heal recipient bone defects. Plastic and Reconstructive Surgery 69: 19

Blair V P 1918 Surgery and diseases of the mouth and jaws, 3rd edn. Mosby, St Louis. p 269

Bos K E 1979 Bone scintigraphy of experimental composite bone grafts revascularized by microvascular anastomoses. Plastic and Reconstructive Surgery 64: 353

Bos K E 1980 Transplantatie van autoloog bot en revascularisatie door middel van microvaatanastomosen. Doctoral thesis, Amsterdam

Bourguet J 1936 La véritable chirurgie esthétique du visage. Plon, Paris, p 55

Brent B 1979 Reconstruction of the ear. In: Grabb W C, Smith J W (eds) Plastic surgery: a concise guide to clinical practice (3rd edn). Little Brown, Boston

Brent B (1980a) The correction of microtia with autogenous cartilage grafts. I. The classic deformity. Plastic and Reconstructive Surgery 66: 11

Brent B (1980b) The correction of microtia with autogenous cartilage grafts. II. Typical and complex deformities. Plastic and Reconstructive Surgery 66: 13

Brent B, Upton J, Ackland R D et al 1986 Experience with the temporoparietal fascial free flap. Plastic and Reconstructive Surgery 78: 300

Brookes M 1971 The blood supply of bone. An approach to bone biology. Butterworth, London

Brookes M, Harrison R G 1957 The vascularization of the rabbit femur and tibiofibula. Journal of Anatomy 91: 61

Byrd H S 1980 The use of subcutaneous axial flaps in reconstruction of the head. Annals of Plastic Surgery 4: 191

Calabrese C T, Winslow R B, Latham R A 1974 Altering the dimensions of the canine face by the induction of new bone formation. Plastic and Reconstructive Surgery 54: 467

Canalis R F, Saffouri M, Mirra J, Ward P H 1977 The fate of pedicle osteocutaneous grafts in mandibulofacial restoration. Laryngoscope 87: 895

Canalis R F, Hemenway W G, Ward P H 1979 Role of periosteum on the fate of pedicle osteocutaneous grafts. Annals of Otology 88: 642

Casanova R, Cavalcante D, Grotting J C et al 1986 The anatomic basis for vascularized outer table calvarial bone flaps. Plastic and Reconstructive Surgery 78: 300

Casson P R, Bonanno P C, Converse J M 1974 The midface degloving procedure. Plastic and Reconstructive Surgery 53: 102

Cestero H J, Salyer K E 1975 Regenerative potential of bone and periosteum. Surgical Forum 26: 557

Cestero H J, Salyer K E, Toranto I R 1974 Role of the periosteum in bone regeneration. Surgical Forum 25: 489

Cestero H J Jr, Salyer K E, Toranto I R 1975 Bone growth into porous carbon, polyethylene and polypropylene prosthesis. Journal of Biomedical Material Research 9: 1

Champy M 1980 Surgical treatment of midface deformities. Head and Neck Surgery 2: 451–465

Charpy A, Poirier P, 1896 Traité d'anatomie humaine. Bataille, Paris

Chase S W, Herndon C H 1955 The fate of autogenous and homogenous bone grafts. Journal of Bone and Joint Surgery 37A: 809

Combelles R, Zadeh J 1984–5 Le lambeau temporal musculoosseux. Etude anatomique technique experimentale et chirurgicate. Revue Stomatologie et de Chirurgie Maxillofaciale 5: 351–354

Conley J 1972 Use of composite flaps containing bone for major repairs in the head and neck. Plastic and Reconstructive Surgery 49: 522

Conley J, Cinelli P B, Johnson P M, Koss M 1973 Investigation of bone changes in composite flaps after transfer to the head and neck region. Plastic and Reconstructive Surgery 51: 658

Conover M A, Kaban L B, Mulliken J B 1985 Antibiotic prophylaxis for major maxillocraniofacial surgery. Journal of Oral and Maxillofacial Surgery 43: 865

Converse J M 1950 Reconstruction of the external ear by prefabricated framework. Plastic and Reconstructive Surgery 5: 148

Converse J M 1958 Reconstruction of the auricle. II. Plastic and Reconstructive Surgery 22: 230

Converse J M 1977 Reconstructive plastic surgery, vol 2, 2nd edn. Saunders, Philadelphia

Converse J M, Telsey D 1971 The tripartite osteotomy of the midface for orbital expansion and correction of the deformity in craniostenosis. British Journal of Plastic Surgery 24: 365–374

Converse J M, and Wood-Smith D 1963 Experiences with the forehead island flap with a subcutaneous pedicle. Plastic and Reconstructive Surgery 31: 521

Converse J M, Wood-Smith D 1971 An atlas and classification of midfacial and craniofacial osteotomies. In: Transactions of the Fifth International Congress of Plastic and Reconstructive Surgery pp. 931–962, Buttersworth, Melbourne. pp 931–962

Converse J M, Ransohoff J, Mathews E S, Smith B, Molenaar A 1970 Ocular hypertelorism and pseudohypertelorism. Advances in surgical treatment. Plastic and Reconstructive Surgery 45: 1

Converse J M et al 1973 The corrective treatment of the skeletal asymmetry in hemifacial microsomia. Plastic and Reconstructive Surgery 52: 221

Converse J M, Wood-Smith D, McCarty J G 1975 Report on a series of 50 craniofacial operations. Plastic and Reconstructive Surgery 55: 283

Converse J M et al 1979 Clinical aspects of craniofacial microsomia. In: Converse J M, McCarthy J G, Wood-Smith D (eds) Symposium on Diagnosis and Treatment of Craniofacial Anomalies. Mosby, St Louis. p 461

Corso P F 1961 Variations of the arterial venous and capillary circulation of the soft tissues of the head of decades as demonstrated by the methyl methacrylate injection technique and their application to the construction of flaps and pedicles. Plastic and Reconstructive Surgery 27: 160

Crockford D A, Converse J M 1972 The ilium as a source of bone grafts in children. Plastic and Reconstructive Surgery 50: 270–274

Cuono C B, Ariyan S 1980 Immediate reconstruction of a composite defect with a regional osteomusculocutaneous flap. Plastic and Reconstructive Surgery 65: 477

Cutting C B, McCarthy J G 1983 Comparison of residual osseous mass between vascularized and nonvascularized onlay bone transfers. Plastic and Reconstructive Surgery 72: 672

Cutting C B, McCarthy J G, Berenstein A 1984 Blood supply of the upper craniofacial skeleton: the search for composite calvarial bone flaps. Plastic and Reconstructive Surgery 74: 603

Dal Pont G 1959 L'osteotomia retromolare per la correzione della progenia. Minerva Chirurgica 18: 1138

Dal Pont G 1961 Retromolar osteotomy for the correction of prognathism. Journal of Oral Surgery 19: 42–47

Daniel R K 1977 Letter to the editor: free rib transfer by microvascular anastomoses. Plastic and Reconstructive Surgery 59: 737

Daniel R K 1978 Mandibular reconstruction with free tissue transfers. Annals of Plastic Surgery 1: 346

De Jonge P 1981 Collagene vezels in het pijpbeen-periosteum in relatie met de mechanische regulatie van de lengtegroei. Medical thesis, Nijmegen

Dobisiková M, Hajniš K 1966 An anthropometric contribution to the determination of reconstruction timing for hypoplastic and aplastic auricles. Anthropogie 4: 1

Dos Santos L F 1980 Retalho circular: um novo retalho livre microcirurgico. Revista Brasileira de Cirugia Cir. 70: 133

Dos Santos L F 1984 The vascular anatomy and dissection of the free scapular flap. Plastic and Reconstructive Surgery 73: 599–603

Epker B N 1964 A modified anterior maxillary osteotomy. Journal of Maxillofacial Surgery 27: 939

Epker B N 1977 Modifications in the sagittal osteotomy of the mandible. Journal of Oral Surgery 35: 155–159

Epker B N, Walford L M 1980 Dentofacial deformities. Surgical orthodontic correction. Mosby, St Louis

Erol O O, Parsa F D, Spira M 1981 The use of the secondary island graft-flap in reconstruction of the burned ear. British Journal of Plastic Surgery 34: 417

Esser J S F 1917 Verschliessung von Larynx und Tracheafisteln oder Defecten mit plastische Operation. Archiv fur Klinische Chirurgie 109: 385–393

Esser J S F 1918 Die Rotation der Wange und allgemeine Bemerkungen bei chirurgischer Gesichtsplastik. Vogel, Leipzig

Finley J M, Acland R D, Wood M B 1978 Revascularized periosteal grafts. A new method to produce functional new bone with bone grafting. Plastic and Reconstructive Surgery 61: 1

Firmin F, Coccaro P J, Converse J M 1974 Cephalometric analysis in diagnosis and treatment of craniofacial dysostosis. Plastic and Reconstructive Surgery 54: 300–311

Flot F, Chassagne F F, Raphael B, Meley M, Brice M, Stricker M 1981 Le peaucier du cou: interet chirurgi cal. Annales de Chirurgie Plastique 26: 52–57

Fonseca J L S 1983 Use of pericranial flap in scalp wounds with exposed bone. Plastic and Reconstructive Surgery 72: 786

Fox J W, Edgerton M T 1976 The fan flap: an adjunct to ear reconstruction. Plastic and Reconstructive Surgery 58: 663

Frost H M 1964 The laws of bone structure. Thomas, Springfield, Ill

Frost H M 1964 The laws of bone structure. Thomas, Springfield Ill

Georgiade N, Nash T 1966 An external cranial fixation apparatus for severe maxillofacial injuries. Plastic and Reconstructive Surgery 38: 142

Gillies H D, Harrison S H 1950 Operative correction by osteotomy of recessed malar maxillary compound in a case of oxycephaly. British Journal of Plastic Surgery 3: 123

Gorlin R J 1976 Maxillonasal dysplasia (Binder's syndrome). In: Gorlin R J, Pindborg J J, Cohen M M (eds) Syndromes of the head and neck. (2nd edn). McGraw-Hill, New York. pp 463–464

Green M F, Gibson J R, Bryson J R, Thomson E 1981 A one-stage correction of mandibular defects using a split sternum pectoralis major osteomusculotaneous transfer. British Journal of Plastic Surgery 34: 11

Guyuron B 1985 Retroauricular island flap for eye socket reconstruction. Plastic and Reconstructive Surgery 76: 527

Habal M B, Maniscalco J E 1981 Observations on the ultrastructure of the pericranium. Annals of Plastic Surgery 6: 103

Harii K, Yamada A, Ishihara K, Miki Y, Itoh M 1982 A free transfer of both latissimus dorsi and serratus anterior flaps with thoracodorsal vessel anastomoses. Plastic and Reconstructive Surgery 70: 620

Hata Y, Ohmori S 1979 On the experiences of periosteoplasty for the closure of the maxillary cleft. Chirurgica Plastica 5: 33

Hauben D J, Van der Meulen J C 1984 Use of temporal musculoperiosteal flap in the treatment of craniofacial abnormalities: experimental study. Plastic and Reconstructive Surgery 74: 355

Hellquist R 1971 Early maxillary orthopedics in relation to maxillary cleft repair by periosteoplasty. Cleft Palate Journal 8: 36

Hendel P M 1985 The harvesting of cranial bone grafts: a guided osteotome. Plastic and Reconstructive Surgery 76: 642

Hill E G, McKinney W 1981 Vascular anatomy and pathology of the head and neck: method of corrosion casting. Advances in Neurology 30: 191

Holmes R E, Salyer K E 1973 Aleveolar augmentation with hydroxyapatite: a preliminary study. Presented at the American Association for Dental Research, Las Vegas

Holmstrom H Surgical correction of the nose and midface in maxillonasal dysplasia (Binders syndrome)

Horowitz J H, Persing J A, Nichter L S, Morgan R E, Edgerton M T 1984 Galeal pericranial flaps in head and neck reconstruction. American Journal of Surgery 148: 489

Hrivnakova J, Fara M, Mullerova Z 1981 The use of periosteal flaps for bridging maxillary defect in facial clefts. Acta Chirurgiae Plasticae 23: 130

Ivy R H 1951 Bone grafting for restoration of defects of the mandible. Plastic and Reconstructive Surgery 7: 333

Jabaley M E, Edgerton M E 1969 Surgical correction of congenital midface retrusion in the presence of mandibular prognathism. Plastic and Reconstructive Surgery 44: 1–8

Jackson I T 1981 Reconstruction of the lower eyelid defect in Treacher Collins syndrome. Plastic and Reconstructive Surgery 67: 365–368

Jackson I T, Hide T A H 1981 Further extensions of cranial facial surgery. Recent Advances in Plastic Surgery 2: 241

Jackson I T, Hide T A H, Barker D 1978 Transposition cranioplasty to restore forehead contour in craniofacial deformities. British Journal of Plastic Surgery 31: 127–130

Jackson I T, Moos K F, Sharpe D T 1981 Total surgical management of Binder's syndrome. Annals of Plastic Surgery 7: 25

Jackson I T, Munro I, Whitaker L, Salyer K 1982 Atlas of craniofacial surgery. Mosby, St Louis.

Jackson I T, Laws E R Jr, Martin R D 1983 A craniofacial approach to advanced recurrent cancer of the central face. Head and Neck Surgery 5: 474

Jackson I T, Tanner N S, Hide T A 1983 Frontonasal encephalocele — 'long nose hypertelorism'. Annals of Plastic Surgery 11: 490–500

Jackson I T, Marsch W R, Hide T A H 1984 Treatment of tumors involving the anterior cranial fossa. Head and Neck Surgery 6: 901

Johanson B, Andersson H, Friede H, Lauritzen C, Lilja J 1981 Treatment of premature sutural synostosis. Scandinavian Journal of Plastic Surgery 15: 213–216

Jurkiewicz M 1973 The voice of polite dissent. Plastic and Reconstructive Surgery 52: 79

Kaban L B, Mulliken J R, Murray J E 1981 Three dimensional approach to analysis and treatment of hemifacial microsomia. Cleft Palate Journal 18: 90–99

Kazanjian V H 1946 Repair of nasal defects with the median forehead flaps. Surgical Gynecology and Obstetrics 83: 37

King K F 1976 Periosteal pedicle grafting in dogs. Journal of Bone and Joint Surgery 58b: 117

Knize D M 1974 The influence of periosteum and calcitonin on onlay bone graft survival. Plastic and Reconstructive Surgery 53: 190

Köle H 1958 Corticalisschwachung zur Unterstutzung bei der kieferorthopadischen Behandlung. Fortschritte der Kiefer-und Gesichts-Chirurgie 4: 208

Köle H 1959 Surgical operations on the alveolar ridge to correct occlusal abnormalities. Journal of Oral Surgery 12: 515–529

Köle H 1965 Results, experience and problems in the operative treatment of anomalies with reserve overbite. Oral Surgery 19: 427

Konig F 1890 Der knocherne Ersatz grosser Schadeldefkte. Zentralblatt fur Chirurgie 17: 65

Lachard J, Gola R, Grisoli F 1974 Traitement chirurgical des sequelles maxillaires des fentes labio-palatines. La disjonction pterigo-maxillaire. Revue de Stomatologie 75: 77–82

Lalonde D H, Williams H B, Rosenthall L, Viloria J B 1984 Circulation, bone scans, and tetracycline labeling in microvascularized and vascular bundle implanted rib grafts. Annals of Plastic Surgery 13: 366

Lasjaunias P 1981 Craniofacial and upper cervical arteries. Williams & Wilkins, Baltimore

Le Fort R 1901 Etude experimental sur les fractures de la machoire superieure. Revue de Chirurgie 23: 208

Le Fort R 1972 Experimental study of fracture of the upper jaw. Plastic and Reconstructive Surgery 50: 497–506

Leriche R, Policard A 1928 The normal and pathological physiology of bone. Mosby, St Louis

Longacre J J 1973 Craniosynostosis and its relation to craniofacial defects: rehabilitation of the facially disfigured. Thomas, Springfield. p 65

Lovie M J, Duncan G M, Glasson D W 1984 The ulnar artery forearm free flap. British Journal of Plastic Surgery 37: 486

Lozano A J, Cestero H J, Salyer K E 1976a A comparative study of the early vascularization of porous carbon and bone as a graft. Journal of Biomedical Materials Research 7: 545

Lozano A J, Cestero H J, Salyer K E 1976b The early vascularization of onlay bone grafts. Plastic and Reconstructive Surgery 58: 302

McCarthy J G, Zide B M 1984 The spectrum of calvarial bone grafting: introduction of the vascularized calvarial bone flap. Plastic and Reconstructive Surgery 74: 10

McCarthy J G, Coccaro P J, Epstein F, Converse J M 1978 Early skeletal release in the infant with craniofacial dysostosis: the role of the sphenozygomatic suture. Plastic and Reconstructive Surgery 62: 335

McCarthy J G, Lorencz Z P, Cutting C, Rachesky M 1985 The median forehead flap revisited: the blood supply. Plastic and Reconstructive Surgery 76: 866

McGregor I A, Morgan G 1973 Axial and random pattern flaps. British Journal of Plastic Surgery 26: 202–213

McKee D M 1978 Microvascular bone transplantation. Clinics in Plastic Surgery 5: 283

Manders E K, Graham W P, Davis T S 19xx Skin expansion to eliminate large scalp defects. Annals of Plastic Surgery 12: 305

Mangold U, Lierse W, Pfeiffer G 1980 The arteries of the forehead as the basis of nasal reconstruction with forehead flaps. Acta Anatomica 107: 18

Marchac D 1978 Radical forehead remodeling for cranio-stenosis. Plastic and Reconstructive Surgery 61: 823

Marchac D, Renier D 1979 Le front flottant, traitement precoce des facio-craniostenoses. Annales de Chirurgie Plastique 24: 121

Marchac D, Bryant T 1985 The axial frontonasal flap revisited. Plastic and Reconstructive Surgery 76: 686–694

Maruyama Y, Urita Y, Ohnishi K 1985 Rib–latissimus dorsi osteomyocutaneous flap in reconstruction of a mandibular defect. British Journal of Plastic Surgery 38: 234

Medgyesi S 1973 Observation on pedicle bone grafts in goats. Scandinavian Journal of Plastic and Reconstructive Surgery 7: 110

Mehnert H 1976 A variation in the vertical osteotomy of the rami for correction of retrognathism. Journal of Maxillofacial Surgery 4: 210

Melcher A H, Accursi G E 1971 Osteogenic capacity of periosteal and osteoperiosteal flaps elevated from the parietal bone of the rat. Archives of Oral Biology 16: 573

Millard D R Jr 1974 Reconstructive rhinoplasty for the lower half of a nose. Plastic and Reconstructive Surgery 53: 133–139

Millard D R Jr 1976–1980 Cleft craft. The evolution of its surgery, vols 1–3. Little, Brown, Boston

Mitz V, Peyronie M 1976 The superficial musculoaponeurotic system (SMAS) in the parotid and cheek area. Plastic and Reconstructive Surgery 58: 80

Montaut J, Stricker M 1977 Dysmorphies craniofaciales — Les synostoses prematurees (craniostenoses et faciostenoses) (Vol 1). Masson et Cie, Paris.

Mulliken J B, Glowacki J 1980 Induced osteogenesis for repair and construction in the craniofacial region. Plastic and Reconstructive Surgery 65: 553–559

Mulliken J B, Kaban L B, Evans C A, Strand R D, Murray J E 1986 Facial skeletal changes following hypertelorbitism correction. Plastic and Reconstructive surgery 77: 7–16

Munro I 1980 One stage reconstruction of the temporo-mandibular joint in hemifacial microsomia. Plastic and Reconstructive Surgery 66: 699

Munro I R, Hoffman H J, Hendrick E B 1975 Total cranial vault reshaping in cranio-facial surgery. In: Transactions of the Sixth International Congress of Plastic and Reconstructive Surgery. Paris. Masson et Cie, Paris. p 158

Murray J E, Swanson L T 1968 Mid-face osteotomy and advancement for craniosynostosis. Plastic and Reconstructive Surgery 41: 299

Murray J E, Kaban L B, Mulliken J B 1984 Analysis and treatment of hemifacial microsomia. Plastic and Reconstructive Surgery 74: 186–199

Murray J E, Kaban L B, Mulliken J B, Evans C A 1985 Analysis and treatment of hemifacial microsomia. In: Caronni E P (ed) Craniofacial surgery. Little, Brown, Boston. pp 377–391

Mustardé J C 1966 Repair and reconstruction in the orbital region. Churchill Livingstone, Edinburgh

Nassif T M, Vidal L, Bovet J L, Baudet J 1982 The parascapular flap: a new cutaneous microsurgical free flap. Plastic and Reconstructive Surgery 69: 591–600

Nelson R L 1977 Quantification of blood flow after Le Fort I osteotomy. Journal of Oral Surgery 55: 10–16

Neuman C G 1957 The expansion of an area of skin by progressive distension of a subcutaneous balloon. Plastic and Reconstructive Surgery 19: 124

Obwegeser H L 1957 Surgical correction of mandibular prognathism, with consideration of genioplasty. Oral Surgery 10: 677

Obwegeser H L 1964 The indications for surgical correction of mandibular deformity by the sagittal splitting technique. British Journal of Oral Surgery 1: 57

Obwegeser H L 1974 Correction of skeletal anomalies of otomandibular dysostosis. Journal of Maxillofacial Surgery 2: 73

Obwegeser H L, Trauner R 1955 Zur operationstechnik bei der Progenie und anderen Unterkieferanomalien. Zahn-, Mund-, und Kieferheilkunde 23: 1

Ollier L 1859a Recherches expérimentales sur la production artificielle des os, au moyen de la transplantation du périoste et sur la régénération des os, après les résections et les ablations complètes. Comptes Rendus Des Séances et Mémoires De la Société De Biologie (Paris) 5

Ollier L 1859b De la production artificielle des os au moyen de la transplantation du périosts des greffes osseuses. Gazette Médicale 14: 212

Ollier L 1867 Traité expérimental et clinique de la Régénération des os et de la production artificielle du tissue osseux (Part 2). Masson, Paris. p 461

Onur E O, Spira M 1980 Complete periosteal bone regeneration after subtotal tibial ostectomy in pigs. Experimental investigation. Acta Chirurgiae Plasticae 22: 200

Ortiz-Monasterio F 1982 Early mandibular and maxillary osteotomies for the correction of hemifacial microsomia. A preliminary report. Clinics in Plastic Surgery 9: 509–517

Ortiz-Monasterio F, Fuente Del Campo A 1981 Nasal correction in hyperteleorbitism. The short and the long nose. Scandinavian Journal of Plastic and Reconstructive Surgery 15: 277–286

Ortiz-Monasterio F, Fuente Del Campo A, Limon-Brown F 1976 Mechanism and correction of V syndrome in craniofacial dysostosis. In: Tessier et al (eds) Symposium on plastic surgery in the orbital region. Mosby, St Louis. pp 246–254

Ortiz-Monasterio F, Fuente Del Campo A, Carrillo A 1978 Advancement of the orbits and midface in one piece combined with frontal repositioning for the correction of Crouzon's deformities. Plastic and Reconstructive Surgery 61: 507

Ousterhout D K, Tessier P 1981 Closure of large cribriform defects with a forehead flap. Journal of Maxillofacial Surgery 9: 7

Panje W, Cutting C 1980 Trapezius osteomyocutaneous island flap for reconstruction of the anterior floor of mouth and the mandible. Head and Neck Surgery 3: 66

Peer L A 1954 Extended use of diced cartilage grafts. Plastic and Reconstructive Surgery 14: 178

Popescu V C 1974 Advancement of the middle third of the face without bone in a case of Crouzon's disease. Journal of Maxillofacial Surgery 2: 219

Psillakis J M, Lapa F, Spina V 1973 Surgical correction of midfacial retrusion (nasomaxillary hypoplasia) in the presence of normal dental occlusion. Plastic and Reconstructive Surgery 51: 67

Psillakis J M 1984 Nova tecnica para o tratamento da microssomia hemicraneofacial. Ann 1st Jornada Sul-Brasileira de Cirurgia Plastica (Florianopolis) 321

Psillakis J M, Zanini S A, Godov R, Cardim V L 1981 Orbital hypertelorism: modification of the craniofacial osteotomy line. Journal of Maxillofacial Surgery, 9: 10–14

Puckett C L, Hurvitz J S, Metzler M H, Silver D 1979 Bone formation by revascularized periosteal and bone grafts compared with traditional bone grafts. Plastic and Reconstructive Surgery 64: 361

Radovan C 1979 Development of adjacent flaps using a temporary expander. ASPRS Plastic Surgery Forum 2: 62

Reid C A, McCarthy J G, Kolber A B 1981 A study of regeneration in parietal bone defects in rabbits. Plastic and Reconstructive Surgery 67: 591

Rhinelander F W, Phillips R S, Steel W M, Beer J C 1968 Microangiography in bone healing: II. Displaced closed fractures. Journal of Bone and Joint Surgery 50A: 643

Richards M A, Poole M D, Godfrey A M 1982 The serratus anterior/rib composite flap in mandibular reconstruction using the latissimus myoosteocutaneous free flap. American Journal of Surgery 144: 470

Rieger R A 1967 A local flap for repair of the nasal tip. British Journal of Plastic Surgery 40: 147

Rintala A, Soivio A, Ranta R, Oikari T, Haataja J 1974 On the bone forming capacity of periosteal flap in surgery for cleft lip and palate. Scandinavian Journal of Plastic and Reconstructive Surgery 8: 58

Risdon F 1933 Ankylosis of the temporomandibular joint. Journal of the American Dental Association 21

Ritsila V, Alhopuro S, Rintale A 1972a Bone formation with periosteum. An experimental study. Scandinavian Journal of Plastic Surgery 6: 51

Ritsila V, Sakari A, Gylling U, Rintala A 1972b The use of free periosteum for bone formation in congenital clefts of the maxilla. Scandinavian Journal of Plastic and Reconstructive Surgery 6: 57

Ritsila V, Alhopuro S, Rintala A 1976 Bone formation with free periosteal grafts in reconstruction of congenital maxillary clefts. Annales Chirurgiae et Gynaecologiae 65: 342

Robinson D W, cited by O'Brien B McC, Morrison W A, Macleod A M, Dooley B J 1979 Microvascular osteocutaneous transfer using the groin flap and iliac crest and the dorsalis pedis flap and second metatarsal. British Journal of Plastic Surgery 32: 188

Rougerie J, Derome P, Anquez L Craniostenoses et dysmorphies cranio-faciales. Principes d'une nouvelle technique de traitement et ses resultats. Neurochirurgie 18: 429–440

Rowsell A R, Davies D M, Eisenberg N, Taylor G I 1984 The anatomy of the subscapular-thoracodorsal arterial system: study of 100 cadaver dissections. British Journal of Plastic Surgery 37: 574

Sabattini P 1838 Cenno storico sull'origine e progressi della rinoplastica e cheiloplastica. Belle Arti, Bologna

Salyer K E 1978 Osseous wound healing and craniofacial surgery. Annals of Plastic Surgery 1: 439

Salyer K E 1981 Recent developments in bone grafting. In: Jackson I T (ed) Recent Advances in Plastic Surgery (No. 2). Churchill Livingstone, Edinburgh

Salyer K E, Holmes R E, Cestero H J Jr 1978 Hard tissue growth and repair. In: Whitaker L A, Randall P (eds) Symposium on Reconstruction of Jaw Deformity (Vol 16) Mosby, St Louis pp 33–42

Schendel S A, Eisenfeld J, Bell W H, Epker B N, Mishelevich D J 1976 The long face syndrome: vertical maxillary excess. American Journal of Orthodontics 70: 398

Schenk A K, Merz W A, Muller J 1969 A quantitative histological study on the bone resorption in human cancellous bone. Acta Anatomica 74: 44

Schmidt D R, Robson M C 1982 One-stage composite reconstruction using the latissimus myoosteocutaneous free flap. American Journal of Surgery 144: 470

Schuchardt K 1942 Ein Beitrag zur chirurgischen Kieferorthopadie unter Berucksichtigung ihrer Bedeutung fur die Behandlung angeborener und erworbener Kieferdeformationen bei Soldaten. Zahn-, Mund-, und Kieferheilkunde 2: 73

Schuchardt K 1954 Die Chirurgie als Helferin der Kieferorthopadie. Fortschritte der Kieferorthopadie 15: 1

Schuchardt K 1955 Formen des offenen Bisses und ihre operativen Behandlungsmoglichkeiten. In: Schuchardt K, Wassmund M (eds) Fortschritte der Kiefer- und Gesichts-Chirurgie 1: 222–230

Schuchardt K 1959 Plastische Operationen in Mund und Kiefer Bereich. Urban & Schwarzenberg, Berlin. p 45

Schuchardt K 1961 Experiences with the surgical treatment of some deformities of the jaws: prognathia, microgenia and open bite. In: Wallace A B (ed) Transactions of the International Society of Plastic Surgeons, Second Congress. Williams & Wilkins, Baltimore. pp 73–78

Serafin D, Villarreal-Rios A, Georgiade N G 1977 A rib containing free flap to reconstruct mandibular defects. British Journal of Plastic Surgery 30: 263

Serafin D, Riefkohl R, Thomas I, Georgiade N G 1980 Vascularized rib periosteal and osteocutaneous reconstruction of the maxilla and mandible. An assessment. Plastic and Reconstructive Surgery 66: 718

Siemssen S O, Kirkby B, O'Connor T P F 1978 Immediate reconstruction of a resected segment of the lower jaw using a compound flap of clavicle and sternomastoid muscle. Plastic and Reconstructive Surgery 61: 724

Skoog T 1965 The use of periosteal flaps in the repair of clefts of the primary palate. Cleft Palate Journal 2: 332

Smith R 1983 The free fascial scalp flap. Plastic and Reconstructive Surgery 72: 786

Song R, Ling Y, Wang G, Yang R 1982 One stage reconstruction of the nose: the island frontal flap and the 'conjoined' frontal flap. Clinics in Plastic Surgery 9: 37

Soutar D S, Scheker L R, Tanner N S B, McGregor I A 1983 The radial forearm flap: a versatile method for intra-oral reconstruction. British Journal of Plastic Surgery 36: 1

Souyris F, Caravel J B, Raynaud J F 1973 Ostéotomie intermédiaire de l'étage moyen de la face. Annales de Chirurgie Plastique 18: 149–154

Stricker M, Montaut J, Hepner H, Flot F 1972 Ostéotomies du crâne et de la face. Annales de Chirurgie Plastique 17: 233

Stricker M, Chancholle A R, Flot F, Malka G, Montoya A 1977 La greffe périostée dans la reparation de la fente totale du palais primaire. Annales de Chirurgie Plastique 22: 117

Tajima S et al 1980 Temporal double inversion method in reshaping the temporal bulging in a case of Apert's syndrome. Journal of Maxillofacial Surgery 8: 125–130

Takayanagi S, Tsukie T 1982 Free serratus anterior muscle and myocutaneous flaps. Annals of Plastic Surgery 8: 277

Tanzer R C 1959 Total reconstruction of the external ear. Plastic and Reconstructive Surgery 23: 1

Tanzer R C 1971 Total reconstruction of the auricle. The evolution of a plan of treatment. Plastic and Reconstructive Surgery 47: 523

Taylor G I, Watson N 1978 One-stage repair of compound leg defects with free, revascularized flaps of groin skin and iliac bone. Plastic and Reconstructive Surgery 61: 494–506

Taylor G I 1982 Reconstruction of the mandible with free composite iliac bone grafts. Annals of Plastic Surgery 9: 361

Tessier P 1967 Ostéotomies totales de la face. Syndrome de Crouzon. Syndrome d'Apert, oxycephales. Scaphocephalies. Turricephalies. Annales de Chirurgie Plastique 12: 273

Tessier P 1969a Expansion chirrurgicale de l'orbite. Annales de Chirurgie Plastique 14: 208–214

Tessier P 1969b Fentes orbito-faciales et obliques et verticales (colobomas) completes et frustres. Annales de Chirurgie Plastique 14: 301–311

Tessier P 1971a The definitive plastic surgical treatment of the severe facial deformities of cranio-facial dysostosis. Crouzon's and Apert's diseases. Plastic and Reconstructive Surgery 48: 419

Tessier P 1971b The scope and principles, dangers and limitations and the need for special training in orbitocranial surgery. In: Hueston J T (ed) Transactions of the 5th International Congress of Plastic and Reconstructive Surgery Melbourne. Butterworth, Melbourne. pp 903–929

Tessier P 1971c Total osteotomy of the middle third of the face for faciostenosis or for sequelae of Le Fort III fractures. Plastic and Reconstructive Surgery 48: 533–541

Tessier P 1971d Traitement des dysmorphies faciales propres aux dysostoses crâniofaciales (DCF), maladies de Crouzon et d'Apert. Neurochirurgie 17: 295–322

Tessier P 1971e Relationship of craniostenoses to craniofacial dysostosis and to faciostenoses. A study with therapeutic implications. Plastic Reconstructive Surgery 48

Tessier P 1972a The conjunctival approach to the orbital floor and maxilla in congenital malformation and trauma. Journal of Maxillo-facial Surgery 1

Tessier P 1972b Orbital hypertelorism: successive surgical attempts. Material and methods. Scandinavian Journal of Plastic and Reconstructive Surgery 6: 135–155

Tessier P 1973 The definitive treatment of orbital hypertelorism by craniofacial or extracranial osteotomies. Scandinavian Journal of Plastic and Reconstructive Surgery 7: 39–58

Tessier P 1974 Le systeme musculoaponeurotique superficiel de la face et ses applications chirurgicales. Presented at the Annual Meeting of the French Society of Plastic Surgeons, Paris, October

Tessier P 1976 Recent improvements in treatment of facial and cranial deformities of Crouzon's disease and Apert's syndrome. In: Symposium on Plastic Surgery in the Orbital Region (Vol 12). Mosby, St Louis. p 271

Tessier P 1976 Atlas of orbital surgery. In: Symposium on plastic surgery in the orbital region (Vol 12, Part IV) p 295

Tessier P 1977 Le telorbitisme. Hypertelorisme orbitaire (oculaire). In Rougier J, Tessier P, Hervouet F, Woillez M, Lekieffre P, Derome P (eds) Chirurgie plastique orbito-palpebrale Masson, Paris p 305

Tessier P 1980 Present status and future prospects of craniofacial surgery. In: Ely J F (ed) Transactions of the 7th International Congress of Plastic and Reconstructive Surgery, Rio de Janeiro. May 20–25, 1979. Cartgraf, Sao Paulo

Tessier P 1982 Inferior orbitotomy: a new approach to the orbital floor clinics in plastic surgery. Clinics in Plastic Surgery 9: 569–576

Tessier P 1982 Autogenous bone grafts taken from the calvarium for facial and cranial applications. Clinics in Plastic Surgery 9: 531–538

Tessier P 1987 Facial recontouring in the Treacher Collins–Franceschetti syndrome, The artistry of reconstructive surgery (Vol 44). Mosby, St Louis, p 343

Tessier P, Delbet J P 1971 Le diadème: nouveau fixateur facial universel a ancrage crânien. Annales de Chirurgie Plastique 16: 12–20

Tessier P, Guiot G, Rougerie J, Delbet J P, Pastoriza J 1967 Osteotomies cranionaso-orbital-faciales. Hypertelorisme. Annales de Chirurgie Plastique 12: 103

Tessier P, Guiot G, Rougerie J, Delbet J P, Pastoriza P 1969 Hypertelorism: cranio-naso-orbito-facial and subethmoid osteotomy. Panminerva Medica 11: 102–116

Tessier P, Rougier J, Hervouet F, Woillez M, Lekieffre M, Derome P 1977 Chirurgie plastique orbito-palpebrale 1977, Rapport de la Societe Francaise d'Ophthalmologie. Masson, Paris

Tessier P, Rougier J, Hervouet F, Woillez M, Lekieffre M, Derome P 1981a Plastic surgery of the orbit and eyelids. Translated by Wolfe S A, 1977. Report of the French Society of Ophthalmology. Masson, USA

Tessier P, Tulasne J F, Delaire J, Resche F 1981b Therapeutic aspects of maxillonasal dysostosis (Binder's syndrome). Head and Neck Surgery 3: 207

Tetsut L, Jacob O 1909 Traité d'anatomie, Octobe Doin, Paris

Trauner R 1959 Kiefer- und Gesichts-Chirurgie. Munchen, Urban & Schwarzenberg, Munchen

Trauner R, Obwegeser H 1957a The surgical correction of mandibular prognathism and retrognathia with consideration of genioplasty. I. Surgical procedures to correct mandibular prognathism and reshaping of the chin. Oral Surgery 10: 677–689

Trauner R, Obwegeser H 1957b The surgical correction of mandibular prognathism and retrognathia with consideration of genioplasty. II. Operating methods for microgenia and distocclusion. Oral Surgery 10: 787–792

Tulasne J F, Tessier P 1981 Analysis and late treatment of plagiocephaly unilateral coronal synostosis. Scandinavian Journal of Plastic and Reconstructive Surgery 15: 257–263

Uddstromer L 1978 The osteogenic capacity of tubular and membranous bone periosteum. Scandinavian Journal of Plastic and Reconstructive Surgery 12: 195

Uddstromer L, Ritsila V 1978 Osteogenic capacity of periosteal grafts. Scandinavian Journal of Plastic and Reconstructive Surgery 12: 207

Urist M R 1965 Bone formation by autoinduction. Science 150: 893

Urist M R, Sato K, Brownwell A G et al 1983 Human bone morphogenetic protein (hBThP). Proceedings of Experimental Biology and Medicine 173: 194

Van den Wildenberg F A 1982 Free revascularized autologous periosteum transplantation. An experimental study. Doctoral thesis, Nijmegen

Van der Meulen J C 1974 Craniofacial surgery in unilateral deformities. Paper presented to the Winter Meeting of the British Association of Plastic Surgeons

Van der Meulen J C 1976 The pursuit of symmetry in cranio-facial surgery. British Journal of Plastic Surgery 29: 85–91

Van der Meulen J C 1979 Medial faciotomy. British Journal of Plastic Surgery 32: 339–342

Van der Meulen J C H 1982 The use of mucosa-lined flaps in eyelid reconstruction: a new approach. Plastic and Reconstructive Surgery 70

Van der Meulen J C 1984 Reconstruction of a socket using a retroauricular temporal flap. Plastic and Reconstructive Surgery 75: 112

Van der Meulen J C 1985 Discussion of retroauricular island flap for eye socket reconstruction. Plastic and Reconstructive Surgery 76

Van der Meulen J C 1987 Surgery of median and paramedian clefts. In: Marchac D (ed) Proceedings of the First International Congress of the International Society of Cranio-Maxillo-Facial Surgery. Craniofacial Surgery. Cannes-La Napoule, 1985. Springer, Berlin. pp 210–216

Van der Meulen J C H, Hauben D J, Vaandrager J M, Birgenhager-Frankel D H 1984 The use of a temporo-osteoperiosteal flap for reconstruction of malar hypoplasia in Treacher Collins syndrome. Plastic and Reconstructive Surgery 74: 687

Vandervord J G, Watson J D, Teasdale G M 1982 Forehead reconstruction using a bi-pedicled bone flap. British Journal of Plastic and Reconstructive Surgery 35: 75

Van der Werf M A J 1966 Role de la dure-mere dans la reossification des breches de la voute cranienne. Neurochirurgie 12: 524–527

Van der Werf M A J 1971 Ten year experience with a new method in the treatment of craniostenosis. Journal of Neurology, Neurosurgery and Psychiatry 34: 105

Warrel E, Taylor J F 1979 The role of periosteal tension in the growth of long bones: Journal of Anatomy 128: 179

Wassmund M 1927 Frakturen und Luxation des Gesichtsschadels. Meusser, Leipzig

Wassmund M 1935 Lehrbuch der praktischen Chirurgie des Mundes und der Kiefer. Meusser, Leipzig

Watson-Jones R 1933 The repair of skull defects by a new pedicle bone graft operation. British Medical Journal 1: 780

Watzek G, Grundschober F, Plank H, Eschberger J 1982 Experimental investigations into the clinical significance of bone growth and viscero-cranial sutures. Journal of Maxillofacial Surgery 10: 61

Whitaker L A 1978 Evaluation and treatment of upper facial asymmetry. In: Whitaker L A, Randall P (eds) Symposium on reconstruction of jaw deformity. Mosby, St Louis. pp 160–170

Whitaker L A, Munro I R, Jackson I T, Salyer K E 1976a Problems in cranio-facial surgery. Journal of Maxillofacial Surgery 4: 131

Whitaker L A, Schut L, Randall P 1976b Craniofacial surgery: present and future. Annals of Surgery 184: 558

Whitaker L A, Munro I R, Sayer K E, Jackson I T, Ortiz-Monasterio F, Marchac D 1979 Combined report of problems and complications in 793 craniofacial operations. Plastic and Reconstructive Surgery 64: 198

Whitaker L A, Broennle A M, Kerr L P, Herrlich A 1980 Improvements in craniofacial reconstruction: methods evolved in 235 consecutive patients. Plastic and Reconstructive Surgery 65: 561

Wolfe S A 1978 The utility of pericranial flaps. Annals of Plastic Surgery 1: 146

Wolfe S A 1982 Autogenous bone grafts versus alloplastic material in maxillofacial surgery. Clinics in Plastic Surgery 9: 539

Wood M B 1983 Canine vascularized bone segment transfers — quantitation of blood flow. Orthopedic Transactions 7: 354

Wunderer S 1963 Erfahrungen mit der operativen Behandlung hochgradiger Prognathien. Zahn-, Mund-, und Kieferheilkunde 39: 451

Zins J, Whitaker L 1983 Membranous versus enchondral bone: implications for craniofacial reconstruction. Plastic and Reconstructive Surgery 72: 778

Indications

CRANIO-ORBITOMAXILLARY

Anderl H, Muhlbauer W, Twerdy K, Marchac D 1983 Fronto facial advancement with bony separation in cranial dysostosis. Plastic and Reconstructive Surgery 71: 303

Anderson F M, Gwinn J L, Todt J C 1962 Trigonocephaly: identity and surgical treatment. Journal of Neurosurgery 19: 723

Anderson F M 1981 Treatment of coronal and metopic synostosis: 107 cases. Neurosurgery 8: 143

Barlett S P, Whitaker L A, Marchac D 1986 A comparison of treatment methods in plagiocephaly. Presented at Craniofacial

Surgery: An International Symposium on Long term Results, 43rd Anniversary Meeting of the American Cleft Palate Association. New York, May 17

Converse J M, McCarthy J G, Wood-Smith D 1975 Orbital hypotelorism. Pathogenesis associated facio cerebral anomalies, surgical correction. Plastic and Reconstructive Surgery 56: 389

Converse J M, McCarthy J G, Wood-Smith D, Coccaro P J 1977 Principles of craniofacial surgery. In: Converse J M (ed) Reconstructive plastic surgery (Vol 4). Saunders, Philadelphia

David D J, Poswillo D E, Simpson D A 1982 The craniosynostoses: causes, natural history and management. Springer, Berlin

Delaire J 1971 Considerations sur la croissance faciale. Deductions therapeutiques. Revue de Stomatologies 72: 57–76

Edgerton M T, Udvarhelyi G B, Knox D L 1970 The surgical correction of ocular hypertelorism. Annals of Surgery 172: 473

Edgerton M T, Jane J A, Berry F A, Fisher J C 1974 The feasibility of craniofacial osteotomies in infants and young children. Scandinavian Journal of Plastic Surgery 8: 164

Edgerton M T, Jane J A, Berry F A, Fisher J C 1974 Cranio-facial osteotomies and reconstruction in infants and young children. Plastic and Reconstructive Surgery 54: 13–27

Edgerton M T, Jane J A, Berry F A, Marshall K A 1975 New surgical concepts resulting from cranio-orbito-facial surgery. Annals of Surgery 9: 228

Freihofer H P M 1982 The timing of facial osteotomies in children and adolescents. Clinics in Plastic Surgery 9: 445

Firmin F, Coccaro P J, Converse J M 1974 Cephalometric analysis in diagnosis and treatment of craniofacial dysostosis. Plastic and Reconstructive Surgery 54: 300–311

Gillies H, Harrison S H 1951 Operative correction by osteotomy of recessed malar maxillary compound in a case of oxycephaly. British Journal of Plastic Surgery 3: 123–127

Hoffman H J, Mohr G 1976 Lateral canthal advancement of the supraorbital margin: a new corrective technique in the treatment of coronal synostosis. Journal of Neurology 45: 376

Jabaley M E, Edgerton M E 1969 Surgical correction of congenital midface retrusion in the presence of mandibular prognathism. Plastic and Reconstructive Surgery 44: 1

Jackson I T 1978 Transposition cranioplasty to restore forehead contour in craniofacial deformities. British Journal of Plastic Surgery 31: 127–130

Jackson I T 1981 Aesthetic correction of coronal craniostenosis. Clinics in Plastic Surgery 8: 317–326

Jackson I T, Munro I R, Salyer K E, Whitaker L A 1982 Atlas of Craniomaxillofacial Surgery. Mosby, St Louis

Kreiborg S, Aduss H 1986 Pre- and post-surgical facial growth in children and adolescents with Crouzon's and Apert syndromes. Presented at Craniofacial Surgery: An international Symposium on Long-term Results, 43rd Anniversary Meeting of the American Cleft Palate Association. New York, May 17

Lannelongue M 1890 De la crâniéctomie dans la microcéphalie. Comptes Rendus de l'Académie des Sciences 110: 1382

Lewin M L 1952 Facial deformity in acrocephaly and its surgical correction. Archives of Ophthalmology 47: 321

McCarthy J G, Coccaro P J, Epstein F, Converse J M 1978 Early skeletal release in the infant with craniofacial dysostosis. Plastic and Reconstructive Surgery 62: 335

McCarthy J G, Coccaro P J, Epstein F T 1979 Early skeletal release in the patient with craniofacial dysostosis. In: Converse J M, McCarthy J G, Wood-Smith D (eds) Symposium on diagnosis and treatment of craniofacial anomalies. Mosby, St Louis. p 295

McCarthy J G, Epstein F, Sadova M, Grayson B, Zide B 1984a Early surgery for craniofacial synostosis: an 8-year experience. Plastic and Reconstructive Surgery 73: 521–533

McCarthy J G, Grayson B, Bookstein F, Vickery C, Zide B 1984b Le Fort III advancement osteotomy in the growing child. Plastic and Reconstructive Surgery 74: 343–354

McNamara J A, Carlson D S, Ribbens K A 1982 The effect of surgical intervention on craniofacial growth. Ann Arbor, Center for Human Growth and Development, the University of Michigan

Marchac D 1978 Radical forehead remodelling for craniostenosis. Plastic and Reconstructive Surgery 48: 419

Marchac D 1979 Forehead remodelling for craniostenosis. In: Converse

J M, McCarthy J G, Wood-Smith D (eds) Symposium on Diagnosis and Treatment of Cranio-facial Anomalies. Mosby, St Louis. pp 323–335

Marchac D, Renier D 1979 Le front flottant, traitement précoce des faciocrâniostnoses. Annales de Chirurgie Plastique 24: 121

Marchac D, Renier Đ 1981 Craniofacial surgery for craniosynostosis. Scandinavian Journal of Plastic and Reconstructive Surgery 15: 235–243

Marchac D, Renier D 1982 Craniofacial surgery for craniosynostosis. Little, Brown, Boston. p 88

Marchac D, Renier D 1985 Early frontofacial monobloc advancement. Presented at the 1st International Congress, International Society of Cranio-Maxillo-Facial Surgery. Cannes-La Napoule, September 8

Marchac D, Cophignon J, Achard E, Dufourmentel C 1977 Orbital expansion for anophthalmia and micro-orbitism. Plastic and Reconstructive Surgery 59: 486–491

Mohr G H, Hoffman I R, Munro I R et al 1978 Surgical management of unilateral and bilateral coronal craniostenosis: 21 years of experience. Neurosurgery 2: 83

Muhlbauer W, Anderl H 1983a Totale Hirn- und Gesichtsschadelmobilisierung im Sauglingsalter. In Kraniofaziale Fehlbildungen und ihre operative Behandlung. Thieme, Stuttgart. pp 91–102

Muhlbauer W, Anderl H 1983b Miniplattenosteosynthese in der Craniofacialen Chirurgie Handchir. Mikrochir Plast Chir 15: 77–82

Muhlbauer W, Anderl H 1985 Early facial advancement in craniofacial stenosis. Presented at the 1st International Congress, International Society of Cranio-Maxillo-Facial Surgery, Cannes-La Napoule, September 8

Muhlbauer W, Anderl H, Marchac D 1982 One-stage fronto-facial advancement in infants via the coronal approach only. Presented at the 9th Alpine Workshop for Plastic and Reconstructive Surgery. Zuers, Austria, Feb 27–March 6

Muhlbauer W, Anderl H, Marchac D 1983 Plastische Chirurgie komplexer Gesichts- und Schadelmissbildungen. Chirurgica Praxis 32: 89–110

Munro I R 1977 Reshaping the cranial vault. In: Converse J M (ed) Reconstructive Plastic Surgery (Vol 4). Saunders, Philadelphia

Munro I R 1981 Current surgery for craniofacial anomalies. Otolaryngologic Clinics of North America 14: 157

Murray J E, Swanson L T 1968 Mid-face osteotomy and advancement for craniosynostosis. Plastic and Reconstructive Surgery 31: 299–306

Murray J E, Swanson I E, Cohan M 1971 Correction of midfacial deformities. Surgical Clinics of North America 51: 341

Obwegeser H L 1969 Surgical correction of small or retrodisplaced maxillae: the 'dishface' deformity. Plastic and Reconstructive Surgery 43: 351–365

Ortiz-Monasterio F, Fuente Del Campo A, Carrillo A 1978 Advancement of the orbits and midface in one piece combined with frontal repositioning for the correction of Crouzon's deformities. Plastic and Reconstructive Surgery 61: 507

Ousterhout D, Mellsen B, 1985 Anatomy and growth of the pterygomaxillary region in relation to Le Fort procedures. Presented at the 1st International Congress, International Society of Cranio-Maxillo-Facial Surgery, Cannes-La Napoule, September 8

Raulo Y, Tessier P 1981 Fronto-facial advancement for Crouzon's and Apert's syndromes. Scandinavian Journal of Plastic and Reconstructive Surgery 15: 245–250

Renier D, Marchac D 1988 Intracranial pressure recordings. Analysis of 300 cases. In: Marchac D (ed) Craniofacial surgery, Proceedings of the First International Congress on Cranio-maxillo-facial Surgery. Springer, Heidelberg

Renier D, Sainte-Rose c, Marchac D, Hirsch J F 1982 Intracranial pressure in craniosynostosis. Journal of Neurosurgery 57: 370

Renier D, Brunet M, Marchac D 1987 IQ and craniostenosis: evolution in treated and untreated cases. In: Marchac D (ed) Craniofacial surgery, Proceedings of the 1st Congress of the International Society of Craniomaxillofacial Surgery. Springer, Heidelberg. p 114

Rougerie J, Derome P, Anquez L 1972 Crâniostenoses et dysmorphies crâniofaciales. Principles d'une nouvelle technique de traitement et ses resultats. Neurochirurgie 18: 429–440

Rougier J, Tessier P, Hervouet F, Woillez M, Lekieffre M, Derome P

1977 Les cranio faciostenoses: maladie de Crouzon et d'Apert. In: Chirurgie plastique orbito palpebrale (Ch 21). Masson, Paris. p 27

Stricker M, Montaut J, Hepner H, Flot F 1972 Les osteotomies du crâne et de la face. Annales de Chirurgie Plastique 17: 233–244

Tajima S et al 1980 Temporal double inversion method in reshaping the temporal bulging in a case of Apert's syndrome. Journal of Maxillofacial Surgery 8: 125–130

Tessier P 1967 Ostéotomies totales de la face. Syndrome de Crouzon, syndrome d'Apert, oxycéphalies. Scaphocéphalies. Turricéphalies. Annales de Chirurgie Plastique 12: 273–286

Tessier P 1971a The definitive plastic surgical treatment of the severe facial deformities of cranio-facial dysostosis. Crouzon's and Apert's diseases. Plastic and Reconstructive Surgery 48: 419

Tessier P 1971b The scope and principles, dangers and limitations and the need for special training in orbitocranial surgery. In Hueston J T (ed) Transactions of the 5th International Congress of Plastic and Reconstructive Surgery. Butterworth, Melbourne. pp 903–929

Tessier P 1971c Total osteotomy of the middle third of the face for faciostenoses or for sequellae of Le Fort III fractures. Plastic and Reconstructive Surgery 48: 533–541

Tessier P 1971d Traitement des Dysmorphies Faciales Propres aux Dysostoses Craniofaciales (DCF), Maladies de Crouzon et d'Apert. Neurochirurgie. Paris, tome 17, u. 4, pp 295–322, 1971

Tessier P 1971e Relationship of craniostenosis to craniofacial dysostosis and to faciostenosis. Plastic and Reconstructive Surgery 48: 224

Tessier P 1980 Present status and future prospects of craniofacial surgery. In Ely J F (ed) Transactions of the 7th International Congress of Plastic and Reconstructive Surgery, Rio de Janeiro, May 20–25, 1979. Cartgraf, Sao Paulo

Tessier P 1985 Apert's syndrome: acrocephalosyndactyly. Type I. In: Caronni E (ed) Craniofacial surgery. Little, Brown, Boston

Tessier P 1986 Craniofacial surgery in syndromic craniosynostosis. Craniosynostosis, diagnosis, evaluation and management (Vol 12). Raven Press, New York. p 321

Van der Meulen J C H 1976 Medial faciotomy. British Journal of Plastic Surgery 32: 339–342

Whitaker L A, Schut L, Kerr L 1977 Early surgery for isolated craniofacial dysostosis. Plastic and Reconstructive Surgery 60: 575–581

Whitaker L A, Munro I R, Salyer K E et al 1979 Combined report of problems and complications in 793 craniofacial operations. Plastic and Reconstructive Surgery 64: 198

Whitaker L A, Boennle A M, Kerr L P, Herlich A 1980 Improvements in craniofacial reconstruction: methods evolved in 235 consecutive patients. Plastic and Reconstructive Surgery 65: 561

Whitaker L A, Shut L, Rosen H M 1981 Congenital craniofacial asymmetry: early treatment. Scandinavian Journal of Plastic and Reconstructive Surgery 15: 227–233

Wood-Smith D 1976 Reconstruction of the orbital skeleton in anophthalmos. In: Symposium on plastic surgery in the orbital region (Vol 12) p 177

CRANIO-ORBITONASAL

Converse J M, Smith B 1962 An operation for congenital and traumatic hypertelorism. In: Trostman R C, Converse J M, Smith B (eds) Plastic and Reconstructive Surgery of Eye and Adnexa. Butterworth, Washington DC

Converse J M, Telsey D 1971 The tripartite osteotomy of the midface for orbital expansion of the deformity in craniostenosis. British Journal of Plastic Surgery 24: 365

Converse J M, Ransohoff J, Mathews E S, Smith B, Molenaar A 1970 Ocular hypertelorism and pseudohypertelorism. Advances in surgical treatment. Plastic and Reconstructive Surgery 45: 1

David D J, Sheffield L, Simpson D et al 1984 Frontoethmoidal meningoencephaloceles: morphology and treatment. British Journal of Plastic Surgery 37: 271–284

Edgerton M T, Udvarhelyi C B, Knox D L 1970 The surgical correction of ocular hypertelorism. Annals of Surgery 172: 473

Edgerton M T, Jane J A, Berry F A 1974 Craniofacial osteotomies and reconstruction in infants and young children. Plastic and Reconstructive Surgery 54: 13–27

Esser E 1939 Median fissure of nose; surgical therapy of cases. Plast Chir 1: 40–50

Firmin F, Coccaro P J, Converse J M 1974 Cephalometric analysis in diagnosis and treatment planning of craniofacial dysostosis. Plastic and Reconstructive Surgery 54: 300

Gillies H, Harrison S H 1951 Operative correction by osteotomy of recessed malar maxillary compound in a case of oxycephaly. British Journal of Plastic Surgery 3: 123

Hemmy D C, David D J 1985 Skeletal morphology of anterior encephalocele defined through the use of three-dimensional reconstruction of computed tomography. Paediatric Neuroscience 12: 18–22

Hemmy D C, David D J, Herman G T 1983 Three-dimensional reconstruction of craniofacial deformity using computed tomography. Neurosurgery 13: 534–541

Hoffman H J, Mohr G 1976 Lateral canthal advancement of the supraorbital margin in the treatment of coronal synostosis. Journal of Neurosurgery 45: 376

Jabaley M E, Edgerton M T 1969 Surgical correction of congenital midface retrusion in the presence of mandibular prognathism. Plastic and Reconstructive Surgery 44: 1

Jackson I T 1984 Orbital hypertelorism. In: Serafin D, Georgiade N G (eds) Pediatric plastic surgery. Mosby, St Louis. pp 467–498

Jackson I T, Munro I R, Salyer K E, Whitaker L A 1982 Atlas of craniomaxillofacial surgery. Mosby, St Louis

Jackson I T, Smith J, Mixter R C 1983 Nasal bone grafting using split skull grafts. Annals of Plastic Surgery 11: 533

Lannelongue M 1890 De la crâniectomie dans la microcéphalie. Comptes Rendus de l'Académie de Science 110: 1382

McCarthy J, Coccaro P J, Epstein F, Converse J M 1978 Early skeletal release in the infant with craniofacial dysostosis. Plastic and Reconstructive Surgery 62: 335

McCarthy J G, Coccaro P J, Wood-Smith D, Converse J M 1979 Longitudinal cephalometric studies following surgical correction or orbital hypertelorism: a preliminary report. In: Converse J M, McCarthy J E, Wood-Smith D (eds) Symposium and diagnosis and treatment of craniofacial anomalies. Mosby, St Louis. 229

McGabe B F 1976 The osteo-mucoperiosteal flap in repair of cerebrospinal fluid rhinorrhea. Laryngoscope 86: 537

Mclaurin R L, Matson D D 1952 Importance of early surgical treatment of craniosynostosis. Pediatrics 10: 637

Marchac D 1978 Radical forehead remodelling for craniostenosis. Plastic and Reconstructive Surgery 61: 823

Marchac D, Dufourmentel C 1974 A propos des ostéotomies d'advancement du crâne et de la face. Annales de Chirurgie Plastique 19: 311

Marchac D, Renier D 1979 Le front flottant. Trraitement précoce des faciocrâniostenoses. Annales de Chirurgie Plastique 24: 121

Marchac D, Renier D 1982 Craniofacial surgery for craniosynostosis. Little, Brown, Boston. p 104

Marchac D, Cophignon J, Achard E et al 1977 Orbital expansion for anophthalmia and micro-orbitism. Plastic and Reconstructive Surgery 59: 486

Marino H, Davis J 1954 Hipertelorismo tratamiento quirurgico. Revista Latino-Americana de Cirugia Plastical 1: 58

Milton T, Edgerton J A, Jane J A, Berry F A, Marshall K A 1975 New surgical concepts resulting from cranio-orbito-facial surgery. Annals of Surgery Sept: 228–239

Montaut J, Stricker M 1977 Dysmorphies crâniofacial: les synostoses prématurées (crâniostenoses et faciocrâniostenoses) Masson, Paris. p 249

Mulliken J B, Kaban D M D, Evans C A, Strand R D, Murray J E 1986 Facial skeletal changes following hypertelorbitism correction. Plastic and Reconstructive Surgery 77: 7–16

Munro I R 1975 Orbito-cranio-facial surgery: the team approach. Plastic and Reconstructive Surgery 55: 170

Munro I R, Chir B, Das S K 1979 Improving results in orbital hypertelorism correction. Annals of Plastic Surgery 2: 6

Murray J E, Swanson L T 1968 Midface osteotomy and advancement for craniosynostosis. Plastic and Reconstructive Surgery 41: 299

Murray J E, Swanson L T, Strand R D, Hricko G M 1975 Evaluation of craniofacial surgery in the treatment of facial deformities. Annals of Surgery

Naim-Ur-Rahman 1979 Nasal encephalocele: treatment by transcranial operation. Journal of Neurological Science 42: 73–85

Ortiz-Monasterio F, Fuente-del-Campo A 1979 Hiperteleorbitismo Cirugia Plastica Ibero-Latinoamericana special number

Ortiz-Monastro F, Fuente-del-Campo A 1981 Nasal correction in hypertelorbitism: the short and the long nose. Scandinavian Journal of Plastic and Reconstructive Surgery 15: 277

Psillakis J M, Zanini S A, Godoy R, Cardim V L N 1981 Orbital hypertelorism: modification of the craniofacial osteotomy line. Journal of Maxillofacial Surgery 9: 10

Reilly W A 1931 Hypertelorism; four cases. Journal of the American Medical Association 1929–1933

Rosasco S A, Massa J L 1968 Frontonasal syndrome. British Journal of Plastic Surgery 21: 244

Schmid E 1968 Surgical management of hypertelorism. In: Longacre J J (ed) craniofacial anomalies: pathogenesis and repair. Lippincott, Philadelphia. p 155

Simpson D A, David D J, White J 1984 Cephaloceles; treatment outcome and antenatal diagnosis. Neurosurgery 15: 14–21

Suwanwela C 1972 Geographic distribution of frontoethmoidal encephalomeningocele. British Journal of Preventive and Social Medicine 26: 193–198

Suwanwela C, Sukabote C, Suwanwela N 1971 Frontoethmoidal encephalo-meningocele. Surgery 69: 617–625

Tessier P 1970 Treatment of facial dysmorphia peculiar to cranio facial dysostosis. Chirurgia 96: 667

Tessier P 1971a Traitement des dysmorphies faciales propes aux dysostoses crânio-faciales (DCF). Maladies de Crouzon et d'Apert. Neurochirurgie 17: 295–322

Tessier P 1971b The scope and principles, danger and limitations and the need for special training in orbitocranial surgery. In: Transactions of the Fifth international Congress of Plastic Surgeons. Butterworth, Melbourne. p 903

Tessier P 1971c The definitive plastic surgery treatment of the severe facial deformities of craniofacial dysostosis. Plastic and Reconstructive Surgery 48: 419

Tessier P 1972 Orbital hypertelorism I. Scandinavian Journal of Plastic and Reconstructive Surgery 6: 135

Tessier P 1973 Orbital hypertelorism. II. Scandinavian Journal of Plastic and Reconstructive Surgery 7: 39

Tessier P 1974 Experiences in the treatment of orbital hypertelorism. Plastic and Reconstructive Surgery 53: 1

Tessier P 1977 Le telorbitisme, hypertelorisme orbitaire (oculaire). In: Tessier P, Hervouet F, Voillez M, Lekieffre, Derome P (eds) Chirurgie plastique orbito-palpebrale. Masson, Paris

Tessier P, Guiot G, Rougerie J, Delbet J P, Pastoriza J 1967 Hypertelorism: cranio-naso-orbito-facial and subethmoid osteotomy. Annales de Chirurgie Plastique 12: 103

Tulasne J F 1985 Maxillary growth following total septal resection in telorbitism. In: Caronni E P (ed) Craniofacial surgery. Little, Brown, Boston. pp 176–189

Van der Meulen J C 1976 The Pursuit of symmetry in craniofacial surgery. British Journal of Plastic Surgery 29: 85–91

Van der Meulen J C 1979 Medial faciotomy. British Journal of Plastic Surgery 32: 339

Van der Meulen J C 1987 Surgery of median and paramedian Clefts. In: Marchac D (ed) Proceedings of the First International Congress of the International Society of Cranio-Maxillo-Facial Surgery, Cannes-La Napoule, 1985. Springer, Berlin. pp 210–216

Van der Meulen J C, Moscona A R, Vaandrager J M, Hirshowitz B 1982 Pathology and treatment of nasoschizis. Annals of Plastic Surgery 8: 474

Van der Meulen J C, Vaandrager J M 1983 Surgery related to the correction of hypertelorism. Plastic and Reconstructive Surgery 71: 6

von Meyer E 1890 Ueber eine basale Hirnhernie in der Gegund der Lamina Cribosa. Virchows Archiv Abteilung A 120: 309

Webster J P, Deming E G 1950 The surgical treatment of the bifid nose. Plastic and Reconstructive Surgery 6: 1

Wheeler E S, Kawamoto H K, Zarem H A 1981 Bone grafts for nasal reconstruction. Plastic and Reconstructive Surgery 69: 9

Whitaker L A, Shut L, Kerr L 1977 Early surgery for isolated craniofacial dysostosis. Plastic and Reconstructive Surgery 60: 575

NASOMAXILLARY

Atherton J D 1970 Histological changes following the surgical closure of a canine cleft palate. British Journal of Plastic Surgery 23: 365–370

Atherton J D 1974 The growth of the bony palate of the pig consequent to transpositioning the oral and nasal mucoperiosteum. Cleft palate Journal 11: 429–438

Barro W B, Latham R A 1981 Palatal, periosteal response to surgical trauma. Plastic and Reconstructive Surgery 67: 6–16

Chancholle A R 1980 Le voile du palais existe-t-il Plaidoyer anatomique pour le velo-pharynx. Annales de Chirurgie Plastique 25: 5–14

Davis J S, Ritchie H P 1922 Classifications of congenital clefts of the lip and palate. Journal of the American Medical Association 70: 1323

Dunn F S 1952 Management of cleft palate cases involving the hard palate so as not to interfere with the growth of the maxilla. Plastic and Reconstructive Surgery 9: 108

Enlow D H 1975 Handbook of facial growth. Saunders, Philadelphia

Fogh-Andersen P 1942 Inheritance of harelip and cleft palate. Busck, Copenhagen

Grabb W C 1972 Communicative disorders related to cleft lip and palate. Little, Brown, Boston

Grunewald J 1979 La greffe périostée. Ses répercussions sur la croissance faciale des enfants porteurs de fentes labio-alveolo-palatines opérées. Thèse de médecine, Nancy

Hata Y, Ohmori S 1979 On the experiences of periosteoplasty for the closure of the maxillary cleft. Chirurgia Plastica 5: 33

Harkins C S, Berlin A, Harding R, Longacre J J, Snodgrass R A 1962 A classification of cleft lip and cleft palate. Plastic and Reconstructive Surgery 29: 31

Hellequist R 1971 Early maxillary orthopedics in relation to maxillary cleft repair by periosteoplasty. Cleft Palate Journal 8: 36

Hrivnakova J, Fara M, Mullerova Z 1981 The use of periosteal flaps for bridging maxillary defect in facial clefts. Acta Chirurgiae Plasticae 23: 130

Kriens O 1969 An anatomical approach to veloplasty. Plastic and Reconstructive Surgery 43: 29–31

Malek R, Psaume J 1983 Nouvelle conception de la chronologie et de la technique chirurgicale du traitement des fentes labio-palatines. Résultat sur 220 cas. Annales de Chirurgie Plastique 28: 237–247

Millard D R Jr 1976–1980 Cleft craft. The evolution of its surgery, vols 1–3. Little, Brown, Boston

Ollier L 1867 Traité expérimental et clinique de la régénération des os et de la production artificielle du tissu osseux. Masson, Paris

Ollier L 1891 Traité des résections et des opérations conservatrices qu'on peut pratiquer sur le système osseux. Masson, Paris

Perko M A 1979 Two-stage closure of cleft palate. Journal of Maxillofacial Surgery 7: 76–80

Psaume J, Malek R 1977 Must cleft palate be repaired before cleft lip? 3rd International Congress on Cleft Palate, Toronto, June.

Raphael B 1981 La fonction labiale. Son rôle dans la morphogenèse facial. Annales de Chirurgie Plastique 26: 107–111

Raphael B, Stricker M 1983 La réparation primaire dans les fentes. Philosophie Therapeutique. I. Orthodontie Française 54: 463–479

Raphael B, Labboz P, Lebeau J 1980 L'étape orthopédique dans le traitement primaire des fentes labio-maxillo-palatines. Annales de Chirurgie Plastique 25: 217–224

Raphael B, Lebeau J, Antoine P 1982 Réflexion ou parti-pris dans le traitement des fentes labio-maxillo-palatines. Annales de Chirurgie Plastique 27: 232–238

Ritsila V 1972a The use of free periosteum for bone formation in congenital clefts of the maxilla. Scandinavian Journal of Plastic Surgery 6: 57–60

Ritsila V 1972b Bone formation with free periosteum. Scandinavian Journal of Plastic Surgery 6: 51

Ritsila V, Alhopuro S, Rintala A 1976 Bone formation with free periosteal grafts in reconstruction of congenital maxillary clefts. Annales de Chirurgiae et Gynaecologiae 65: 342

Robertson N R E, Jolleys A 1979 The timing of hard palate repair. Scandinavian Journal of Plastic and Reconstructive Surgery 8: 49–51

Ross R B, Johnston M C 1972 Cleft lip and palate. William & Wilkins, Baltimore. p 319

Ruding R 1964 Cleft palate anatomic and surgical considerations. Plastic and Reconstructive Surgery 32: 132–147

Schuchardt K (ed) 1964 Treatment of patients with cleft of lip, alveolus and palate. 2nd Hamburg International Symposium. Grune & Stratton, Hamburg

Skoog T 1965 The use of periosteal flaps in the repair of the primary palate. Cleft palate Journal 2: 332

Skoog T 1967 The use of periosteum and surgical for bone restoration in congenital cleft of the maxilla. Scandinavian Journal of Plastic Surgery 1: 113–130

Stenstrom S, Thilander B 1974 Management of cleft palate cases. Scandinavian Journal of Plastic Surgery 8: 6–72

Stricker M, Raphael B 1983a Le périoste dans les fentes labio-palatines. Chirurgie Pédiatrique 24: 4–5, 274–281

Stricker M, Raphael B 1983b La réparation primaire dans les fentes. Philosophie therapeutique II. Orthontie Française 54: 481–496

Stricker M, Chancholle A R, Flot F, Malka G, Montoya A 1977a La greffe périostée dans la reparation de la fente totale du palais primaire. Annales de Chirurgie Plastique 22: 117–125

Stricker M, Chassagne J F, Pabst A, Malka G, Flot F, Raphael B 1977b L'équilibre labial et sa rupture dans les fentes. Annales de Chirurgie Plastique 22: 109–115

Tessier P 1969a Colobomas: vertical and oblique complete facial clefts. Panminerva Medica 11: 95

Tessier P 1969b Fentes orbito-faciales verticales et obliques (colobomas), complètes et frustes. Annales de Chirurgie Plastique 14: 301

Trauner R 1948 Lippen-Kiefer-Gaumen-Spalten. In: Pichler H, Trauner R (eds) Mund- und Kieferchirurgie (Vol II, Part 2). Urban & Schwarzenberg, Vienna. p 704

Van der Meulen J C 1976 The pursuit of symmetry in craniofacial surgery. British Journal of Plastic Surgery 29: 85–91

Van der Meulen J C H 1985 Oblique facial clefts: pathology, etiology and reconstruction. Plastic and Reconstructive Surgery 76: 213

Van der Meulen J C 1987 Surgery of median and paramedian clefts. In: Marchac D (ed) Proceedings of the First International Congress of the International Society of Cranio-Maxillo-Facial Surgery, Cannes-La Napoule, 1985. Springer, Berlin. pp 210–216

Van der Meulen J C, Hauben D J, Vaandrager J M, Birgenhager-Frenkel D H 1984 The use of a temporal osteoperiosteal flap for the reconstruction of malar hypoplasia in Treacher Collins syndrome (Vol 74, No. 5). pp 687–693

Veau V 1931 Division palatine. Masson, Paris. p 568

Veau V 1938 Bec le lievre. Masson, Paris. p 326

Weiffenbach J M 1972 Infants with clefts of lip and palate: observations of touch, elicited oral behavior. In: Bosma J F (ed) Oral sensation and perception. Thomas, Springfield. pp 391–399

Zuckerkandl E 1882 Normale u. pathologische Anatomie der Nasenhöhle. Braumüller, Vienna

LATERAL FACIAL

Anderl H 1969 Free vascularized groin fat flap in hypoplasia and hemiatrophy of the face: a three year observation. Journal of Maxillofacial Surgery 7: 327

Antia N H, Buch V I 1971 Transfer of an abdominal derma-fat graft by direct anastomosis of blood vessels. British Journal of Plastic Surgery 24: 15

Arnold R S 1971 Defects of the first branchial cleft. South African Journal of Surgery 9: 93–98

Avelar J 1977 Total reconstruction of the auricular pavilion in one stage. Revista Brasileira de Cirugia 67: 139

Belenky W M, Medina J E 1980 First branchial anomalies. Laryngoscope 90: 28–39

Bellucci R J 1972 Congenital auricular malformations. Indications, contraindications and timing of middle ear surgery. Annals of Otology, Rhinology and Laryngology 81: 659

Bennun R D, Mulliken J B, Kaban L B, Murray J E 1985 Microria: a microform of hemifacial microsomia. Plastic and Reconstructive Surgery 76: 859

Brent B 1971 Ear reconstruction with an expansile framework of autogenous rib cartilage. Plastic and Reconstructive Surgery 53: 619

Brent B 1979 Reconstruction of the ear. In: Grabb W C, Smith J W (eds) Plastic Surgery, 3rd edn. Little, Brown, Boston. pp 299–320

Brent B 1980 The correction of microtia with autogenous cartilage grafts. II. Atypical and complex deformities. Plastic and Reconstructive Surgery 66: 1

Brent B, Byrd H S 1983 Secondary ear reconstruction with cartilage grafts covered by axial, random, and free flaps of temporoparietal fascia. Plastic and Reconstructive Surgery 72: 141

Burston W R 1969 Mandibular retrognathia. In: Rickham P P, Johnston J H (eds) Neonatal Surgery. Butterworths, London, p. 137

Byars I T, Anderson R 1951 Anomalies of the first branchial cleft. Surgical Gynecology and Obstetrics 93: 755

Caldarelli D D, Hutchinson J C, Gould H J 1980 Hemifacial microsomia: priorities and sequence of comprehensive otologic management. Cleft Palate Journal 17: 111–115

Champy M, Petrovic A 1982 In: Besson J C (ed) Greffe autologue costale osteo-chondrale de allongement de la branche montante de la mandibule. Thèse Strasbourg, no. 247

Combelles R, Zadeh J 1984–85 Le lambeau temporal musculo-osseux. Etude anatomique, technique experimentale et chirurgicale. Revue Stomatologie et de Chirurgie Maxillo-faciale 85: 351–354

Converse J M 1958 Reconstruction of the auricle. Part 1. Plastic and Reconstructive Surgery 22: 150, 230

Converse J M 1963 Construction of the auricle in congenital microtia. Plastic and Reconstructive Surgery 32: 425

Converse J M, Rushton A M 1957 In: Gillies H, Millard D R (eds) The principles and art of plastic surgery (Vol 1). Little, Brown, Boston

Converse J M, Shapiro H H 1952 Treatment of developmental malformations of the jaws. Plastic and Reconstructive Surgery 19: 173

Converse J M, Shapiro H H 1954 Bone grafting in malformations of the jaws. Cephalographic diagnosis in the surgical treatment of malformations of the face. American Journal of Surgery 88: 858

Converse J M, Wood-Smith D 1971 Corrective and reconstructive surgery in deformities of the auricle in children. In: Mustardé J C (ed) Plastic surgery in infancy and childhood. Churchill Livingstone, Edinburgh. p 274

Converse J M, Coccaro P J, Becker M H, Wood-Smith D 1973a On hemifacial microsomia. Plastic and Reconstructive Surgery 51: 268

Converse J M, Horowitz S L, Coccaro P J, Wood-Smith D 1973b The corrective treatment of the skeletal asymmetry in hemifacial microsomia. Plastic and Reconstructive Surgery 52: 221

Converse J M, Wood-Smith D, McCarthy J G, Coccaro P J, Becker M H 1974 Bilateral facial microsomia. Plastic and Reconstructive Surgery 54: 413

Converse J M, McCarthy J G, Coccaro P J, Wood-Smith D 1979 Clinical aspects of craniofacial microsomia. In: Converse J M, McCarty J G, Wood-Smith D (eds) Symposium on diagnosis and treatment of craniofacial anomalies. Mosby, St Louis

Cosman B, Crikelair G F 1972 Mandibular hypoplasia and the late development of glossopharyngeal airway obstruction. Plastic and Reconstructive Surgery 50: 573

Cosman B, Keyser J J 1975 Eye abnormalities and skeletal deformities in Pierre Robin syndrome. Plastic and Reconstructive Surgery 56: 109

Cronin T D 1979 Reconstruction of the ear with a silastic framework and facial flap. Presented at the annual meeting of the California Plastic Surgery Society, Monterey, California, March 9

Davis W B 1968 Reconstruction of hemiatrophy of face. Plastic and Reconstructive Surgery 42: 489

Delaire J 1970 De l'intérêt des ostéotomies sagittales dans la correction des infragnathies mandibulaires. Annales de Chirurgie Plastique 15: 104

Dingman R O, Grabb W C 1963 Mandibular laterognathism. Plastic and Reconstructive Surgery 31: 563

Dingman R O, Grabb W C 1964 Reconstruction of both mandibular condyles with metatarsal bone grafts. Plastic and Reconstructive Surgery 43: 441

Dufourmentel C 1958 La greffe cutanée libre tubule. Nouvel artifice technique pour la réflection de l'helix au cours de la reconstruction du pavillon de l'oreille. Annales de Chirurgie Plastique et Estetique 3: 311

Dupertuis S M 1950 Growth of young human autogenous cartilage grafts. Plastic and Reconstructive Surgery 5: 486

Dupertuis S M, Musgrave R H 1959 Experiences with the reconstruction of the congenitally deformed ear. Plastic and Reconstructive Surgery 23: 361

Edgerton M T, Bachetta C A 1974 Principles in the use and salvage of implants in ear reconstruction. In: Tanzer R C, Edgerton M T (eds) Symposium on reconstruction of the auricle. Mosby, St Louis. pp 58–68

Edgerton M T, Marsh J L 1977a Surgical reconstruction for congenital auriculomandibular deformities. Clinics in Plastic Surgery 4: 587

Edgerton M T, Marsh J L 1977b Surgical treatment of hemifacial microsomia (first and second branchial arch syndrome). Plastic and Reconstructive Surgery 59: 653

Edgerton M T, Jane J A, Berry F A 1974 Craniofacial osteotomies and reconstruction in infants and young children. Plastic and Reconstructive Surgery 54: 13

Eitner E 1920 Uber Unterpolstering der Gesichtshaut. Medizinische Klinik 16: 93

Entin M A 1958 Reconstruction in congenital deformity of the temporomandibular component. Plastic and Reconstructive Surgery 21: 461

Fischer J C, Edgerton M T 1974 Timing for reconstruction of the child born with facial deformity. Pediatrics 3: 183

Flot F, Chassagne J F, Raphael B, Meley M, Brice M, Stricker M 1981 Les peauciers du Cou interet chirurgical. Annales de Chirurgie Plastique 26: 52–75

Fujino T, Rytinzaburo T, Sugimoto C 1975 Microvascular transfer of free deltopectoral dermal-fat flap. Plastic and Reconstructive Surgery 55: 428

Glahn M, Winther J E 1967 Metatarsal transplants as replacement for lost mandibular condyle (3 year follow-up). Scandinavian Journal of Plastic and Reconstructive Surgery 1: 97

Hart K 1967 Free omental transfer. Transactions of the 6th International Congress of Plastic Surgery Masson, Paris. p 61

Harvold E P 1975 Centric relation. A study of pressure and tension systems in bone modeling and mandibular positioning. Dental Clinics of North America 19: 473

Harvold E P 1983 Treatment of hemifacial microsomia. Liss, New York

Jabaley M E, Edgerton M E 1969 Surgical correction of congenital midface retrusion in the presence of mandibular prognathism. Plastic and Reconstructive Surgery 44: 1

Kaban L B, Mulliken J B, Murray J E 1981 Three-dimensional approach to analysis and treatment of hemifacial microsomia. Cleft Palate Journal 18: 90

Kiehn C I, DesPrez J D, Converse C F 1979 Total prosthetic replacement of the temporomandibular joint. Annals of Plastic Surgery 2: 5

Knowles C C 1966 Cephalometric treatment, planning and analysis of maxillary growth following bone grafting to the ramus in hemifacial microsomia. Dental Practitioner 17: 28

LaRossa D, Whitaker L, Dabb R, Mellissinos E 1980 The use of microvascular free flaps for soft tissue augmentation of the face in children with hemifacial microsomia. Cleft Palate Journal 17: 138

Lauritzen C, Munro I R, Ross R B 1985 Classification and treatment of hemifacial microsomia. Scandinavian Journal of Plastic and Reconstructive Surgery 19: 33

Longacre J J, Gilby R F 1951 The use of autogenous cartilage graft in arthroplasty for true ankylosis of temporomandibular joint. Plastic and Reconstructive Surgery 7: 271

Longacre J J, deStefano G A, Holmstrand K 1961 The early versus the late reconstruction of congenital hypoplasias of the facial skeleton and skull. Plastic and Reconstructive Surgery 27: 489

Longacre J J, DeStefano G A, Holmstrand K E 1963 The surgical management of first and second branchial arch syndromes. Plastic and Reconstructive Surgery 31: 507

Manchester W M 1965 Immediate reconstruction of the mandible and temporomandibular joint. British Journal of Plastic Surgery 18: 291

Manchester W M 1972 Some technical improvements in the reconstruction of the mandible and temporomandibular joint. Plastic and Reconstructive Surgery 50: 249

Meurman Y 1957 Congenital microtia and meatal atresia. Archives of Otolaryngology 66: 443

Millard D R 1969 The crane principle for the transport of subcutaneous tissue 43: 451

Moyson F 1961 A plea against tracheotomy in the Pierre Robin's syndrome. British Journal of Plastic Surgery 14: 187

Munro I R 1980 One-stage reconstruction of the temporomandibular joint in hemifacial microsomia. Plastic and Reconstructive Surgery 66: 699

Munro I R, Lauritzen C G K 1985 Classification and treatment of hemifacial microsomia. In: Caronni E (ed) Craniofacial surgery. Little, Brown, Boston

Munro I R, Chen Y R, Park B Y 1986a Simultaneous total correction of temporomandibular ankylosis and facial asymmetry. Plastic and Reconstructive Surgery 77: 517

Munro I R, Phillip J, Griffen G et al 1986b Long-term growth in costochondral grafts after temporomandibular reconstruction. Presented at the Canadian Society of Plastic Surgeons Meeting, Toronto, May

Murray J E, Mulliken J B, Kaban L B, Belfer M L 1979 Twenty-year experience in maxillofacial surgery. An evaluation of early surgery on growth function and body image. Annals of Surgery 190: 320

Murray J E, Kaban L B, Mulliken J B 1984 Analysis and treatment of hemifacial microsomia. Plastic and Reconstructive Surgery 74: 186

Murray J E, Kaban L B, Mulliken J B, Evans C A 1985 Analysis and treatment of hemifacial microsomia. Craniofacial Surgery 33: 377

Neuman C G 1953 The use of a large buried pediculated flap of dermis and fat. Clinical and pathological evaluation in the treatment of progressive facial hemiatrophy. Plastic and Reconstructive Surgery 11: 315

Obwegeser H L 1957 The surgical correction of mandibular prognathism and retrognathism with consideration on genioplastic. Oral Surgery 10: 77

Obwegeser H L 1970 Zur korrektur der Dysostosis otomandibularis. Schweizerische Monatsschrift fur Zahnheilkunde 80: 331

Obwegeser H L 1974 Correction of the skeletal anomalies of otomandibular dysostosis. Journal of Maxillofacial Surgery 2: 73

Ohmori S 1978 Reconstruction of microtia using the silastic frame. Clinics in Plastic Surgery 5: 379

Ortiz-Monasterio F 1982 Early mandibular and maxillary osteotomies for the correction of hemifacial microsomia. Clinics in Plastic Surgery 9: 509

Ortiz-Monasterio F, Del Campo A F 1985 Early skeletal correction of hemifacial microsomia. VIII. Otocranial and hemifacial syndromes. Chirurgia Plastica Ibero-Latinoamericana 35: 401

Pearl R M, Laub D R, Kaplan E N 1978 Complication following silicon injection for augmentation of the contours of the face. Plastic and Reconstructive Surgery, 61: 888

Pickerill H P 1942 Ankylosis of the jaw: cartilage graft restoration of the joint. A new operation. Australian and New Zealand Journal of Surgery 11: 197

Poswillo D E 1974 Otomandibular deformity: pathogenesis as a guide to reconstruction. Journal of Maxillofacial Surgery 2: 64

Pruzansky S 1969 Not all dwarfed mandibles are alike. Birth Defects 1: 120

Pruzansky S 1980 The experiment on the experiments of nature. Presented at the 56th Congress of the European Orthodontic Society, Paris

Psillakis J M 1984 Nova tecnica para o tratamento da microssomia hemicraneofacial. Ann 1st Jornada Sulbrasileira de Cirurgia Plastica (Florianopolis) 321

Raulo Y, Tessier P 1981 Mandibulo-facial dysostosis. Scandinavian Journal of Plastic and Reconstructive Surgery 15: 251–256

Rees T D 1976 Facial atrophy. Clinics in Plastic Surgery 3: 637

Rogers B O 1976 Surgical treatment of mandibulofacial dysostosis. Clinics in Plastic Surgery 3: 653

Rowe N L 1972 Surgery of the temporomandibular joint. Proceedings of the Royal Society of Medicine 65: 383

Sanvenero Rosselli G 1960 Microgenia e Palatoschisi. Minerva Chirurgica 15: 956–964

Sarnat B G, Laskin D M Surgery of the temporomandibular joint. In: Sarnat B G (ed) The temporomandibular joint. Thomas, Springfield, Ill

Shambaugh G E 1959 Surgery of the ear. Saunders, Philadelphia

Smith D W 1982 Recognizable patterns of human malformation, 3rd edn. Saunders, Philadelphia

Snyder C C 1956 Bilateral facial agenesis (Treacher Collins syndrome). American Journal of Surgery 92: 81

Snyder C C, Levine G A, Dingman D L 1971a Trial of a sternoclavicular whole joint graft as a substitute for the temporomandibular joint. Plastic and Reconstructive Surgery 48: 447

Synder C C, Benson A K, Slater P V 1971b Construction of the temporomandibular joint by transplanting the autogenous sternoclavicular joint. Southern Medical Journal 64: 807

Souyris F 1976 Surgical treatment of facial asymmetry by bilateral upper and lower osteotomy. Transactions of the 6th International Congress of Plastic Surgery Masson, Paris. p 276

Stenstrom S J, Sundmark E S 1966 Contribution to the treatment of the eyelid deformities in dysostosis mandibulofacialis. Plastic and Reconstructive Surgery 38: 567

Swanson L T, Murray J E 1974 Mandibular reconstruction in hemifacial microsomia. In: Tanzer R C, Edgerton M T (eds) Symposium on reconstruction of the auricle. Mosby, St Louis. p 270

Swanson I, Murray J E 1978 Asymmetries of the lower part of the face. In: Whitaker I A, Randall P (eds) Symposium on reconstruction of jaw deformity. Mosby, St Louis. p 171

Tajima S, Aoyagi E, Maruyama Y 1978 Free perichondrial grafting in the treatment of temporomandibular joint ankylosis. Plastic and Reconstructive Surgery 61: 876

Tanzer R C 1959 Total reconstruction of the external ear. Plastic and Reconstructive Surgery 23: 1

Tanzer R C 1971 Total reconstruction of the auricle. The evolution of a plan of treatment. Plastic and Reconstructive Surgery 47: 523

Tessier P 1980 Utilisation du muscle temporal en chirurgie faciale. Conference held at the Sanvenero Rosselli Milan Foundation

Tessier P 1987 Facial recontouring in the Treacher Collins — Franceschetti syndrome. The Artistry of Reconstructive Surgery 44: 343

Treacher Collins E 1900 Case with symmetrical congenital notches in the outer part of each lower lid and defective development of the malar bones. Transactions of the Ophthalmological Societies of the UK 20: 109

Upton J, Mulliken J B, Hicks P D, Murray J E 1980 Restoration of facial contour using free vascularized omental transfer. Plastic and Reconstructive Surgery 66: 500

Van der Meulen J C H, Hauben D J, Vaandrager J M, Birgenhager-Frankel D H 1984 The use of a temporo-osteoperiosteal flap for reconstruction of malar hypoplasia in Treacher Collins syndrome. Plastic and Reconstructional Surgery 74: 687

Wells J H, Edgerton M T 1977 Correction of severe hemifacial atrophy with a free dermis-fat flap from the lower abdomen. Plastic and Reconstructive Surgery 59: 223

Whitaker L A 1978 Evaluation and treatment of upper facial assymetry. In: Whitaker L A, Randall P (eds) Symposium on the reconstruction of jaw deformity. Mosby, St Louis

Williams H B, Crepeau R J 1979 Free dermal fat flaps to the face. Annals of Plastic Surgery 3: 1

Wood-Smith D 1967 Surgical treatment of the eyelid defect in the Treacher Collins syndrome: a preliminary report. In Smith B, Converse J M (eds) Plastic and reconstructive surgery of the eye and adnexa. Mosby, St Louis. p 334

Wynn-Williams D 1963 Antogenous rib graft in unilateral aplasia of the mandible. Transactions of the 3rd International Congress of Plastic Surgery (in press).

21. Postoperative care

D. Tibboel

INTRODUCTION

After correction of craniofacial anomalies, monitoring in a well-equipped intensive care unit is essential. The complications that may occur after extensive operations of long duration are related to the respiratory tract, such as upper airway obstruction in case of bleeding or soft tissue oedema, as well as pneumothorax. A rise in intracranial pressure, epi- and subdural haematoma, infections and leakage of CSF are all serious complications in the postoperative phase. Severe disturbances in the serum electrolyte levels may occur in relation to the clinical picture of diabetes insipidus or inappropriate ADH secretion.

For continuous monitoring an indwelling arterial catheter is essential in all patients for registration of blood pressure and heart rate, and it offers the possibility to analyse intra-arterial blood gas values. A central venous catheter as well as a urinary catheter with monitoring of the urinary volume per hour is a reliable aid in evaluating the circulating volume of the patient. A stomach tube is used to prevent postoperative dilatation of the stomach. Thorough knowledge of the different syndromes which come to operation for correction is essential for the paediatric intensivist, because in a number of patients congenital heart anomalies (Goldenhar's syndrome) or anomalies of the urinary tract exist.

Monitoring of patients by means of physiological parameters (Yeh et al 1984) such as blood pressure, heart rate, breathing frequency and especially the Glasgow coma scale is the keystone for postoperative treatment. In this way extensive laboratory investigation is not necessary.

Evaluation of our patient's proved that after admittance to the intensive care unit no laboratory measurements other than Hb, haematocrit and serum sodium and potassium, as well as osmolality, were necessary. Evaluation of blood loss in case of wound drains can be monitored by regular haematocrit measurements in the drainage fluid.

Only in cases where polyuria exists, defined as urine production of more than 5 ml kg^{-1} per hour, both serum and urine measurements of sodium and potassium, as well as osmolality, are necessary to evaluate fluid overload or dehydration of the patient. One has to be aware of hyperglycaemia in the postoperative phase, especially in combination with polyuria. In these cases osmotic diuresis occurs, due to glucosuria. Only on strict indication, such as persistent bleeding from the operative area or the occurrence of petechiae, is haemostatic evaluation needed.

RESPIRATORY TRACT

In almost all cases patients are admitted to the intensive care unit without an endotracheal tube. Even children, who have an intermaxillary fixation, only need prolonged endotracheal intubation or a tracheostomy in case an occluding intraoral prosthesis was placed during the operation (Delegue & Gilbert 1985). Intermaxillary fixation alone does not hamper a normal mechanism of swallowing or coughing. When children are able to breathe spontaneously without an artificial airway, secondary pulmonary infections will be prevented.

Regulary monitoring both of the breathing frequency, as well as the way of breathing (intercostal retractions, stunting) in combination with continuous non-invasive monitoring of the oxygen saturation by means of pulse oxymetry, makes regular blood gas analysis almost unnecessary. Only in case of doubt is blood gas analysis to detect carbon dioxide retention and metabolic acidosis needed, because in this way elevated intracranial pressure may be prevented.

INTRACRANIAL PRESSURE MONITORING

The most serious complication after craniofacial corrections is an increase in intracranial pressure and brain oedema. Headache, vomiting and, in later phases, loss of consciousness may all fit in with the diagnosis of raised intracranial pressure. Regular control of the Glasgow coma scale is essential in these patients. One has to be aware of the fact that, while children are younger who come to operation in recent years, the Glasgow coma scale has to be adjusted to the age of the child.

In children having an orbital advancement or midfacial correction, pupillary reactions cannot be followed after 24–36 hours due to collateral oedema of the soft tissues, leading to serious swelling of the eyelids. Regular application of Duratears ® to prevent corneal lesions is essential in this phase. On suspicion of raised intracranial pressure reintubation and artificial ventilation are required. A combination of hyperventilation (pCO_2 between 25 and 30 mmHg) and use of osmotic diuretics (mannitol $0.3–1$ g kg^{-1} infusion over a period of 20 min) may lower intracranial pressure. Application of mannitol has to be repeated every 4–6 hours because of the well-known rebound phenomenon, resulting in an increase in intracranial pressure. Monitoring of serum osmolality may be of help in these cases. Rapid lowering of intracranial pressure can be achieved by furosemide $1–2$ mg kg^{-1}, followed by the above-mentioned measurements. The use of corticosteriods in the treatment of raised intracranial pressure is still under discussion.

Fontanelle pressure monitoring in young children or intracranial pressure monitoring through a bone defect using the epidural method for intracranial pressure monitoring offers nowadays new possibilities to detect raised intracranial pressure at an early stage (Plandsoen et al 1987). In those patients who have epileptic insults and use medication before the operation, blood levels have to be known in the preoperative phase. Especially in these children convulsions may occur in the postoperative phase owing to pressure on the brain during the operation, or wash-out of the medication during the operation caused by changing large volumes of blood. To prevent this complication new loading doses have to be given to those patients in which the circulating volume is changed more than once.

INFECTIONS

All patients are operated on under prophylactic use of broad-spectrum antibiotics (Cefamandol) for 2–5 days. In many patients a rise in temperature occurs 6–18 hours after operation, which is not due to a severe bacterial infection. Although minor clinical symptoms of meningitis exist cultures of blood and CSF are always negative.

This so-called aseptic meningitis is the result of accumulation of blood in the CSF. No therapy is needed. Although infection is rare in the postoperative phase of these patients one has to be aware that postoperative bacterial meningitis, a brain abscess, as well as osteomyelitis, may occur. Especially in those cases in which there is leakage of CSF, bacterial infections may easily appear.

VOLUME AND ELECTROLYTE DISTURBANCES

Disturbances in circulating volume, in combination with electrolyte disturbances, can be related to the operative procedure as such. In the first 24 hours after operation fluid therapy has to be guided by the amount of blood and CSF losses, diuresis and drainage from the stomach tube. Dehydration or fluid overload can be judged on the combination of measurements of arterial blood pressure, heart rate, CVP value and haematocrit, as well as volume and specific gravity of the urine. In patients in which a supraorbital or orbital advancement has taken place, diabetes insipidus or inappropriate ADH syndrome may occur, owing to pressure on the hypothalamic–hypophyseal area (Perkin & Levin 1980, Gruskin et al 1982).

In patients with diabetes insipidus large amounts of urine are produced with a very low specific gravity near 1.000, and a low excretion of sodium and potassium. These patients may dehydrate in a couple of hours, especially in the very young age group (less than 1 year). All urinary losses have to be replaced in the form of glucose, 5% in water, under regulatory control of the serum sodium levels. Pitressine tannate in oil intranasally (Minrin) should only be given under very excessive circumstances, because anuria may occur, with a resulting rise in intracranial pressure and severe brain oedema. Without treatment and prevention of dehydration diabetes insipidus disappears spontaneously in 24–72 hours.

In patients with inappropriate ADH syndrome there is always low urinary output. Blood chemical analysis reveals low serum sodium and osmolality levels, while in the urine much sodium is excreted and the osmolality of the urine is very high. When serum sodium is as low as 120 meq l^{-1} these patients become agitated as well as convulsive, which may have dramatic effects on intracranial pressure. In these children restriction of fluid intake in combination with an adequate amount of sodium chloride is the treatment of choice. We have the impression that restriction of fluid to two-thirds to three-quarters of the normal fluid intake in the first hours after the operation is of value in the prevention of inappropriate ADH syndrome. In Table 19.1 a summary of the complications during and after anaesthesia is given.

CONCLUSIONS.

Correction of rather complicated craniofacial anomalies is a safe procedure once children can be monitored in the postoperative phase in a well-equipped specialized paediatric surgical intensive care unit.

REFERENCES

Delegue L, Guilbert M 1985 Management of airway problems during the repair of craniofacial anomalies in children. In: Caronni E P (ed) Craniofacial surgery. Little, Brown, Boston. pp 141–154

Gruskin A B, Balnarte H J, Predis J W et al 1982 Serum sodium abnormalities in children. In: Fine R N (ed) Pediatric nephrology. Saunders, Philadelphia. pp 907–932

Perkin R M, Levin D L 1980 Common fluid and electrolyte problems in the pediatric intensive care unit. In: Orlowski J P (ed) Pediatric intensive care. Saunders, Philadelphia pp 567–586

Plandsoen W C G et al 1987 Fontanel pressure monitoring in infants with the Rotterdam teletransducer: a reliable technic. Medical Progress through Technology 13: 21–27

Yeh T S, Pollack M M, Ruttiman V E et al 1984 Validation of a physiologic index for use in critically ill infants and children. Pediatric Research 18: 455–451

Complications

22. Complications

I. T. Jackson, W. R. Marsh

INTRODUCTION

In spite of the fact that there are many complications which can result from craniofacial surgery, this has received scant attention in the literature. What is even more disturbing is a lack of detailed analyses of how to prevent complications and how to cope with them when they occur (Converse et al 1975, Matthews 1979).

It is hoped to rectify this situation in this chapter. When the term craniofacial is used, it will include cranio-, orbital and major orbitomaxillary procedures. The most minor procedure will be a Le Fort II osteotomy and these are relatively few in number. Localized orbital surgery, Le Fort I, onlay bone grafts and cleft and mandibular surgery are not included. These latter categories are not considered to be craniofacial procedures.

Although the author has previously been involved in reviews of combined series of craniofacial cases (Whitaker et al 1976, Whitaker et al 1979) only a personal series will be used as a basis for discussion. This provides uniformity, thus trends and developments are easier to follow. The results of the first 1000 craniofacial procedures have already been published (Jackson 1985).

This consists of a mixture of tumours, acute trauma and deformities resulting from congenital defects, trauma and tumour excision. The incidences of the more major complications have been given; this has not been possible with the less severe problems (Table 22.1).

INTRACRANIAL COMPLICATIONS

Dural Tear

This is not uncommon, especially with trauma and tumour cases. Dural tears should not be neglected. Many can be repaired directly with silk or nylon sutures, while others require a graft. If the tear occurs in relation to a small skull defect giving poor exposure, the first move in repair should be to enlarge the bony opening to facilitate suturing. Where there is no nasopharyngeal or sinus connection,

Table 22.1 Complications of craniofacial procedures (1969–1984, 1000 patients).

Complication	Number	Percentage
Deaths	2 (1970, 1971)	0.2
Blindness	0	0
Severe infection	10	1
Minor infection	8	0.8
Frontalis palsy, permanent	2	0.2
Meningitis (not included in severe infection)	2	0.3
CSF leak, reoperation	3	0.3

Orbital dystopia, extraocular muscle function, diplopia, enophthalmos, canthal deformity, palpebral shape, bone graft resorption, relapse, speech problem, asymmetry, bad scars, airway problems

lyophilized dura can be used; if a connection is present fascia lata repair is preferred. Interrupted sutures are employed and an effort is made to ensure that the repair is as watertight as possible. A connection with the nasopharynx is worrisome from the infection point of view and the possibility of subsequent meningitis.

Partial dural tear — arachnoid cyst

This has been seen on two occasions. The first was a plagiocephaly correction referred from elsewhere, presenting with a soft tissue swelling in the temporal area. The second was the result of harvesting of a full-thickness skull graft, this being the only occurrence of this complication in 365 cases of cranial bone grafting (Fig. 22.1).

The partial thickness tear exposes the intact arachnoid and an arachnoid cyst forms. Any overlying bone graft is resorbed by the pressure of the cyst. Thus the presentation is one of a skull defect with a soft tissue swelling coming through. Treatment is by dural repair and bone grafting of the cranial defect.

CSF leak

Although CSF leak is frequently reported by the nursing

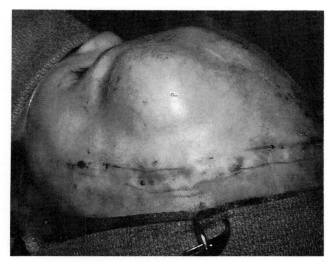

Fig. 22.1 Arachnoid cyst presenting through skull defect following harvesting of full-thickness vascularized skull graft.

staff, this is a rare complication. If it does occur, it usually ceases within a few days. Continuation of leakage for 7–10 days calls for once or twice daily spinal taps. If after 3–4 days there has been no improvement in the leak, then an exploration and formal repair should be performed. If there is any doubt as to the site of the leak, a metrizamide CT scan can be performed to identify the involved area. This has been necessary on two occasions. One is worthy of note: a hypertelorism correction was performed in a child under 1 year of age. What became apparent on re-exploration was that the thin lateral edge of the ethmoid resection, in the floor of the anterior fossa, had sliced through the dura as the orbits were moved medially.

Subdural haematoma

This has been encountered on one occasion during surgery and resulted from traumatization of a dural vessel during the dural repair. The diagnosis is made by observing an enlarging blue discoloration under the dura. The treatment involves opening of the dura, aspiration of blood and coagulation of the bleeding vessel.

If this were to occur postoperatively, it would be manifest by signs of increasing intracranial pressure. This situation calls for immediate re-exploration with removal of haematoma and coagulation of the bleeding point.

Intracerebral haematoma

This is unlikely to occur unless cerebral tissue is being resected. Aspiration and coagulation are the required treatment. Depending on where this occurs in the brain, so the neurological deficit varies.

ORBITAL PROBLEMS

Blindness

This probably results from vascular injury due to traction on the vessels, or rarely from direct trauma during orbital nerve decompression. It is much less likely to result from direct optic nerve or globe injury.

During surgery, the tension in the globe should be constantly assessed. The pupil must be observed, but it should be noted that a fixed dilated pupil is not unusual in major orbital procedures. Should there be any cause for worry, the globe should be decompressed by incision of the periorbitum, decompression of the orbit and the drug treatment outlined in Table 22.2 commenced. It is recommended that this treatment plan be posted in a conspicuous place in the operating room. It is also important to ensure that the drugs required are always immediately available.

Table 22.2 Instructions if concerned about eye (posted in operating room)

1. Call ophthalmologist
2. Acetazolamide (Diamox) 500 mg i.v., then 1000 mg orally in divided doses over 24 hours
3. Mannitol 20%, 2 g kg^{-1} body weight up to 125 mg i.v., over 3–4 min
4. Solumedrol 100 mg i.v.
5. Canthotomy

Postoperative

Immediately after surgery in the operating room, by prior arrangement with the anaesthetist, the patient should be conscious enough to be able to distinguish light. The eyes should be inspected and tested for light every 30 minutes in the recovery and intensive care areas. In the context of blindness, patients 'at risk', e.g. glaucoma, retinal detachment, visual acuity defects, should be identified and any eye prosthesis carefully documented by a preoperative ophthalmological examination.

Dangerous surgical procedures are also recognized and modified; these are hypertelorism correction, tumour surgery, enophthalmos correction, Le Fort III and monobloc osteotomies. It is for this reason that the last procedure is avoided if at all possible — during the operation, there comes a time when the only posterior connections of the monobloc are the optic nerves.

Should blindness occur after surgery, all sutures are removed from any incisions around the eyes, the orbit is decompressed, the drug treatment mentioned above is instituted and a lateral canthopexy may be performed. If there is thought to be a definite causation, e.g. reduced cranial capacity, excessive orbital bone grafting, the patient is returned to the operating room and the suspected cause corrected. One case of blindness occurred immediately after an orbital osteotomy. This was associated with hardness and proptosis of the globe. It responded rapidly to orbital decompression in the recovery room with no residual ill effects.

Corneal abrasion

This may occur during surgery, or postoperatively. The incidence of the former may be lessened by inserting ophthalmic ointment, establishing a temporary complete tarsorrhaphy during surgery or using scleral shields. Unfortunately, these measures interfere with assessment of eye position, pupil size and pupil reaction to light. It is our custom to use scleral shields and remove them as necessary.

Postoperatively, there may not be complete lid closure; this, coupled with relative immobility of the globes, places the cornea at risk. If this situation is established it can be managed by frequent insertion of eye ointment, a temporary total tarsorrhaphy or an airtight plastic dome over the eye. Pain due to a corneal abrasion is treated with atropine drops.

Using these measures ensures that serious corneal injury can be prevented. An established erosion is again treated by atropine drops, ointment, temporary total tarsorrhaphy or a plastic eye dome.

Orbital dystopia

This is particularly liable to occur after trauma or tumour resection. The congenital cases at risk are those in which one orbit is moved or both are moved independently. Measurements on preoperative facial bone X-rays and life-size black and white photographs allow more accurate orbital positioning. Perhaps the single most important advance in correct orbital positioning has been the retention of the orbital bar in hypertelorism correction. When the condition is present, it calls for a total orbital repositioning; in more minor cases, in the interest of safety the orbital roof can be contoured and the orbital floor bone grafted.

Diplopia

This can occur as a result of orbital dystopia, orbital floor damage, extraocular muscle dysfunction or change in eye position. It has been disappointing to note that diplopia resulting from orbital trauma is rarely completely cured even when eye and orbit malposition is corrected. There is much about this condition which has yet to be elucidated. A sagittal CT scan of the orbit is useful in showing the exact area of orbital floor involved.

Enophthalmos

This condition may occur after trauma, resection of tumour or less commonly after correction of congenital anomalies. It is due to an increase in orbital volume (Bite et al 1985). A coronal and sagittal CT scan will be helpful in determining the site of enlargement of the orbit. A three-dimensional CT scan with a volume-measuring programme quantifies the volume increase. If there is an identifiable area involved, e.g. medial, lateral orbital wall or floor, this region is selectively bone grafted. If there is a generalized orbital enlargement, all walls are grafted far posteriorly behind the globe meridian. Correction can be complete after one procedure but this may have to be repeated.

Extraocular muscle dysfunction

This may be due to direct trauma to the muscles; fortunately it usually resolves completely. If there is fibrosis in the muscle, the problem may be permanent and may require direct muscle surgery to re-establish muscular balance. Sixth nerve trauma is a frequent cause of lateral rectus dysfunction (see Fig. 22.10b). This occurs following orbital osteotomies and orbital trauma. The great majority of these palsies resolve spontaneously in six months. If this does not occur, muscular surgery is performed. Rarely, a superior fissure syndrome with an immobile eye and ptosis may be seen. This is usually a result of trauma and in our experience has always shown spontaneous resolution. However, this happy outcome is not always the case.

Eyelid ptosis

There are several causes of upper eyelid ptosis. In many of the congenital syndromes involving the orbit, especially Crouzon's and Saethre–Chotzon, there is a slight preexisting ptosis which is made more obvious by the corrective surgery. This is due to an increased length of the levator aponeurosis and weakness of the levator muscle (Fig. 22.2).

After severe fronto-orbital trauma, there may be a resulting ptosis. This may be caused by several mechanisms. The levator aponeurosis may be torn or stretched, the levator muscle may be encased in scar tissue adherent to the orbital roof, or there may be a superior fissure syndrome. Similar problems may result after excisional surgery for tumours in this region.

Treatment involves careful analysis of the situation, and according to the findings the most appropriate operation is undertaken. This may be levator shortening, levator freeing, lid resection, frontalis sling or frontalis muscle advancement. If the eye is anaesthetic or if there is no Bell's phenomenon, a decision to operate is made with

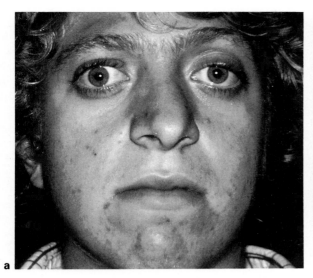
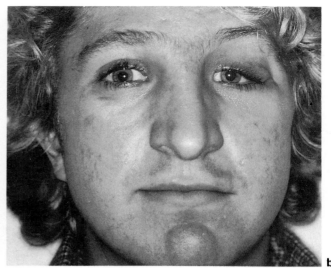

Fig. 22.2 Crouzon's disease: (a) preoperative — note ptosis, left upper eyelid; (b) postoperative — note ptosis, left upper eyelid increased.

great care. In some cases, surgery can only be contemplated if the eye is covered with protective contact lens. In others, it may be wiser not to operate.

Epiphora

This may result from congenital absence of the lacrimal system or blockage of the system owing to trauma or surgery. When the system is absent, for whatever reason, the likelihood of establishing effective drainage is not high. A conduit for tears can be formed using a buccal mucosal tube, a lateral nasal mucosa upper lateral cartilage tube or a Lester–Jones type glass or plastic tube (Jackson 1982) (Fig. 22.3). Unfortunately, tear drainage is a dynamic phenomenon due to a pumping action of orbicularis fibres

around the upper part of the lacrimal sac. Without this, epiphora may be improved but is rarely eliminated. Where there is blockage in the region of the sac, a dacryocysto-rhinostomy can be performed. Provided care is taken with this procedure the results are usually excellent (Jackson 1986).

Canthal position

MEDICAL CANTHUS

When procedures involve reattachment of the medial canthi, there may be problems postoperatively with canthal asymmetry, canthal drift or anterior placement of the ligaments.

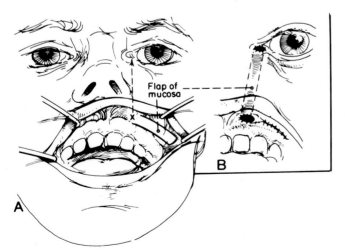
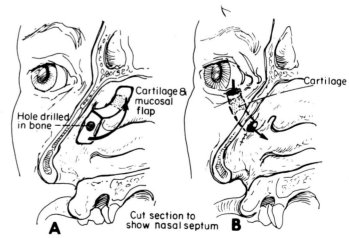

Fig. 22.3 (a) Formation of lacrimal conduit using tubed flap of buccal mucosa; (b) formation of lacrimal conduit using lateral nasal mucosa with portion of upper lateral cartilage. This is taken through a hole drilled in the medial orbital wall.

If the canthi are asymmetrical, repositioning is performed by local skin rearrangement if possible, e.g. Z-plasty. If the ligament is displaced then it will require repositioning with a transnasal canthopexy. Canthal drift can be prevented by secure initial canthal positioning; each canthus is inserted individually into a hole in the nasal bone and wired onto thick frontal bone (Jackson 1984, Jackson et al 1982). If there are associated epicanthal folds, or excess skin medial to the canthus, this is dealt with by the Mustarde 'jumping man' technique (Mustarde 1980) (Fig. 22.4). Anterior placement of the medial canthi is a common error. They must be detached and reinserted at the posterior lacrimal crest.

LATERAL CANTHUS

It is not uncommon after correction of Apert's and Crouzon's by maxillary advancement that there may be a postoperative downward slant of the lateral canthi (anti-mongoloid slant) (Fig. 22.5). This can be prevented by positioning the canthi high on the lateral orbital rim at the

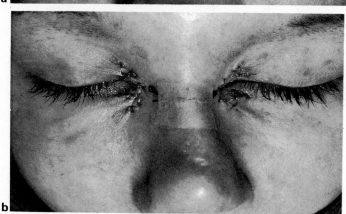
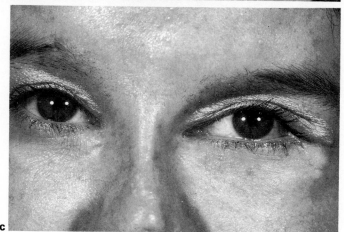

Fig. 22.4 (a) Epicanthal folds following on hypertelorism correction being corrected by Mustarde 'jumping man' technique; (b) immediately postoperatively; (c) 2 years following epicanthal fold correction.

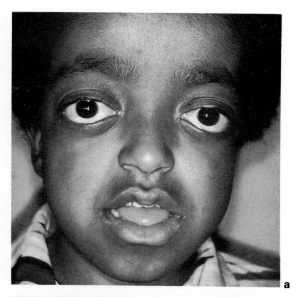
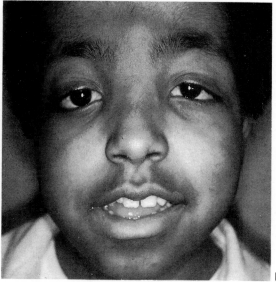

Fig. 22.5 Crouzon's disease: (a) Preoperative appearance; (b) postoperative appearance, showing antimongoloid slant of palpebral fissures owing to low positioning of lateral canthal ligaments.

time of the osteotomy. In the postsurgical situation this can be done as a separate procedure.

Palpebral fissures

On many occasions after maxillary advancement or hypertelorism correction, the palpebral fissures may be almond-shaped (Fig. 22.6). Many patients do not like this appearance but there is nothing to be done to improve it.

Transorbital constriction

In wide hypertelorism with a considerable medial shift of

the orbits, the 'hour glass' deformity may be produced (Fig. 22.7). This can be prevented by using the sagittal split approach rather than total osteotomy. The choice between these procedures requires considerable judgement and experience.

ANOSMIA

Many patients presenting for craniofacial surgery, e.g. midline clefts, hypertelorism, post-traumatic deformity, have absent or diminished sense of smell. If possible this should be determined preoperatively.

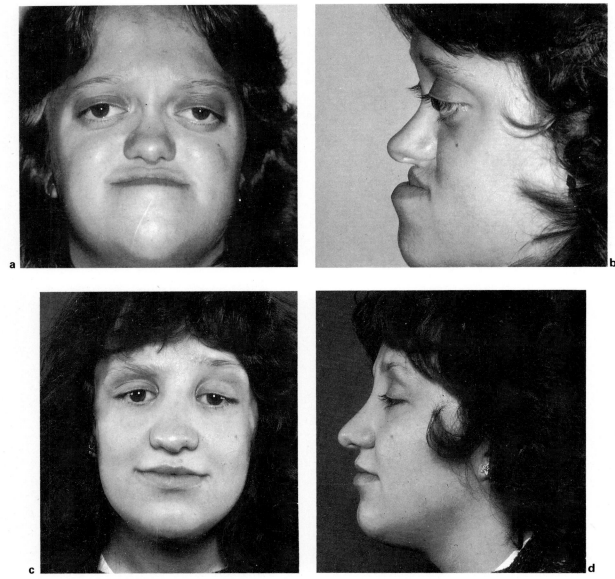

Fig. 22.6 Crouzon's disease: (a) preoperative; (b) postoperative, showing almond-shaped palpebral fissures; (c) preoperative profile; (d) postoperative profile.

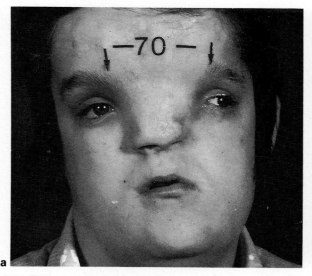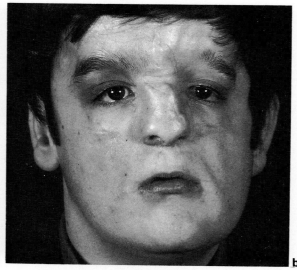

Fig. 22.7 (a) Wide asymmetrical hypertelorism with orbital dystopia; (b) post-hypertelorism correction and nasal reconstruction. 'Hour glass' deformity of face due to transorbital constriction.

The correction of hypertelorism may result in complete anosmia, as may certain tumour resections. The patient is made aware of this before surgery and told that there is no treatment for the established condition should it occur (McCarthy 1979, 1984).

COMPLICATIONS OF THE CORONAL INCISION

These are four in number: sensory disturbance, wide scar, hair loss and frontalis palsy.

Sensory disturbance

This may be present in the flap or in the scalp posterior to the incision line. It appears as though this is usually temporary, with a gradual return to normal sensation over a period of three to six months. Undoubtedly, in some patients it is permanent; there is no treatment for this.

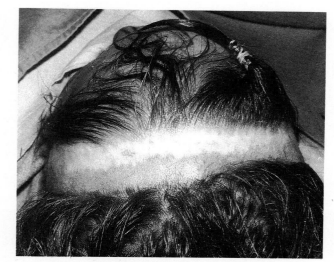

Fig. 22.8 Wide coronal incision scar following hypertelorism correction.

Wide scar

This is probably related to the transverse tension on the scar or initial healing problems rather than to the method of closure. It may also be more apparent than real; there may be some hair loss at the edge of the scar. This is usually a temporary phenomenon. Often the significant area is in the temporal region (Fig. 22.8). Certainly this is the most difficult region to hide. The most successful scar revisions in this area have been with a W-plasty technique.

Hair loss

If the coronal flap is lifted at a plane which is too super-

ficial, the hair roots may be traumatized, causing alopecia. A similar situation may occur with ischaemia due to closure of the coronal suture under tension. Only small areas are involved and this has never been a permanent hair loss. On one occasion with a frontal advancement, a strip of alopecia occurred over a round Jackson–Pratt drain (Fig. 22.9). This was permanent and required excision. Since then, the flat, softer variety of Jackson–Pratt drain has been used and no problems have been seen.

SKIN NECROSIS

This has been seen in two areas: the forehead and the nose.

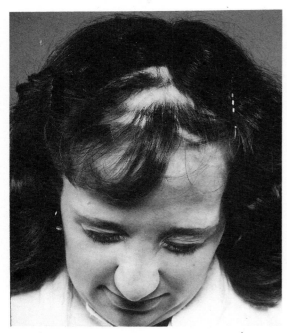

Fig. 22.9 Area of alopecia overlying drainage tube. This recovered spontaneously with time.

Forehead

On two occasions, a central area of full-thickness skin necrosis was seen on the forehead owing to the overzealous application of a head dressing. One case was a hypertelorism correction with a frontal advancement (Fig. 22.10) and the other was following excision of a midface and anterior cranial fossa chondrosarcoma. The former was excised and closed directly after mobilization of the posterior scalp. Treatment was delayed for 14 days to ensure better vascularity of the area of scalp between the necrosis and the coronal incision. In the latter, it was necessary to use a posterior scalp rotation flap and skin-graft the resulting occipital defect.

This complication is less likely to occur if the individual performing the surgery applies the dressing. The latter should be well padded. There are individuals who feel that it is unwise to apply a dressing because of the possibility of this serious complication.

On one occasion, a round Jackson–Pratt drain placed under the forehead almost resulted in full-thickness skin loss. As mentioned earlier, the soft, flat variety of drain is now used.

Nose

In two patients the nasal bone graft has eroded though the nasal tip. When this occurs, the bone should be rongeured until bleeding occurs and the nasal skin can be closed over the graft. If there is no infection, the graft should always be left in position.

BLOOD LOSS

In congenital deformity, trauma and post-traumatic deformity correction, this is rarely a significant problem. In infants blood loss must be assessed and minimized carefully. It has been found useful to place a small graduated container within the suction line in a position easily seen by both anaesthetist and surgeon. All bleeding should be aspirated if possible, since significant volumes can be hidden under the head and posterior chest.

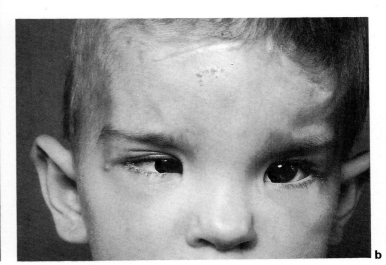

Fig. 22.10 Area of full-thickness forehead and scalp skin loss due to tight bandaging on a forehead advancement in hypertelorism correction; (b) corrected by excision and advancement of scalp, 14 days later. Note lateral rectus weakness.

The coronal flap is raised with bleeding in mind. Firstly, the area is infiltrated with 0.5% Xylocaine and 1:400 000 adrenaline with the patient in a reversed Trendelenburg position. The scalp incision is made in stages, placing Reyne clips anteriorly and Dandy's forceps posteriorly. In this way the procedure is almost bloodless.

During surgery bleeding in the temporal area must be controlled; it is possible to have a significant ooze from this region in prolonged procedures.

In Le Fort III osteotomies, bleeding may occur on mobilization of the maxilla. This usually settles very quickly and is not severe. If there was significant bleeding packing could be inserted into the area responsible until bleeding ceased. This would probably follow secure stabilization of the maxilla. Bleeding of this magnitude is not a problem which has been encountered. When the scalp is closed, this again should be done in segments. The clips and forceps are removed and a haemostatic running suture inserted. This is repeated until the total incision is closed. A flat, soft suction drain is inserted to prevent accumulation of postoperative blood loss. This is important in young children and infants.

VELOPHARYNGEAL INCOMPETENCE

This may occur after maxillary advancement. We, like others (Witzel & Munro 1977), have noted that this is only seen if there was a degree of velopharyngeal incompetence (VPI) prior to surgery. Only in Le Fort I osteotomies are the numbers sufficient to draw any conclusions; in these VPI increased in 10% of patients who had a degree of escape beforehand. The treatment is pharyngoplasty or modification of a pre-existing pharyngeal flap or pharyngoplasty.

PHARYNGEAL FLAP

In some patients with midface retrusion having a previous pharyngeal flap, this structure can become tight and pale following maxillary advancement. If the tension is judged to be significant the flap is divided and the resulting VPI is treated when the situation has stabilized, i.e. after six months. A pharyngeal flap or a pharyngoplasty is performed according to the analysis of the causation of the VPI.

RELAPSE

Orbits

In hypertelorism correction, especially in young patients, there is a distinct possibility of relapse. There are probably several reasons for this:

1. Insufficient correction
2. New subperiosteal bone formation

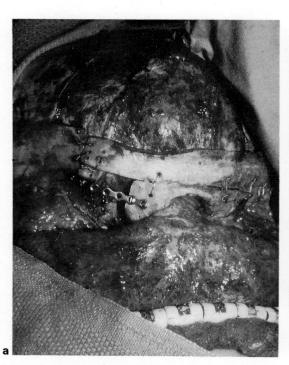 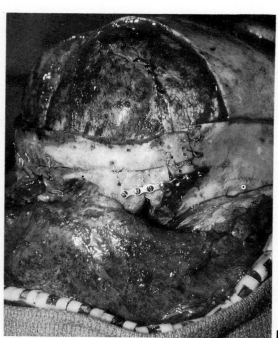

Fig. 22.11 (a) Hypertelorism correction. Orbits stabilized with Champy plate; (b) insertion of bone graft into the lateral defect, held in position with screws through the central portion of the plate.

3. Regrowth of ethmoidal air cells
4. Frontal lobes between the medial orbital walls
5. Medial orbital walls convex into orbit.

It is probable that insufficient correction and poor mobilization account for most relapse, although Mulliken et al (1986) in a recent review stated that an intraorbital distance of 32 mm produced a good result, i.e. relapse less than 5 mm. When the average intraorbital distance was over 40 mm, there was a relapse of more than 5 mm. They also suggested that correction at an early age may retard anterior maxillary growth and they therefore advise postponing surgery for as long as possible. It is our custom to remove all bone between the anterior lacrimal crests and to pay little attention to measurements; this had greatly decreased relapse. The use of Champy plate fixation has further improved results (Figs. 22.11, 22.12). New subperiosteal bone formation is possible but unlikely, as is regrowth of ethmoidal sinus air cells if these have been removed completely.

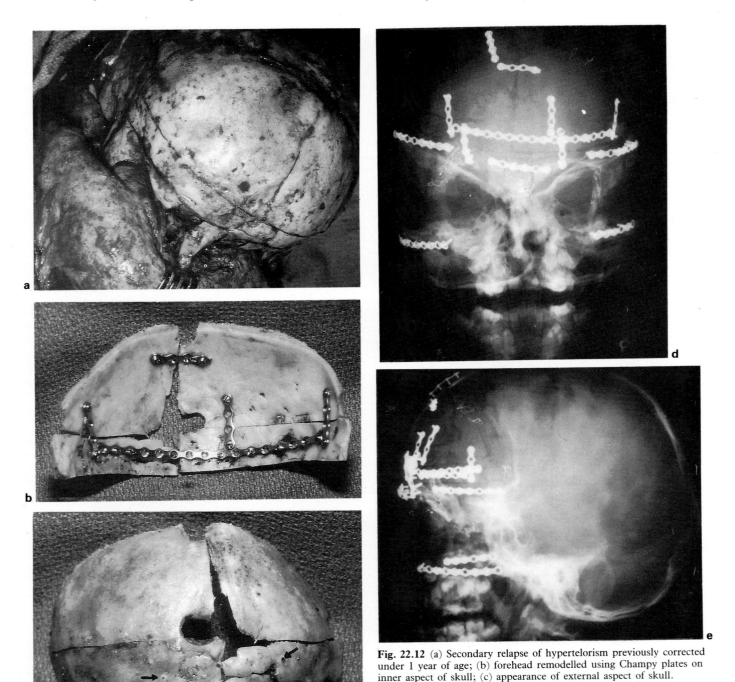

Fig. 22.12 (a) Secondary relapse of hypertelorism previously corrected under 1 year of age; (b) forehead remodelled using Champy plates on inner aspect of skull; (c) appearance of external aspect of skull. Perforating portions of screws reduced with contouring burr (arrows); (d, e) postoperative radiographs to show multiple Champy plate fixation for stability.

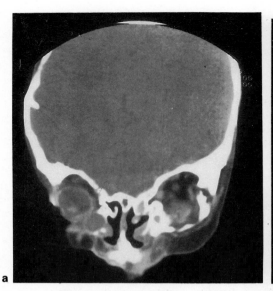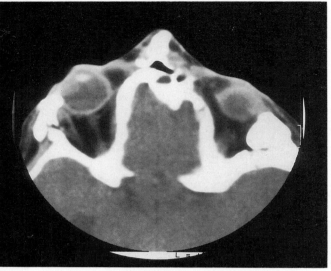

Fig. 22.13 Coronal CT scan showing low-lying cribriform plate with convex medial orbital walls. Low position of frontal lobes; (b) axial CT scan to show brain far down between orbits and convex appearance of medial orbital walls.

The presence of frontal lobes between the orbits results form a low-lying cribriform plate. This also produces upper medial orbital walls convex into the orbit (Fig. 22.13). This should be diagnosed on CT scan in the initial assessment or in the assessment of the recurrent case. The central area of the anterior cranial fossa is raised with a skull bone graft and the convex orbital walls are replaced with concave bone grafts. In this way, the frontal lobe is elevated and one of the most potent causes of relapse can be eliminated.

Maxilla

Poor fixation occurs for several reasons: poor surgery, excessive forward movement of the maxilla, the primary pathology, e.g. clefts. In addition to this, there is what might be termed pseudorelapse. This is where maxillary advancement is performed at an early age. The maxilla remains static in terms of growth, the mandible grows and a class III skeletal and dental situation recurs (Fig. 22.14).

POOR SURGERY

If the osteotomy is not mobilized properly, then relapse is inevitable. It should be possible to move the maxilla into the correct preplanned position without a great deal of effort. Bone grafts should fit accurately into residual defects and it is best to fix them with miniplates (Jackson & Adham 1986) (Fig. 22.15).

POOR FIXATION

Secure fixation of the advanced maxilla is one of the keys

to a good result. The interdental splint should be accurately fashioned and the teeth should seat securely into the splint.

If possible, a self-locking osteotomy is designed, but this is determined by the extent and type of deformity. Similarly, whenever possible, miniplates are used to hold the maxilla in its advanced position. These are applied at the root of the nose, lateral orbital wall and zygomatic arch. At the time of surgery, this gives the most secure fixation possible (Jackson et al 1986a). Fixation is further helped by the accurate bone grafting described above.

MAXILLARY OVERADVANCEMENT

When a maxillary advancement of 20 mm or more is necessary, it may be wise to split this between the maxilla and mandible. The maxilla is advanced and the mandible is set back. This manoeuvre may not give the ideal cephalometric result, but it may well prevent maxillary relapse due to overadvancement.

PRIMARY PATHOLOGY

Where there is a lot of scarring posterior to the maxilla as in old trauma cases and previously repaired maxillary clefts, the tendency for relapse is undoubtedly higher. This is especially so if the patient has few teeth or is edentulous. In these cases, every possible trick is used to prevent relapse: good mobilization, secure fixation with plates, accurate bone grafting and shared mandibular/maxillary osteotomies.

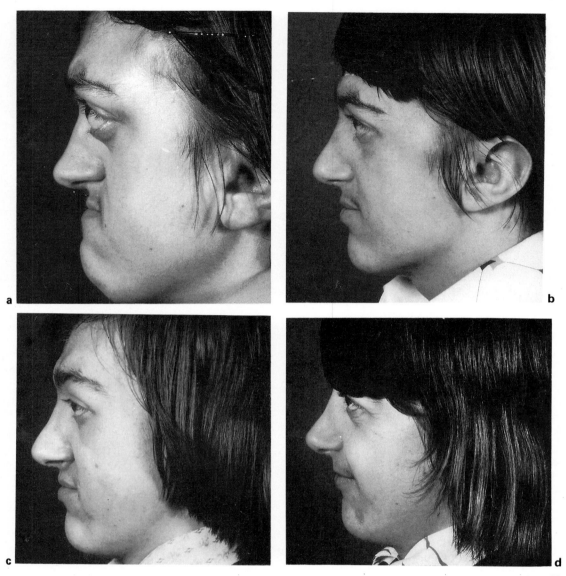

Fig. 22.14 (a) Crouzon's disease, aged 14; (b) postoperative result 1 year later, aged 15; (c)postoperative result at 2 years, aged 16. Note what appears to be midface retrusion recurring. Cephalometrically this was due to continued growth of the mandible; (d) patient aged 18 following Le Fort I advancement of the maxilla.

PSEUDORELAPSE

Ideally, midface advancement should be postponed until facial growth is complete (Freihofer 1973). However, in many patients the advancement cannot be delayed. What has emerged form this is that the upper face, i.e. the orbital area, usually achieves a permanent and acceptable correction, whereas the dentoalveolar region reverts to a class III situation. Fortunately, the majority of these patients can be later rehabilitated with a Le Fort I advancement.

BONE GRAFTING

In this area, many changes have taken place. The traditional sites — rib and iliac crest — are used less and less, with the skull being used more and more (Tessier 1982, Jackson et al 1983, Jackson et al 1986b; 1987). Because of this, there is shorter operating time, less pain, fewer scars and reduced donor site morbidity. Resorption of cranial bone grafts has been shown experimentally to be less (Zins & Whitaker 1983) and this seems to be the case on follow-up of clinical cases. In many patients, e.g. Treacher Collins', the resorption of free bone grafts presented a

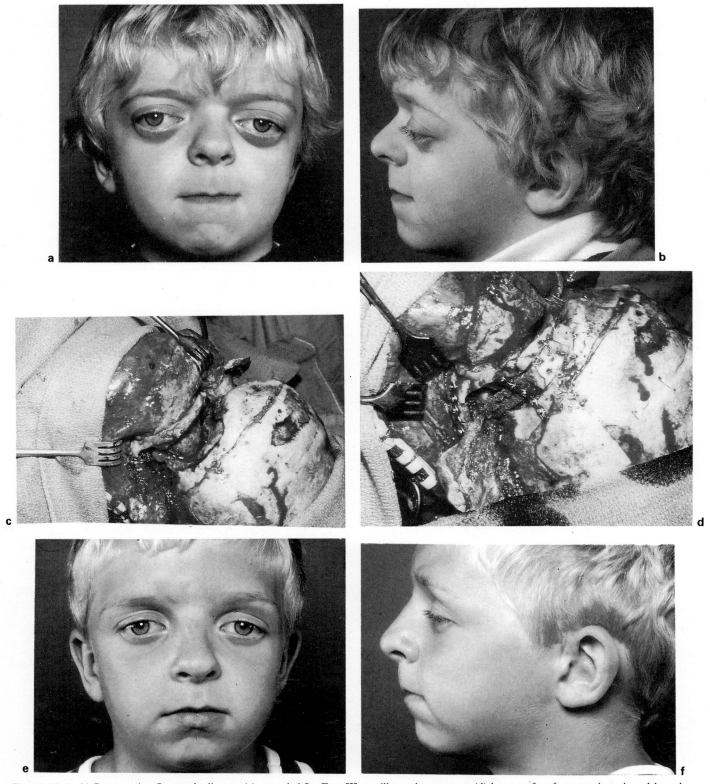

Fig. 22.15 (a, b) Preoperative Crouzon's disease; (c) extended Le Fort III maxillary advancement; (d) bone grafts of zygomatic arch and lateral orbital wall held in position with Champy plates; (e, f) postoperative result at 2 years.

considerable problem and required multiple grafting procedures. This situation has been helped greatly by vascularized, pedicled bone grafts of skull based on known vascular territories (Cutting et al 1984, McCarthy & Zide 1984, Van der Meulen 1984, Cassanova et al 1986, Psillakis et al 1986).

These osteomuscular and osteogaleal flaps all show good blood flow and survive (Bite et al 1987). This has greatly decreased the problem of bone graft resorption and reoperation. Accordingly, it is recommended wherever possible.

INFECTION

This is the most significant problem in craniofacial surgery, causing great distress to surgeon and patient alike and occasionally becoming the subject of medicolegal disputes.

Minor infection

This is classified as an infection which does not significantly prolong the patient's hospitalization and does not require a major operative procedure to deal with it. Into this category would fall wound infections, small infected haematomas and infections around small onlay bone grafts. These situations are easily dealt with by incision and drainage, usually without a visit to the operating room, and rarely does the patient require (Fig. 22.16) hospitalization. The incidence of this problem in our series was 0.8% (Table 22.1).

Major infection

In this type of infection, the patient has a major systemic upset, requires prolongation of hospitalization and a significant surgical procedure. Some individuals will have a residual deformity requiring a major reconstruction.

Fortunately, the incidence of severe infection has decreased with experience, reduced operating time and the introduction of techniques to counteract the occurrence of infection. Perhaps the most significant advance has been the recognition of the 'at risk' patient.

AT RISK PATIENT

Basically, this is the patient who has a frontal advancement, trauma or tumour resection and who then has a connection between the extradural space and the nasopharynx. If there has been a dural repair there is a risk of meningitis. In this type of patient, the potential problem should be recognized preoperatively and the surgery modified accordingly. There is a powerful argument for undertaking all frontal and fronto-orbital advancements in infancy. In this age group, the brain will fill the dead space, whereas in the older patient this does not occur and the stage is set for a disaster.

SIGNS AND SYMPTOMS

An 'abcess type' temperature chart with swelling around the eyes and temporal region which does not show signs of resolving within four to five days postoperatively is extremely significant. The temporal swelling has a very distinct boggy, oedematous quality. The presence of fluid under the coronal flap, any discharge from the wound and fluid other than blood in the suction drain are further causes for concern.

TREATMENT

When the above signs are present, the coronal incision

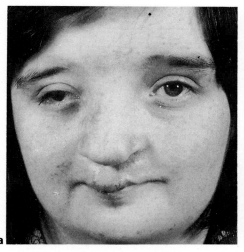 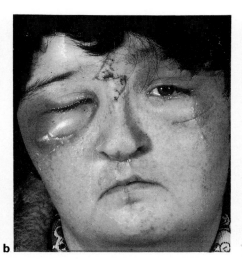 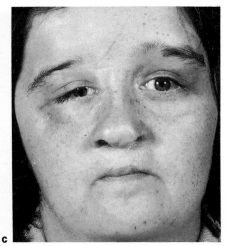

Fig. 22.16 (a) Patient with hypertelorism, orbital dystopia and old cleft lip deformity; (b) following hypertelorism correction, localized infection around rib graft to right malar area; (c) postoperative result after removal of rib grafts.

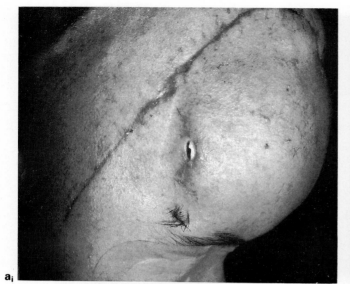

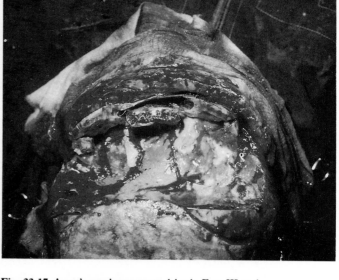

Fig. 22.17 Apert's syndrome treated by le Fort III and simultaneous forehead advancement; (a) Obvious extradural infection with frontal bone presenting through defect on right side of forehead. After removal of the frontal bone, the extradural abscess is obvious. Upper portions of orbits debrided; (b) extensive lateral defect is shown.

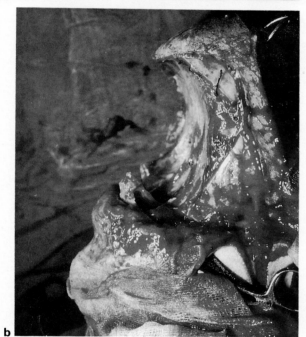

which will be reconstructed at a later date (Figs. 22.17, 22.18). Again, the irrigation and suction treatment together with the indicated systemic antibiotics are instituted. These measures are essential where there has been a previous dural repair or graft.

If there is an open nasopharyngeal connection, either direct or through the frontal or ethmoidal sinuses, this must be repaired by vascularized tissue. Where the brain can expand the galeal frontalis flap is used and has been proved to be a life-saving procedure (Jackson et al 1986c). Where the brain cannot expand and there is a chance of saving the frontal bone flap, then a free muscle graft (Guelinckx & Lejour 1986) or a free omental transfer (Fisher & Jackson 1989) is performed (Fig. 22.19). These two procedures have been two of the most important contributions to the treatment and prevention of major craniofacial infections.

PROPHYLAXIS

This involves recognition of the 'at risk' patient and acting accordingly. Any patient over the age of 5 or 6 years requiring a frontal advancement may have a dead space between the frontal bone and the dura. If this persists, there may be fluid accumulation and infection, or there may be slow loss of the frontal bone, since contact with the dura is required for adequate vascularization. Serial CT scans are necessary and if the defect persists, or if there is evidence of infection, the area is explored and omentum vascularized from the external carotid and internal jugular

should be reopened and the operated area inspected as soon as possible. Better an early negative exploration than a delayed exploration; this may make the difference between a retrievable and an irretrievable situation. If exploration is early, it may be possible to perform irrigation, minimal debridement and set up a suction irrigation system. The fluid used for irrigation is gentamicin 80 mg, polymyxin B sulphate 100 mg and neomycin sulphate 500 mg/l of saline. Usually within 48 hours the situation has settled and all is well. If this happy outcome does not occur, or if exploration is delayed, all non-viable bone and foreign material, e.g. wires and plates, must be removed. This will frequently result in an enormous bony defect

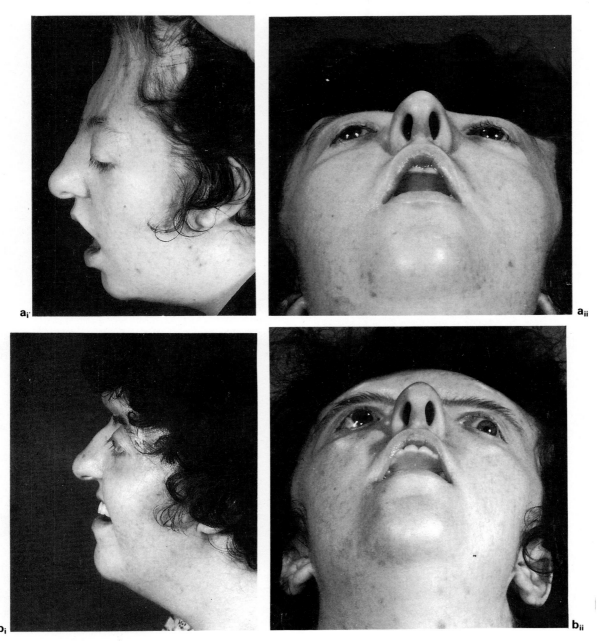

Fig. 22.18 (a) Fronto-supraorbital defect following extensive debridement shown above; (b) result following split-rib reconstruction of frontal area 1 year later.

is inserted. Where a skull reconstruction is being performed, and the dura is scarred and unlikely to expand, especially in the presence of a nasopharyngeal connection, a primary insertion of free vascularized muscle, e.g. latissimus or omentum, is strongly advised.

It should be recognized that certain operations place the patient at risk. Any procedure which moves the frontal area and the midface produces an extradural nasopharyngeal connection and is associated with a greater risk of infection. For this reason, we avoid this if possible, prefer-

ring to split the procedure into two stages: frontal advancement and, at a later date, maxillary advancement. This is against a background of having been the initial group after Tessier to describe the monobloc procedure (Jackson, 1978). It was later presented by Ortiz-Monasterio et al (1978). It is possible to modify the frontal advancement to minimize the extradural nasopharyngeal connection. This modification maintains the integrity of the skull base, but allows a high Le Fort III to be performed (Jackson 1978, Anderl et al 1983). When a single-stage procedure is

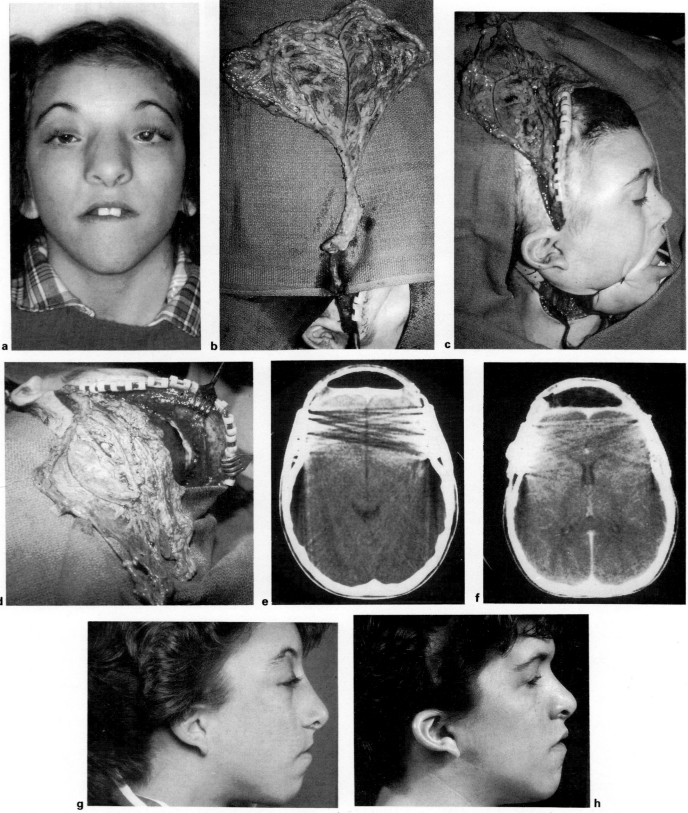

Fig. 22.19 (a) Preoperative appearance, Saethre–Chotzen's syndrome. This was treated with forehead and supraorbital advancement. The brain failed to expand, resulting in an extradural dead space which became infected; (b) omentum with gastroepiploic vessels anastomosed to the external carotid artery and internal jugular vein; (c, d) omentum being placed into extradural dead space; (e) axial CT scan showing the lack of brain expansion and extradural dead space behind the frontal bone; (f) axial CT scan showing omentum in the extradural dead space; (g) preoperative profile of forehead; (h) postoperative profile $2\frac{1}{2}$ years following omental free flap to show good retention of forehead contour owing to satisfactory survival of underlying frontal bone.

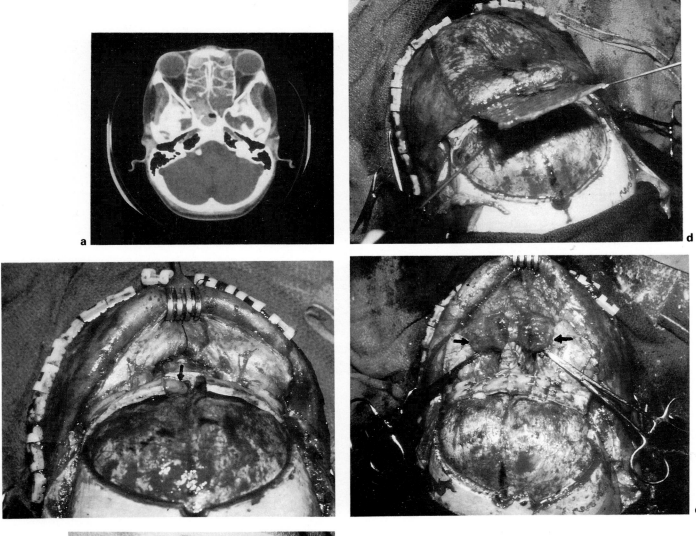

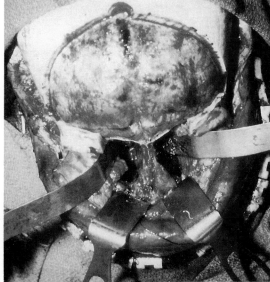

Fig. 22.20 (a) Mucocele of ethmoid sinuses, sphenoid sinuses with pneumotization of the clivus. The frontal and maxillary sinuses were also involved. The patient had hypertelorism resulting from this, since the mucocele had occurred at an early age; (b) mucocele of frontal sinus (arrow); (c) appearance after removal of ethmoid sinuses, frontal sinuses, sphenoid sinus and exploration and removal of mucocele from maxillary sinuses; (d) elevation of large galeal frontalis flap to close off the extradural nasopharyngeal and sinus connection; (e) following hypertelorism correction and bone grafting to nose, the galeal frontalis was divided into two parts and is effectively closing off the nasopharyngeal opening from the extradural space (arrows). The haemostats have been applied to the medial canthal ligaments.

indicated, it is best to perform the standard advancement in a step wise fashion — frontal, supraorbital rim, maxilla — and close the nasopharyngeal defect with a galeal frontalis flap (Fig. 22.20). Any tear of nasal mucosa, e.g. in hypertelorism, must be carefully repaired. If the frontal sinus is traumatized, it should have the mucosa removed and should be obliterated with a galeal frontalis flap, especially in trauma with a connection into the nose. Dural replacement in a compromised situation should be with fascia lata rather than lyophilized dura. Scalp wounds should be drained to prevent haematoma and firm bandaging is advised for the same reasons.

Antibiotics are given before, during and after surgery; rarely is this prolonged for more than 48 hours postoperatively. Undoubtedly, one of the main factors in the decrease in major infections has been the reduction in operating time; this comes with experience.

Using the measures described above, the major infection rate in craniofacial procedures has been reduced to a very acceptable level. The overall incidence in the 1000 patients reviewed between 1969 and 1984 was 1%. Bony reconstruction after infection should not be undertaken for at least six months and preferably between nine and twelve months.

VASCULAR COMPLICATIONS

These are of two types: soft tissue and bone.

Soft tissue

When a large frontal advancement has been performed, the scalp closure may be tight, in spite of wide mobilization of the scalp and galeal scoring. This can induce ischaemia of the wound edges, poor healing and a resulting wide scar which requires later revision.

If head bandages are applied too tightly without regard to the inevitable postsurgical swelling and in cases with previous surgical scars in that area as mentioned earlier, skin necrosis may occur (see Fig. 22.10). It is a matter of urgency to get these covered with viable skin because of the underlying frontal bone flap which is devascularized.

Bone necrosis

Bone necrosis due to ischaemia is rare in the larger osteotomies. It has occurred once in our practice in a Le Fort I osteotomy for a post-cleft retrusion (Fig. 22.21). Since this is not a craniofacial procedure, it was not included in the series reviewed. However, in a cleft patient treated elsewhere by Le Fort III advancement, a considerable loss of maxilla was seen. This was treated by observation, sequestrectomy, subsequent bone grafting and dental

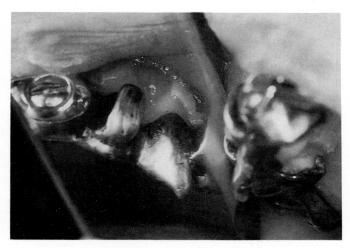

Fig. 22.21 Mirror showing anterior necrosis on the greater segment of a maxilla advanced at the Le Fort I level in a cleft lip and palate case.

rehabilitation using osseointegration techniques (Branemark 1983).

ANAESTHETIC AND AIRWAY PROBLEMS

With an experienced craniofacial team, airway problems are anticipated and measures taken to prevent them from occurring (Davies & Munro 1975, Ferguson et al 1983, McMichan 1988). Trauma, post-traumatic and tumour patients may require tracheostomy for very specific reasons, such as mandibular fracture, severe trismus and floor of mouth and mandibular resection. In the rare cases of bilateral Goldenhar's syndrome, hemifacial microsomia or Treacher Collins' syndrome, this may be necessary. Actually most of these patients have had their tracheostomies (usually unnecessarily) performed elsewhere. The reason for the demise of the tracheostomy has been fourfold: increased anaesthetic experience, the flexible fiberoptic bronchoscope, prolonged postoperative endotracheal intubation and the improvement of intensive care facilities. Recently Lauritzen et al (1986) and Munro & Sabatier (1985) have advised tracheostomies for children requiring Le Fort III osteotomies and forehead advancement. This has not been our experience so far.

In our own series, there have been no significant intraoperative misadventures. Postoperatively, the patients are in the neurosurgical or general surgical intensive care facility. The only problem that has occurred in this area has been the occlusion of a nasotracheal tube with mucus. This situation was relieved by removing the tube.

With the advent of miniplates for stabilization of maxillary osteotomies and fractures, intermaxillary fixation is often removed at the conclusion of the surgical procedures. In this way, there is considerably less compromise of the airway postoperatively.

CONCLUSION

Craniofacial surgery is now a safe procedure in experienced hands. The series reported here has value in that it has been performed by one surgeon. It illustrates an evolution of thought and experience and it is composed of a significant group of purely major craniofacial procedures.

Other reports have been from multiple centres (Whitaker et al 1979; Whitaker et al 1976); a recent report by Munro & Sabatier (1985) presents skewed statistics, since less than half of the cases would fulfil the definition of a craniofacial case outlined in this chapter. The orthognathic surgery, onlay bone grafts and secondary procedures following on craniofacial corrections represent an entirely different group with different problems. Inclusion of these artificially improve results and could cause significant future problems of all kinds, both clinical and medicolegal.

We must strive for further improvement in our results. Uppermost in our minds as craniofacial surgeons should be the concept of safe surgery rather than spectacular surgery. The acceptance of this concept is closely related to surgical maturity. Having satisfied ourselves that a second anaesthetic is safe, we should not hesitate to perform two-stage surgery if this will result in fewer surgical complications. As has been stated many times in the past, craniofacial surgery should be performed by specialized teams. These teams should be composed of individuals who have had extra training in this speciality and who devote the major part of their time to it.

REFERENCES

Anderl H, Muhlbauer W, Twerdy K, Marchac D 1983 Frontofacial advancement with bony separation in craniofacial dysostosis. Plastic and Reconstructive Surgery 71: 303

Bite U, Jackson I T, Forbes G S, Gehring D G 1985 Orbital volume measurements in enophthalmos using three-dimensional CT imaging. Plastic and Reconstructive Surgery 75: 502–507

Bite U, Jackson I T, Wahner H W, Marsh R W 1987 Vascularized skull bone grafts in craniofacial surgery. Annals of Plastic Surgery 19: 3–15

Branemark P I 1983 Osseointegraton and its experimental background. Journal of Prosthetic Dentistry 50: 399

Casanova R, Cavalcante D, Grotting J C, Vasconez L O, Psillakis J M 1986 Anatomic basis for vascularized outer-table calvarial bone flaps. Plastic and Reconstructive Surgery 78: 300–308

Converse J M, Wood Smith D, McCarthy J B 1975 Report on a series of 50 craniofacial operations. Plastic and Reconstructive Surgery 55: 283

Cutting C B, McCarthy J G, Berenstein A 1984 Blood supply of the upper craniofacial skeleton: the search for composite calvarial bone flaps. Plastic Reconstructive Surgery 74: 603

Davies D W, Munro I R 1975 The anesthetic management and intraoperative care of patients undergoing major facial osteotomies. Plastic and Reconstructive Surgery 55: 50

Ferguson D, Barker J, Jackson I T 1983 Anesthesia for craniofacial osteotomies. Annals of Plastic Surgery 10: 333–338

Fisher J, Jackson I T 1989 Microvascular surgery as an adjunct to craniomaxillofacial reconstruction. British Journal of Plastic Surgery (in press)

Freihofer H P M Jr 1973 Results after midface osteotomies. Journal of Maxillofacial Surgery 1: 30

Guelinckx P, Lejour M 1986 Free muscle transplants in chronic infections of the frontocranial region. European Journal of Plastic Surgery 9: 88–93

Jackson I T 1978 Midface retrusion. In: Whitaker L A (ed) Symposium on Reconstruction of Jaw Deformity. Proceedings of the Symposium of the Educational Foundation of the American Society of Plastic and Reconstructive Surgeons, vol. 16. Mosby, St Louis. Ch 23, pp 276–310

Jackson I T 1982 Nasolacrimal duct reconstruction. In: Aston S J, Hornblass A, Meltzer M A, Rees T D (eds) Third International Symposium of Plastic and Reconstructive Surgery of the Eye and Adnexa. Williams & Wilkins, Baltimore. Ch 12, pp 59–63

Jackson I T 1984 Orbital hypertelorism. In: Serafin D, Georgiade N (eds) Pediatric plastic surgery, vol 1. Mosby, St Louis. Ch 28

Jackson I T 1985 Advances and innovations in craniofacial surgery. Plastic Surgery Nursing 5: 22–25

Jackson I T 1988 Trauma to the lacrimal system. In: Hornblass A (ed) Oculoplastic, orbital and reconstructive surgery (in press)

Jackson I T, Adham M N 1986 Metallic plate stabilisation of bone grafts in craniofacial surgery. British Journal of Plastic Surgery 39: 341–344

Jackson I T, Munro I R, Salyer K E, Whitaker L A 1982 Atlas of craniomaxillofacial surgery. Mosby, St Louis

Jackson I T, Pellett C, Smith J M 1983 The skull as a bone graft donor site. Annals of Plastic Surgery 11: 527–523

Jackson I T, Somers P C, Kjar J G 1986a The use of Champy miniplates for osteosynthesis in craniofacial deformities and trauma. Plastic and Reconstructive Surgery 77: 729–736

Jackson I T, Helden G, Marx R, Nellen R, Bite U 1986b Skull bone grafts in maxillofacial and craniofacial surgery. Journal of Oral and Maxillofacial Surgery 44: 949–955

Jackson I T, Adham M N, Marsh W R 1986c Use of the galeal frontalis myofascial flap in craniofacial surgery. Plastic and Reconstructive Surgery 77: 905–910

Jackson I T, Adham M N, Bite U, Marx R 1987 Update on cranial bone grafts in craniofacial surgery. Annals of Plastic Surgery 18: 37–40

Lauritzen C, Lilja J, Jarlstedt J 1986 Airway obstruction and sleep apnea in children with craniofacial anomalies. Plastic and Reconstructive Surgery 77: 1

McCarthy J G 1979 A study of gustatory and olfactory function in patients with craniofacial anomalies. Plastic and Reconstructive Surgery 64: 52

McCarthy J G 1984 Gustatory and olfactory function in patients with craniofacial anomalies. In: Caronni E P (ed) Craniofacial surgery. Little, Brown, Boston. p 27

McCarthy J G, Zide B M 1984 The spectrum of calvarial bone grafting: introduction of the vascularized calvarial bone flap. Plastic and Reconstructive Surgery 74: 10

McMichan J 1988 Anesthesia for paediatric plastic surgery. In: Mustardé J C, Jackson I T (eds) Plastic surgery in infancy and childhood, 3rd ed. Churchill Livingstone, Edinburgh.

Matthews D 1979 Craniofacial surgery — indications, assessment and complications. British Journal of Plastic Surgery 32: 96

Mulliken J B, Kaban L B, Evans C A, Strand R D, Murray J E 1986 Facial skeletal changes following hypertelorism correction. Plastic and Reconstructive Surgery 77: 7

Munro I R, Sabatier R E 1985 An analysis of 12 years of

craniomaxillofacial surgery in Toronto. Plastic and Reconstructive Surgery 76: 29

Mustarde J C 1980 Repair and reconstruction in the orbital region. Churchill Livingstone, Edinburgh

Ortiz-Monasterio F, Fuente del Campo A, Carillo A 1978 Advancements of the orbits and midface in one piece combined with frontal repositioning for the correction of Crouzon deformities. Plastic and Reconstructive Surgery 61: 4

Psillakis J M, Grotting J C, Casanova R, Cavalcante D, Vasconez L O 1986 Vascularized outer-table calvarial bone flaps. Plastic and Reconstructive Surgery 78: 309–317

Tessier P 1982 Autogenous bone grafts taken from the calvarium for facial and cranial applications. Clinics in Plastic Surgery 9: 531

Van der Meulen J C H, Hauben D J, Vaandrager J M, Birgenhager-Frenkel D H 1984 The use of a temporal osteoperiosteal flap for the reconstruction of malar hypoplasia in Treacher Collins syndrome. Plastic and Reconstructive Surgery 74: 687

Whitaker L A, Munro I R, Jackson I T, Salyer K E 1976 Problems in craniofacial surgery. Journal of Maxillofacial Surgery 4: 131–136

Whitaker L A, Munro I R, Salyer K E, Jackson I T, Ortiz-Monasterio F, Marchac D 1979 Combined report of problems and complications in 793 craniofacial operations. Plastic and Reconstructive Surgery 64: 198–203

Witzel M A, Munro I R 1977 Velopharyngeal insufficiency after maxillary advancement. Cleft Palate Journal 14: 176

Zins J E, Whitaker L A 1983 Membranous versus endochondral bone: implications for craniofacial reconstruction. Plastic and Reconstructive Surgery 72: 778

Index